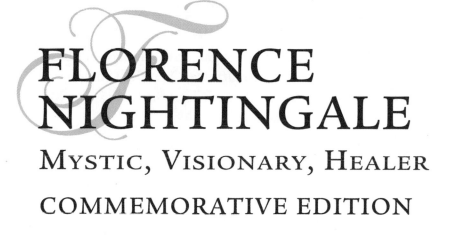

FLORENCE NIGHTINGALE

Mystic, Visionary, Healer

COMMEMORATIVE EDITION

Florence Nightingale

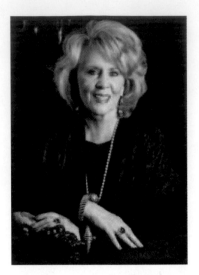

Barbara Dossey, PhD, RN, AHN-BC, FAAN
International Co-Director, Nightingale Initiative for Global Health,
Washington, DC and Ottawa, Ontario, Canada
Director, Holistic Nursing Consultants, Santa Fe, New Mexico

Barbara Dossey, PhD, RN, AHN-BC, FAAN, is internationally recognized as a pioneer in the holistic nursing movement. She is International Co-Director and board member of the Nightingale Initiative for Global Health (NIGH), Washington, DC and Ottawa, Ontario, Canada, and Director, Holistic Nursing Consultants in Santa Fe, New Mexico. She is a Florence Nightingale scholar and an author or co-author of 23 books. Her most recent include *Holistic Nursing: A Handbook for Practice* (5th ed., 2008), *Being with Dying: Compassionate End-of-Life Care Training Guide* (2007), *Florence Nightingale Today: Healing, Leadership, Global Action* (2005), and *Florence Nightingale: Mystic, Visionary, Healer* (2000; Commemorative Edition, 2010).

Barbara's Theory of Integral Nursing (2008) is considered a grand theory that presents the science and art of nursing. It includes an integral process, integral worldview, and integral dialogues that is Praxis—theory in action. It also focuses on compassionate care of the dying, and nurses' roles as 21st century Nightingales. Her collaborative global nursing project, the Nightingale Declaration Campaign (NDC) has developed two UN Resolution proposals for adoption—2010: International Year of the Nurse and 2011-2020: UN Decade for a Healthy World.

Barbara is a Fellow of the American Academy of Nursing. She is certified in holistic nursing. She is a eight-time recipient of the prestigious *American Journal of Nursing Book of the Year* Award. She was awarded the 1985 Holistic Nurse of the Year by the American Holistic Nurses' Association; the 1998 Healer of the Year by the Nurse Healers Professional Associates International, Inc.; the 1999 Pioneering Spirit Award by the American Association of Critical Care Nurses; the 1999 Scientific and Medical Network Book of the Year by the Scientific and Medical Network, United Kingdom. In 2001 she was recognized as TWU 100 Great Nursing Alumni, Texas Woman's University, Denton, Texas. In 2003 she received the Distinguished Alumna Award from Baylor University, Waco, Texas. With her husband, Larry, she received the 2003 Archon Award from Sigma Theta Tau, International, the international honor society of nursing, honoring the contributions that they have made to promoting global health. In 2004, Barbara and Larry also received the Pioneer of Integrative Medicine Award from the Aspen Center for Integrative Medicine, Aspen, Colorado.

For the 72nd General Episcopal Church Convention in Philadelphia July 1997, Barbara wrote three of five documents to accompany the Resolution Proposal to request the reconsideration of Nightingale's commemoration and for her name to be placed on the church calendar list of Lesser Feast and Fasts in the Book of Common Prayer. The official vote to accept Nightingale to the church calendar occurred in July 2000. The inaugural Florence Nightingale Commemorative Service was held on August 12, 2001, at the Washington National Cathedral, Washington, D.C. The Florence Nightingale Centennial Service will be held April 25, 2010 at the Washington National Cathedral.

See Web sites: http://www.dosseydossey.com & http://www.NightingaleDeclaration.net

FLORENCE NIGHTINGALE

MYSTIC, VISIONARY, HEALER

COMMEMORATIVE EDITION

Barbara Montgomery Dossey

F.A. Davis Company • Philadelphia

BP45

To my colleagues in nursing, who understand
Florence Nightingale's vision and the
role of spirituality in healing.

F. A. Davis Company
1915 Arch Street
Philadelphia, PA 19103
www.fadavis.com

Printed in the United States of America

Last digit indicates print number: 10 9 8 7 6 5 4 3 2 1

Publisher, Nursing: Joanne P. DaCunha, RN, MSN
Project Editor: Kim DePaul
Art and Design Manager: Carolyn O'Brien
Cover Design: Mary Ludwicki; Kris Magyarits, first edition

ABOUT THE COVER: The collage illustrates the mystic, visionary, and healer aspects of Florence Nightingale's life. Centered over her left eye is her famous wedge diagram indicating the causes of death of British soldiers in the Crimean War. The nurses at the bottom, from the Army Nursing Service at Royal Victoria Hospital, Netley, illustrate Nightingale's role as the founder of modern secular nursing. Nightingale's distinctive script floats in the background, with her signature at the bottom, a symbolic foundation on which modern nursing rests. Overseeing all is Nightingale's penetrating gaze, from a photograph taken at age 37.

As new scientific information becomes available through basic and clinical research, recommended treatments and drug therapies undergo changes. The author(s) and publisher have done everything possible to make this book accurate, up to date, and in accord with accepted standards at the time of publication. The author(s), editors, and publisher are not responsible for errors or omissions or for consequences from application of the book, and make no warranty, expressed or implied, in regard to the contents of the book. Any practice described in this book should be applied by the reader in accordance with professional standards of care used in regard to the unique circumstances that may apply in each situation. The reader is advised always to check product information (package inserts) for changes and new information regarding dose and contraindications before administering any drug. Caution is especially urged when using new or infrequently ordered drugs.

Library of Congress Cataloging-in-Publication Data

Dossey, Barbara Montgomery.
 Florence Nightingale : mystic, visionary, healer / Barbara Montgomery Dosse.--
Commemorative ed.
    p. ; cm.
 Originally published: Springhouse, PA : Springhouse Corp., c2000.
 Includes bibliographical references and index.
 ISBN-13: 978-0-8036-2169-5
 ISBN-10: 0-8036-2169-8
 ISBN-13: 978-0-8036-2282-1 (special ed.)
 ISBN-10: 0-8036-2282-1 (special ed.)
 1. Nightingale, Florence, 1820-1910. 2. Nurses--England--Biography. I. Title.
 [DNLM: 1. Nightingale, Florence, 1820-1910. 2. Nurses--England--Biography. 3. History of
Nursing England--Biography. WZ 100 N688D 2000a]
 RT37.N5D67 2010
 610.73092--dc22
 [B]
                                        2009021268

7 / 7 / 10

Contents

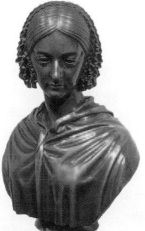

Preface

Nursing is an art; and if it is to be made an art,
requires as exclusive a devotion, as hard a preparation,
as any painter's or sculptor's work;
for what is the having to do with dead canvas or cold marble,
compared with having to do with the living body —
the temple of God's spirit?
It is one of the fine arts;
I had almost said, the finest of the Fine Arts.

— Florence Nightingale, "Una and the Lion," 1868

Like a fiery comet, Florence Nightingale streaked across the skies of 19th-century England and transformed the world with her passage. She was a towering genius of both intellect and spirit, and her legacy resonates today as forcefully as during her lifetime.

We know Nightingale best as the founder of modern secular nursing, but that is only one side of her many-faceted life. The source of her strength, vision, and guidance was a deep sense of unity with God, which is the hallmark of the mystical tradition as it is expressed in all the world's great religions. This aspect of her life has been vastly underestimated, yet we cannot understand her legacy without taking it into account.

Evelyn Underhill, one of the most respected authorities on Western mysticism, described Nightingale as "one of the greatest and most balanced contemplatives of the nineteenth century." This conclusion was based on Nightingale's life work of social action, which she considered her way of honoring "God's laws in nature."

Although Nightingale was deeply religious, she was extremely tolerant and honored the beliefs, rituals, and practices of all cultures under the British Empire. Her embrace of cultural diversity was ahead of its time and is particularly apparent in her 40 years of work to improve sanitary conditions in India. She stressed that all the world's great religions should be studied because, as she put it, this gave "unity to the whole — one continuous thread of interest to all these pearls."

Like most of my colleagues in nursing, I gained only a meager and essentially trivialized picture of Nightingale during my professional education. When my interests led me to explore her life more deeply, I was awed by what I found. I realized that her legacy was far more magnificent — and that she, as an individual personality, was much more complex — than I had ever imagined. The further my research took me, the larger Nightingale loomed — not just in nursing but in other fields as well, such as public health, statistics, hospital design, philosophy, and spirituality. By any measure, she is one of the most towering figures in the Victorian age, which her long life spanned. Indeed, it is difficult to find her equal on the entire canvas of 19th-century Western civilization.

As a nurse, my interests have naturally centered on how Nightingale integrated the art and science of nursing. But I am also fascinated by her concept of healing and how one can become an instrument of healing. Nightingale's vision has inspired in me a deeper, richer, and more compassionate view of nursing than I had ever conceived. I believe this awareness is valuable not only for nurses, but for anyone who has ever been drawn to ease the pain and suffering of another.

In today's specialized world, we are often tempted to compartmentalize our lives, assigning our professional interests to one corner and our spiritual lives to another. To Nightingale, such fragmentation would have been unthinkable. As she put it, her work was her "must" — her spiritual vision and her professional identity were seamlessly combined. Nightingale is therefore an icon of wholeness, an emblem of a united, integrated life. By her uncompromising, shining example, she invites each of us to find our meaning and purpose — our own "must" — in our individual journey through life.

May Florence Nightingale change your life, as she has mine.

Barbara Montgomery Dossey, PhD, RN, AHN-BC, FAAN

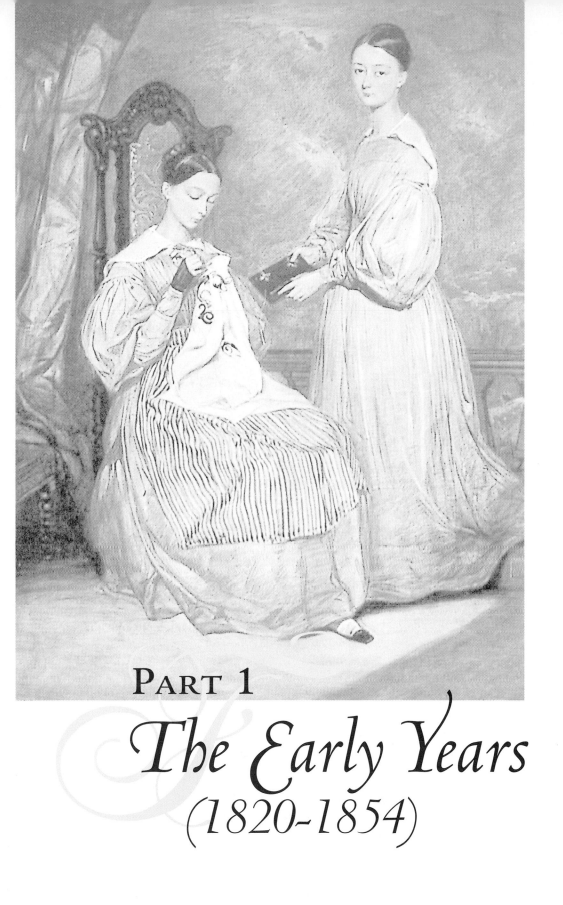

PART 1

The Early Years
(1820-1854)

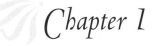

Chapter 1

A Different Kind of Child

*G*od has always led me of Himself ... the first idea I can recollect when I was a child was a desire to nurse the sick. My day dreams were all of hospitals and I visited them whenever I could. I never communicated it to any one, it would have been laughed at; but I thought God had called me to serve Him in that way.

— *Florence Nightingale, Curriculum Vitae, 1851*[1]

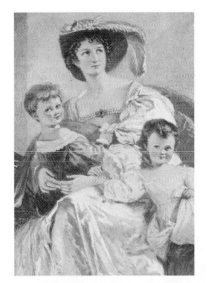

Frances (Fanny) Nightingale with her two daughters, Florence (in mother's lap with book in hand) and Parthenope, c. 1824

When Florence Nightingale was 6 years old, she was sick throughout the year with whooping cough, colds, and other related illnesses. Yet she remembered it as the happiest time of her life. For her, the days and weeks of illness and infirmity were times of heightened peace and quiet, which she always craved. In the serenity of the sick room, away from the bustling of family and servants and the constant stream of visitors to her country home, she had a deeper sense of the spiritual world that she was drawn to at an early age.

She recalled being sickly throughout her childhood. She had a weakness in her hands and didn't begin to write in cursive script until age 10 (although she was printing in a fine hand by age 7). She often wore steel-lined boots for a similar weakness in her ankles. At times, the whole household seemed to be bedridden with colds, coughs, or influenza. Florence's childhood letters are dotted with constant references to sickness — a part of everyday life.

Florence — known to her family as Flo — always felt that the cold and wet English climate didn't suit her because she had been born in sunny, warm Florence, Italy, the city for which she was named. She was born on May 12, 1820, at the Villa Colombaia near the Porta Romana and was christened Florence on July 4.

Florence's sister, Frances Parthenope, had been born a year earlier in Naples and was named after the old Greek village on that site; her nickname was Parthe or Pop. The girls' charming, cultivated father, who was nearly always called W.E.N., for William Edward Nightingale, and their beautiful mother Frances, called Fanny, had enjoyed a grand honeymoon in and around Florence, Italy, that lasted over 3 years. Naming their daughters for the foreign cities of their birth was unheard of at the time; it was one of the few unconventional things that Fanny Nightingale ever did.

The Nightingales belonged to the "upper ten thousand," the social, political, and economic class that ruled England. Although they enjoyed a life of relative luxury, they also had to contend with sickness and disease to a degree that is now forgotten. Lingering illness and sudden death were facts of life for everyone — rich or poor — in the era before modern medicine. Without antibiotics or antiseptic practices, any infection could become life-threatening, especially for women in childbirth and anyone who suffered a wound that broke the skin. Contagion and disease were a threat to all; among the poor and lower working classes, scrofula (tuberculous cervical lymphadenitis) and consumption (tuberculosis) were endemic.

A distinguished family

The Nightingales had two country homes: Lea Hurst, a summer estate located some 150 miles northwest of London in Derbyshire, and Embley, their estate in southern England where they spent most of the year. Flo's favorite home was Lea Hurst — or "the Hurst," as she called it — because of its warm childhood memories and pastoral beauty:

> ... Such country! ... a garden with stone terraces and flights of steps ... gorgeous with masses of hollyhocks, dahlias, nasturtiums, geraniums ... then a sloping meadow losing itself in a steep wooded descent (such tints over the wood!) to the river Derwent, the rocks on the other side ... of a red colour streaked with misty purple. Beyond this, interlacing hills ... the first, deep brown with decaying heather, the next in some purple shadow, and the last catching some pale watery sun-light ... In every direction the walks are most beautiful; old English ... villages are hidden in the moorland hills about here.[2]

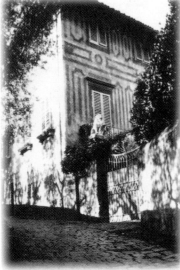

Villa Colombaia in Florence, Italy, where Florence Nightingale was born on May 12, 1820, and christened in the drawing room on July 4

RIGHT: *Lea Hurst in Derbyshire, the Nightingales' summer residence*

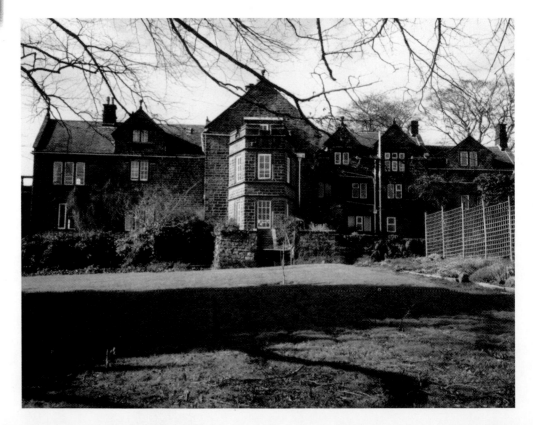

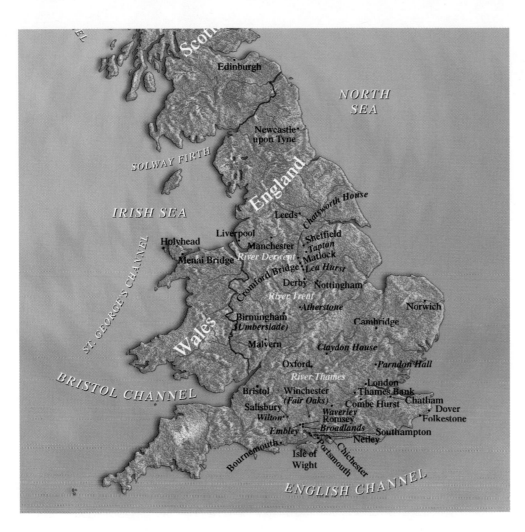

Florence Nightingale's England, showing the major towns and estates that were important in her life

Lea Hurst had been inherited by Florence's father, who was born William Edward Shore, of the old Shore family of Sheffield, Yorkshire. Under the then-existing laws that governed the transmission of property to lineal descendants, he changed his name to Nightingale at age 21 as heir to the properties of his mother's childless uncle, Peter Nightingale of Lea.

Florence had been born into a man's world: The heir to land was usually the eldest son, a practice which kept the large estates intact down through succeeding generations. If a son died before his father, the inheritance usually passed to the next eldest brother and then to nephews, as in the case of Florence's father. It was a rare occasion when a woman received the primary inheritance.

Florence's paternal grandfather, William Shore, had been a long-standing, successful banker in Sheffield, one of the early industrial and commercial centers of England. Like his father, W.E.N. was a prudent manager of money and property his entire life. When he went to college — first to Edinburgh, and then to Cambridge — W.E.N. had an annual income of £7,000 to £8,000 (approximately £267,000 to £306,000 and US$444,000 to $507,000 in today's values).[3]

When Fanny and W.E.N. returned to England in 1821 with their two young daughters, they lived in Herefordshire while awaiting the completion of their new home. The old, tumbled-down Lea Hall of Peter Nightingale had proved too small and rustic for

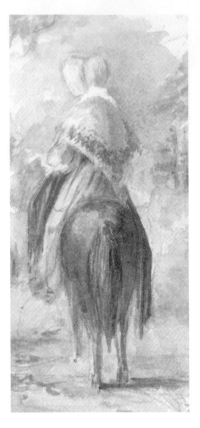

Flo, astride her favorite pony, Peggy, at Embley, in a watercolor by her beloved first cousin Hilary Bonham Carter

the family. W.E.N., who counted architecture among his talents, designed a handsome three-story mansion perfectly situated on a hillside overlooking the River Derwent. They called their new home Lea Hurst.

Florence was close to her father's family, most of whom lived nearby. W.E.N.'s sister, Mary Shore, whom the girls called Aunt Mai (pronounced "my"), spent much of her time with the Nightingales and took an early interest in Florence. Also nearby were Florence's two darling "old people": Great Aunt Elizabeth Evans, known as Aunt Evans, who lived within walking distance in Cromford Bridge, and Aunt Evans's sister Mary, Florence's Grandmother Shore, who lived at the old family home in Tapton, only a day's carriage ride from Lea Hurst.

In later years Florence's reminiscences of her visits to Aunt Evans evoked the quiet beauty of the English countryside:

> *The greatest delight of those child days was our visits to my dear old Aunt in the Valley. She was the very emblem, the spirituality of tenderness and sweetness, complete abnegation of Self — the gentlest of God's creatures — & dearly we loved her, tho' I cannot say we valued all this at the worth we now do, certainly did not so formularize our belief. She lived in the most perfect of Derbyshire old Houses, with its paved terrace & its flights of stone steps overlooking the dashing River — with a Virginian Creeper over its roof, which in Autumn was a perfect sheet of fire twisting with a broad leaved Vine in & out of the old mullioned windows, shutting out light as none in these days would be allowed to do uncropped.*
>
> *It was always hot & dusty, I recollect on the days of those much expected visits, & as we two little maidens [Florence and Parthe] with a Poney's help made our way along the valley, we always loaded ourselves with enormous bunches of Campanulas and blue geraniums which were sure, when wearily we had convoyed them home, to be thrown remorselessly away by tidy housemaids![4]*

Those were the joys of summer. During the first winter, however, it became apparent that there were problems with Lea Hurst. The new house was very cold, and both Florence and Parthe developed bronchitis. For Florence's mother Fanny, the greater problem was that the house was poorly located and too small for serious entertaining. While the setting and countryside were beautiful, the Derbyshire hills were too distant from London — in the decade before railroads — to attract many guests.

Fanny was a great beauty who possessed the vitality, willfulness, and practical intelligence characteristic of her family. Her grandfather had come up to London in the mid-1700s from a small estate on the Isle of Wight and made a fortune in the grocery business. Her father, William Smith, was a Member of Parliament for over 40 years, during which time he was a leader for religious freedom and humanitarian reform, a stalwart in the antislavery movement, and an advocate for the disenfranchised and poor.

Fanny grew up at Parndon Hall, Essex, with her four sisters and five brothers, amid a constant stream of scintillating guests, including the political and cultural leaders of the day. When she failed to gain her father's financial support for marriage to a poor but respectable suitor, she quickly married familiar young William Nightingale, a schoolmate of her brother Octavius and 6 years her junior. The newlyweds left for Italy soon after.

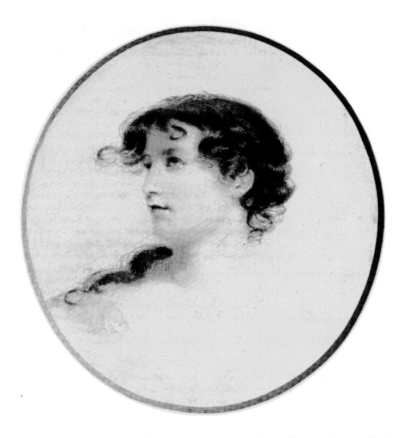

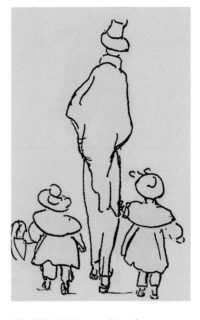

Flo (left), W.E.N., and Parthe, out for a stroll, c. 1825, in a sketch drawn by Fanny's sister, Julia Smith ("Aunt Ju")

LEFT: *Frances (Fanny) Smith Nightingale (1788-1880), Florence's mother*

The same ambition that had brought success to her father and grandfather ran in her blood but, unlike them, Fanny was a woman and totally conventional. The only avenue to success for a conventional married woman, and the only one she desired, was social success: a great house in the style of her childhood; visitors and guests of political, intellectual, and artistic note; travels to and from the great country estates of England; the London social season each spring; and excellent marriages for her daughters.

W.E.N. began a search for a second home, and a letter to Fanny discussing their priorities reflected the life of relative ease that the wealthy upper class led: "The difficulty is, where is the country that is habitable for twelve successive months? ... I think that, provided I could get about 2,000 acres and a house ... where sporting and scenery were in tolerable abundance, and the visit to Lea Hurst were annually confined to July, August, September, and October, then all would be well."[5]

In 1825, W.E.N. found the perfect neighborhood for his needs and Fanny's dreams in Embley Park, a 4,000-acre estate of park and farmland in warmer southern England, near the village of Romsey in Hampshire. It was only a few miles from Southampton; on a clear day, the English Channel could be seen as a distant glint. Situated on the edge of the New Forest, Embley was majestic with its old oaks, beeches, cedars of Lebanon, flowering laurels, gardens, fields of wildflowers, and thickets of rhododendrons lining the long road to the mansion. At both estates, the Nightingales lived amid great natural beauty: The moors and hilltops of England's first national park, Peak District National Park, are visible from the Lea Hurst hillside and the New Forest is now a national forest.

Family, friends, and many of the "right people" of county society lived near Embley Park. Fanny's married sisters were close by, with scads of cousins for Florence and

Parthe to play with. Joanna Smith married John Carter (later Bonham Carter) and lived at Fair Oaks, about 10 miles away near Winchester. Just over the county border at Waverley Abbey in Surrey was Anne, wed to George Thomas Nicholson. London itself was within comfortable distance, and upstream from London lived Uncle Octavius and Aunt Jane Smith at Thames Bank, near present-day Kingston. After Flo's paternal Aunt Mai married her maternal Uncle Sam Smith, their home was at Combe Hurst, also in Surrey. The oldest and youngest of Fanny's sisters — Patty and Julia — remained unmarried. Fanny's brother William Adams remained a bachelor and was a frequent visitor in Florence's childhood. There was one brother — Benjamin — with whom Fanny forbade any contact. After his first wife died, leaving him with one daughter, Benjamin lived with a woman he didn't marry and had other children out of wedlock.

The pattern of the Nightingales' life was established. They spent the summer and early fall at Lea Hurst. They spent the rest of the year at Embley, with trips to London for the spring social season and special events. Amid these seasonal migrations were a wide variety of visits and trips to family and friends that lasted from days to months. Sometimes Florence and Parthe would visit cousins separately or together; or Fanny and W.E.N. might be away while other relatives were staying at Embley or Lea Hurst with the two young sisters.

Letters & sermons

LEFT: *Parthe Nightingale with her young cousins Alfred, Alice, and Harry Bonham Carter in a sketch made at Lea Hurst in 1834 (artist unknown)*

RIGHT: *Laura, Alice, and Hugh Nicholson (to left of table) with Harry and Mrs. Bonham Carter in a drawing dated 1847*

Flo was a serious little girl who liked to write and showed a remarkable independence at an early age. By the age of 7, she was a serious and prolific letter-writer who showed powers of observation and analysis far beyond her years. Letters were the only method of communication possible among the extended family, outside of first-hand reports by visitors and travelers. Florence's letters as well as her journals and the autobiography she wrote in French between the ages of 8 and 10, called *La Vie de Florence Rossignol*, provide the most vivid picture of her daily life.

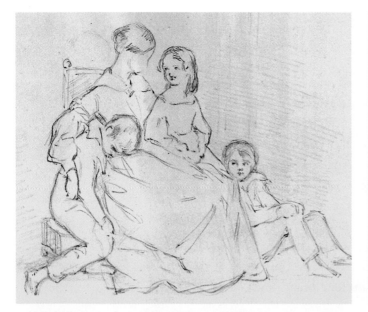

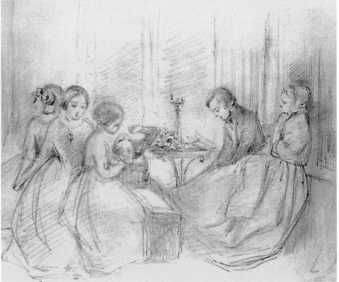

A DIFFERENT KIND OF CHILD

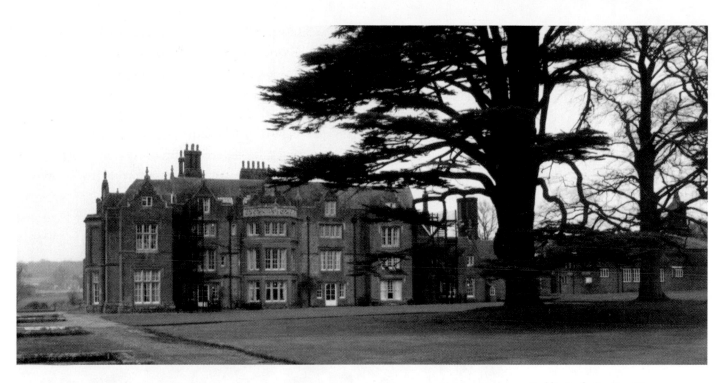

Embley Park, Romsey, Hampshire, the Nightingales' main residence

One of her early journal entries recorded an event of great importance to her and the whole family. In Florence's 7th year, Aunt Mai, her favorite aunt and special friend, married Uncle Sam, her mother's brother, at the Shores' ancestral home in Tapton. In her journal entry for the wedding day, August 26, 1827, Flo wrote:

> *On Wednesday Aunt Mai was married to Uncle Sam. I, Papa, Uncle Sam, Pop and Mr. Bagshaw [the clergyman], went first. Mama and Aunt Mai in the bride's carriage. Aunt Julia and Miss Bagshaw came last. When they were married we were all kneeling on our knees except Mr. Bagshaw. Papa took Aunt Mai's hand and gave it to Uncle Sam. We all cried except Uncle Sam, Mr. Bagshaw and Papa.[6]*

After the wedding, the family returned to Embley at a leisurely pace, stopping along the way to stay with friends. They visited old castles and abbeys, and Flo wrote in her autobiography about the ruins of Tintern Abbey, immortalized in Wordsworth's poem. She also recorded that, unlike other visitors, "Mama did not give anything to the beggars" who milled about when they came out of the abbey.[7]

In the fall of 1827, Miss Sara Christie came to Embley to be the girls' governess. Flo had learned how to read and write from previous governesses, her parents, and the host of relatives who filled the house, but now she became more serious about her lessons. In addition to academic work, Miss Christie gave Florence and Parthe daily lessons in voice, music, piano, and the social arts, such as needlework, dancing, flower arranging, proper manners, and congenial conversation. She traveled with the family on nearly all of their visits.

A letter that 7-year-old Flo wrote to her Grandmother Shore in March 1828 provides a telling glimpse of what upper-class women did with their time. Florence writes of a visit by two distant relatives, Mrs. Sydney Shore and Miss Lydia Shore, during which Mrs. Shore had been ill. She writes, "Mrs. Sydney is better here. She draws. She takes her luncheon with us. She walks better. She is merriest. She paints. She plays on the piano." Then Flo, showing the inclinations of the future woman, continued with a rigorous, factual analysis, "She does not look much better. She goes to bed early. She sleeps better. She was not very well yesterday. She does not go out on cold days."[8]

During a visit to the Carters at Fair Oaks in April 1828, Florence wrote to Fanny that "our sick house has begun again, now the cold weather is come on, for Rebecca, [a servant], miss Wood [governess to the Carter children], Alfy, Harry, and Alice [Carter children] have all very bad colds. I have taken to my steel boots, again, for my feet were very cold again these last days."[9]

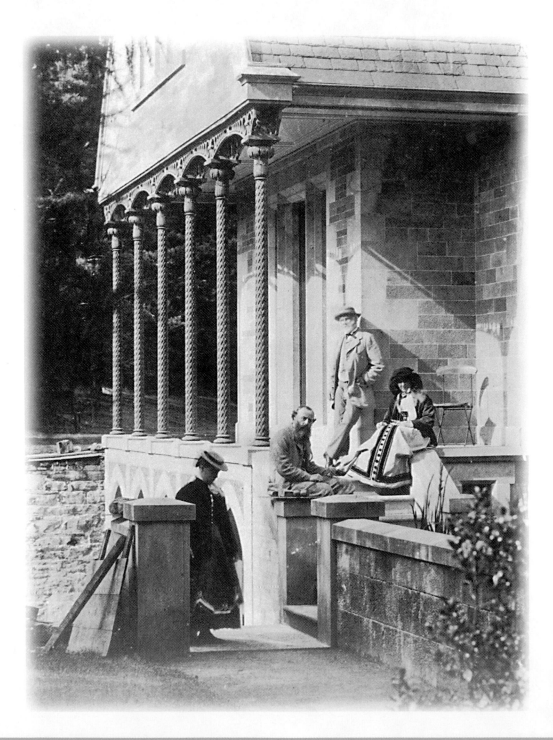

Aunt Mai and Uncle Sam Smith (couple at left) with friends

A DIFFERENT KIND OF CHILD

Dear Parthe,   April 4th 1828

You have not sent "God is good".

Here is a new game for you. Take any word, and see how many words you can make out of the letters. The best way to do those words I told you, is to cut out the letters. There is a box of letters at Embley, so you need not take that trouble.

Mrs. Nightingale. Emily Romsey Hurst

Here are five words for you to make a words out of them of the same quality of being but changing the places of them. Gay and GREAT HELP Try, the first is very easy. I have found it out, the last I have not. Your sister.

I took "breath," and I made 40 words. You need not take all the letters, you know, but as many as you please. You must not double, a letter, that is, putting in two of the same kind in one word. Is it not a nice game.

Dear Mama

I finished my housewife at the forest (that is to say, put on the strings and cassimere,) and I began another. We bought a skein of red silk at Southampton, and yesterday, the day before Gale and Kitty went to Rom...

P.S. Do you know where my smallest Indian Cabinet is? What fine days you have had!

...sey, and bought us some flannel, and some cambric muslin, to make us flannel-petticoats, and night-gowns for our dolls, and a yard and a half of red ribban. Give my love to Papa, Miss Christie is going to send... him on my letter a Sheriff's writ. Good-bye, ever your affectionate child Florence Nightingale

LEFT: *Flo's letter to her sister, dated April 4, 1828, in which she describes a new word game*

RIGHT: *Flo's letter to her mother, dated August 11, 1828, written around a legal paper of her father's because paper and postage were expensive*

Like many children, Florence's life was busy, even when her parents were away, as this letter she wrote at age 8 makes clear:

> Dear Mama , I have got a little cold, but it is so little, that I hopes [sic] it will be well before you come back. I don't go to church to-day because of that. I did figures very well yesterday. Then we went to poor Mrs. Bungy's, she had a bad head-ache. We dined in the Piano drawing room; and I did music, Latin, French reading, and walzing [sic], Miss Christie played. This morning I did everything as usual, except that I have not written my copy, and that I have learnt more poetry and read in the Bible the XVII chapter of the I book of Kings (about Elijah being fed by ravens and being supported by the Sareptan [Zarephathan] woman and raising her son to life again), and the IV chapter of the II book (about Elisha). Yesterday, we went to Mrs. Staples, (besides Mrs. Bungy's) and she _be'es_ very well, and he (her leg) _be'es_ very well too. [Florence had underlined Mrs. Staples's vernacular.] Ask poor dear Bon [cousin Bonham "Bonny" Carter] whether he would like any-thing besides the books that I could give him. Do it secretly, because I want to surprise him with something. Buy the knife for miss Christie; I asked her to tell me everything she buys, so I shall know if she buys a knife, or not, and then I shall present it. I play better at battledore and shuttlecock, we are going to have a game now, I and miss Christie, as we cannot go out. Goodbye. Your affec^te Flo N.[10]

One of Miss Christie's exercises was to develop ladylike handwriting in her charges by making copies of moral sentiments, one for each letter of the alphabet. Florence began with "Avoid lying: it leads to every other vice." However, by the time she got to the T's with "Temperance in prosperity indicates wisdom," her intuitive preference for the

Dear Papa   Sunday Embley 11 o'clock
        I played with Miss Christie at battledore and
shuttlecock yesterday, and I got once 9 once 8 and several times
I got seven. We were very much tempted to send our letters
in the Duke's frank, but we thought we might make some
mistake. Has Pop had many teeth out at Mr Dumergue's? Flo—
Dear Mama — I have got a little cold, but it is so little,
that I hopes it will be well before you come back. I
don't go to church to-day because of that. I did figures
very well yesterday. Then we went to poor Mrs. Bungy's, she
had a bad head-ache. We dined in the Piano drawing room,
and I did music, Latin, French reading, and valzing, and Miss
Christie played. This morning I did everything as usual, except that I have not written my copy, and that I have learnt
more poetry, and read in the Bible the XVII chapter of
the I book of Kings (about Elijah being fed by ravens and being
supported by the Sareptan woman, and raising her son to life
again, and the IV chapter of the II book (about Elisha) Yesterday, we went to Mrs Staples, (besides Mrs. Bungy's) and
she bees very well, and he (her lee) bees very well too.
Ask poor dear Bon whether he would like any-thing
besides the books that I could give him. Do it secretly, because I want to surprize him with something. Buy the knife for miss Christie; I asked
                                        turnlegover

her to tell me everything she buys, so I shall know if she
buys a knife, or not, and then I shall prevent it.
I play better at battledore and shuttle cock, we are
going to have a game now, I and Miss Christie,
as we cannot go out Goodbye. Your affec.te Flo N.

The Duke and Duchess of
Wellington present their com-
pliments to Mr. Nightingale
and request the Honor of His
Company to dine and sleep
at Hatfield Saye on Sunday
the 1st March, to meet My
Lords the Judges.
London Feb. 13 — 18[   ]

The front and back of a letter
from Flo to her parents, written
on an invitation the Nightingales received from the Duke
and Duchess of Wellington

practical application of ideas became apparent; humdrum rote learning was not for her.
At the end of this line she wrote: "Stupid Copy." Then at the bottom of the page she
continued, "The good of this copy I never could see and I do not like it, I never wish to
write it and I never will if I can help it." Miss Christie immediately understood her exceptional student's need for meaning and function. Rather than write "Unity is the necessary condition of success," she let Florence write "Uxbridge near which are the remains
of an ancient camp."[11] Writing about real things was much more sensible to Flo.

Another exercise was to record the lives of real people such as their French maid,
Selina Clémence Coulbeaux, who had had an exciting childhood. During the French
Revolution, her father had been a footman to Louis XIV, and she had had many adven-
tures while escaping from France to England. Flo also learned geography and English
history and could answer questions like "What is the first unfeeling circumstance of
Henry I as King? What was Caesar's favourite Legion?"[12]

In a letter to Parthe at age 8, Flo described a new game: Take the letters of any word
and see how many new words you can make out of the letters. She had made 40 words
from "breath." Flo included the rules as well as advice on the best way to proceed; such
protocols were second nature to her, reflecting the passion for systemization that would
become her hallmark in later years.[13]

An instinct for nurturing

In a tiny notebook made out of W.E.N. and Fanny's old letters, Flo's innate and deepest interest surfaced. In her schoolgirl handwriting is a medical prescription for how many grains of James' powder, a common remedy for various ailments at the time, people of different ages should take: "16 grains for an old woman, 11 for a young woman, and 7 for a child."[14] While staying with her cousins, the Nicholsons, she began thinking about helping sick people. Her grandmother noted that conscientious Flo was "both Martha and Mary, two excellent characters blended in one."[15]

In June of 1829, her cousin "Bonny" Carter died after a half year's illness. Flo's description of his last days revealed the hardy spirit in which persons of her class — even children — were expected to endure pain. It also reveals Flo's powers of observation and ability to focus on details of illness and suffering. She wrote to a friend that her cousin was a:

> dear, kind boy ... He was kind to every body to the last, and so very patient, he was never cross. Half an hour before his death, he asked to see Aunt Patty, and he was looking about the room for a sofa for her. We left [Nurse] Gale in London to help to take care of him, but nothing would do: His complaint had got so much the better of medecine [sic], doctors, nursing and all, that all hope was given up. He had a great deal of pain, throughout his illness. Mama saw him once, he talked to her a great deal, and was so anxious to give her everything she liked. Gale slept by his side. One night, she got up to do something for him and he said to her, "Come, it will do very well, there's a good creature, go to bed now, go to sleep." One day, he said to his papa, when in great pain, "I will bear it as well as I can, but if I were strong, I think I should leap about the room with this pain."[16]

Flo's instincts for nurturing and healing appeared early in her life. Like many young girls, she nursed sick dolls but her instincts for caring were on a different scale than most. At one time she had "her 18 dolls *all* ill in rows in bed, when she was quite a little thing."[17] In her ninth summer at Lea Hurst, when the family made visits to the villagers and received guests, Flo carefully and systematically wrote down the illnesses of all the people she met, especially the children, noting the circumstances and nature of each person's condition.

Doing God's work

The world in which Florence came of age was deeply religious; the church and religion were an integral part of everyday life. In her childhood letters and other writings, Flo frequently referred to various duties she had completed, which reflected the wide range of obligations expected of upper class children. In the fall of 1829, she inscribed on the inside cover of one of her journals reminders of things that were important to a nine-year-old girl and that would remain important all her life: "Allowed 6 pence a week/ Journal of Flo/Embley/The Lord is with thee/Wherever thou art."[18]

Doing God's work on earth included an emphasis on spiritual things as well as attention to budgetary items, a natural attitude for a child whose grandfathers both were Unitarian — exemplars of Protestant thrift and industry. A list of physical, moral, and educational goals from January 1830 (possibly written for her mother or governess) provides a clear indication of the dutiful, thoughtful girl Flo already was by age 9. Two items — "to pray regularly" and "to visit the poor people and take care of those who are sick" — were harbingers of the life-work to come:

> I promise to take run before breakfast to gate ... ½ an hour's walk before dinner, long walk after, or if cold & damp long walk before & ½ an hour's after ... to do 20 arms [exercises] before I dress, 10 minutes before breakfast & 10 after exercises, if ill done 10 more ... to practice 1 hour a day ... to draw ½ an hour regularly ... not to lie in bed ... to go to bed in proper time ... to read the Bible & pray regularly before breakfast & at night ... to visit the poor people & take care of those who are sick ... to take medicine when I want it ... to go regularly after breakfast on Sundays to church when there is any one to go with me, to read, write & do the Bible ... to read my books you put out for me ... to read to Aunt Mai & save her trouble ... to read this paper every day ... to write to you. I think I should be much better here than elsewhere. I should have fewer temptations. FN.[19]

During a 2-month stay with the Carters at Fair Oaks, from February to April 1830, 9-year-old Flo's letters paint a vivid picture of her rich and varied childhood in a large and happy family. (Around this time, the Carters became the "Bonham Carters," when John Carter inherited some property and had to change his name, as W.E.N. had years earlier.) In these narratives, glimmers of her talent for methodically organizing information begin to emerge. She begins to number items sequentially by category, to develop lists and tables, and to assign names and headings to diagrams. An example is reflected in a letter to Parthe about the play house she was building with cousins Jack and Hilary:

> We stick little sticks in the ground in our larder, and interlace them with rushes, making a little enclosure, in which we keep potatos etc. We have made 2 sofas in our parlour; we have dragged up several boughs of laurel, and are going to make a bower with it in the dining-room, and have made a little tool-house in our larder, in which we keep, viz. 1 spade, 2 rakes, 2 hoes, 4 baskets.[20]

For a little girl away from home, without her own personal servants to perform every task, the incipient craving for independence and meaningful work began to find expression:

> I say my prayers to myself morning and night ... I keep all my clothes myself. I make out my own washing-bills myself, and fold up all my things. All of which I like extremely ... I dress and undress, and put in my curl-papers all myself, and manage all my clothes myself ...[21]

A letter to her mother in March 1830 about a sermon she had just heard shows an impressive display of memory and sequencing for a 9-year-old. It also reveals the increasing intimations of the spiritual world that began to appear in her writings at this time:

> Dear Mama, I am just come from church. Mr. Green preached from Luke, Chap. XV, Verse 10, "There is joy in heaven over one sinner that repenteth"... I had no pencil with me, but I recollect he said, that it is not in the resolution, but in the doing of a thing, that we must rejoice over. And he gave us three examples. First, in the parable of the man having 100 sheep, losing 1, leaving the 99 in the wilderness, and going to seek the one he had lost. Then, and not till then,

Feb 24th Wednesday. Fair-Oak.

Dear Papa

I have not put your Scrap-Book any-where, but one day I saw it in the drawer in the Music-room, next to the bow-window; and I think it very odd, you did not think of looking for it there!!! We have banked up the kitchen-door, (at our house) and made a new one. We have made a sofa of sand in the kitchen, covered with heather. Our moss-beds are so wet, we cannot sleep in them. We have filled up our potato-holes in the kitchen, and made a larder. We have made a great addition to our provisions, viz.

Vegetable		Fruits	
little Cones	Potatos	Horse Chestnut	Peaches
		Dif-te-rent Kinds of	Pine-apples
ons Cones	Cucumbers		Pears
			Strawberries
			Goose-berries
Kind of Painting Peas	Cones	Currants	

We intend to make another larder. We have made 3 other paths to different parts of our house. We have made a parlour, and a summer-house, and are making

did he send for his neighbours to rejoice with him. The same with the woman and her ten pieces of silver. She did not call her neighbours to rejoice with her, till she had found her silver, not when she was resolving she would sweep her house and look for it. The same with the prodigal son. He says, I will arise and go to my father, and say, I have sinned, and am not worthy to come into thy presence, and the Scriptures add immediately after, that he did do it. Then, and not till then, did his father come, and fall on his neck, and kiss him, and order the best robe to be brought, and the fatted calf to be killed, to make him a feast. Good-bye, dear Mama. Your affec^te Flo.[22]

During a visit to Uncle Octavius and Aunt Jane in July 1830, Flo — now 10 years old — wrote her mother about another sermon she had heard, "a very pretty one, on the text I Corinthians, Chap XIII, verse 9th 'for we know in part, and we prophesy in part,' our favourite chapter, you know." Although Fanny often seemed more concerned with social matters, the chapter that Flo remembered as their favorite ends with "And now abideth faith, hope, charity, these three; but the greatest of these is charity."[23]

She continued her letter with an enchanting word picture of a sunset over the river Thames that reflected her appreciation of the divine presence in nature:

> *I had a very nice quiet little row with miss Southwood, [possibly governess to the Smith children] by ourselves except 2 men to row us. We went up to Battersea Bridge ... The sunset was particularly beautiful. On one side, the golden clouds shed such a beautiful tinge on the water, and on the other, it looked so dark and stormy, and there were 2 sweet little ends of a rainbow on each side the sky, & 2 windmills against it, & little boats gliding up and down the river, Oh! so beautiful! and there were 2 steam boats just seen in the distance, that had passed us, with the smoke curling up. I felt so happy, mama, I thought I loved God then ... Uncle and Aunt Oc and miss Southwood are all very kind, and so am I, I hope, to my cousins. I do not eat too much, I assure you, and I do not play too much. I lie down sometimes. I have found a very pretty book here, called The Christian's Friend, consisting of short Sermons, and Stories showing the shortness of life, and suddenness of death.[24]*

She concluded her letter with a practical application of her spiritual impulse — something she would later take to much higher levels: "How do you find the poor people? Have they suffered much in the flood?"[25]

Florence's autobiography and letters from this period show that she was thinking seriously about life and trying hard to be good. A letter to her sister reveals the inner workings of a young girl with a powerful predilection for carrying out her moral obligations: "Dear Pop, I think of you, pray let us love one another more than we have done. Mama wishes it particularly, it is the will of God, and it will comfort us in our trials through life."[26]

A need to be useful

In 1831, the girls' governess, Miss Christie, left the family to marry. The emptiness left by this departure was soon relieved by the birth of a little boy, William Shore Smith (nicknamed Shore), to Flo's dear Aunt Mai. Shore joined his older sister Blanche just as Flo was becoming old enough to help with the babies; now she could be really useful, as she had always wanted. From the first time Shore was put in Flo's arms, she claimed him as "my boy Shore" and from then on he was.

Now with a "baby of her own," Flo could write to her favorite cousin, Hilary Bonham Carter, about babies. Hilary was the oldest child in her family and had lots of little brothers and sisters. In March 1832, Flo wrote, "I am very sorry to hear that your Baby is still so poorly, but our Baby is much better for he has got two teeth through." When Aunt Mai left Shore at Embley, and Nurse Gale became ill, Flo was elated when she became the one to take care of Shore full time. [27]

Flo found another grown-up way to be useful when Grandmother Smith visited Embley in the spring. She wanted to read to her every day, but Parthe also wanted to read and, being older, got that job. However, Grandmama liked to walk a little every day, up and down the room, and Flo was delighted to find that she was now tall and strong enough to help. She reveled in her new duty, which she called "walking Grandmama." While Parthe read, Flo provided Grandmama with a strong young arm to lean on each day.[28]

There were also hard lessons to learn from life. First came the news that Miss Christie had died after childbirth. Then Hilary's little brother Hugh died, the second Bonham Carter child to die. Flo wrote at this time that she felt the uncertainty of all earthly ties. She wrote to Hilary and Grandmama that she pictured Hugh as a little angel with his older brother, Bonny, as well as Miss Christie, all in heaven. She also thought to herself that perhaps Miss Christie would not have died had she not married and had a baby.[29]

Now Florence's contemplative, spiritual instincts were about to be wedded to mature knowledge, and the concerns of a little girl were about to be put behind her. For, after the departure of Miss Christie, the Nightingales found no tutors who met both Fanny's lofty requirements in the social graces and W.E.N.'s exacting standards for academic excellence. Consequently, W.E.N. took charge of Florence and Parthe's academic instruction, and a tutor was hired for music and drawing.

At a time when universities were for men only and the belief in an equal education for women was rare, W.E.N.'s initiative was extraordinary and the best thing that could have happened in young Florence's life. She would receive a young man's education at home. If she couldn't go to university, Edinburgh and Cambridge would come to her.

A Cambridge home education

Of the day that the serious, 12-year-old Florence first entered her father's library to begin her home education, she later wrote, "I had the most enormous desire of acquiring. For 7 years of my life I thought of little else but cultivating my intellect."[30] Her education, combined with her drive for perfectability to accomplish God's will on earth, would help to crystallize her moral world view.

As a teacher, W.E.N. could do what he loved most with his younger daughter — explore the world of ideas. Florence became a companion to him in the intellectual world. In a letter to a friend, novelist Elizabeth Gaskell described the essential W.E.N.: "He is a very superior man; full of great interests; took high honors at college — and worked away at classics and metaphysics, and mathematics." [31]

In addition to W.E.N.'s great love of the classics and scholarship, he was also steeped in the reform traditions of his Unitarian family and was an adherent of Jeremy Bentham, the chief architect of modern government. At the heart of Florence's great gifts to nursing and public health would be her synthesis of the classical and modern worlds that her education bridged.

Florence's classical education emphasized Platonic thought, with its underlying concept of the Good, and pure and perfect form. This study enabled her to examine the accumulated wisdom of the ancient world and western civilization to her time, to distill from it the moral tenets that underlie these worlds, and to apply these guides to her thought and work. Her modern outlook was first shaped by her father's world view; then informed by her own genius and practical understanding of the emerging fields of social science, statistics, and public administration; and finally driven by the needs of women and the world.

W.E.N.'s hidden bookcase door in the library at Embley, through which he would sometimes emerge disguised as a ghost to delight his daughters

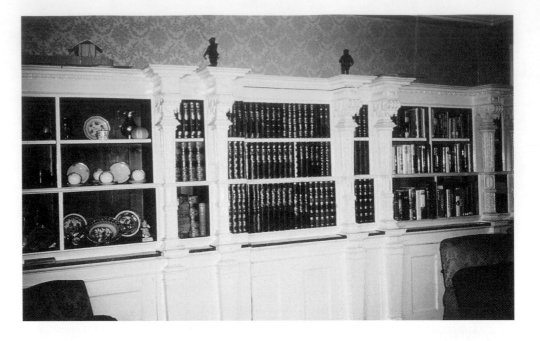

W.E.N. provided for Florence the home equivalent of an Edinburgh and Cambridge education, in which she was first in a class of two. The hours were long, the work hard. As the years progressed, Florence emerged as a serious scholar; Parthe increasingly opted to join Fanny in the drawing room and the garden. The family preferences established at this time remained for the rest of their lives: Fanny and Parthe, the extroverted traditionalists, immersed in their social whirl and absorbed by daily conventions; W.E.N. and Florence, the two introverts — he the firm, exacting professor who preferred "the quiet and the shadows"[32] and she the brilliant, intuitive student — sharing journeys of the mind.

At times, the library became a sort of theater. W.E.N.'s elaborately carved bookcase contained a hidden door leading to his study, from which he sometimes emerged draped in a ghostly white sheet to delight Flo and Parthe. The books on these shelves were fakes — wooden dummies with elegant bindings — and the titles held clues to the spoof. For example, there were volumes titled "Leather on Woods," "History of Morocco" (leather), "Optical Delusions," "Tales of the Doorway," and "Oaths Not Binding." [33]

Florence studied Roman, French, German, Italian, and Turkish history — unknowing preparation for her future travels — as well as English political and constitutional history, philosophy, ethics, grammar, composition, mathematics, and the Bible. Always organized, she kept her books alphabetized by headings, for example, the Age of Reason, Bigotry, Creeds, Death, and Education. She annotated and copied her favorite passages, and accumulated a huge storehouse of information and ideas for contemplation. She began to rise early before the household awoke, between 4 a.m. and 6 a.m., to prepare for her daily lessons.

Florence shared with her father a natural gift for language. She became fluent in Latin, Greek, French, German, and Italian and was reading Homer at age 16. She translated parts of Plato's *Phaedo, Crito,* and *Apology.* In later life, she would help the master of

Balliol College, Benjamin Jowett, by critiquing the summaries and introductions in his translations of Plato. In her late 20s, when traveling through Austria-Hungary with family friends, she would speak Latin, sometimes the only common language shared with the monks and nuns, to arrange lodging at abbeys and monasteries.

Two early influences: Plato & Stewart

Among the great thinkers whose works Florence read, two in particular captured her interest: the ancient Greek philosopher Plato and Dugald Stewart, a popular lecturer in moral philosophy and political economy at the University of Edinburgh from 1785 to 1809.

Florence was captivated by Plato because he proposed a society in which women could have roles of action and responsibility equal to those of men. In *The Republic,* written in the 4th and 5th centuries B.C., Plato maintained that men and women should be educated equally for the good of the State and that women's perceived inferiority was a perversion of nature and a waste of resources of half the population.

Plato had two basic assumptions about human nature — first, that each person is born with a specific aptitude for one task above all others; second, that a division of labor among the people was necessary for the State to prosper. Plato identified three basic divisions of labor: artisan, auxiliary, and ruler. A person's natural ability determined the category for which he was best suited. Artisans (craftsmen and shopkeepers) carried out the physical maintenance of the State; the auxiliary classes were the soldiers who defended the State; and the rulers were the wisest elders, those who led the State.

In addition to these three categories, Plato also described an elite group known as Guardians, who could come from either the auxiliary or ruler class. The Guardians were people of rare gifts who had a command of many kinds of knowledge. Focusing solely on philosophical and intellectual pursuits, they were to be free from the practical concerns of daily life such as caring for children. Although Plato knew that the female sex was generally considered inferior to the male, he believed that certain women could possess the qualities necessary to be a Guardian.

The characteristics of the Guardians with Florence and were reflected in her writings throughout her life. Guardians should be "brave and high-spirited, because a high spirit makes the soul fearless."[34] They must love wisdom and be rational thinkers, able to argue their case according to facts rather than opinions.

On a practical note, Plato said the best natures must be trained in mathematics. To avoid being confused by a plurality of issues or objects, and to always be able to determine absolute unity, the principal men of the State must study arithmetic "until they see the nature of numbers with the mind only ... Arithmetic has a very great and elevating effect, compelling the soul to reason about abstract number." The philosophers must master mathematics and abstract numbers because they have "to rise out of the sea of change and lay hold of true being."[35] Plato could well have been writing about the situations that Florence would face in later life.

It's easy to understand why Dugald Stewart's *Elements of the Philosophy of the Human Mind* commanded Florence's attention. Stewart shared with Plato the belief that people

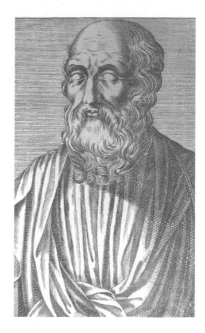

Plato (427?-347 B.C.), the Greek philosopher whose belief in the importance of mathematics and the need to allow women a meaningful role in society profoundly influenced Florence

have certain gifts and should be educated accordingly. His concept of "enlightened conductors" paralleled Plato's concept of Guardians. Stewart wrote:

> The most essential objects of education are ... to cultivate all the various principles of our nature, both speculative [mind] and active [body], in such a manner as to bring them to the greatest perfection of which they are susceptible.
>
> Surely the great aim of an enlightened and benevolent philosophy is not to rear a small number of individuals, who may be regarded as prodigies in an ignorant and admiring age, but to diffuse, as widely as possible, that degree of cultivation which may enable the bulk of a people to possess all the intellectual and moral improvement of which their nature is susceptible.
>
> If the multitude must be led, it is of consequence, surely, that it should be led by enlightened conductors; by men who are able to distinguish truth from error.[36]

The phrase "truth from error" would be a recurring theme in Florence's mature written works. To distinguish truth from error and to write it down as an example or path for the collective good was also a way of putting into everyday practice the spiritual values of the Good and the Divine that she already felt so deeply inside.

Bentham & utilitarianism

Another pivotal influence in the development of Florence's world view was the fact that her father, in theory and practice, was a follower of Jeremy Bentham, founder of the principle of utilitarianism, the concept of "the greatest good for the greatest number." Bentham opposed the old notion of the "social contract," the idea that all of society was an organic whole created by God and that all individuals should stay in their place and class — an idea accepted and promulgated as absolute truth by the ruling European nobility and established churches. His *Fragment on Government*, written in 1776, was "the first publication by which men at large were invited to break loose from the trammels of authority and ancestor wisdom on the field of law."[37]

Bentham's utilitarian principle was instrumental in laying the foundations of modern government and social science. Following the Newtonian concept of a mechanistic universe that resembled a big clock, in which everything was fixable and capable of perfection, the Benthamites believed in the existence of immutable laws of human behavior.

Utilitarianism provided a formula for deciding on a choice of action by using the "pleasure vs. pain" principle. This formula weighed six categories of anticipated effects: intensity, duration, certainty, propinquity (closeness of effect), fecundity (secondary effects), and purity. These six qualities were to be taken into account in making individual choices; if more than one person were involved, then a seventh factor, the total number affected, would be added to the equation. The "good" results, or pleasure, were described by Bentham as "profit ... or convenience, or advantage, benefit, emolument, happiness, and so forth." These were compared with the painful results, described as "mischief, or inconvenience, or disadvantage, or loss, or unhappiness, and so forth." The determination of public and political issues, according to the greatest good for the greatest number, was to come through universal suffrage.[38]

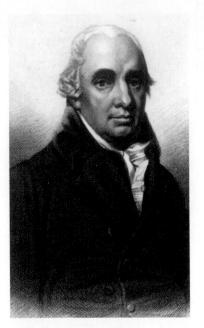

Dugald Stewart (1753-1828), popular lecturer in moral philosophy at the University of Edinburgh whose concept of "enlightened conductors" made a lasting impression on Florence

Bentham was a prodigious intellect whose work primarily involved the fields of jurisprudence, government, political philosophy, and ethics. His true legacy is the whole of British (and to a great extent American) executive government, both national and local. He was a founder of the science of public administration, in which nonpartisan, tenured professionals put legislation into action and constantly supervise the results, thereby achieving uniform standards and relatively efficient operation, ensured by inspection. His influence ranged far beyond the British Isles in the development of democratic constitutions and governments around the globe.

Bentham's lifelong ambition had been the complete overhaul of English law and administration, which was a hodgepodge of custom, practice, and anachronism inherited from Roman and medieval times. For instance, as late as the 1820s, more than 200 offenses in the English penal code were punishable by death. But after 1825, as a result of the growing influence of Bentham's followers, the death penalty ceased for such crimes as forgery, sheep-stealing, damaging Westminster Bridge, stealing more than five shillings' worth of goods from a shop, and impersonating an inmate of the Chelsea Hospital for old and disabled soldiers.

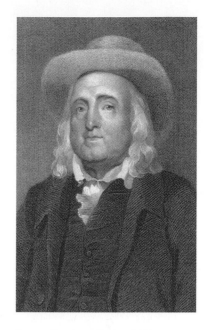

Jeremy Bentham (1748-1832), English jurist and philosopher whose utilitarian principles drove the reform legislation of Florence's time

Learning to be comfortable in a man's world

Just as important as the content of Florence's education was her professor — her father. She and her father had great affection for each other and shared interests that they discussed until his death. Through the give and take of philosophical discussions with him, she learned early on to ask questions openly and to develop and defend her positions. She became emotionally and psychologically comfortable in the man's world of business, politics, and power and was effective all her life in working with men in a businesslike manner. She would never be fazed by the "power and pervasiveness of male fantasy structures" that nearly always bedevilled early women professionals.[39]

Although Florence and her father agreed on much, there was, even at this time, a fundamental difference in their natures. At one point in 1832, W.E.N. wrote a note to Fanny on some point of contention, "Ask Flo if she has lost her intellect. If not, why does she grumble at troubles which she cannot remedy by grumbling?"[40] For her father, inquiry and speculation were largely an end in themselves. At heart he was a man of ease, determined to enjoy life. For Florence, the "grumbling" was a prelude to her future life of action. Lessons learned were to be translated into action according to God's plan; her internal visions demanded external form.

The Nonconformist conscience

Florence was always familiar with the intricate relationship between politics, business, and religion that characterized the England of her time. Her extensive family — consisting of merchants, bankers, and landowners — were among the Nonconformists, or Dissenters, who were largely responsible for the inexorable tide of reform that shaped modern England. Their moral beliefs and concept of duty came to be known as the "Nonconformist conscience." They were "patient men and such as believe that labour and industry is their duty to God."[41]

Dissenters were groups that separated from or developed independently of the Church of England (Anglican Church) and who were persecuted or denied full equality under various Parliamentary laws having to do with religion. (Technically, "dissent" pertains to disagreement with Church doctrines; "nonconformity" to the refusal to comform to Church ritual.)[42] In earlier times, Dissenters were penalized mainly by being excluded from many professions and trades, which were controlled by the Church and State. However, as commerce and trade increased with the Industrial Revolution, a middle class of merchants began to emerge, and families such as the Smiths and Shores parlayed their entrepreneurial talents into wealth and political power.

Men of independent means, such as William Edward Nightingale and others of his class, supplanted many of the squires and gentry who had lived solely as farmers and stockmen off their smaller land-holdings. They brought with them a higher level of culture to the small towns and countryside. Those with wealth from commerce, mining, and manufacturing — derived from the beginnings of the industrial revolution — speeded the process of consolidation of estates that had begun in earnest during the previous century. They infused their modern outlook and progressive politics into local and county government and, in doing so, contributed to the growing movement for religious, political, and legal reform.

In Florence's time, politics in England were as much a matter of denomination as class and party. The Church of England was established in 1534 by Henry VIII. It was not just the king's desire for an heir that precipitated the split; Henry wanted the church wealth that flowed to Rome to remain in England. At the time, the Catholic church controlled about one-fourth of the land and one-half the income in England. After Henry VIII, the Church of England grew rich and worldly as the official State church.

By the mid-1700s, the number of Dissenters and Nonconformists rapidly began to increase as the Church of England paid little attention to the spiritual needs of a growing and changing population. As a result, many denominations grew and multiplied: Methodists, Baptists, Presbyterians, Unitarians, Roman Catholics, Quakers, Jews, and others. Over the years, the governing classes, who were usually of the Tory political party, came to associate Roman Catholics with disloyalty to England (because of their loyalty to the Pope in Rome) and Protestant Dissenters with disloyalty to the king (because the king was the titular head of the Church of England).[43] Dissenters, however, pointed out that they merely sought complete freedom of religion — their right to determine their own spiritual affairs with God alone, without interference by the state or the state-sanctioned church.

By the 1830s, the Dissenters had five main grievances against the Church of England:

• A man and woman could be legally married only in the parish church, unless they were Quakers or Jews.

• The government registered births only in baptismal registers of the parish churches.

• Except in larger cities, the cemetery was church property and often Dissenters were buried with rites they disapproved of or in silence.

• Every citizen (unless too poor) had to pay a tax to repair the local parish church.

The Dissenter was thus compelled by law to support a religion he rejected.

• To obtain a degree from Oxford or Cambridge as well the newer University of Durham, a Dissenter had to sign a document called the Thirty-Nine Articles, which declared his allegiance to the Church of England.[44]

For members of the upper class, a great deal of the bias against Dissenters was a form of social snobbery. To ensure her family's social standing in the Hampshire establishment, Fanny had quietly departed from the Smith family's religious tradition of Unitarianism in favor of the more socially acceptable Church of England, raising her daughters as Anglicans. Dissent wasn't fashionable in southern England, where, as Florence would later write, "Unitarians and other Atheists" were universally banned. In her immediate family, Florence was alone in her quest for religious experience that went beyond the conventional Anglican formalities of the day. For these discussions in her early years, she could turn only to her closest cousin Hilary Bonham Carter and her Aunt Julia and Aunt Mai, who shared her spiritual concerns.

Florence's family had been directly involved in these political and religious issues for over two generations, especially on her mother's side, among her aunts, uncles, cousins and, of course, her grandfather William Smith, Member of Parliament for over 40 years. Because W.E.N. was a magistrate for many years, like many country gentlemen of his class, and served a term as High Sheriff of Hampshire, local politics and legal proceedings were familiar to Florence. She had written letters on copies of W.E.N.'s sheriff's writs and often watched her father ride off with an assemblage of 24 shiremen to meet the judges at the Winchester cathedral for the official court sessions. At one trial she attended, she heard a servant who had stolen some beans from his master sentenced to 14 years' imprisonment in Australia.

In addition, Florence's uncle John Bonham Carter, Hilary's father, was active in reform committee affairs in Hampshire. He would serve as the member for Portsmouth in the first Parliament formed after the Reform Bill of 1832. His eldest son, Jack, one of Flo's childhood playmates, would become a member of Parliament from Winchester in the 1860s. Uncle Adams, her mother's brother, also stood for Parliament at Sudbury. Even the uncle whom Fanny shunned, Benjamin Smith, was a member of Parliament in the 1840s. His daughter, Barbara Leigh Smith (later Bodichon), would emerge as one of the leaders of the organized women's rights movement that took form in the 1850s.

Evangelical influence

From the day she was born, Florence was immersed in and molded by the two great streams of political and religious ideas that shaped reform and social action in 19th-century England: utilitarianism and Evangelicalism. The influence of utilitarianism was largely due to W.E.N.'s belief that "Bentham has taught great moral truth more effectually than all the Christian divines." That of Evangelicalism stemmed from her family's Unitarian background, which shared the Evangelicals' great moral passion in the fight for religious freedom and against slavery. Their protest resulted in the abolition of British participation in the slave trade in 1807 and in the abolition of slavery in all British possessions in 1833.

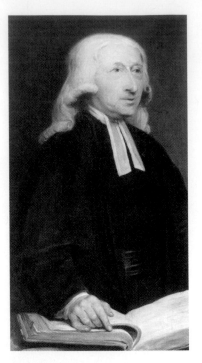

John Wesley (1703-1791), the great English Evangelical preacher and founder of Methodism

Although the origins of these movements were entirely different — one based on a belief in "the greatest good for the greatest number" to be attained through social legislation and the other based on a spiritual concern for man's immortal soul — they shared humanitarian concerns. Together, they drove the great tide of social reform that arose in response to the unchecked abuses of urbanization and the Industrial Revolution, reforms that were the lasting legacy of Victorian England and that helped set the stage for Florence Nightingale's life work.

For the village poor and the urban masses who felt ignored by the Church of England, the Evangelical churches provided a true religious experience and a gateway to heaven from the bottom rung of the social ladder. The greatest of the Evangelical preachers, John Wesley, the founder of Methodism, discovered that the "unadorned gospel of atonement preached to laboring crowds converted on the instant."[45] Evangelical fervor touched all denominations, including elements of the Anglican church.

During Florence's early years, Evangelicalism was the strongest religious force in British life and a principal influence on what has come to be called Victorianism:

Men of letters disliked the Evangelicals for their narrow Puritanism, men of science for their intellectual feebleness. Nevertheless during the nineteenth century Evangelical religion was the moral cement of English society. It was the influence of the Evangelicals which invested the British aristocracy with an almost Stoic dignity, restrained the plutocrats newly risen from the masses from vulgar ostentation and debauchery, and placed over the proletariat a select body of workmen enamoured of virtue and capable of self-restraint.[46]

A tradition of reform

Florence's father, her maternal grandfather, and all her uncles in Parliament were active members of the Whig party, which generally stood for tolerance of Dissenters, policies promoting commercial expansion, increased authority for Parliament, strict control of royal power, and guarantees for the "rights of the subject" against the government. The Whig party was composed mainly of the landowning class — the upper tier of country gentlemen — and the rapidly expanding merchant class whose growing wealth and power made them a progressive political force.

Opposing the Whigs were the deeply conservative Tories, who supported the monarchy and the established church. The Tory party consisted mainly of smaller landowners — the squires and the gentry — who, in the social hierarchy of the time, ranked just below the nobility and were tied to the agrarian economy. Together with the Anglican clergy, they resisted change and distrusted the more progressive Whig nobility, many of whom were already participants in the new mercantile economy or relied on credit from this emergent wealthy class.

Florence's great-grandfather, Samuel Smith, had been an eminent member of the new merchant class. Originally from the Isle of Wight, where his family had owned a small estate, Samuel made a fortune in London as a grocery merchant. He exhibited an independence and humanitarianism that would also be apparent in several other Smiths and a Nightingale. With his brother, he was landlord for a large part of the city of Savannah, Georgia, but was such a strong supporter of the American colonists that after the Declaration of Independence, he made no claim for his loss of property.[47]

William Smith, Florence's maternal grandfather, was an exemplar of the Nonconformist conscience; his political career mirrored the progress of reform in his lifetime. He expanded and gave political form to his father's impulses, and personified the Unitarian creed of good works determined by reason and conscience. For 44 years as a radical member of Parliament, Smith was a leader for religious freedom, an activist for reform, and an advocate for the disenfranchised and poor. In 1790, he spoke in defense of the radical scientist Joseph Priestley, discoverer of oxygen and outspoken Dissenter, whose house and scientific instruments were burned by a "Church and State" mob in Birmingham, forcing Priestley to flee to the United States.[48]

Smith sponsored and saw passed in 1813 the Unitarian Toleration Act, after which nonbelief in the divinity of Christ (one of the tenets of Unitarianism) was no longer a crime, a major step toward full equality for Dissenters. He participated in nearly every debate on religious issues until the repeal of the Test Act in 1828, which allowed Dissenters to sit in Parliament. (Prior to this date, an Act of Indemnity was passed each year to pardon Dissenters of any violations of religious laws, thus allowing them to serve in Parliament.) He also worked to curb the power of the King and pushed for reform of the electoral process, municipal governments, the criminal code, and archaic economic and commercial regulations.

The family was proud of the role that Grandfather Smith had played in the abolition of the slave trade — "the open sore of the world."[49] Smith was one of the inner circle of activists who, under the leadership of William Wilberforce, campaigned for four decades to end slavery under the British flag, an achievement that has been termed "one of the turning events in the history of the world."[50] John Wesley had voiced the moral imperative of the moment when he wrote to Wilberforce, "But if God be for you who can be against you."[51]

After retiring in 1830, it was written of him that "if he had gone mourning all his days, he could scarcely have acquired a more tender pity for the miserable, or have laboured more habitually for their relief."[52] Grandfather Smith died when Florence was 15, but his example of social action fired by religious belief would be taken to new heights by his granddaughter.

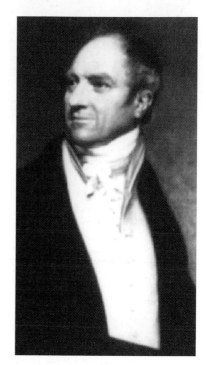

William Smith (1756-1835), Florence's maternal grandfather, a radical member of Parliament and a leading activist for religious reform and the abolition of slavery

A valuable lesson in politics

The steady, inexorable campaign for religious freedom to which William Smith had devoted so much of his life paved the way for the drastic wave of change that swept over England in the aftermath of the French Revolution and Napoleonic Wars. In 1832, Parliament passed the Great Reform Bill, which cautiously expanded the right to vote and established new electoral districts that provided more equal representation to the rapidly growing industrial areas in the Midlands and North.

Florence got her first taste of a real political campaign in the same year. In the new constituency of South Hampshire, her father and Uncle John Bonham Carter headed the reform committee and led the campaign to secure a seat in Parliament for their friend and neighbor, Lord Palmerston. Palmerston had lost his old seat under the Reform Bill and had to stand for popular election for the first time. He had entered Parliament in 1807 at age 23, served as Secretary at War from 1809 to 1829, and been appointed Secretary of State for Foreign Affairs in 1830. Bonham Carter was also running for a seat in Parliament from Portsmouth.

Florence's first political campaign was victorious. In the historic first election after the Reform Bill, both Palmerston and Uncle Carter won their seats, and a heavy Whig majority was returned to Parliament. Florence would always carry with her the advantage that children of successful political families often develop: an early understanding of local and national political processes, the psychology of the people involved, where the levers of power are, and how to win.

Cholera & the miasma theory of disease

In May of 1832, Florence wrote to her mother about a sermon she had heard on a topic that had aroused fear in England as nothing had since the black plague — the first appearance of Asiatic cholera. "It was a sort of Cholera Sermon, I think, talking about the Uncertainty of [and] the only Use of life being to prepare for heaven, a very good sermon."[53] This sermon reflected the conventional wisdom of the time — that the ultimate purpose of life on earth was to prepare for heaven.

The cholera pandemic that blanketed England and all of Europe in the early 1830s, killing more than 52,000 people in the British Isles alone, had its roots in Britain's widening control of the Indian subcontinent. The disease had been endemic in India since ancient times; Hindu physicians first mentioned cholera in about 400 B.C. When the British gained military control over all of India in 1817, routine troop movements rapidly spread the disease to the frontiers. In the same year, carried by traders and religious pilgrims, cholera suddenly appeared in Persia, Turkey, southern Russia, parts of southeast Asia, and Japan. Between 1826 and 1829, it spread to European Russia, northern Europe, and Sweden. Quebec and New York City were infected by 1832, and the contagion finally extended south to Cuba and Mexico.

An acute infectious disease of the intestines, cholera results when food and water supplies are contaminated with feces containing the bacterium *Vibrio cholerae*. Its main characteristic is overwhelming dehydration and severe muscle cramps brought on by severe diarrhea and vomiting, which is usually the cause of death. The death rate is high, usually 50% in untreated cases, and as high as 90% in epidemics.

Whereas consumption, typhus, and other diseases had been largely limited to the poor, cholera cut across social, economic, class, and geographic lines, striking down the rich as well as the poor, the parliamentarians as well as the disenfranchised. Death often came within 3 days.

The causes of cholera and other infectious diseases were unknown in the 1830s, and there were no laws or sanitary regulations to deal with such an outbreak. The government responded as well as it could. The Privy Council issued an order to make cholera subject to rules under the Quarantine Act. A royal proclamation notified the public of the threat and established a temporary consultative Board of Health, which had no binding powers over localities. In November 1831, King William ordered a Form of Prayer against the disease. When the cholera continued to spread "in defiance of winter,"[54] the King declared a national day of fasting and humiliation in March 1832.

The cholera sermon that Florence reported to Fanny reflected the religious acceptance of disease as punishment for sin. If the only purpose of life was to prepare for heaven, then many saw the cholera epidemic as God's judgment on a sinful nation; there were "cries to close theatres and ballrooms, to destroy card-tables, to remedy breaches in keeping the Sabbath, to end parsons who hunted."[55] Preachers throughout the land spoke of the judgment of God, the need for national penitence and, among the Evangelicals, the necessity to better the lot of the poor.

Ancient Greek theory of disease

In the early 1800s, disease was understood in the paradigm known as the miasma theory, which had been inherited from the ancient Greeks. The word *miasma* is derived from the ancient Greek word *miainein*, to pollute. The Greeks believed that disease resulted from atmospheric corruption, or vaporous exhalations, arising from organic matter, usually decayed or putrefied substances.

This theory, originally propounded by the Greek physician Galen in the 2nd century A.D., had endured for 1,600 years with few changes. Galen taught that atmospheric corruption might arise from a "multitude of unburned corpses as may happen in war; or the exhalations of marshes and ponds in the summer; sometimes it is immoderate heat of the air itself as in the pestilence which Thucydides describes." He believed that malnutrition was a likely predisposing factor for disease: "No cause can be sufficient without an aptitude of the body; otherwise all who are exposed to the summer sun, move about more than they should, drink wine, grow angry, grieve, would fall into a fever."[56]

The extent to which the miasma theory persisted unchanged up to Florence's time can be seen in the authoritative work *A Treatise on Fever*, published by Dr. Southwood Smith in 1830. Smith, the chief physician of the London Fever Hospital, who was regarded as a forward-thinking man, wrote:

> *The immediate ... cause of fever is a poison formed by the corruption or the decomposition of organic matter. Vegetable and animal matter, during the process of putrefaction, give off a principle, or give origin to a new compound, which, when applied to the human body, produces the phenomena constituting fever ... The room of a fever-patient, in a small and heated apartment of London, with no perflation of fresh air, is perfectly analogous to a stagnant pool in Ethiopia, full of the bodies of dead locusts. The poison generated in both cases is the same; the difference is merely in the degree of its potency. Nature, with her burning sun, her stilled and pent-up wind, her stagnant and teeming marsh, manufactures plague on a large and fearful scale: poverty in her hut, covered with her rags, surrounded with her filth, striving with all her might to keep out the pure air and to increase the heat, imitates Nature but too successfully; the process and the product are the same, but the only difference is in the magnitude of the result. Penury and ignorance can thus at any time, and any place, create a mortal plague.* [57]

In keeping with this outdated theoretical framework, the cholera regulations advanced by the Board of Health voiced a special concern for "the poor, ill-fed, unhealthy parts of the population, especially those who are of drunken irregular life, and for districts which are unclean, ill-ventilated and crowded." These regulations called for quarantining the sick and maintaining extreme cleanliness and adequate ventilation in all houses. The houses and furniture were to be thoroughly cleaned and purified, and left open to fresh air for at least 1 week.[58]

The medical establishment was ill-equipped to deal with the outbreak and simply let it run its course. The cause of cholera, and disease in general, wasn't understood; the microscopic world was known or imagined by only a few. Pasteur's first published work on fermentation, which would lead to the germ theory of disease, was still more than 25 years away. Medical education and research lagged far behind the advances being made in chemistry, electricity, and physics. A unified medical profession didn't exist.

The cholera epidemic, arriving at the same time as the first great reform successes, helped trigger a new wave of research that jump-started the fledgling field of sanitation, now known as public health. "Many intelligent persons throughout the United Kingdom had occasion to become more critically cognisant than they had ever before been of the sanitary conditions under which the mass of the people was living."[59] For a few doctors with inquiring minds and a modernist understanding of the experimental method, the cholera epidemic was a superb research opportunity.

John Snow: Medical pioneer

In the coal pits of Newcastle-on-Tyne in northern England, near where the first cholera case had appeared in 1831, a young medical apprentice named John Snow was investigating an alarming number of cholera cases among miners. The 19-year old Snow was at the beginning of a distinguished career in which he would come to be regarded as perhaps the greatest British medical scientist and doctor in the first half of the 19th century. Quiet, brilliant, and indefatigable, he was one of the few Englishmen at the time to conduct original medical research and to possess the talents and qualities necessary for meaningful outcomes and real success. He had "a shrewd perception of facts, a capacity for the dispassionate sifting of evidence, a resolution for comprehensive enquiry,"[60] and an utter disregard for traditional and religious rationalizations of disease.

Snow was one of the first to realize that the spread of cholera had something to do with contaminated water — in combination with the intractable diarrhea, unwashed hands, and shared food. One response to his inquiries illustrated this specific link and testified to horrible working conditions in general:

> The average time spent in the pit is eight to nine hours. The pitmen all take down with them a supply of food, which consists of cake, with the addition, in some cases, of meat; and all have a bottle, containing about a quart of 'drink'. I fear that our colliers are no better than others as regards cleanliness. The pit is one huge privy, and of course the men always take their victuals with unwashed hands.[61]

The cholera outbreak also spurred the development of medical cartography. This field had begun with general descriptions of health problems in specific regions.

However, after the cholera epidemic broke out, its distribution among the population was mapped for the first time.

The period from 1835 to 1855 has come to be regarded as the "golden age" of medical cartography.[62] Although there had previously been scattered observations on the correlation between rapidly increasing urban overcrowding and industrialization, and poverty and disease, the mapping of the cholera epidemic brought a critical mass of information to the forefront. For instance, in the factory town of Leeds, about 45 miles north of Lea Hurst, 1% of the population of 76,000 died between May and November, 1832. What before had been mere notions and vague correlations were now blatant facts — the beginnings of accepted social and medical realities. The 1833 Report of the Leeds Board of Health, one of the earliest disease-mapping projects, noted "how exceedingly the disease has prevailed in those parts of the town where there is a deficiency, often an entire want of sewerage, drainage, and paving."[63]

"Want of sewerage" fostered not just the spread of cholera but the whole spectrum of disease. Although sewers existed in the larger towns and cities, they had been built only for purposes of flood control from sea or river. Almost all houses of the upper classes had cesspools, which usually leaked and stank. It was the owner's responsibility to have them periodically emptied and the contents carted away. There were no laws to correct any of the many nuisances that abounded.

Even so, the critical problem was in the mushrooming urban factory areas across England. In the days before building codes, thousands of workers' tenements were being constructed side to side and back to back with no air vents, sewers, or running water. Garbage and human excrement were dumped in room-sized courtyards or in the street and then removed by cart. The poorest people lived in cellars, sometimes several families to a room, where the ooze from the dung heaps permeated basement walls. Disease and fever were endemic. Smokestacks from the factories spewed clouds of smoke, hiding the midday sun. Rivers ran like open sewers.

Although there had been large cities in earlier times, the world had never seen such a concentration of human and industrial waste:

> *Almost nowhere had any competent engineering skill been brought to bear on the sewerage of towns; and town-sewers, retaining large proportions of whatever solid filth passed into them, and often letting more liquid sewage escape into surrounding soil and house-basements than they transmitted to their proper outfall, were among the worst of nuisances to the neighbourhoods which they pretended to relieve. No doubt there existed in each town more or less of pavement, more or less of sewering, more or less of public water-supply: but in each of those respects the standard of quantity and quality did not pretend to be a sanitary standard ... probably very few of our towns ... recognised nearly as high a standard of requirement as had been recognised, two thousand years before, in Rome.[64]*

The Nightingales and their extended family — the Smiths, Bonham Carters, and Nicholsons — were among the lucky ones. All of their country and city homes were either on high ground with safe water supplies or off the path of infected travelers, or both. However, Florence could see these sanitary problems with her own young eyes among the cottages and huts of the "poor people" for whom she was always concerned.

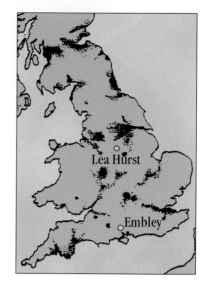

Augustus Petermann's cholera map of the British Isles showing areas affected by the epidemic of 1831-1833, one of the earliest maps to indicate the actual distribution of a disease

The problems described in the cholera reports existed in the small villages around Lea Hurst and Embley.

She also saw the problems from the perspective of her father. W.E.N. also served as county administrator, working with his fellow landowners and appointees to govern on such issues as road repair, care of the poor, conditions of hospitals and asylums, and the growing public sanitation problems of human waste and garbage. From early childhood Florence became familiar not only with national electoral and parliamentary politics but also with the relationship of policy to action and outcomes at the local level.

Florence & the philanthropic impulse

By the time she was a teenager, Florence's life had already begun to revolve around helping her poor and ill neighbors. As a girl of 15 or so, she often disappeared in the evening, only to be found by her mother at the bedside of an ailing villager, saying "she could not sit down to a grand 7 o'clock dinner while this was going on ..."[65] Looking back, Florence wrote that she had always been in the habit of visiting the poor at home: "I longed to live like them and with them and then I thought I could really help them. But to visit them in a carriage and give them money is so little like following Christ, who made Himself like His brethren."[66]

Florence had been elated when she first became responsible for caring for her nephew Shore when Nurse Gale fell ill. As she began to grow in size and strength and flourish in her education, her innate gifts as a healer and her desire to be of service began to find expression in caring for her extended family and the larger world.

When Aunt Julia visited Lea Hurst, Florence went with her to visit the poor people in the nearby villages. Florence admired Aunt Julia, who not only did good, but also had an efficient system for doing so. Julia kept track of who was sick and needed return vis-

Florence's father, W.E.N., and Fanny's sister, Julia Smith ("Aunt Ju"), in a sketch drawn by Hilary Bonham Carter in the early 1840s

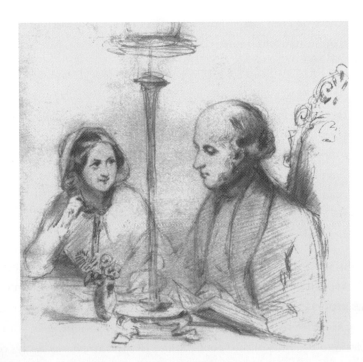

A DIFFERENT KIND OF CHILD

its; which families needed clothing, shoes, blankets, or food; and which mothers needed help tending their flocks of children amidst the filth and poverty.

Although Florence's mother also paid visits to villagers, usually to distribute food from the Nightingale's table or to offer practical advice, "poor-peopling" was only a sidelight in her life; she was consumed with ambition for social success — not social service — for herself and her daughters.

Pioneers in the women's movement

During her visits to help the poor, Florence didn't realize that she was already an activist in her first social reform movement — the philanthropic movement, a female response to the horrors of 18th-century English life. In the years after Napoleon's defeat, England's old organic structure, in which every person had a place in the village or on the estate, began to break apart as a result of the massive dislocations of the Industrial Revolution, population growth, and urban migration. The philanthropic movement was the direct forerunner of the feminist movement, which would emerge in Britain at mid-century, with Florence's cousin Barbara Leigh Smith (later Bodichon), in the forefront:

> On the surface things were unaltered; but across the apparently immutable state of society there flowed the searchlight of the philanthropic movement, and this illumination left behind it not only movements to improve the social and material conditions of the people, but also a great awakening of conscience. The young women who lived under its influence saw that the world was unsatisfactory in a great many ways: they saw that old people were poor and hungry, that children were wild and ragged, and that rain came in through the cottage roofs; and then they realised that they themselves, being 'only women,' were powerless to do any substantial good. And from that illumination the Women's Movement sprang.[67]

Among the women who rejected the idea of "powerlessness" and helped build the "awakening of conscience" in the generation that preceded Florence Nightingale, were two women with whom she would later work — Caroline Chisholm in her emigration program in 1852 and Aunt Julia's friend, Harriet Martineau, the most noted woman writer and journalist of her day, who would become Florence's valuable colleague after the Crimean War. These women pushed their way into unknown psychological terrain with no maps to guide them save their innate wisdom and instincts. Their work in the philanthropic movement provided a training ground for the first organized feminist committees of the 1850s.

A growing desire to serve

Florence's philanthropic impulse was informed by her political training and strengthened by her developing sense of duty. Her father, heartened by the recent passage of the Reform Bill and the success of Lord Palmerston's campaign, decided to stand for Parliament from Andover in 1834. Upon hearing the news for the first time, Florence wrote that she "slept so lightly" that she had the feeling that something "very extraordinary or dreadful" had happened and she kept waking to find out what it was. However, the next day she soberly appraised the situation. With her intuition for seeing cause and effect in larger scenarios and her emerging concept of duty to country, she wrote to her mother:

I am so sorry we shall not see half so much of dear Papa and he will not be able to teach us as he did and we shall live half the year in London and will be like Uncle Carter and say 'Pooh Posh' because he is a great man. I had much rather he should be a little one ... but I suppose I must be a patriot too in my small way and give up a man like Papa (who cannot fail to do good, because he is so disinterested [unselfish]) to the country instead of having him kept in his family.[68]

However, in the end, Florence had little to fear; W.E.N. was an idealist and the rough and tumble of electoral politics was not for him. He refused to bribe voters (in some districts, votes could be bought for £15 to £100[69] [approximately £600 to £4,000 and US$1,000 to $6,300 in today's values[70]]), a normal and pervasive practice, and consequently lost the election; thereafter he was content to concentrate on local politics.

The constant awareness of the sick and the poor that was reflected in young Florence's letters now became the focal point of her life. In the winter of 1837, a great influenza epidemic swept London as well as Embley and the nearby villages. Florence's parents and sister were away visiting, and Florence was tending Shore and his younger sister, Bertha. Shore was the only household member untouched by the flu. Florence wrote to Parthe that "the whole parish here is one mass of illness" and followed with a detailed report of a neighborhood beset by widespread sickness.[71] Another letter reflects the state of medicine at the time: "All the parish here is ill of Influenza & 300 people ditto at Romsey. They have used up all the leeches [a common treatment] & cannot get any in the country for love or money."[72]

Increasingly aware of a world in need of service everywhere she turned, Florence at this time began a work habit that was to be a refuge as she grew to womanhood — she began to rise extremely early. Inundated by the work of minding the children and helping with the sick household and villagers, she wrote that "I find the going to bed at 8 & getting up proportionately early a very agreeable plan as I was always partial to early rising & never liked the long evening hours solitary."[73]

Though energized by the thrill and challenge of work in the real world, Florence still managed to continue her home education in the midst of the epidemic:

It is incredible what some people's industry will perform, e.g., the piles of manuscripts which have arisen like mushrooms under my pen during this last month, while I have been nurse, governess, assistant curate & doctor ... at all events I have killed no patients though I have cured few. But the lives of British Worthies, the histories, the analyses which I have achieved, enough to smother Papa when he returns.[74]

A family friend, Fanny Allen, later wrote her impression of Florence at this stage of her life:

"When I look back on every time I saw her after her sixteenth year, I see that she was ripening constantly for her work, and that her mind was dwelling on the painful differences of man and man in this life. A conversation on this subject between the father and daughter made me laugh at the time, the contrast was so striking; but now, as I remember it, it was the Divine Spirit breathing in her."[75]

Chapter 2

Call & Awakening

I never pray for anything temporal ... but when each morning comes, I kneel down before the Rising Sun, & only say, Behold the handmaid of the Lord — give me this day my work to do — no, not my work, but thine.

— Florence Nightingale to Aunt Hannah, September 24, 1846[1]

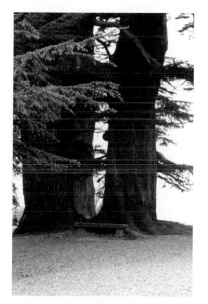

The bench under the cedars of Lebanon at Embley, where Florence felt was a sacred place

In the first stage of the mystic's spiritual development, there is an awakening of the Self to the Divine Consciousness, to the direct, immediate presence of God. This event is nearly always abrupt and well-marked — a "road-to-Damascus" experience. It triggers a complete shift of consciousness to a higher level. Often, it's preceded by a period of restlessness, uncertainty, or any activity that readies the person for this encounter with the Divine to which they are drawn — such as Florence's selfless immersion in nursing during the influenza epidemic of 1837.

Florence Nightingale's awakening, late in her 16th year, was just such a striking event. She experienced a sudden inner "knowing" that is characteristic of the mystic's calling. At the time, she had no clear idea of the exact meaning of this vision or what her path would be. She shared her revelation with no one, not even her cousin Hilary, with whom she shared so much.

In an autobiographical note written in 1867, Florence records her revelation, which she referred to as her "Call from God," that took place at Embley. For an instant, the door to the spiritual world to which she always had been drawn was cracked open. She had clearly known the direct presence of God, if only for a moment. Like nearly all other mystics at this initial stage, she did not yet know how, or have the capacity, to sustain the experience. She had received only the first instruction: "That a quest there is, and an end, is the single secret spoken."[2] Energized by this contact with the Divine Reality, Florence "worked very hard among the poor people" with "a strong feeling of religion" for the next 3 months.[3]

The coming of spring and the waning of the influenza epidemic brought other changes. Ever since Florence's father had lost his bid for a seat in Parliament in 1835, he had begun to speak of the possibility of revisiting the continent, now that the girls were older. Among the European upper classes, the English were the most accustomed to traveling; in the years after Waterloo, in particular, Europe became a playground for the wealthy English. Fanny thought her husband's idea was excellent. Everyone in the family would have a chance to regain their health in the sunny south, and a European tour would provide the finishing touches to Parthe and Florence's education. Just as important, Embley might be remodeled and enlarged in their absence so that it would become a proper setting for the grand society that Fanny envisioned.

W.E.N. set to work designing a large traveling carriage and began plans to convert Embley from a plain Georgian house to a much larger and impressive Elizabethan mansion. The carriage, which was the normal conveyance for the wealthy on such trips before the development of the railroads, held up to 12 people, was pulled by 6 horses, and had seats on top for viewing the scenery in nice weather.

As the Nightingales prepared for their European trip in June 1837, King William IV died. His niece, Princess Alexandrina Victoria, a year older than Florence, was heir to the throne. Her life had been a preparation for this moment, yet it still exemplified many of the constraints upon women. When Victoria descended the stairs of Kensington Palace shortly before dawn on June 20 to hear from the Archbishop of Canterbury and the Lord Chamberlain that she was the Queen of England, it was the first time she had walked down the stairs without anyone holding her hand.[4]

The Nightingales' neighbor Lord Palmerston, then Foreign Minister and an astute judge of people in politics, wrote: "Few people have had opportunities of forming a correct judgment of the Princess; but I incline to think that she will turn out to be a remarkable person, and gifted with a great deal of strength of character."[5]

Victoria would prove to be a most serious and dutiful Queen. When she received the news of her uncle's death, she wrote in her diary:

> Since it has pleased Providence to place me in this station, I shall do my utmost to fulfil my
> duty towards my country; I am very young, and perhaps in many, though not in all things,

The four-to-six-horse traveling carriage that W.E.N. designed for the Nightingales' continental tour in 1837-1839, drawn by Sibella Bonham Carter, c. 1858

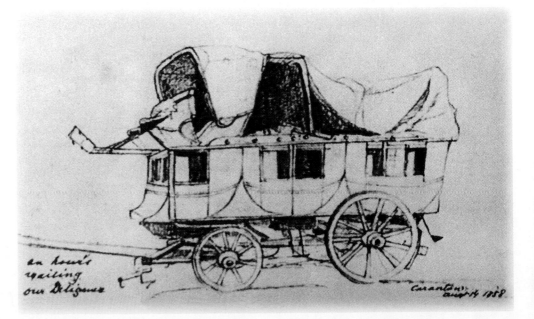

CALL & AWAKENING

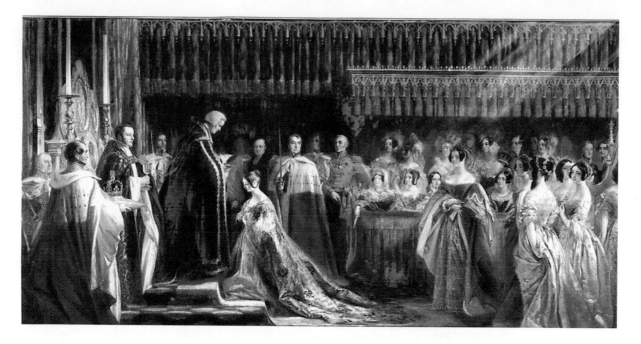

Queen Victoria at her coronation in Westminster Abbey on June 28, 1838

inexperienced, but I am sure that very few have more real good will and more real desire to do what is fit and right than I have.[6]

The Nightingales spent the last days of summer packing and making final plans for the European tour. Discussions went back and forth over which books to include: serious books, guides to flora and fauna, and Milton or Shakespeare for lighter reading. Florence knew she would miss caring for the poor people, but she also thought that in Europe she might learn more about her Call from God.

European tour, 1837-1839

On September 8, 1837, the family sailed from Southampton on the steam passenger boat *Monarch*. Papa, Mama, Parthe, Nurse Gale, and their maid, Thérèse, retired early, but Florence, too excited for sleep, walked the deck in the dark and drizzle, dreaming her visions and talking to one of the mates. As the boat slid into the harbor of Le Havre de Grâce at dawn, both she and Parthe were exhilarated at the newness of being in a foreign country. From the luxury suite of their hotel, they could see the townsfolk carrying on their business on the quays, the women in traditional dress and white caps.

At Rouen, the family's own traveling carriage was waiting and they departed overland. Florence and Parthe took turns sitting beside their father in the box seat as they sped down the poplar-lined roads at full gallop to the jingle of harness bells.

France

The Nightingales' travels took them from Rouen to Chartres and Blois, down the Loire River valley to Tours and Nantes, south to Bordeaux, and then to Biarritz and Bayonne on the Atlantic Ocean. They traveled across the foothills of the Pyrenees to Carcassonne and Narbonne, through the lower Rhone valley via Nimes and Avignon to Toulon, and then along the Riviera to Nice, where they spent December 1837 and the beginning of

January 1838. Between their main destinations, they visited many villages and towns. From Nice they followed the Mediterranean coast to Genoa, where they stayed a month; Pisa; and Florence, where they stayed for 2 months. They visited Northern Italy and the lakes, went on to Geneva for a month, and on October 8, 1838, arrived in Paris, where they stayed until they returned to England in April 1839.

During their European tour, the Nightingales made the most of their social position and extensive network of friends and relatives. Through Fanny's family and social connections and W.E.N.'s intellectual and political interests, they gained access to people in the forefront of French culture and politics, the movement for Italian freedom, and the governmental and cultural affairs of Geneva, which were closely tied to events in France and the states of northern Italy.

Although Fanny envisioned Europe as a finishing school for her daughters, for Florence, it was more like a graduate school abroad. Through W.E.N.'s contacts with like-minded scholarly, cultured, and politically connected friends, Florence was exposed to many of the notable historians, politicians, and academic and literary figures who were interpreting and defining the culture and politics of Europe at the time. She shared with her father a deep interest in politics and the cause of freedom.

Florence's interest in politics began to range much further than the theories and speculations that she and her father had long discussed. She began to observe the effects of politics, laws, and war on the lives of everyday people. She saw old Napoleonic soldiers everywhere; one, who had suffered six wounds, was the caretaker who led them about the Castle at Blaye. In a letter to her cousin Hilary, Florence noted that he seemed to have fought everyone yet felt "rancune [rancor] against none." At Bosuste, a village in the foothills of the Pyrenees ravaged by the Carlist Wars for the Spanish throne in the 1830s, she noted with horror the old women sitting in the sun, covered by flies, and was struck by "the indifference which misery brings."[7]

With her passion for detail, Florence kept elaborate notes on each step of the journey. The format of her entries reflected the developing eye of a born statistician; she recorded, in the columns she had first begun to use in childhood, the day and time of arrival and departure for each destination as well as the distance between cities and towns. She noted the landscape, cathedrals and churches, architecture, and works of art. In the major cities, she compiled details about hospitals and workhouses.

While Parthe filled her sketchbook with detailed illustrations, Florence talked to people whenever possible, making observations that seemed more those of a social scientist than a casual traveler. She wrote about local laws and customs, land systems, social conditions, and benevolent institutions in the various regions. Whenever she could, she visited charitable institutions. She learned as much as she could about the French poor law (the equivalent of today's welfare programs) and its effects on people; she observed the conditions of beggars, the habits of children, and the living arrangements of the residents.

The family's arrival in Nice in December 1837 provided an interlude from the seriousness of Florence's French sojourn. On their first day there, Fanny happily discovered acquaintances from 20 years earlier. The presence of these other English families during the festive Christmas season provided for many visits and expeditions during the day as well as balls in the evenings. There was even an English Protestant church to attend.

For 2 busy months, Florence enjoyed the perfect family vacation "with books and work and healthful play." When the Nightingales left Nice on January 8, 1838, she wrote in her journal that "the worst of travelling is that you leave people as soon as you have become intimate with them and often to never see them again."[8]

Italy

At the head of her second journal, Florence wrote one word, "Italy," which had come to signify for her and many others the aspirations for liberty and freedom of people throughout Europe. After the fall of Napoleon, the Austrian emperor, now the most powerful military despot on the continent, had gained dominion over the eight states of the Italian peninsula. The Austrians governed with a heavy hand, either through direct control or submissive rulers. Napoleon's institution of centralized administration and effective postal systems had helped to develop a unified political consciousness among Italians, who were agreed upon one thing — the desirability of freeing Italy from Austrian influence and governing themselves.

Florence was particularly drawn to the ideas of Giuseppe Mazzini, the great Italian freedom fighter. Mazzini's almost mystical belief in the efficacy of the people working selflessly for the common good fired the imagination of the Italians and other freedom-loving Europeans. He preached republicanism and revolution first, a united Italy second. Florence couldn't have imagined that less than 25 years later, another great Italian patriot, Garibaldi, whom she had not yet heard of, would come to her for advice.

Florence was enchanted with Genoa, which had been, along with Venice, one of the two great seaports and trading centers of medieval Italy. She was captivated by the beauty of the great palaces, which seemed to her like "an Arabian Nights story." Some of the English friends from Nice also were in Genoa and there were more balls, visits, and picnics. After attending the opera, Florence wrote that she would like to see *Lucrezia Borgia* every night of her life, it was "so beautiful, so affecting, so enchanting; how could one ever wish for anything else if one were always looking at that?"[9]

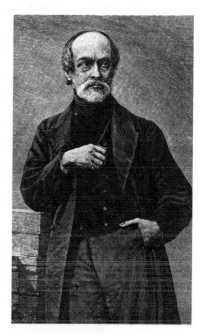

Giuseppe Mazzini (1805-1872), Italian patriot and revolutionary who wove mysticism into politics

Many in Genoa were enchanted by young Florence. At "the most splendid ball of the season," Florence danced with one young man after another. She was more elegant than beautiful, tall and willowy with thick, flowing, golden-red hair; her complexion was smooth with delicate coloring. No pictures have survived of her laughing or smiling broadly, but noted author Elizabeth Gaskell observed that she had "perfect teeth, making her smile the sweetest I ever saw."[10] Her penetrating grey eyes could be pensive or serious but also, in light-hearted moments, "the merriest." Her quiet good looks were enhanced by her most attractive features — the quality of her mind and her otherworldly goodness.

The social whirl couldn't overshadow Florence's serious side for long. In her journal, she noted the King's political and military efforts to control the rising tide of nationalism in the Piedmont. She observed that of the 30,000 inhabitants of Genoa, 8,000 were soldiers and 8,000 were priests, an observation that echoed the words of the youth-

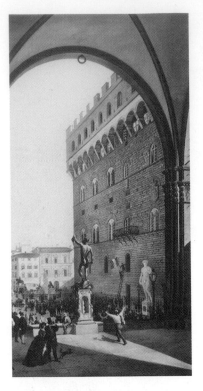

A 19th-century illustration of the Piazza della Signoria in Florence

ful Camillo Benso di Cavour, the future architect of the Italian state, about his native Turin: a "city half-barracks and half-cloister."[11] It seemed to her that the nobles lived in excessive ignorance, while the masses lived in excessive poverty. She visited a school for the "deaf and dumb," noting that while the children looked intelligent, they seemed sickly and depressed, and their rooms were cold and not very clean.

Some three and a half centuries earlier, Genoa had been the home of one of Florence's great spiritual predecessors, Caterina Adorna. In the summer of 1493, the most virulent attack of the plague ever to hit Genoa killed four-fifths of the people who remained in town. As director of the huge Pammetone Hospital, Caterina worked tirelessly to accommodate the large numbers of the sick, who quickly exceeded the hospital's capacity. She created temporary wards by requisitioning canvas from the shipyards and erecting tents in the field behind the hospital. So loving and conspicuous was her service that the townspeople named her Saint Catherine of Genoa.

The Nightingales left Genoa in mid-February 1838, traveling along the rugged coast through Chiavari, the rock quarries of Carrara, and then to Pisa with its famous Leaning Tower. They were among the guests at a great court ball given by the Grand Duke of Tuscany, which lasted through the night and included an inspection of the Duke's camels.

From Pisa the family traveled up the Arno River valley to Florence, where they took a luxurious suite at the Albergo del Arno, near the Ponte Vecchio. The hotel was a former palace, and the rooms were the largest and most magnificent they had seen on their tour, replete with baths. While staying in the city of her birth, Florence took music lessons, and played the piano and sang each day, while Parthe took drawing lessons. The family heard the best European operas and singers of the day. Florence was passionate about every performance, and in her separate music notebooks recorded details on each opera score, libretto, and performer.

The Nightingales stayed in Florence longer than they intended in order to see the events of Holy Week. On the Thursday before Easter, which the Italians kept as the English did Good Friday, the Grand Duke and Duchess led in ceremonies of piety that dated back to medieval times. The Grand Duchess washed the feet of 12 of the oldest and poorest women in the town, "that is to say, she washed a little place on each of their feet for herself to kiss." Florence wrote that although the Duchess did it very gracefully, "it was not much penance, for she had a chamberlain on one side and a lady on the other to help her to kneel down and get up before each of the old women." The Grand Duke, meanwhile, was doing the same at the other end of the room for 12 old men.[12]

After a 2-hour procession in which members of the Court visited seven churches on foot, the city fell silent. Florence wrote that "all the bells are fastened up and no clock strikes nor bell rings from Thursday till Saturday, the time that the Catholics suppose that our Saviour remained in the grave."[13] On Saturday, the period of mourning ended and the quiet was broken by "fire-works and rejoicing." The Holy Week celebrations were followed by a "most brilliant ball in every aspect" at Court.

On April 25, the family left for Bologna on their way to Venice. To their surprise and delight, they found Bologna to have the finest pictures of all the grand cities they had visited. They were also struck by the sight of the domes of Venice rising out of the sea. Leaving their carriage on the mainland, they traveled throughout the city in a gondola. The Nightingales knew many people in Venice. The Contessa Civelli, whose brother-in-law W.E.N. and Fanny knew very well in England, "had been kindness itself," taking them nearly every day to see some site and then to some party at night. Florence wrote to Grandmother Shore that no one could be more hospitable than the Venetians.

The family visited the house of the Austrian governor, where they saw the Vice Queen of Lombardy, who was also the Archduchess of Austria. Most of the splendid old palaces were falling into ruin; only those that the Austrian government had taken for itself were being kept up. On the quay beneath their window, Florence could observe street life, including veiled Turkish women who sang in the street at night and sold bird cages and other objects by day.[14]

Switzerland

From Venice, the Nightingales made their way across northern Italy and through the lake region to Geneva, arriving in September 1838. They knew many people and were received with open arms. Florence wrote:

> They all remembered Papa when he was at Geneva twenty-two years ago in 1816. One family particularly welcomed us in the kindest way for his sake, old Madame Cramer, in whose house he lived for eleven months before he married, she is now grown rather infirm and never stirs out of the house except to church, but she was delighted to see him again and kissed us all round and introduced us to her five sons who had all married ... She was a most anxious mother when Papa knew her last for she had suffered a great deal. In the Revolution of 1792 her father-in-law was shot in the streets when she was only 18 and her husband lost his whole fortune. Then she was obliged to set up a Boarding house and Papa was one of the first boarders she had and she says she never would have got on without him for the other young men were very troublesome ... whereas he ... staid at home all the morning writing French exercises. She taught him French and felt, she says, as if she was his mother.[15]

The Nightingales met the famed historian and political economist Jean Charles Léonard Sismondi, who had married Jessie Allen, a niece of Mrs. Nightingale's old friend, Fanny Allen. Florence was captivated by Sismondi, the Swiss historian who had first gained renown as author of *The History of the Italian Republics*, a 16-volume work in which he asserted that no state can become or remain great without liberty. Sismondi was one of the first thinkers to observe that the Industrial Revolution was dividing society into two classes, the capitalists and the proletariat. (At the time he did not perceive the growth of the middle class.) In the 1820s, he had visited England, which he described as "this astonishing country, which seems to be submitted to a great experiment for the instruction of the rest of the world."[16]

Sismondi's ideas provided a larger context in which Florence could place her perceptions of the village poor around Embley and Lea Hurst, the destitution of war she had seen in France, and her youthful ideas on the disparity between "man and man" in this life. Her personal experience in visiting and nursing the poor was illuminated by

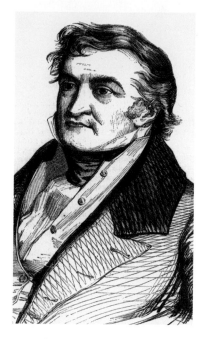

Jean Charles Léonard Sismondi (1773-1842), Swiss historian and political economist whom Florence met in Geneva

Sismondi's scholarly perspective on England and Europe, and she learned that her feelings and notions were historical facts. She made notes as fast as she could write.

Florence was as much moved by Sismondi's compassion as by his intellect. "All Sismondi's political economy seems to be founded on the overflowing kindness of his heart. He gives to old beggars on principle, to young from habit. At Pescia [the family home in northern Italy] he had 300 beggars at his door."[17]

Geneva offered Florence an opportunity to see history in the making. Two events in particular heightened political tensions in the city. The first incident was the amnesty announced by the Austrian emperor for Italian political offenders, which affected the community of exiles and émigrés to whom the Nightingales had been introduced. They gathered at a huge party at Sismondi's, where the amnesty decree was read aloud and followed by excited discussion. Unfortunately, the decree proved to be full of limitations.

The second crisis — a military one — caused the Nightingales to cut short their visit to Geneva. Louis Bonaparte Napoleon, nephew of Napoleon and pretender to the French throne, had fled to Switzerland and been granted asylum. The French government threatened to invade the tiny country, and the Genevans rose to defend their city. For the first time, Florence saw armed troops — and friends — preparing for combat. She wrote that Madame Cramer was very anxious because she had "just seen her youngest sons march by among the troops which were preparing to resist the French." W.E.N. had difficulty finding horses because they were needed for the artillery; when the Nightingales finally departed, with Sismondi seeing them off in tears, Florence wrote that the Genevans were "determined to resist to the utmost ... were arming their soldiers, raising their fortifications and bristling them with stockades. The poor soldiers had been working all Sunday (like tigers) up to their knees in water and planting the cannon on the ramparts. It is hoped, however, that the cause of all these misfortunes, Louis Bonaparte, will move off of his own accord."[18]

After 6 days of traveling from dawn to dark, the Nightingales reached Fontainebleau, where they stopped to see the magnificent royal palace and to arrange lodgings in Paris, which was crowded with English visitors. There, word soon reached them that Louis Napoleon was leaving Switzerland for England with the approval of the French, and the Genevans were dancing in the streets at the news.

Mary Clarke: A new kind of woman

The family's arrival in Paris in October 1838 opened Florence's eyes to an entirely different way for a woman to live, for here she met the extraordinary Mary Clarke, one of the most independent and forward-thinking women in Europe. Clarke's mother Elizabeth was a friend of Florence's Aunt Patty, who had provided a letter of introduction to Mrs. and Miss Clarke. Florence first met "Clarkey," as they came to call her, playing blind man's bluff at a children's soirée to which she had invited the Nightingales.

Mary Clarke was 45 years old, a year older than W.E.N., and had come to Paris in the early 1800s with her mother, whose health required a warmer climate. Her maternal grandmother, Mrs. Hay, was the widow of a Scottish sea captain. Her Irish father had been an architect in Westminster, a man of classical and literary interests who died in 1809. Mary and her mother traveled frequently in Europe and usually returned to England at least once a year.

Clarke's childhood had been well grounded in the intellectual and literary life of England through her grandmother's friends, Hazlitt, Coleridge, Wordsworth, the Lambs, and many others. As a young woman in Edinburgh, Mrs. Hay had been a member of the same intellectual circles as David Hume and Adam Smith.

Even as a child, Clarke had been noted for her independence, originality, and out-spokenness, traits that, when combined with her brilliant mind and gift for language, endeared her to the French. Quick-witted, intelligent, perceptive, and unconventional in manners, dress, and conduct, Clarke broke all the rules of proper Victorian society to which the Nightingales were accustomed. An artist by nature, she had at one time considered portraiture to augment her income but eventually unleashed her creativity in her letters and her salon.

Clarke's fashionable literary salon included scholars and journalists, statesmen and artists, and many persons who sympathized with or were directly involved in the early stages of the women's emancipation movement. At a time when women in England had almost no opportunities for public intellectual discussion, the literary salon, which was a tradition in France, afforded a woman an opportunity to participate in and even lead spirited interchanges among great minds. Clarke had learned the art of the salon from Madame Récamier, one of the great literary salon hostesses; it was her equivalent of a university education.

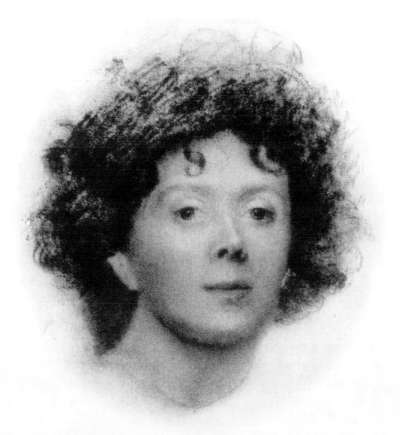

Mary Clarke (1793-1883), the well-known literary salon hostess whom the Nightingales met in Paris in 1838 and who became Florence's lifelong friend and confidante

Nearly all the people in Clarke's circle whom the Nightingales met were not only notables in their field, but also passionate advocates for the liberty of the individual, ideas to which Florence was inherently drawn. There was Alexis de Tocqueville, author of *Democracy in America*, who argued that the drive to democracy was irrevocable; Augustin Thierry, one of the first historians to insist that research should include original documents and accounts of the common people; and Adolphe Thiers, historian and first President of the Third Republic. The Nightingales became friends with François Guizot, who was Professor of Modern History at the Sorbonne and later Minister of Education, Foreign Minister, and Prime Minister. They heard the aging Chateaubriand, the genius of the first wave of Romanticism to sweep Europe, read his memoirs.

Other regulars were the novelist Victor Hugo, the geologist Elie de Beaumont, the naturalist Roulin, the poet Madame Tastu, the great educator Victor Cousin, and Julius Mohl, the leading Orientalist in Europe whom Clarke eventually married. Many of Mary Clarke's English friends were also acquainted, or would be, with the Nightingales and their extended family — among them journalist Harriet Martineau, Elizabeth Gaskell, and the Brownings.

Although Mary Clarke was 27 years older than Florence, the two women developed an instant affinity for each other that evolved into a lifelong friendship. The 4 months in Paris were filled with constant excitement. From their ornate apartment in the Place Vendome, the Nightingales accompanied Clarke to literary gatherings, concerts, picture galleries, and meetings with her friends. Looking back years later, Parthe wrote:

Place Vendome in Paris, where the Nightingales stayed from November 1838 to March 1839

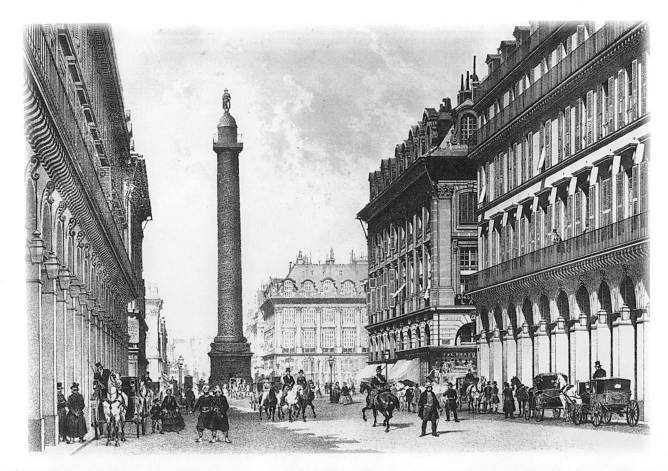

She made us acquainted with all her friends, many and notable, among them Madame Récamier. I know now, better than then, what her influence must have been thus to introduce an English family (two of them girls who, if French, would not have appeared in society) into that jealously guarded sanctuary, the most exclusive aristocratic and literary salon in Paris. We were asked, even, to the reading by Chateaubriand ... of his Mémoires d'Outre Tombe *... a favour eagerly sought for by the cream of the cream of Paris society at that time.*[19]

By the time she left Paris in March 1839, Florence was noted for her quick wit, her vast knowledge, her incisive analysis, her cutting and accurate perception, and her fluency in five languages. She was inadvertently on her way to becoming a light in European society. Even so, she hadn't forgotten her Call from God. She wrote in a private note that, to make herself worthy of God's service, she must overcome "the desire to shine in society."[20]

Society debut

When the family returned to England in April 1839, they stayed at the Carlton Hotel in London for the social season because of the remodeling at Embley. Much of the extended family was also in town, including the Nicholsons and Uncle Sam and Aunt Mai. Some of the cousins were away: Hilary was studying in Liverpool, Henry Nicholson was at Cambridge, and Fred Smith was with the Grey expedition in Western Australia.

While Fanny consulted with her sisters about the interior design for Embley, Florence was drawn again into the social whirl. Her close companion during this period was her beautiful, impulsive, and charming cousin Marianne Nicholson, who was as "music-mad" as she was. Together they went to the opera, private concerts, and parties; played and sang at the Carlton; and endlessly discussed the merits of the great singers of the day. Other annual events of the social season included exhibits at the Royal Academy of Arts, horse racing at Ascot, and the Henley Regatta in July.

The London social season, in addition to providing genuine recreation and entertainment among friends and family, served two important functions in the life of the upper class: arranging suitable marriages between families and promoting contacts and alliances among the elite for affairs of business, politics, and government. When a young woman of the aristocracy or landed gentry approached the age of 18, she would be presented at court. This event marked her "coming out" into fashionable society and announced that she was ready for marriage.

Florence made her formal entrance into society in May 1839, when she was presented at the Queen's Drawing Room. On such occasions, the name of the girl being presented was announced, she approached, curtsied to Queen Victoria, kissed the Queen's hand, and then backed out of the room. For her own presentation, Florence wore a white dress bought in Paris and reported herself "not nearly so much frightened as I expected." Young Queen Victoria, only a year older than Florence, "looked flushed and tired, but the whole sight was very pretty."[21] Florence's presentation was the first in a series of steps that Fanny hoped would result in an excellent marriage for her daughters; Parthe had been presented before the family went to Europe.

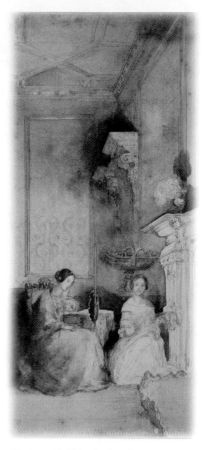

Florence (left) in the drawing room at Embley with her first cousin Marianne Nicholson in a watercolor by her sister, Parthe, c. 1836

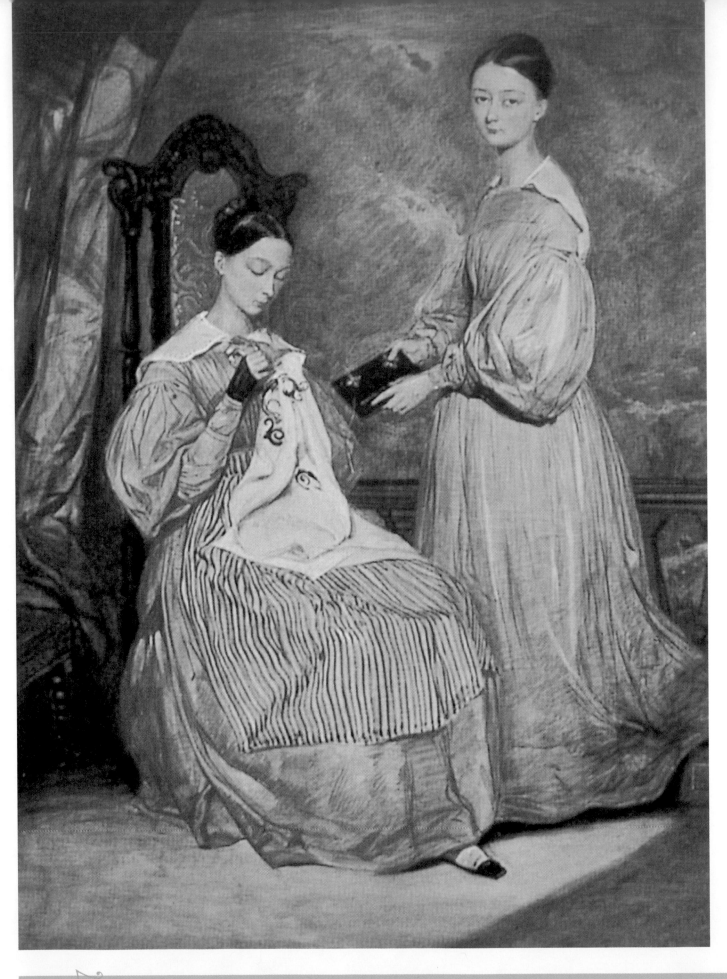

CALL & AWAKENING

The Nightingales were members of society, or the "upper ten thousand," by virtue of their social standing and income, and the fact that they were large landowners. Society, in the strictest sense, was composed of only about 1,500 families drawn from the aristocracy, which was composed of titled persons, or peers, and the substantial gentry, like the Nightingales. The life of this small upper class was vastly different from that of the middle class and the working class. The tiny upper class didn't work for wages; they either owned property or had investments, or both. For many, their "work" was politics and governance. The middle class performed mental labor, and the working class performed the physical labor, an enormous activity in Victorian England.

The London season took place in May through July, when Parliament was in session, and peers were in town for the sessions of the House of Lords. About a third of the members of the House of Commons also had ties to the peerage. The social season officially ended on August 12th, when Parliament recessed and grouse season opened.

An interest in mathematics

As a member of society, Florence had the opportunity to meet many of the notable personages of the day. At one dinner party, she met Charles Babbage, a leading mathematician and scientist who is credited with inventing the forerunner of the modern computer. Around 1812, Babbage had first gotten the idea that lengthy mathematical calculations might be done by machine and spent most of his life working on his inventions.

Brash and outspoken, Babbage had criticized the Royal Society of London in a volume entitled *The Decline of Science in England* (1830), which led to the founding of the British Association for the Advancement of Science the following year. Founded in 1660, the Royal Society was originally intended to provide a platform for the exchange of all forms of knowledge, but as science progressed and became increasingly differentiated, the society's focus became too diffuse. The British Association, in contrast, was better organized and had various subdivisions, such as the Statistical Section, established by Babbage in 1833. W.E.N. attended the British Association's annual meetings, which became a clearinghouse for scientific information, and Florence joined him after the Association opened its doors to women in 1834.

When the 1839 London season ended, the Nightingales went to Lea Hurst for their summer stay, joined by other family members and Mary Clarke. Florence confided to Clarke that mathematics gave her a sense of certainty. Florence's cousin Henry Nicholson was visiting, and he and Florence worked together on their studies, focusing especially on mathematics. Henry's interests had started to turn in another direction as well; he was beginning to fall in love with Florence.

The novelty and excitement of coming out in society were already beginning to wane, and Florence, now a young woman, yearned for experiences wider than the artificial boundaries of her class. Returning to the remodeled Embley in September, Florence found herself bored with the daily routine, perplexed with her ambivalence toward Henry, and frustrated by her inability to further decipher her Call. Much of the family gathered at Embley for Christmas, but a tragic event cast a shadow over the holidays.

News arrived from Australia that Fred Smith, the eldest son of Uncle Octavius and Aunt Jane, had died of starvation and thirst on the Grey expedition.

In February, Florence was back in London, thrilled to attend the wedding of Queen Victoria to Prince Albert. In the spring, the family sent her to be with Aunt Jane, who was expecting a baby and still in mourning for her son. Aunt Jane's comments revealed the level of devotion to duty that ran in the family and in the English character, "I had rather a son die as he has done of exhaustion and exertion, than see one before my eyes always at home without any other object but living from breakfast till dinner."[22]

Amid the sadness at Aunt Jane's house was one bright spot for Florence; an opportunity arose for her to pursue her study of mathematics. Florence had come to realize that music wouldn't fulfill her and had confided to Aunt Mai that she wished to learn more mathematics, that the mastery of numbers gave her a sense of purpose and certainty. Now that Florence was entering womanhood, her relationship with Aunt Mai became a sharing between equals. Like Florence, Aunt Mai possessed the Shore proclivity for the intellectual and spiritual life.

Aunt Mai secured a tutor — a married clergyman and established teacher of young ladies, who had also tutored Fred Smith. Through quiet, unrelenting conversations and letters, Aunt Mai overcame Fanny's objections that mathematics wasn't a preparation for marriage, that Florence was needed for household duties, and that it was not proper for a young lady to meet with a man alone. In a pointed postscript to Fanny, perhaps piqued that Florence's mother couldn't see the obvious, Aunt Mai wrote: "I don't think you have any idea of half that is in her."[23]

Uncle Octavius volunteered his library as a meeting place. In the spring of 1840, Florence wrote that "I have had three charming lessons of Mr. Gillespie, tho' he gives me

Watercolor by Parthe Nightingale of Aunt Mai (second from left) and Florence with two of Aunt Mai's children, Beatrice (left) and Bertha

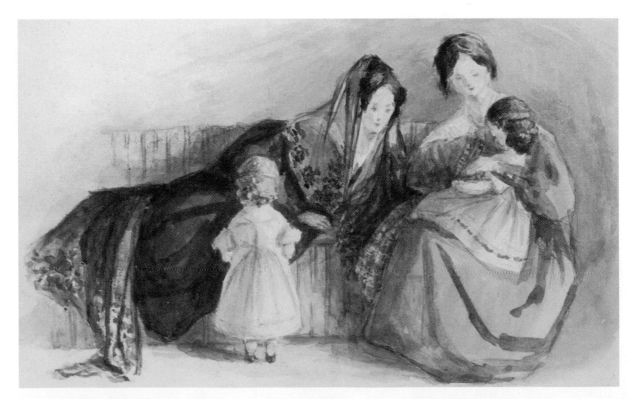

so much work to do that I can hardly find time for it except at night."[24] A great obstacle had been overcome, if only temporarily. The lessons were possible only when Florence was at Aunt Jane's house in Thames Bank or at Aunt Mai's in London, near Mr. Gillespie's home. By the next year, Florence was helping cousins Lothian and Lolly Nicholson with their algebra.

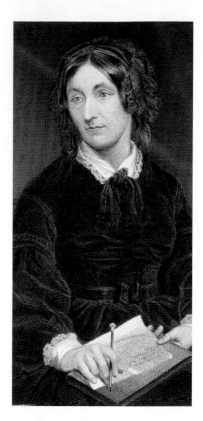

Mary Somerville (1780-1872), one of the early women scientists in England

Florence was lucky that her family, by dint of its Unitarian heritage, was more disposed to the education of women than society at large was at that time. Of the few women who were able to break the mold early, many came from Unitarian or other Dissenter families. Underlying the reluctance to educate women was Victorian society's belief that women were too fragile for difficult mental activity. As late as 1873, Edward C. Clark argued in *Sex and Education* that an overindulgence in matters of the mind would shrivel women's reproductive organs. Such fields of study as mathematics and science were viewed as masculine activities, and the few women who did manage to achieve prominence in these fields had to overcome much bias. Women of great ability who learned largely on their own or were lucky enough to obtain instruction often used male names or initials when corresponding with established mathematicians. The Royal Society didn't admit its first woman member until 1945.

The life of Fanny's acquaintance Mary Somerville (1780-1872) vividly illustrates how women had to struggle for an education. One of the great early women scientists in Britain, Somerville had grown up near Edinburgh, the daughter of a vice-admiral. Her family harbored the same prejudices as the larger society — that a woman's place was in the home and that young girls were fit only to learn domestic arts. In her mid-teens, while leafing through a fashion magazine, Somerville noticed some odd symbols:

> *I read what appeared to me to be simply an arithmetical question, but on turning the page I was surprised to see strange-looking lines mixed with letters, chiefly Xs and Ys, and asked, "What is that?" "Oh," said the friend, "it's a kind of arithmetic; they call it Algebra; but I can tell you nothing about it"... And we talked about other things; but on going home I thought I would look if any of our books could tell me what was meant by Algebra.[25]*

Somerville picked up a few clues to this intriguing world while her younger brother was being tutored in geometry. One day, when he hesitated to answer a problem, she prompted him and startled the tutor by her depth of knowledge. He explained a few basic theorems, and over the next few months Somerville memorized all of Euclid.

After her first husband died, Somerville for the first time had an independent income and was able to pursue her studies. Yet even then the expectations were the same that Florence faced: "I was considered eccentric and foolish, and my conduct was highly disapproved by many, especially by some members of my own family. They expected me to entertain and keep a gay house for them, and in that they were disappointed."[26]

One of Somerville's talents was her ability to present mathematics, physics, and other scientific subjects in plain language for laymen, but she also extolled the virtues of hard work and discipline. Later in life, Florence remembered an occasion when her mother complimented Somerville on her "genius," to which Somerville modestly replied: "Genius, my dear, there is no such thing. There is industry and regularity. I write every morning of my life from 7 to 11. I allow nothing to interrupt me."[27]

Feeling the pain of the world

In the spring of 1840, Florence's eyes were opened even more to the world around her, specifically to the position of women and to the plight of the poor and the suffering. Her Grandmother Smith died at the age of 81, and Aunt Julia, freed from her nursing responsibilities, joined the preparations for the World Anti-Slavery Convention in London, for which Lord Palmerston had been the moving force.

The American delegation, led by the great abolitionist William Lloyd Garrison, included four women and three men. Although women such as Aunt Julia were organizers and financial supporters, they were not allowed to participate in the deliberations. When the American women delegates — including pioneering feminists Elizabeth Cady Stanton and Lucretia Mott — were refused voting privileges, Garrison refused to attend in a show of solidarity. On their way home from the convention, Stanton and Mott resolved to form a society to advocate women's full civic, religious, and domestic freedoms as soon as they returned to the United States; within a decade (1848), they had convened the first women's rights convention at Seneca Falls, N.Y.

In the neighborhood at Embley, the marriage of the Nightingales' friend Lord Palmerston brought the family increased access to the upper echelons of the government and reform movement. Lord Palmerston, in his 10th year as foreign secretary, married Lady Emily Cowper, the widowed sister of the prime minister, Lord Melbourne. A woman of intellect, wide experience, charm, and tact, Lady Palmerston entertained extensively at informal gatherings and salons that provided a powerful support to her

Lord Ashley, later Lord Shaftesbury, (1801-1885) one of the great English humanitarians and reformers whose example of translating his religious beliefs into social reform through political action was a formative influence on Florence

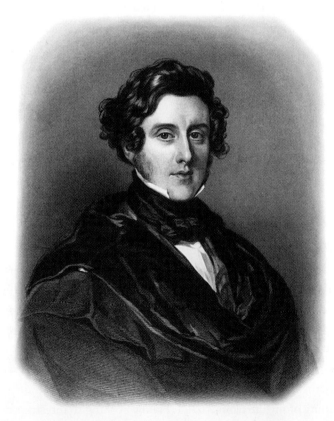

CALL & AWAKENING

husband's official position. The Nightingales were often invited to the Palmerstons' home, Broadlands, to dine, and the Palmerstons became frequent visitors at Embley.

Lady Palmerston's son-in-law was Lord Ashley (later Lord Shaftesbury), who was well on his way to becoming the conscience of English philanthropic reform in the 19th century. Having already helped secure passage of bills to improve the treatment of lunatics, he worked diligently from 1833 to limit child labor, and then all labor, to 10 hours a day, a cause that finally succeeded in 1847 with the passage of the Ten Hours Bill. Lord Ashley's efforts included protection for chimney sweeps, mine workers, and women as well as many other causes. From him, Florence learned of the Royal Commission report looking into the terrible sanitary conditions of towns and cities and another inquiry that was to address the enormous health problems of the working classes and the poor. She quickly became an avid reader of every government Blue Book (government reports on various social problems) that she could find.

The poverty and ill health that Florence had seen among the poor throughout her life were now being chronicled on an official basis and brought to the attention of the country. A new phrase had crept into the language — the "condition of the people." The Reform Bill of 1832 and other measures since then were slowly bringing more reformers into positions of power in national and local government.

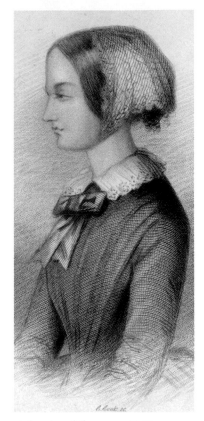

A drawing of Florence, c. 1840 (artist unknown)

The beginning of the 1840s (the "hungry Forties") saw an economic downturn which, combined with several years of a poor agricultural harvest, created hardship throughout the country. Wages were low and food prices were high because of the Corn Laws, which put a tariff on all imported grains — a tariff that was supported by the conservatives and those landowners whose economic success depended on high commodity prices. While visiting the Nicholsons at Waverley, Florence wrote that "there is a dreadful deal of want of work here & beggars."[28]

Around this time, Florence would enter the second stage of the mystic's spiritual development — purgation, a state of great spiritual pain and effort — as she struggled to find the path to her chosen work of nursing. While Florence inwardly longed to find meaningful work, her duty to family continued to dictate her life. As a young lady in society, she was expected to be at the disposal of her parents, available at all times to show guests around the estates and make pleasant conversation. The family received many distinguished visitors, leaving Florence no time for the serious studies she wished to undertake. Although she accompanied the family on the regular round of seasonal visits and parties at Embley, Lea Hurst, and London, her thoughts were far away — with the plight of the women and poor people who were the subject of the debate over Lord Ashley's Ten Hours Bill.

Mrs. Nightingale had no idea of the serious thoughts and desire for a meaningful life that occupied her younger daughter's mind. Fanny's plans for her daughters and her social ambitions were moving forward nicely. Lord Palmerston's marriage and the new contacts developed through Mary Clarke had greatly enhanced life at Embley. The Nightingales were invited to a gala fete at one of the great houses of Derbyshire, Chatsworth, only a few miles from Lea Hurst. Fanny described the scene in a letter to Mary Clarke:

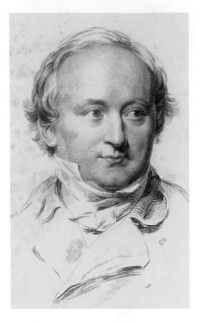

Christian Carl Josias von Bunsen (1791-1860), the Prussian diplomat, scholar, and theologian who first informed Florence about the Kaiserswerth Institution for nurses' training in Düsseldorf

... The Duke of Devonshire with his courteous manners plays the Host well. During the three days we were there we had every variety of amusement ... an omnibus plied at the gates of Chatsworth every morning from eleven till one, to take those who could not walk so far to the monster conservatory which covers an acre of ground, and where groves of palms and bananas are making all haste to grow to their natural size. One evening, we had a promenade in the Statue Gallery and Conservatory, brilliantly illuminated; another, a ball in the Banqueting Room, opened for the first time. You may imagine how our damsels went rejoicing.[29]

One damsel didn't rejoice. Florence thought the festivities as transparent as the Duke's huge glass conservatory (greenhouse), then the largest in England. The bright lights and gay people only made her feel uneasy and suffocated. She had recently begun to read about astronomy, one of the subjects about which Mary Somerville wrote so well, and wanted time alone to explore a few things, such as the Divine presence among the stars that shone above the terrace.

A seed of hope

During the social rounds of 1842, Florence met the new Prussian ambassador to England, Christian Carl Josias von Bunsen. In addition to being a diplomat, Bunsen was a theologian and scholar of international repute in ancient and oriental languages and mythology. He was also a close friend of Queen Victoria and Prince Albert. He had studied Jewish, Christian, Islamic, and Hindu scriptures as well as ancient Egyptian, Chinese, Persian, and Arabic languages. Like Florence, he was very interested in Plato and the Christian mystics.

Bunsen was concerned with more than philosophical and historical understanding; he was exploring the importance of religion and spirituality in the life of human beings. His scholarly and spiritual objectives were to bring into his own life and to German culture the contemplative and spiritual traditions of the East. Since the days of Frederick the Great, German scholars had led the way in Europe in historical criticism of the Bible. Many years before Darwin, new geological evidence and historical and linguistic investigation suggested that the gospels weren't absolute fact, but perhaps parables expressing truths about divine ideas.

The emergence of historical criticism and scientific discoveries, combined with the faith in reform and self-improvement that was a hallmark of Dissenters, led to widespread questioning of religious dogma and structures. Three major theological movements emerged in England during Florence's life: the Low Church, the High Church, and the Broad Church. The Low Church was composed mainly of Evangelicals — both Anglicans and Dissenters — who focused on the scriptures and personal religious experiences. The High Churchmen were those who emphasized the Church's authority on doctrines, as found in the Thirty-Nine Articles (the articles of faith developed in 1563) and the Book of Common Prayer. Followers of the Broad Church, including Bunsen, emphasized Christian ethical principles over doctrines and believed that divine revelation had been given to mankind throughout human history and wasn't exclusive to Christianity. They demanded that the clergy be free to interpret theology and scripture for themselves.

Florence became a frequent visitor to the Bunsen home in Carlton Terrace, a center of intellectual activity. Bunsen had married an Englishwoman of high social standing, and their children adored Florence. One evening she asked him: "What can an individual do towards lifting the load of suffering from the helpless and the miserable?"[30] Bunsen's answer provided the seed of hope that Florence had been seeking. He told her that he would get her information on an experiment recently begun in Germany for training nurses. The place was called Kaiserswerth, near Düsseldorf, and he had gone there to recruit qualified nurses to work at London's German Hospital.

From the beginning, Bunsen was impressed with Florence's sincerity and quiet brilliance. His wife recorded in her memoirs:

> From the first [he] valued her, on a few occasions, when nothing occurred pecularily to rouse and reveal the soul which subsisted in her, in the fullness of its energy, or the powers which only waited for an opportunity to be developed; but her calm dignity of deportment, self-conscious without either shyness or presumption, and the few words indicating deep reflection, just views, and clear perceptions of life and its obligations, and the trifling acts showing forgetfulness of self and devotedness to others, were of sufficient force to bring conviction to the observer, even before it had been proved by all outward experience, that she was possessed of all that moral greatness which her subsequent course of action, suffering, and influential power, has displayed.[31]

A serious suitor and family strife

In the summer of 1842, a new suitor came into Florence's life. Mrs. Nightingale had met a young man whose family she had known in the North, and Florence was soon introduced to the young politician, poet, and philanthropist Richard Monckton Milnes. At age 33, he was a charming fixture in London society who aspired to politics and was devoted to the improvement of mankind. One of his first philanthropic endeavors was to have young offenders separated from adults and placed in juvenile reformatories.

Monckton Milnes was also a scholar who later compiled and edited a memoir and letters by John Keats. However, he was more celebrated in London society for his fabulous breakfasts, to which he invited scholars, politicians, and other notable persons from all walks of life for lively conversation. Thomas Carlyle, when asked what would be the first thing to happen if Christ came back to earth, said "Monckton Milnes would ask him to breakfast."[32]

Florence avoided the obligations of society whenever she could and sought to be of service to her "darling old people," Grandmother Shore and Aunt Evans. She also went to London in 1843 for several weeks to be with a close friend whose sister had died in childbirth. Florence tried to extend her visit as long as possible. It was at this time that Parthe first began to feel threatened by her sister's frequent absences from the family. Florence complained to her mother:

> Parthe's letters are pure misery & if you cannot stop her, I suppose I must come home on Friday. The Horners asked me to their ball, but of course I declined, & Mrs. Austin was most kindly anxious to take me home with her to the Dorking ball ... but of course I did not go.[33]

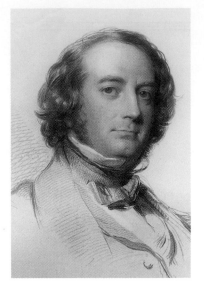

Richard Monckton Milnes (1809-1885), poet, politician, and philanthropist, who remained lifelong friends with Florence Nightingale despite her refusal to marry him

That Christmas the family gathered at the Nicholsons' home, Waverley, where Florence heard her cousin William's stories of life in his regiment in Australia. Florence was surprised to hear of the living conditions in the army, even for officers, who lived in dark huts where there wasn't enough light to read by. No wonder, she thought, that so many took to drink. At the Nicholsons, Florence became too ill to return to Embley, but the illness was a blessing in disguise because she met Uncle Nicholson's sister, Aunt Hannah, who had come to live at Waverley. Aunt Hannah was a deeply spiritual person who became a much needed mentor. The two women began corresponding.

Addled by her inability to find a meaningful path in life, Florence sometimes slipped into what she called her "dreaming" as an escape from her onerous daily routine. She dreamed of doing great things for the glory of God, sometimes even falling into a trancelike state. However, her acquaintance with this older woman of inexhaustible sympathy "to whom all unseen things seemed real, and eternal things near"[34] awakened Florence. In July 1844, she wrote Aunt Hannah a long letter of self-examination:

> *There is nothing I reproach myself more bitterly for, than for my want of faith ... Oh if one did but think one was getting nearer to the divine patience, when to us as to Him a thousand years will appear but as a day ... alas! a moment of discouragement seems a thousand years ... You are afraid, I see, of the 'attractions' of London for me! but I assure you, I never was so glad to leave it. There was not a thing I was sorry <u>not</u> to see again ... I hope, dear Aunt Hannah, that I shall show some day the good you have done me — indeed I think now my pride is falling down about me, like the walls of Jericho, at some unknown voice, & that is worth living for.[35]*

In the summer of 1844, family friends introduced the Nightingales to the famed American educator and philanthropist Dr. Samuel Gridley Howe, and his wife, Julia Ward Howe. Mrs. Howe would later become a well-known suffragette and reformer as well as the composer of the "Battle Hymn of the Republic." The Howes knew England well; as philanthropists, they had previously visited numerous public institutions, including schools, workhouses, prisons, and insane asylums. On a visit to a prison with novelist Charles Dickens, the group watched the prisoners' daily routine of "ungrateful work," and Dickens commented, "My God! if a woman thinks her son may come to this, I don't blame her if she strangles him in infancy."[36]

One morning, Florence asked to meet with Dr. Howe. She came straight to the point: "Dr. Howe, do you think it would be unsuitable and unbecoming for a young Englishwoman to devote herself to works of charity in hospitals and elsewhere as Catholic sisters do? Do you think it would be a dreadful thing?"[37] From his conversations with family friends, Dr. Howe was well aware of Florence's struggles with her parents over her desire for a meaningful vocation, but his answer reflected his own conscience and his American understanding of the strictures of English society:

> *My dear Miss Florence, it would be unusual, and in England whatever is unusual is apt to be thought unsuitable; but I say to you, go forward if you have a vocation for that way of life; act up to your inspiration, and you will find that there is never anything unbecoming or unladylike in doing your duty for the good of others. Choose, go on with it wherever it may lead you, and God be with you.[38]*

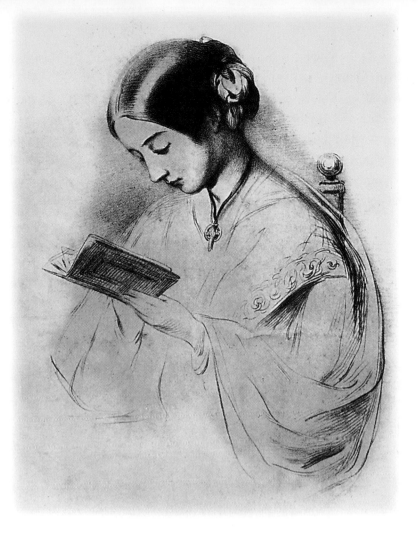

Florence Nightingale in a familiar pose, c. 1839, sketched by her cousin Hilary Bonham Carter

At this time in England, "nurses" were generally drawn from the ranks of the poor and unskilled, and usually remained in that state, with the exception of those women with natural healing instincts and intelligence. They also had a reputation for drunkenness and immoral conduct. This sad state of affairs had evolved for three centuries as nursing passed into its "dark ages" in England. Since the Reformation and the suppression of monasteries, the quality of nursing and hospitals had suffered in all the Protestant European countries but most severely in England.

When Henry VIII established the Church of England in 1534, he seized over 600 charitable institutions and suppressed all religious orders. This seizure of church properties had a direct negative effect on women and nursing — women lost political and administrative control of nursing operations. Inexperienced civil administrators took over from religious professionals who were steeped in a culture of care that had evolved since the beginning of the Christian church. Women lost their voice in both hospital administration and nursing management.[39] The whole medical system began a downward spiral of mismanagement, crowding, filth, and contagion. It was these conditions that prompted Howe to tell Florence that her avocation might be thought "unusual."

Inwardly cheered by Dr. Howe's encouragement, Florence turned to her personal life. Henry Nicholson had at long last proposed, and she declined, not only because she wasn't in love with him, but also because he was her first cousin. The Nicholsons felt that she had led him on, and Marianne broke off their friendship.

In the fall of 1845, Nurse Gale died after a long illness and her passing marked the end of childhood things for Florence, who was holding the hand of her dear old nurse-maid when she died. In a letter to her cousin Hilary, Florence wrote: "How *unheimlich* [disquieting] it is coming out of the room where there is only her and God and me, to come back into the cold and false life of prejudices and hypocrisy and conventionalisms; by which I do not mean to find fault with life but only with the use I make of it."[40]

The first struggle

By late 1845, Florence had come to realize the need for training to learn the rudiments of nursing. After the death of Nurse Gale, she threw herself into her work in West Wel-low village near Embley whenever she had the opportunity. She realized that she and others were limited by their lack of knowledge in the specifics of care, whether it was the preparation of fomentations or treating fever. She could learn to nurse just as she had learned to play the piano or dance quadrilles.

With the agreement of family friend Dr. Richard Fowler, for many years a doctor at Salisbury Hospital, Florence proposed to her family that she go to study under his direction for 3 months. In an era when "doctor" could mean any of several levels of training and knowledge, Dr. Fowler was a man of common sense, original thinking, and fine character. He was trained in the prevailing miasma theory (that disease arises from the decomposition of organic matter), which would endure for another 2 decades, and he believed in fresh air and cold water treatments. Even so, along with a few others of his era, he understood the tentative advances of science and foresaw the revolutionary changes that soon would come in medicine. Each day he walked 3 miles and engaged in 2 or 3 hours of "mental exercise." His own self-treatment had saved his eyesight when 4 years earlier an oculist had said that it would last only a few weeks more.

The plans of the two forward thinkers ran into a wall of absolute conventionality. Mrs. Nightingale was horrified and called Florence "odd"; such a venture was totally beneath their class and unequivocally forbidden. It was unbelievable that Florence would even consider such unladylike behavior. What if men who weren't "gentlemen" made advances to her? Didn't she care what others thought of her? Even Dr. Fowler's wife, upon whose sympathy Florence had depended, felt that conditions at Salisbury Hospital were far too coarse for a lady of Florence's upbringing. At this time in England, as Florence would later write, caregivers were "merely women who would be servants if they were not nurses ... it was as if I had wanted to be a kitchen-maid."[41]

It wasn't just the field of nursing to which the Nightingales so vehemently object-ed; doctors and hospitals were also included in their concerns. A unified medical profession, in the sense now known, didn't exist. The rapid modernization and industrialization that was creating many new professions in England and changing others for the better hadn't begun to reach the medical sector. Doctors were regarded as little better than tradesmen, and hospitals and nursing were little changed from the previous

3 centuries. The filth and stench of hospitals were such that only the poor and the destitute went there; those who could afford it were nursed at home.

Crushed, Florence poured out her feelings to cousin Hilary. In a torrent of emotion, she revealed that she was thinking not only of nursing for herself, but also in terms of plans for an organization:

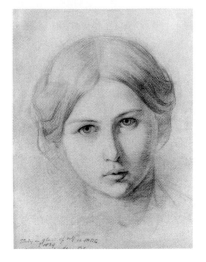

Self-portrait of Hilary Bonham Carter (1821-1865), Florence's favorite first cousin

> *I have always found that there was so much truth in the suggestion that you must dig for hidden treasures in silence or you will not find it; and so I dug after my poor little plan in silence, even for you. It was to go to be a nurse at Salisbury Hospital for these few months to learn the "prax"; and then to come home and make such wondrous intimacies at West Wellow under the shelter of a rhubarb powder and a dressed leg; let alone that no one could ever say to me again, your health will not stand this or that. I saw a poor woman die before my eyes this summer because there was no one but fools to sit up with her, who poisoned her as much as if they had given her arsenic. And then I had such a fine plan for those dreaded latter days (which I have never dreaded), if I should outlive my immediate ties, of taking a small house in West Wellow. Well, I do not like much talking about it, but I thought something like a Protestant Sisterhood, without vows, for women of educated feelings, might be established.*
>
> *But there have been difficulties about my very first step, which terrified Mama. I do not mean the physically revolting parts of a hospital, but things about the surgeons and nurses which you may guess. Even Mrs. Fowler threw cold water upon it; and nothing will be done this year at all events, and I do not believe — ever; and no advantage that I see comes of my living on, excepting that one becomes less and less of a young lady every year, which is only a negative one. You will laugh, dear, at the whole plan, I daresay; but no one but the mother of it knows how precious an infant idea becomes; nor how the soul dies between the destruction of one and the taking up of another. I shall never do anything, and am worse than dust and nothing. I wonder if our Savior were to walk the earth again, and I were to go to Him and ask, whether He would send me back to live this life again, which crushes me into vanity and deceit. Oh for some strong thing to sweep this loathsome life into the past.[42]*

Although she had been thwarted in her initial attempt to study nursing, Florence accepted the reality and moved on. Her correspondence with Aunt Hannah reflected a growing maturity on her path of mystical development. Her self-dialogue was a preparation for the continuing struggles she would face — struggles that would require much discipline:

> *I was almost heart-broken to leave [Lea Hurst]. There are so many duties there, which lie near at hand & I could be well content to do them there all the days of my life ... I have left so many poor friends there ... so much might have been done for them. One's days pass away like a shadow, & how we spend hours that are sacred in things that are profane, which we choose to call necessities, & then say "we cannot" to our Father's business. We think and reason ... We dream our intellectual dreams ... Where will they be when we are gone?... I feel my sympathies all with Ignorance & Poverty — the things which interest me, interest them. We are alike in expecting little from life, much from God ...*
>
> *I never pray for anything temporal, not even for my lad [Shore] — but when each morning comes, I kneel down before the Rising Sun, & only say, Behold the handmaid of the Lord — give me this day my work to do — no, not my work, but thine ...*

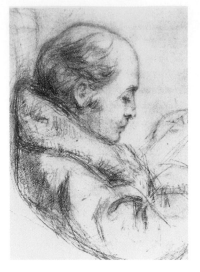

Julius Mohl, the German scholar and translator who married Florence's dear friend Mary Clarke (right) in 1847

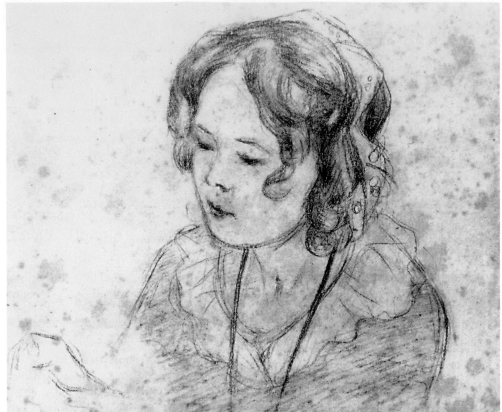

My imagination is too filled with the misery of this world, that the only thing, in which to labour brings any return, seems to me helping or sympathizing there — & all that poets sing of the glories of this world appears to me untrue — all the people I see are eaten up with care or poverty or disease ...

Life is no holiday game, nor is it a clever book, nor is it a school of instruction, nor a valley of tears — but it is a hard fight, a struggle, a wrestling, with the Principle of Evil, hand to hand, foot to foot — every inch of the way must be disputed ...

You say well, in your last dear letter, that I have not found "permanent" peace — but I do feel it sometimes, & can pray now, that such discipline may be appointed me, that soon I may not have one personal feeling left — may be able to say in all things "Not as I will but as thou will" ...[43]

Florence believed that there were great turning points in people's lives, and she now felt she was approaching one. Her intuition was correct. An answer to the question she had posed to Ambassador Bunsen 4 years earlier arrived. The nurses' training center in Düsseldorf of which he had spoken had finally published the *Year Book of the Institution of Deaconesses at Kaiserswerth*. It described the project that had begun in a single house in 1836 and now had 100 beds and had trained 116 deaconesses (Protestant nurses). On reading this report, sent to her by Bunsen, Florence wrote: "There is my home; there are my brothers and sisters all at work. There my heart is, and there I trust one day will be my body ..."[44]

In 1847, the Nightingales attended a British Association meeting at Oxford, accompanied by Florence's suitor, Richard Monckton Milnes. The purpose of the gathering was to honor the codiscoverers of the planet Neptune, John C. Adams, the British mathematician and astronomer, and J.J. Le Verrier, the French astronomer. Florence pressed a white rose in remembrance of her special time with Monckton Milnes, and she wrote in her diary of the enthusiastic, stimulating company she encountered. When they returned from Oxford, a letter was waiting from Mary Clarke ("Clarkey") and Julius Mohl announcing their marriage.

In the wake of Clarkey's wedding, the issue of marriage pressed in on Florence, now age 27. All the conventions of the day decreed that a woman's fulfillment was to be found in marriage; among the upper class, a good marriage was the highest objective for a daughter. Even so, Florence found it hard to visualize life as a proper Victorian wife and mother, with all of its hollow responsibilities and limitations. At the same time, she questioned her motives for the success she craved as a single woman: "Vanity, love of display, love of glory ... Everything I do is poisoned by the fear that I am not doing it in simplicity and godly sincerity."[45] In a long letter to Clarkey, Florence wrote:

> We must all take Sappho's leap, one way or another, before we attain her repose — though some take it to death and some to marriage and some again to a new life even in this world. Which of them is the better part, God only knows. Popular prejudice gives it a favor of marriage ... In single life, the stage of the Present and the Outward World is so filled with phantoms, the phantoms, not unreal tho' intangible, of Vague Remorse, Tears, dwelling on the threshold of every thing we undertake alone, Dissatisfaction with what is, and Restless Yearnings for what is not ... love laying to sleep those phantoms (by assuring us of a love so great that we must lay aside all care for our own happiness ... because it is of so much consequence to another) gives that leisure frame to our mind, which opens it at once to joy.[46]

Roman holiday

In the fall of 1847, a golden opportunity arose that provided relief to all in the family. The Bracebridges, friends of the Nightingales, invited Florence to accompany them on a trip of several months to Rome. She was reluctant to leave because she would have to give up "all my little plans," which would stand still in her absence. Most of her desires were for home and she had prayed earnestly to know exactly what was the will of "that Loving Father" for the proposed trip. She concluded that, because the "wish was not father of the thought," it was right to go.[47]

Florence's parents urged her to take the trip, thinking it would be good for her. The Bracebridges, a childless couple who treated Florence like a daughter, were both energetic travelers but in delicate health, and Florence could minister to their needs. Charles Bracebridge was a sharp businessman and a quintessential English gentleman of many interests. An ardent Hellenist along with his wife, he had even fought with the Greeks in their revolt against Turkish rule in the 1830s. Selina Bracebridge, although much older than Florence, was a kindred spirit whose goodness Florence compared to that of a Protestant saint. The Nightingales called her "Sigma," for the Greek letter Σ, to recognize her love of Greece and her Hellenist traits of character. Of this dear friend and confidante, Florence wrote with appreciation:

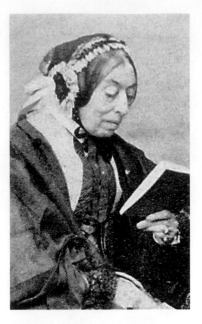

Selina Bracebridge, the kindred soul who rescued Florence more than once from her despair over family constraints, in a photograph taken in 1853

She never told me life was fair and my share of its blessings great and that I ought to be happy. She did not know I was miserable, but she felt it; and to me, young, strong, blooming as I then was, to me, the idol of the man I adored [Milnes], the spoilt child of fortune, she had the heart and the instinct to say, 'Earth, my child, has a grave and in heaven is rest.' [48]

The Bracebridges provided a great window on the world for Florence. Even Parthe favored the trip: "God is very good to provide such a pleasant time and it will rest her mind ... from wearing thoughts, that all men have at home when their duties weigh much on their consciences ..."[49] It wasn't that Parthe didn't understand her sister's unconventional ambitions; she simply couldn't step outside the mold of convention, nor imagine or tolerate her sister doing likewise.

The threesome arrived in Rome at the beginning of November 1847. W.E.N. had poured over his large map of Rome and made an extensive list of attractions that Florence methodically ticked off. They visited the catacombs, the Coliseum, churches, and galleries and enjoyed the full panoply of tours and sightseeing. On December 15, the custodian of the Sistine Chapel left Florence and Selina alone for the afternoon to savor the beauty and genius of Michelangelo. Florence described her reaction to this wonderful day in a letter that reveals her thoughts about her own spiritual journey through references to the Delphic sibyl:

Oh, my dearest, I have had such a day ... of all my days in Rome this has been the most happy and glorious. Think of a day alone in the Sistine Chapel with Σ [Selina Bracebridge], quite alone, without custode, without visitors, looking up into that heaven of angels and prophets ... I did not think that I was looking at pictures, but straight into Heaven itself ... There is Daniel, opening his windows and praying to the God of his Fathers three times a day in defiance of fear. You see that young and noble head like an eagle's, disdaining danger, those glorious eyes undazzled by all the honours of Babylon. Then comes Isaiah, but he is so divine that there is nothing but his own 53rd chapter will describe him ... Next to Isaiah comes the Delphic Sibyl, the most beautiful, the most inspired of all the Sibyls here ... there is an uncertainty, a wistfulness in her eyes; she expects to be rewarded rather in another stage than this for her struggle to gain the prize of her high calling, to reach to the Unknown that Isaiah knows already. There is not uncertainty as to her feeling of being called to hear the voice, but she fears that her earthly ears are heavy and gross, and corrupt the meaning of the heavenly words. I cannot tell you how affecting this anxious look of her far-reaching eyes is to the poor mortals standing on the pavement below ... No one can have seen the Sistine without feeling that he has been very near to God, that he will understand some of His words better for ever after; and that Michael Angelo ... has received as much of the breath of God, and has done as much to communicate it to men, as any Seer of old. [50]

For the rest of her life, Florence kept copies of the Sistine frescoes in her room.

Two life-altering encounters

In Rome, Florence met several people whose sympathy and expertise opened new and wider doors to her dreams of service; two would be of great importance. One was Madre Santa Colomba, who introduced her to the discipline necessary for her mystical development. The other was Sidney Herbert, only 10 years Florence's elder, but already a force in English politics. Herbert, who would become her great political ally, was one of many pragmatic conservatives who, under the leadership of Sir Robert Peel, became more liberal as their careers progressed.

Sidney Herbert and his bride, Elizabeth à Court, who also was like a daughter to Mrs. Bracebridge, were in Rome on holiday and soon became fast friends with Florence. Herbert was the son of the Earl of Pembroke, a great landowner of Wiltshire. After his father's death, Herbert became a conscientious landlord who personally looked after the welfare of his tenants and villagers. His wife worked with him in arranging new cottages for tenants and developing a convalescent home for the poor who had no place to recover from severe illness or surgery.

For Herbert, as for Florence, politics and public affairs were part of everyday life. A steadfast High Churchman, he was concerned with reform and philanthropy, both in his government posts and in his private life. Only 22 years old when he entered Parliament as a Tory member for Wiltshire in 1832, Herbert served as secretary to the Board of Control during Peel's first term as Prime Minister (1834-1835). When Peel returned to lead the government in 1841, Herbert served as Secretary to the Admiralty, in which post he reformed the naval school at Greenwich. Within a year he was promoted to Secretary at War, where he immediately launched a series of educational reforms in the military schools by establishing a system of qualifications for regimental schoolmasters, where none had existed before.

Florence also made the acquaintance of the Rev. Henry Manning, archdeacon of Chichester and a close friend of Sidney Herbert. Unlike many clergymen of his era, Manning had been a model parish priest, ministering to the spiritual and physical needs of his parishioners. Although not an original thinker, he was a superb organizer and had been active in the National Society for Promoting the Education of the Poor. One of the leaders of the Anglican High Church, Manning had begun drifting toward Roman Catholicism in the preceding months during a trip through Belgium and Germany on his way to Rome. In 1851, he would leave the Church of England for the Catholic priesthood, and would later become involved in providing Roman Catholic nurses for Nightingale's historic nursing mission to the Crimea.

A lesser figure on the scene was Mary Stanley, a friend of the Herberts who was 8 years older than Florence. The daughter of the Bishop of Norwich, she had gained some experience in church-related social work and would later lead the second delegation of nurses to the Crimea. Her younger brother, Arthur Stanley, would become Dean of Westminster Abbey.

Of much greater significance was Florence's introduction, in February 1848, to Madre Santa Colomba, the mother superior of the Convent Trinità de Monti, who would become her great teacher. During a 10-day spiritual retreat at the convent, Florence was introduced to the discipline of formal meditation and contemplation, a spiritual practice that would enable her to move forward in her spiritual development. Madre Santa Colomba, who saw something special in the young Englishwoman, believed that the only thing that mattered was to do the will of God and advised Florence

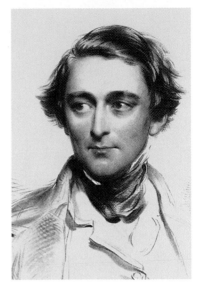

Sidney Herbert (1810-1861), the statesman and reformer who later became Florence's indispensable friend and political colleague in the battle for army, medical, and nursing reform

to "turn her whole heart to God that she might be ready to do his work."

At the end of the retreat, Florence recorded this dialogue:

C. Did not God speak to you during this retreat? Did he not ask you anything?

F. He asked me to surrender my will.

C. And to whom?

F. To all that is upon the earth.

C. He calls you to a very high degree of perfection ...[51]

She vowed to devote every 7th day of the month, the date of her Call from God, to reflection and prayer. Madre Santa Colomba emphasized to her the importance of maintaining the discipline of this practice. Once again, Florence expressed the universality of her religious impulse, writing:

I do not feel though Pagan in the morning, Jew in the afternoon, and Christian in the evening, anything but a unity of interest in all these representations. To know God we must study Him as much in the Pagan and Jewish dispensations as in the Christian (though that is the last and most perfect manifestation), and this gives unity to the whole — one continuous thread of interest to all these pearls.[52]

No to marriage

Florence's 6 months in Rome with the Bracebridges were inspiring and invigorating; she recalled them as some of the happiest days of her life. Full of enthusiasm, she returned to England and the sobering prospect of her unchanged family environment. Even so, her new friends the Herberts were a joy; she often visited them and their children at Wilton House near Salisbury. She had great hopes of visiting Kaiserswerth in the fall of 1848, when her mother was planning a trip to the Carlsbad baths near Frankfurt, but was crushed when the trip was precluded by the European revolutions of that year.

Instead, Florence found great pleasure in teaching at one of London's "ragged schools" (so named for the poor condition of the childrens' clothes), one of several hundred charity schools for the poor across England and Scotland. Family friend Lord Ashley was president of the Ragged School Union, which was staffed by volunteers like Florence and some paid teachers. She spoke of the children as her "little thieves of Westminster" and called them her greatest joy in London. In her diary she wrote:

Life is seen in a much truer form in London than in the country. In an English country place everything that is painful is so carefully removed out of sight, behind those fine trees, to a village three miles off. In London, at all events if you open your eyes, you cannot help seeing in the next street that life is not as it has been made to you. You cannot get out of a carriage at a party without seeing what is in the faces making the lane on either side, and without feeling tempted to rush back and say, "Those are my brothers and sisters."[53]

Although still deeply unhappy, Florence felt that she was finally creating some new possibilities for meaningful work. With determination and strength, she proceeded in silence. Her family wasn't aware of the depth of knowledge that she was developing

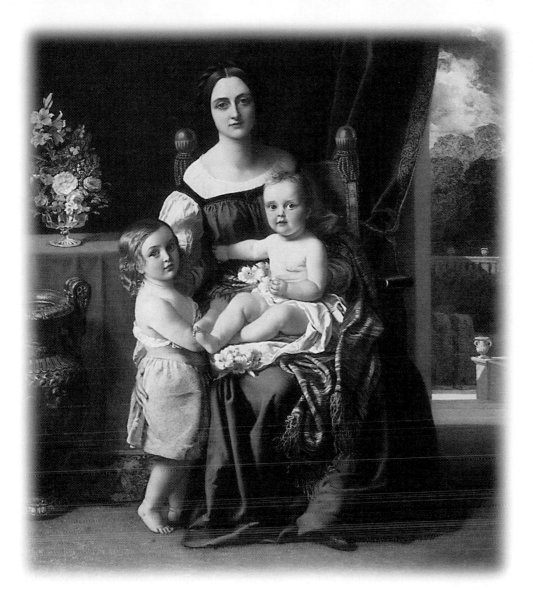

about hospitals and nursing. She would rise at 4 a.m., according to her custom. Now a careful reader of the government's Blue Books, she was amazed at the lack of careful statistical details, the usefulness of which was becoming clear to her. She resolved to compile her own data and tabulate facts with more precision. In so doing, she was laying the foundation for the work that would soon make her the first expert on hospitals in all of Europe.

In 1849, Richard Monckton Milnes asked Florence to marry him. She rejected the proposal, which only exacerbated family tensions. In her private notes, she methodically analyzed the reasons for her refusal:

> *I have an intellectual nature which requires satisfaction, and that would find it in him. I have a passionate nature which requires satisfaction, and that would find it in him. I have a moral and active nature that requires satisfaction, and that would not find it in him ... I could be satisfied to spend a life with him combining our different powers in some great object. I could not satisfy this nature by spending a life with him in making society and arranging domestic things ... To be nailed to a continuation and exaggeration of my present life, without the hope*

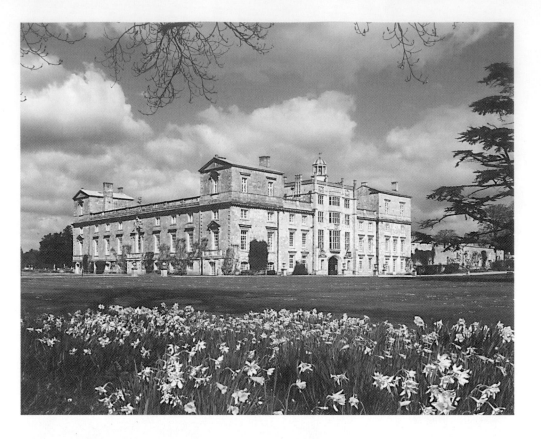

of another, would be intolerable to me. Voluntarily to put it out of my power never to be able to seize the chance of forming for myself a true and rich life would seem to me like suicide ...

I think that [God] has clearly marked out some to be single women as He has others to be wives, and has organized them accordingly for their vocation. I think some have every reason for not marrying, and that for these it is much better to educate the children who are already in the world and can't be got out of it, than to bring more into it.[54]

After 7 years of courtship, Monckton Milnes could hardly be accused of impatience but he was unwilling to court Florence forever. Shortly after her refusal, he married Annabel Crew. At first, Florence was miserable, feeling he was now truly lost to her. For the next few months, she pined for him and the rapport they had shared. The relationship did not end, however; Monckton Milnes and Florence remained lifelong friends. She was a godparent to his son and he named a daughter after her. He wrote or advised her on many subjects throughout his life, spoke on her behalf at public meetings, and encouraged her to meet influential people outside her circle who could help her further her mission.

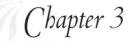

Chapter 3

Egypt, Greece, & Kaiserswerth

I *look back with pity & shame upon my former self, when I attached importance to my life & labours. It is because I am one with Christ that I am so wounded. Because we have the Spirit of the Father — what he wishes, we wish, what he hates, we hate. I could not be happy if God was not glorified & if I had not the enjoyment of his presence, for which I felt that I was now educating. I had rightfully no other business each day but to do God's work as a servant constantly regarding his pleasure. A despicable indulgence in lying in bed gave me such a view of the softness of my character that I resolved on knees to live a life of non self. The views of my own heart have produced, not humility but discontent. I pass so many hours as if there were no God at all. Setting a watch over my first thoughts on awaking ... I find to be an excellent preparation for a right spirit during the day.*

— *Florence Nightingale, Private Note, May 1850*[1]

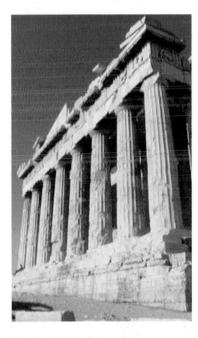

The Parthenon, the temple to Athena built in the 5th century B.C., which Florence visited in 1849

Once again, Mr. and Mrs. Bracebridge came to the rescue. Unsettled by Florence's decision to refuse marriage to Richard Monckton Milnes, the Nightingales easily agreed to the Bracebridges' invitation for Florence to accompany them on a tour of Egypt, Greece, and Europe in 1849. They planned to spend several months in Egypt, then move on to Greece, where they owned property in Athens, and return through central Europe.

Florence was delighted at the opportunity. Writing a last note from Folkestone before departing for France, she thanked her parents "more than I can say — bless you more than I can bless you. I hope I shall come back to be more of a comfort to you than ever I have been. Thank you all a thousand times."[2]

British scholars, collectors, and tourists had enthusiastically traveled to Egypt in the years after Nelson's defeat of the French fleet at Aboukir Bay in 1801. When Napoleon invaded Egypt in 1798, his army was accompanied by scholars who sketched and described in detail all the pyramids, temples, and sites known at the time. In 1809, the monumental work *Description de l'Egypte,* the first extensive study that opened the field of Egyptian antiquities to the West, was published.

Egypt

Traveling by rail across France to Marseilles, the trio arrived in Cairo on November 27. On December 4, they started their Nile voyage in a dahabiah, a large river sailing boat, that Florence christened "Parthenope" in a tribute to her sister. She made a cloth pennant for the boat from her petticoat tape and carefully stitched on it the Greek word ΠΑΡΘΕΝΟΠΗ (Parthenope). Sailing past the beautiful landscape with temples, villages, and the changeable desert, flat and low in the delta, high-banked and fading away to the mountains in the south, Florence had a great deal of time to reflect.

Wherever they stopped, the Bracebridges and Florence did everything they could to avoid "society's superficial chatter;" Florence thought it was hard to be among the remains of a great ancient civilization all day and come home and talk about quails or London. She took every opportunity to search for artifacts to send home to her family but was very disappointed when she discovered only small bits of Egyptian "rubbish." In the years since Napoleon's defeat, many precious Egyptian antiquities had been plundered and sold to individuals or collectors for private museums and collections abroad.

For much of the trip Florence was deep in contemplation. However, she frequently left the dahabiah to wander about the desert on her own, poking her nose into the villages to see how people lived. She was struck by how intact the villages were, practically unchanged since ancient times. Wherever she went she was accompanied by the Bracebridges, by her maid, or by an Egyptian attendant — her efreet, or demon, as she called him. As a white Christian woman, she was an odd yet fascinating sight for the villagers. At the sacred mosques in Cairo, her efreet was forced to beat back with a whip worshippers who protested her presence, an incident that greatly saddened her. She saw great suffering and poverty everywhere. For example, at the slave markets, she saw young girls and boys being sold for £2 to £9 per head.

Florence's correspondence with her family while in Egypt reveals her grasp of both ancient and modern religions. She had read the work of the French Egyptologist, Jean François Champollion, who deciphered Egyptian hieroglyphics in 1822 with the help of the Rosetta Stone. She was also familiar with the hermetic writings, Latin and Greek texts from the 2nd and 3rd centuries that contain elements of Egyptian theology and emphasize the knowledge (*gnosis*) of God. The hermetic idea — that divine knowledge is a way for man to achieve an ultimate union with God — was another reflection of the universal nature of mysticism. Florence analyzed the leading ideas of Egyptian scholars, studied Egyptian mythology, made tables of dynasties, and copied plans of temples.

The pennant embroidered with the Greek name "Parthenope," which Florence made from her petticoat tape to christen the sailboat on which she and the Bracebridges toured the Nile in 1849

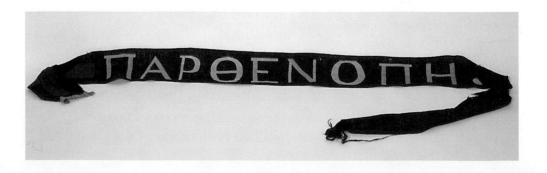

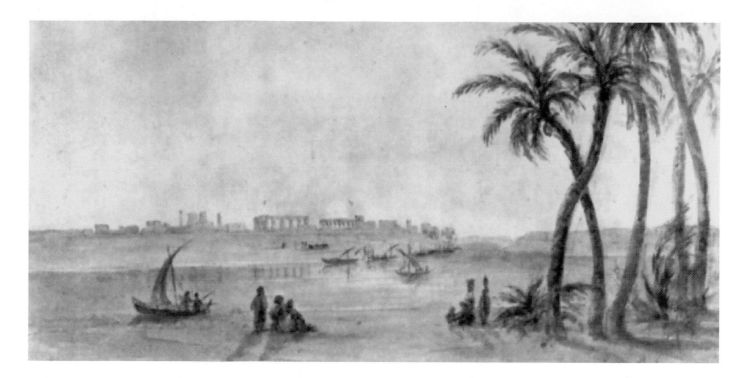

The trio's 3½-month Nile expedition took them some 900 miles upriver to Ipsamboul, near today's Aswan High Dam. On the return leg downstream, they spent several days at Thebes. They visited the pyramids, the Valley of the Kings, and many other archeological sites, sometimes crawling from one tomb or chamber to another. It was an adventurous journey with real risk. They endured gales and water spouts on the Nile, sandstorms and enervating heat, and brawls among the crew, all under the watchful eyes of basking crocodiles.

Another Call from God

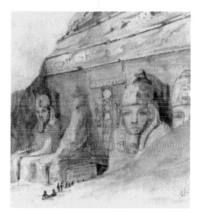

Sketches by Selina Bracebridge of Thebes (top), the ancient city on the Nile in southern Egypt (now the site of Luxor and Karnak), and the Great Temple of Abu Simbel at Ipsamboul, Egypt

Florence's days and nights on the Nile, where one seemed to lose all feeling of identity and everything became supernatural, evolved into a reverie of inner questing — a spiritual and intellectual retreat from the demands of everyday life. In this phase of her spiritual development, her path paralleled that of many other mystics in the Western tradition: a withdrawal from the world for the purpose of reevaluating the beliefs, goals, and values of the originating society, a sojourn in the spiritual wilderness from which the mystic returns intent on his or her mission in the world. The progress of Florence's spiritual journey was reflected in her diary entries:

> *March 3. Sunday. Did not get up in the morning but God gave me the time afterwards, which I ought to have made in the morning — a solitary 2 hours in my own cabin, to "meditate" on my Madre's [Madre Santa Colomba] words.*
>
> *7. Thursday. Gale all night & all day … God called me in the morning & asked me "Would I do good for Him, for Him alone without the reputation [self-interest]."*
>
> *8. Friday. Thought much upon this question. My Madre said to me, Can you hesitate between the God of the whole Earth & your little reputation?*

9. Saturday. During half an hour I had by myself in the cabin ... settled the question with God.

11. Monday. Thought how our leaving Thebes was quite useless owing to this contrary wind ... but without it I might not have had this call from God.

12. Tuesday. Very sleepy. Stood at the door of the boat looking out upon the stars & the tall mast in the still night against the sky ... & tried to think only of God's will — & that every thing is desirable only as He is in it or not in it — only as it brings us nearer or farther from Him. He is speaking to us often just when something we think untoward happens.

15. Friday. Such a day at Memphis & in the desert of Sakkara ... God had delivered me from the great offense — & the constant murderer of my thoughts [her "dreaming"].

16. Saturday – 17. Sunday. Tried to bring my will one with God's ... Can I not serve God as well in Malta as in Smyrna, in England as at Athens? Perhaps better — perhaps it is between Athens & Kaiserswerth — perhaps this is the opportunity my 30th year was to bring me. Then as I sat in the large dull room waiting for the letters, God told me what a privilege he had reserved for me, what a preparation for Kaiserswerth in choosing me to be with Mr. B. during his time of ill health & how I had neglected it — & had been blind to it. If I were never thinking of the reputation, how I should be better able to see what God intends for me ...[3]

In her diary at Cairo she wrote: "Oh God, thou puttest into my heart this great desire to devote myself to the sick and sorrowful. I offer it to thee. Do with it what is for thy service."[4] Florence described her last day in Egypt as perhaps the "most curious" of her life." She had received introductions to the nuns of St. Vincent de Paul in Alexandria, who operated a school and offered medical services from their dispensary. Welcomed as a visitor, Florence found other visitors there: the Reverend Mother of the Good Shepherdesses, whom she had met in Cairo, and a group of Sisters of Mercy from Australia, who were passing through. Florence was struck by the spirit of cooperation and mutual sympathy, rather than jealousy, among the various orders.

After their farewells, Florence was off with another new friend from Cairo, the wife of the Tuscan consul. Madam Rosetti had arranged a surprise visit to the harem of Said Pasha, eldest son of the ruler of Egypt. Florence was stunned by the dreadful ennui of the harem, the women lying about with no work or even play to engage in. She wrote: "If heaven and hell exist on this earth, it is in the two worlds I saw on that one morning — the Dispensary and the Hareem."[5]

Greece

Florence and the Bracebridges arrived in Athens in mid-April 1850 at the height of a diplomatic incident involving the Nightingales' neighbor and family friend, Lord Palmerston, the British Foreign Secretary. By virtue of her family's social and political position, Florence had a front-row seat to the high-level diplomatic and military maneuvers that ensued. The conflict, known as the Don Pacifico incident, had arisen out of the claims against the Greek government of a Portuguese-Jewish native of Gibraltar (thus a British subject) named Don Pacifico, who lived in Athens. Pacifico contended that the Greek government was responsible for property he lost during anti-Semitic riots at Easter of 1847.

Although the complete truth was never fully established, Palmerston sent a naval squadron to enforce the claims, a move that aroused the ire of the French, who were always concerned about the spread of British influence in the Mediterranean. The conservative House of Lords passed a vote of censure, and when debate opened in the House of Commons, it appeared that all the forces of opposition, roused by what they considered the nonsense of the Don Pacifico affair, would turn Palmerston out. On the second day of the debate, Palmerston spoke for 4 hours, brilliantly winning the day.

Florence was dining aboard the warship H.M.S. *Howe,* anchored in the port of Piraeus on April 26, when the Greek government's message of submission was brought to Mr. Wyse, the Minister to Greece, who had invited her to dinner. Palmerston had turned a small, messy, and ambiguous affair into a great victory by rendering the issue in essential political and moral terms that the people could easily understand. Twenty-nine-year-old Florence Nightingale, who only months before had written that she "never expected nor intended to leave England again," would never forget this lesson learned abroad.

At the Bracebridges' house in Athens, Florence slept in the library, which overlooked the rear of the Acropolis. True to form, she kept elaborate notebooks about Greek mythology and the spiritual concepts that were embodied in the worship of the Greek gods. She was absorbed by how the soul of the Greek people was expressed in their sculpture, art, and architecture. She most loved the Doric columns and described their simplicity, severity, and perfection of proportion as the image of an ideal republic. Viewing the Parthenon by moonlight, she observed that it is "impossible that earth or heaven could produce anything more beautiful."[6] On one visit to the Parthenon, she purchased from some Greek boys a baby owl that had fallen from its nest. She named this owlet Athena, and it became her constant companion, riding on her shoulder or in her pocket and eating from her hand.

Florence met friends of the Bracebridges, the American missionaries John and Frances Hill, whose school for girls and orphanage were considered the best in Greece. Florence wrote that the couple had "the real missionary in them," as they were purely devoted to "God & their fellow-creatures" and not "to some fid-fad or other."[7] She saw in Mrs. Hill the same spiritual qualities possessed by Madre Santa Colomba, qualities that were eternal and the same regardless of the person's country or religion:

> It is interesting to me to see the "same mind as it was in Christ Jesus," clothed in a different coat, in different parts of the world — my Madre at Rome, whose mind was dressed in black & white nun's robes even more than her body — & the Evangelical American here, Mrs. Hill, my true missionary, are so alike — & both I see, are always listening for the voice of God, looking for His will.[8]

On April 30, Florence noted in her diary Mrs. Hill's account of how she began her missionary life. "It was always God who made the initiative never she ... Let God show the way by the circumstances."[9] On May 12, 1850, her 30th birthday, Florence took her spiritual vow of obedience and chastity, like many mystics, and wrote in her diary: "Today I am 30 — the age Christ began his Mission. Now no more childish things, no more vain things, no more love, no more marriage. Now, Lord let me only think of Thy will, what Thou willest me to do. O, Lord, Thy will, Thy will."[10]

A week later, her diary entry reflected her clearer understanding of the mystic's path when she wrote that the privilege of knowing the Hills had turned her to "the will of God — to show me what was the true end of my life — not to be useful nor to accomplish this or that mission, but to find out as they do, what is the will of God for me."[11]

Florence and the Bracebridges left Athens in mid-June, making their way across Europe via Trieste, Vienna, Prague, Berlin, and Hamburg. Her mood rose and fell with the turning of the carriage wheels, reflecting the mystic's process of developing the character, discipline, and capacity required to sustain an increasingly high level of mental intensity and expanding consciousness — a process that is necessary to achieve each step upward toward Divine Union.

Now that she had fully learned to open herself to God's will after years of struggle, one of her most ardent wishes was about to be fulfilled. In Berlin on July 11, Mrs. Bracebridge made arrangements for Florence to visit Kaiserswerth, the German training school for nurses that she had been hoping to attend for several years. True to her pattern, Florence also visited different charitable institutions in Berlin and Hamburg.

While in Hamburg, Florence met with her former suitor, Richard Monckton Milnes, who was on his way to Marienbad. Although her refusal of his marriage proposal the year before had been difficult for both of them, their meeting now had a graceful symmetry: Florence, about to embark on her spiritual mission to Kaiserswerth, meeting once more in friendship with the man she'd had to deny for her life's work. There is only a short entry in her diary, reflecting their visit to a boy's school: "Well satisfied with our lark — & Richard was himself again."[12]

First visit to Kaiserswerth

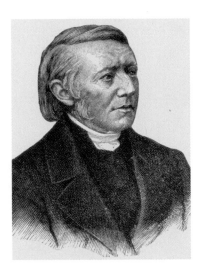

Pastor Theodor Fliedner, founder of the Institution of Deaconesses at Kaiserswerth in Düsseldorf, which Florence first visited in 1850

Florence arrived at Kaiserswerth on July 31, 1850, and was shown around the next morning by Pastor Theodor Fliedner, the founder. During her 2-week stay, she received an overview of all the operations of the Protestant institute, which served 100 patients and had 116 deaconesses, 67 of whom had been placed in hospitals, parishes, and poorhouses after completing their nurses' training. Upon leaving Kaiserswerth on August 13, Florence wrote that she felt "so brave as if nothing could ever vex me again."[13]

In a farewell note to Fliedner's eldest daughter, Luise, she quoted from an Arabic proverb:

> *Four things, O God, I have to offer Thee, which Thou hast not in all Thy treasury: my Nothingness, my sad Necessity, my fatal Sin and earnest Penitence. Receive these gifts and take the giver hence Florence Nightingale, who, with an overflowing heart, will always think of the kindness of all her friends at dear Kaiserswerth. I was a stranger and ye took me in. Kaiserswerth August 13, 1850.[14]*

Before Florence left Kaiserswerth, Fliedner asked her if she would write an informational piece on the institute and she agreed on the condition that she remain anonymous. (Both she and the Bracebridges wished to keep the visit to Kaiserswerth a secret from her family.) Florence wrote the 32-page pamphlet, her first literary work, in 5 days; after Mr. Bracebridge edited it, she sent a copy to Fliedner on August 19, 1850. In the pamphlet, entitled *The Institution of Kaiserswerth on the Rhine for the Practical Training of Deaconesses under the Direction of the Rev. Pastor Fliedner, Embracing the Support and Care of a Hospital, Infant and Industrial Schools, and a Female Penitentiary*, Florence presented the basic information requested by Fliedner but, more important, she forcefully addressed the misconception that had long stifled the development of nursing in England — the idea that nursing was a Roman Catholic institution and that nurses were therefore dangerous because of their proselytizing tendencies and ultimate loyalty to Rome.

In a definitive, scholarly passage, she traced the roots of nursing to the "very first times of Christianity... for the employment of women's powers directly in the service of God." She pointed out that the office of "deaconess," or nurse, had existed along with "deacon" in the early church. The importance of deaconesses "had been recognized by all divisions of Christians; and they accordingly existed, *free from vows or cloistered cells ...* long previous to the establishment of the Order of Sisters of Mercy in 1633."[15]

The Kaiserswerth pamphlet, which she had printed anonymously in 1851, remains a hidden gem in the literature of the women's movement — a self-dialogue in which Florence was working out the larger issue of her own liberation as a woman. If nursing was appropriate in a Protestant context, "free from vows or cloistered cells," a logical next step would be for a "handmaid of the Lord" to have a professional career in a secular institution. This specifically applied to "unmarried women and widows."

Florence's intuition was leading her to the awareness that the main obstacle to nursing progress in England was not only the issue of training, but also that of administration — that nursing must be freed from the political tangle between government and the Anglican church, in which nursing itself wasn't the main priority but subsidiary to other agendas. Florence Nightingale alone was beginning to understand that for nursing to flourish as a spiritual vocation in England, it must be separated from religion.

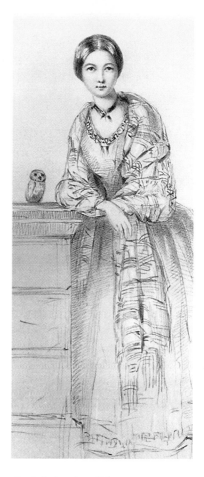

Parthe's drawing of Florence with her pet owl, Athena, c. 1850, the first drawing in which she is looking squarely at the viewer and the world, eyebrows arched, her steel grey eyes fixed on the prize ahead

Return to a world unchanged

Florence arrived home on August 21, 1850. In spite of feeling "so brave" upon leaving Kaiserswerth, she now felt herself in need of every bit of her discipline and resolve. Her secret visit to the nursing institution had somehow been revealed to her family, triggering Fanny's anger and Parthe's fears. The next months passed for Florence in an agony of family routine: carriage rides with her father; an endless stream of visitors, parties, and dinners; and constant companionship to the fragile Parthe, whose health had deteriorated as her anxiety increased during her sister's absence.

Among her family duties were some welcome respites — visits to her darling "old people," with whom she felt the deep sympathy she craved and where she could collect her thoughts. In October, she and Aunt Mai went to stay with 88-year-old Aunt Evans, whose housekeeper had gone away for a rest. They then went to Tapton to nurse Grandmother Shore but there received word that cousin Henry Nicholson had drowned while traveling in Spain. Florence was asked to go to London with Aunt Anne and Marianne to gather Henry's things. Florence alone saw Henry's death in a different light from the others, as part of a greater plan — to her, his life on earth had been only a stopping place on the road to a higher spiritual destination.

Watching the family assemble in their grief and being drawn into endless discussions on such trivial matters as the proper evening dress for mourning had a suffocating effect on Florence, dispelling the hope and clarity she had experienced at Athens and Kaiserswerth. She once again despaired of ever breaking free from her family's hold.

As the winter wore on, she became even more introspective. One of her few escapes was being allowed to teach at an adult evening school for factory girls, which she considered "the most satisfactory thing" she had ever done. However, Parthe, alarmed by yet another threat to her ordered existence, became hysterical. Fanny asked Florence to abstain "from doing anything" that Parthe disliked for 6 months and "to give up that time entirely to her."[16] With W.E.N. remaining indifferent, the tension in the household became unbearable for Florence. On December 30, 1850, she wrote:

> I have no desire but to die. There is not a night that I do not lie down in my bed, wishing that I may leave it no more. Unconsciousness is all that I desire. I remain in bed as late as I can, for what have I to wake for? I am perishing for want of food — & what prospect have I of better? While I am in this position, I can expect nothing else. Therefore I spend my days in dreams of other situations which will afford me food … for how many long years I have watched that drawing room clock & thought it never would reach the ten & 20 or so more years to do this. It is not the misery, the unhappiness that I feel so insupportable, but to feel this habit, this disease gaining power upon me — & no hope, no help. This is the sting of death.[17]

As was her custom, she turned to self-dialogue and exhaustively wrote out her innermost thoughts, an action that served not only as a therapy but as a means of analyzing her complex problem, considering options, and distilling strategies to escape the labyrinth of custom and sexism that oppressed her. In analyzing her father, she may have been overly critical, but she was describing the life that she feared for herself:

> My father is a man who has never known what struggle is … Effleurez, n'appuyez pas [touch lightly, do not dwell on them] has been not the rule but the habit of his life, liberal by instinct, not by reflection. But not happy, why not? He has not enough to do — he has not enough to fill his faculties — when I see him eating his breakfast as if the destinies of a nation depended upon his getting done, carrying his plate about the room, delighting in being in a hurry, pretending to himself week after week that he is going to Buxton or else where in order to be in legitimate haste, I say to myself how happy that man would be with a factory under his superintendence — with interest of 2 or 300 men to look after.[18]

In the same private note she described her mother:

> My mother … has the Genius of Order, to make a place, to organize a parish, to form Society. She has obtained by her own exertion the best society in England — she goes into a school & can put this little thing right which is wrong — she has a genius for doing all she wants to do & has never felt the absence of power. She is not happy. She has too much fatigue & too much anxiety — anxiety about Papa, about Parthe's health, my duties, about the Servants, the parish

... when I feel her disappointment in me, it is as if I was becoming insane. When she has organized the nicest Society in England for us & I cannot take it as she wishes.[19]

And on Parthe:

She wants no other religion, no other occupation, no other training than what she has — she is in her unison with her age, her position, her country. She has never had a difficulty, except with me — she is a child playing in God's garden and delights in the happiness of all his works, knowing nothing of human life except the English drawing-room, nothing of struggle in her own unselfish nature — nothing of want of power in her own Element. And I, what a murderer I am to disturb this happiness.[20]

Florence continued with a summary of her own dilemma:

What am I that I am not in harmony with all this, that their life is not good enough for me? Oh God, what am I? The thoughts & feelings that I have now I can remember since I was 6 years old. It was not I that made them. Oh God, how did they come? Are they the natural cross of my father and mother? What are they? A profession, a trade, a necessary occupation, something to fill & employ all my faculties, I have always felt essential to me, I have always longed for, consciously or not ... The first thought I can remember & the last was nursing work & in the absence of this, education work, but more the education of the bad than of the young.

But for this, I have had no education myself — & when I began to try, I was disgusted with my utter impotence. I made no improvement ... This nobody could understand. You teach better than other people, was the desperate answer always made me — they had never wanted instruction, why should I? The only help I ever got was a week with my Madre at Rome, which I made use of directly & taught my girls at Holloway [village near Lea Hurst] always on that foundation & my fortnight at Kaiserswerth. Still education I know is not my genius — tho' I could do it if I was taught, because it is my duty here.

But why, oh my God, cannot I be satisfied with the life which satisfies so many people? I am told that the conversations of all these good clever men ought to be enough for me — why am I

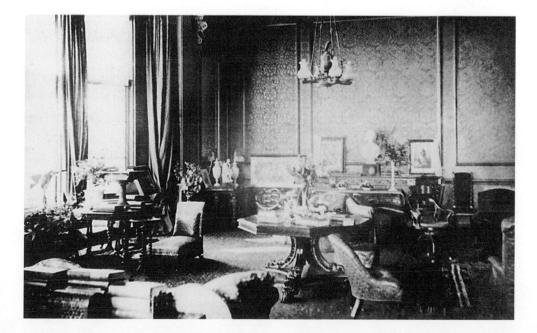

The drawing room at Embley, where Florence spent long social hours marking the slow passage of time on the mantel clock

RETURN TO A WORLD UNCHANGED

71

starving, desperate, diseased upon it? … My God, what am I to do? teach me, tell me, I cannot
go on any longer waiting till my situation sh'd change … [21]

Then, just as she had done on the Nile and in Athens, she listened to her Divine
inner voice and mapped her own plan for a way out:

All that you want, will come — in one stage or another you (& all the rest of God's creatures)
will have all food, all training, all occupation necessary to make you one with God. You have
already learnt something; with this certainty, cannot you wait? …You say yourself, "what do
they know who have never suffered?" Had you not rather have had all your experience than
not? … Remember that you know what is the real object of life better than you did, better than
many who have not suffered and, if you like, sinned. Remember that you believe in God, that
all will become one with Him.[22]

Elizabeth Blackwell's example

Early in the winter of 1851, a role model and catalyst appeared on the scene. Through
the Bracebridges, Florence met Dr. Elizabeth Blackwell, who had achieved a great breakthrough in becoming the first woman doctor in the United States. Blackwell was a year
younger than Florence, and their meeting began an amicable relationship that would
last until their deaths in the same year, 1910. They shared similar philosophical, political, and reform ideas and were a source of moral support and inspiration for each other.
Both were destined to change the course of modern medicine and nursing — especially
for women — although neither could then have conceived the impact of their eventual
contributions.

Despite differences in class and social position, common threads ran through both
women's lives. Both were shy yet headstrong as children and would overcome severe illness and physical hardship to realize their dreams. Both had mystical experiences and
would remain unmarried, wed to their work. Both had fathers who were independent
thinkers who provided an excellent classical education for their daughters. Both came
from families that were stalwarts for reform and the abolition of slavery and both would
travel extensively, gaining experience that shaped their future.

Blackwell's father, Samuel, was a successful and respected Bristol sugar merchant
who emigrated with his family to America in 1832, partly because he had become increasingly disenchanted with the limited educational and professional opportunities for
his children, especially his daughters. A disciple of the British abolitionist William Wilberforce, he had long wrestled with his conscience over his profession, whose single
commodity — sugar — depended on slavery in the British colonies.

Elizabeth Blackwell had supported herself as a teacher since the age of 17, when
her father died. Despite the hardships she had endured while living in the frontier towns
of Cincinnati and Louisville, she enjoyed one blessing that Florence could only wish
for — all her family had supported her on every inch of her journey with love, enthusiasm, and generosity. All of Blackwell's siblings became successful in their own right, and
they supported each other emotionally, intellectually, and financially.

By the summer of 1847, Blackwell had saved enough money to begin medical school. She first knocked on the doors of leading doctors in Philadelphia, then the seat of American medicine, but couldn't gain admission to a major medical school. Persistent and resourceful, she sent out applications to 12 "country schools" and finally was admitted to Geneva College of Medicine, a small school in upstate New York.

The faculty and staff were supportive and friendly, and the behavior of the 150 young male students during the 2 years Blackwell was with them was "admirable," she later wrote.[23] Between terms, she worked in a women's syphilitic ward in Philadelphia and saw firsthand the horrors that would propel her crusade for women's health. Medical school then was rudimentary by today's standards; she finished the 2-year term at Geneva and graduated with honors, obtaining her M.D. degree in January 1849.

Even with her medical degree in hand, Dr. Blackwell knew she needed far more training than could be found in the United States, where the medical establishment still viewed her as a curiosity. She went to Europe and found that only La Maternité, the state school for midwifery in Paris, would accept her for further studies. Here she pursued her training in obstetrics and surgery at an institution that cared for thousands of pregnant women each year.

In November 1849, her 5th month of study, while she was "syringing" the eye of a newborn for purulent ophthalmia, some of the water spurted into her own eye, result-

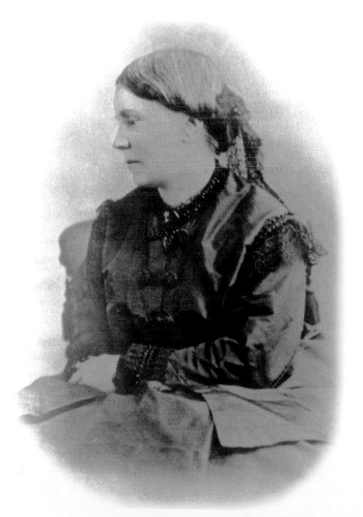

Elizabeth Blackwell (1821-1910), the first woman doctor to graduate in the United States, who became friends with Florence while studying in London in 1850-1851

ing in an infection.[24] Racked by pain and loss of vision in her left eye, she withdrew from her studies. Neither water cures nor time brought healing; in August 1850, her left eye was removed and she was fitted with a glass eye.

While recuperating, Blackwell happily received word that she had been fully admitted to St. Bartholomew's Hospital in London with the help of an English cousin who had written on her behalf to the famous dean, Dr. James Paget. She would study at St. Bartholomew's for a year, then begin a practice in New York City, where she later would be joined by her younger sister, Dr. Emily Blackwell, and Dr. Marie Zakrzewska. Together, they would open the New York Infirmary for Women and Children in 1857.

Fully recovered from her injury and undaunted, Blackwell moved to London in October 1850. It was here, in the winter of 1851, that her friendship with Florence flourished. Years later, she wrote in her autobiography:

> One of my most valued acquaintances was Miss Florence Nightingale, then a young lady at home, but chafing against the restrictions that crippled her active energies. Many an hour we spent by my fireside ... discussing the problems of the present and hopes of the future. To her, chiefly, I owed the awakening to the fact that sanitation is the supreme goal of medicine, its foundation and its crown.[25]

In the spring, Florence invited Blackwell to Embley, where the two shared their ideas about women and medicine. Florence spoke of the new role she envisioned for women — trained and educated nurses. Blackwell later recalled:

> As we walked on the lawn in front of the noble drawing-room she said, "Do you know what I always think when I look at that row of windows? I think how I should turn it into a hospital ward and just where I should place the beds!" She said she should be perfectly happy working with me, she should want no other husband.[26]

Blackwell's experiences and actions galvanized Florence. Now her notes began reflecting ideas and plans — the necessary practical steps to actually separate from her family, who were her prison. She finally realized that she had to free herself of the need for their approval because she would never receive it:

> ... I must place my intercourse with those three [her parents and sister] on a true footing ... I must expect no sympathy or help from them. I have so long craved for their sympathy that I can hardly reconcile myself to this. I have so long struggled to make myself understood ... insupportably fretted by not being understood (at this moment I feel it when I retrace these conversations in thought) that I must not even try to be understood ... Parthe says that I blow a trumpet — that it gives her indigestion — that also is true. Struggle must make a noise — and everything that I have to do that concerns my real being must be done with a struggle.[27]

Training at Kaiserswerth

Florence's parents eventually agreed to allow their daughter to spend 3 months at the Institution of Deaconesses at Kaiserswerth while Parthe and Fanny took the water cure at Carlsbad and traveled in Europe. However, they instructed her not to tell anyone lest any family members or friends should find out. The nurses' register at Kaiserswerth records that Florence entered the institution on July 6, 1851, and was discharged on October 7, 1851. At the age of 32, Florence donned the blue print deaconess dress and joined the German girls, most in their early twenties. On July 24, 1851, she wrote her curriculum vitae:

> My life was so wholly unpractical that I never did my own hair til I came here ... We always had company, from 10 to 15 people staying in the house in the country, and I was always expected to be in the drawing-room. Our society consisted of clever intellectual men, all very good society, that I allow they never talked gossip or foolishly. But they took up all our time ... I had always been in the habit of visiting the poor at home. But it was so unsatisfactory — for me to preach patience to them, when they saw me with what they thought every blessing (ah how little they knew) seemed to me such an impertinence and always checked me. I longed to live like them and with them and then I thought I could really help them. But to visit them in a carriage and give them money is so little like following Christ, who made Himself like His brethren.[28]

For Florence, Kaiserswerth was a home, where she connected body, mind, and soul. It was a smoothly managed institution with goals, rules, and an organizational structure — advanced for its day — that ensured quality care for very sick patients as well as rehabilitation for orphans, prostitutes, and others, teaching them the skills needed to lead a useful life.

During her 3 months at Kaiserswerth, Florence wrote over 100 pages of detailed notes about her activities and observations, a record that also reveals her profound

Institution of Deaconesses at Kaiserswerth, where Florence received her first training in nursing during a 3-month stay in 1851

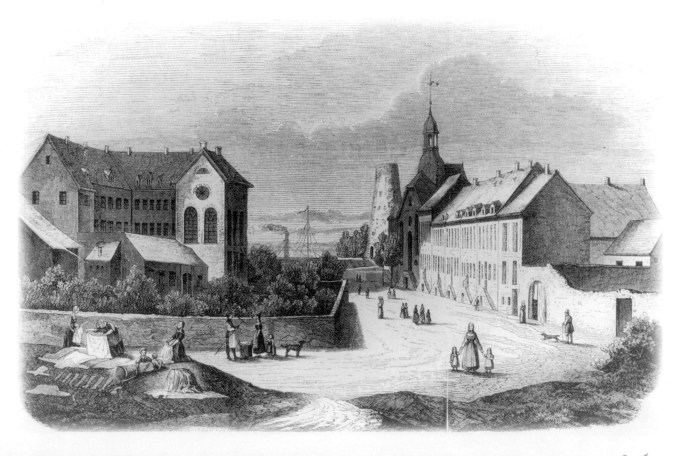

Orphanage at Kaiserswerth,
where Florence helped care for
and tutor the children

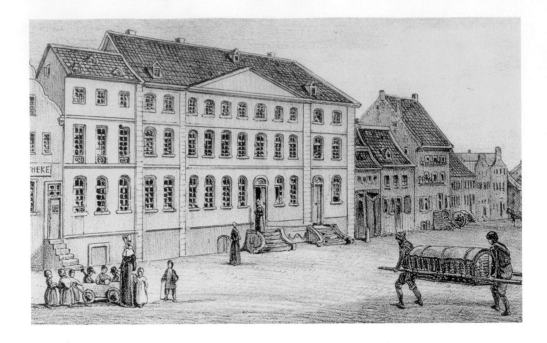

awareness of the sacredness of her work. She often recorded her bedside nursing activities at 15- to 30-minute intervals, describing the patients' physical changes in response to the illness, surgical procedures, and treatments as well as their emotional and spiritual responses. She cared for patients with major problems, observed numerous therapies, and assisted in surgical procedures that employed the newly discovered anesthetic, chloroform.

Consistent with the miasma theory, which remained the medical paradigm, the most frequently used therapies were fomentations, poultices, stupes, and leeches. Fomentations were hot, wet applications used to relieve pain or inflammation. Poultices were hot, moist masses of linseed, mustard, or soap and oil placed between two pieces of muslin and applied to the skin to relieve congestion or pain, to stimulate absorption of inflammatory products, and to act as a counterirritant. Stupes were hot, wet medicated cloths applied externally for various purposes, such as counterirritation or to stimulate circulation. Leeches were bloodsucking water worms used for centuries to induce bleeding, which was thought to cure various symptoms.

Florence's bedside notes reveal her astute observations and an impressive command of procedures, as seen in the following excerpts from July, August, and September 1851 (dates show the day first followed by the month and hour):

Thursday 31/7: 9-11   The two doctors arrived — room prepared for Meurer's amputation — leg taken off as high up as possible. Chloroform acted well. Dressing difficult — it was 10½ before I left the room ... A beautiful operation. Patient suffered much in the afternoon — cold water compresses every 5 minutes — one of us always with him

7-8 ... Patient quiet. Prayed with him — Catholic. What made the operation so difficult was the adhering of the skin to the flesh from disease, which prevented the surviving skin enough to foldover the wound which was draped with Collodium strips, but these not being enough, were taken off — & the wound sewed with three stitches — then the Collodium strips replaced —

& a Maltese cross bandage put on — Taking up of the arteries beautiful. Sawing of the bone momentary.

Saturday 2/8 ... The amputated man going on well — much with him — wet compresses every 10 min. He was never left alone — read with him.[31]

Tuesday 5/8: 10-6 ... Sat up with Meurer, a short night it seemed to me ... Meurer slept much, compressing every ¼ hour — Moved part of the night — Night watching is always pleasant ...

Thursday 7/8: ... Meurer, who had been going on perfectly well, began to be delirious — bleeding at the nose & then stupor — the 8th day doctor came 3 times to see him — bladder [cold pack] on the head — every hour renewed cold water compresses back of the neck & on temples, hands, chest & frequently washed — pulse 130

3-10 ... Sister Sophie & I putting leeches on his temple — [he is] occasionally audible.

Friday 8/8: 6-8 ... With Meurer — bleeding at the temple continues, held dry compresses strongly pressing upwards with my flat hands, upon the places ...

7 ... Extreme unction was administered — as he was too unconscious to communicate — the old priest prayed beautifully ...

9 ... Doctor came & checked & declares it typhus ... the tongue & teeth were black, every half hour 30 drops of ether on the head -- every 2 hours the ice bladder removed ... anxiety all along has been his symptom ... Chamomile tea compresses to the stump every hour... the stump was healing nicely. Strong [illegible] & acids every hour internally — & as much water as he could drink mixed with raspberry vinegar.

Saturday 9/8: ... Meurer still alive.

9 ... Doctor saw him & did not strip the stump.

10 ... He was just breathing & in a few minutes without any struggle he died.

1 ... The body removed with all possible precautions, chloride of lime & Vitriolic Acid fumigating the room, to the chamber of the dead where it was sprinkled with chloride of lime & no one allowed to go in.

Sunday 10/8: 1-2 ... The poor sisters of Meurer came, not knowing even of his amputation & wanted to see him. They had to be told first of the amputation, then that he was ill & that they could see not see him & lastly that he was dead. Sister Amelia told them & did it beautifully. The doctor would not let them see the body & they went away broken hearted.[29]

An eye for administration

The one indispensable model Florence required for her future career was a working knowledge of the most modern hospital management system of her day. The model at Kaiserswerth was one of centralized administration; the institute's superintendent was a woman with complete control of operations, who reported to one superior only (the pastor's wife). Florence recorded as much information as possible about this woman's responsibilities. Her pages of notes reveal her organizational mind absorbing every administrative detail pertaining to staff motivation, effective delegation of responsibility, meaningful controls, and measurable outcomes:

I. 3 times in the week she gives an account of the events of the house to the Pastoress & he [Pastor Fliedner] talks much with her… once a week she gives an account to the Pastor of the spiritual state of the sick & sends the "station sisters" to him to give an account of their sick.

II. All the sisters give her obedience — an account of their office & have to take her counsel thereupon — & to be appointed by her — which she however only does by guidance of the Pastor. Every sister may however take counsel with the Pastor on pastoring directly … [30]

Among the superintendent's primary responsibilities were welcoming new deaconesses, acquainting them with the rules of the house and their duties, seeing that they had the necessary clothes, registering new patients, coordinating the laundering of bed linens, consulting about and sometimes leading family prayers, making daily rounds with the surgeon, arranging for and keeping accounts of money spent on repairs, conducting visitors through the facility, and overseeing family visits. The superintendent also informed the Pastoress when any deaconess became ill and helped Pastor Fliedner correspond with sisters abroad. Finally, Florence concluded:

XX. She has to consider herself as the mother of the house who has at least the welfare of every member, & cares for it with zeal & love & power. She should help every sister find her heart, & seek the confidence of the [nurses in training] to make their abode in the house as pleasant as possible & make them love their chosen vocation & become capable of it.[31]

A change in the wind

After she returned to England from Kaiserswerth, Florence's self-dialogues contained a spirit of optimism, even a newfound brashness, as if deep inside she intuited the first ripples of a coming change in family attitudes. In early December 1851, she wrote this imaginary conversation with Fanny:

Why, my dear, you don't think that with my "talents" and my "European reputation" & my "beautiful letters and all that," I'm going to stay dangling about my mother's drawing room all my life — I shall go & look out for work, to be sure. You must look upon me as your son, your vagabond son, without his money. I shan't cost you near so much as a son would have done. I haven't cost you much yet — except my visits to Egypt and Rome. Remember I should have cost you a great deal more if I had married or been a son — Well, you must now consider me married or a son — You were willing to part with me to be married.[32]

At the beginning of 1852, Florence had an opportunity to put her Kaiserswerth training into practice on her father, a milestone that marked the onset of a slow change in his attitude toward her dream of a vocation. W.E.N. was having a variety of health problems, including a recurring eye inflammation and a serious bout of constipation. She accompanied him for a month's water cure at Umberslade, near Birmingham. The water cure, a state-of-the-art medical treatment at the time, consisted of six vigorous walks per day, baths and "can douches" (water poured out of cans), a healthy diet, recreation, and intellectual entertainment, such as reading the classics. Florence made a point of meeting with W.E.N.'s doctor and enlightening him about her father's case.

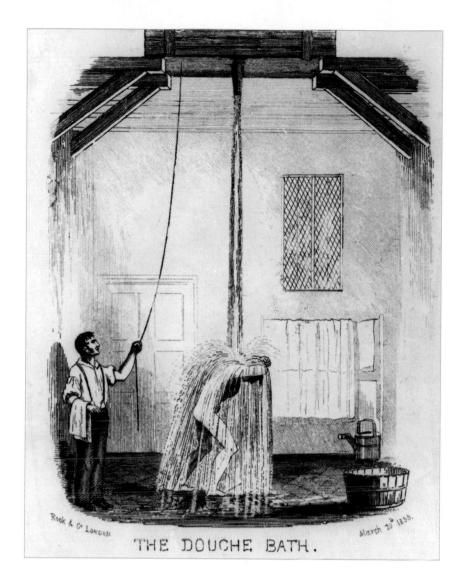

THE DOUCHE BATH.

Illustration of a man having a "douche bath" at Malvern spa, c. 1855. Florence's father took the popular "water cure" at Umberslade, another popular spa, in 1852.

W.E.N. was in excellent spirits; his health was improving and the amenities were pleasant. He and Florence were delighted to be staying in a beautiful old house designed by the famous architect Inigo Jones, and Florence wrote that "Papa's architectural feelings are so strong that he has no others & they keep him warm."[33] The food was sensible by today's standards: "Papa says capital mutton & potatoes, beautiful brown bread pudding & today a beautiful apple Charlotte."[34] W.E.N.'s doctor recommended brown bread and vegetables in abundance, and corrected an earlier prescription for quinine, which was prescribed for nearly everything. Although W.E.N.'s condition improved temporarily, he continued to have relapses, and a few months later Florence mentioned to Fanny: "I wonder whether Papa would try Homeopathy for his eyes."[35]

A note from W.E.N. to Fanny in his shorthand style reflected his easy-going manner and the beginnings of a new awareness about his younger daughter:

> *Well, we've no grievances — plenty of fires — good rooms, small party — attentive people ... Flo is a good right hand & is quite full of work & preparation. We have 3 hours of the Doctor in the house. apparently good man. he is very lavish of his time & conversation. full of small advice & common sense.*[36]

Suggestions for Thought & "Cassandra"

Florence was indeed very much "full of work and preparation." After leaving Umberslade in early February 1852, she spent most of late winter and spring with Aunt Mai, away from the tensions at Embley. Aunt Mai, who had the same interest in theology and philosophy as Florence and W.E.N., had recognized her niece's exceptional qualities early on and had frequently been an effective behind-the-scenes family mediator on her behalf. At this point, as Florence developed and refined her religious philosophy, she became even more influential as a companion and spiritual colleague.

Ever since her first Call at age 16, Florence had been examining spiritual and theological questions at length in her letters, journals, and notes. As she often did before a major transition in her life, she now sought to clarify her thoughts on the personal and national religious issues before her. In this effort, she generated piles of manuscript that she eventually had privately printed in a three-volume work entitled *Suggestions for Thought to the Searchers After Truth Among the Artizans of England,* which included her classic feminist essay, "Cassandra."

Her original impetus in beginning the work was her concern about the rising agnosticism and lack of spiritual values among skilled working people, or "artizans," across England. She was not the only person concerned about this; all the organized churches — Anglican, Protestant Dissenter, and Roman Catholic — were struggling to cope with a population that had doubled in the first half of the century from 9 million to 18 million people, most of whom lived in the cities and had no access to churches or chapels. Many educated and religious citizens feared that this alienation of the urban masses from church and religion, which was perceived as infidelity, would create political instability and threaten the nation's very existence. The census of 1851 made public knowledge what the clergy had known for 50 years:

> Between 1780 and 1860 a large number of Englishmen, whose families worked upon the land since families existed, moved into towns and cities ... So far as the churches or chapels possessed the allegiance of the working class of England and Wales, they lost that allegiance when the country labourer became a town labourer ... In the industrial city was no squire, no parson, no tradition, no community. Instead there was a proletariat ... The parish churches, the dissenting chapels, the Roman Catholic chapels, were not equipped to cope with this tide of immigrants. The churches and chapels were not unique. Nothing in the cities was equipped to cope.[37]

The underlying themes in Florence's *Suggestions* were that "mankind must discover the organization by which [it] can live in harmony with God's purpose" by seeking out the will of God and that "the world never makes much progress except by saviors."[38] Florence's definition of "savior" was one who saves from error — a concept she developed not only from Plato's "guardians" and Dugald Stewart's "enlightened conductors" but, more important, from the example of Christ. A law was nothing more than a thought of God; every human being had an inner divine nature that would be realized through an application of the laws of God. These applications extended to man's endeavors in the fields of government, legislation, institutions, and churches. Making

God's laws manifest would lead to perfection because human consciousness would become one with the consciousness of God.

Although she was profoundly critical of and disenchanted with the Church of England, Florence never seriously considered leaving it because it was her home; some of her most precious moments had been receiving communion when visiting Aunt Evans and Grandmother Shore. Her great frustration lay in the fact that the Anglican church gave her no work to do — it had no established nursing system like the Catholic church and had virtually abdicated its responsibility to the poor and the suffering. When Henry Manning, the Anglican archdeacon who had converted to Catholicism, asked why she didn't convert, she replied that she couldn't belong to the Catholic church which "insists peremptorily upon my believing what I cannot believe."[39]

Suggestions for Thought was in the mainstream of Western mystical writings in its cry for reform and true religious experience, and critical of the established church, which poorly served the spiritual needs of the lower classes. Florence, who didn't care to know a thing unless she could understand it thoroughly, resolved for herself in this exhaustive self-dialogue not only the theological, ethical, and social questions that her alienation from her class and the Church of England had provoked, but also the equally important issue of her liberation as a woman. The completion of *Suggestions for Thought* and her classic feminist essay, "Cassandra," marked a turning point in Florence's thinking about family, class, religion, and gender.

"Cassandra" took its title from a character in Greek mythology, the daughter of Hector and Hecuba, who was gifted with the power of prophecy. In this powerful essay, considered an early landmark of feminist thought, Florence argued for the liberation of upper-class Victorian daughters from the prison of the drawing room. She condemned society's insistence that privileged young women must spend their days in endless trivial occupations instead of being allowed to pursue meaningful vocations. "Why have women passion, intellect, moral activity — these three — and a place in society where no one of the three can be exercised?"[40]

She compared young women's idleness to a kind of mental and spiritual starvation. "To have no food for our heads, no food for our hearts ... is that nothing? ... One would think we had no heads or hearts, by the total indifference of the public towards them."[41] Florence saw clearly the fundamental problem between her and the family she loved; theirs wasn't just a generation gap, it was a century gap: "My people were like children playing on the shore of the eighteenth century. I was their hobby-horse, their plaything; and they drove me to and fro, dear souls! never weary of the play themselves, till I, who had grown to woman's estate and to the ideas of the nineteenth century, lay down exhausted, my mind closed to hope, my heart to strength."[42]

Illumination

Working away at her writing desk on the draft of *Suggestions,* her liberation theology, Florence broke through her final psychological barrier by virtue of her spiritual strength, her courage, and her genius. Her strength and peace of mind reflected the mystic's progress to the stage of illumination, the halfway point in the upward path

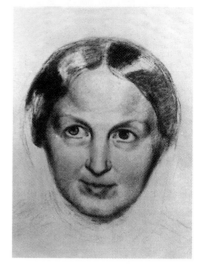

Florence's beloved Aunt Mai (1798-1889), who recognized her niece's exceptional talents early on and was instrumental in helping her finally break free of family constraints

toward the Unitive life (becoming one with the Divine Reality, or God). At this point, the Self is becoming more detached from "things of sense" and enjoys a sense of the Divine Presence but not true Union with it. In this state, the mystic draws strength and peace from a new level of consciousness.[43]

On May 7, 1852, Florence experienced another "voice," a conscious Call from God to be a "savior." On May 12, she wrote to her father:

> *I am glad to think that my youth is past, and rejoice that it can never, never return ... When I speak of the disappointed inexperience of youth, of course I accept that, not only as inevitable, but as the beautiful arrangement of Infinite Wisdom, which cannot create us gods, but which will not create us animals, and therefore wills mankind to create mankind by their own experience — a disposition of Perfect Goodness which no one can quarrel with. I shall be very ready to read you, when I come home, any of my "Works," in your own room before breakfast, if you have any desire to hear them.*[44]

Parthe's illness & breaking free

Florence's increasingly lengthy absences from home and her inexorable drift toward independence were having an adverse effect on her older sister. Parthe, self-absorbed and unable to fathom the cause of her own discontent, had worked herself into a nervous breakdown over Florence's increasing independence. She was sent for rest and observation to stay with family doctor and friend Sir James Clark at his home in Scotland.

In August 1852, Florence accompanied Dr. Fowler, of the Salisbury Hospital, and his wife to Ireland to attend the British Association meeting in Belfast and to visit hospitals in Dublin. Returning from Ireland in early September, Florence set off for the Clark home in Scotland at the family's request to accompany Parthe back to Embley. Sir James Clark was much more than a doctor and family friend — he was also Queen Victoria's personal doctor and a quiet advocate for sanitation reform.

The visit to Clark's house was a blessing in disguise: It marked the beginning of a personal and professional relationship between Florence and Clark in the cause of reform. Clark recognized in Florence the same talent for administration and political action at which he himself excelled. Their common ground would eventually grow to encompass the health of the British Army and public health in England. From this time on, Florence could count on his support and action.

In the near future, Florence would also benefit from Clark's direct access to Queen Victoria, a relationship that only few in the kingdom enjoyed. The Queen's Scottish residence, Balmoral Castle, was just 5 miles from Clark's home. In addition to his medical duties, Clark served the royal family as a trusted confidant on personal and professional matters.

However, it was Clark's medical opinion about Parthe that had the most immediate effect on Florence, acting as the springboard for her subsequent course of action to gain her independence. For years, family members and friends had gently hinted to W.E.N. and Fanny that Florence should be able to pursue her dream of finding a meaningful vocation. However, it was Clark's medical opinion that Florence's presence at

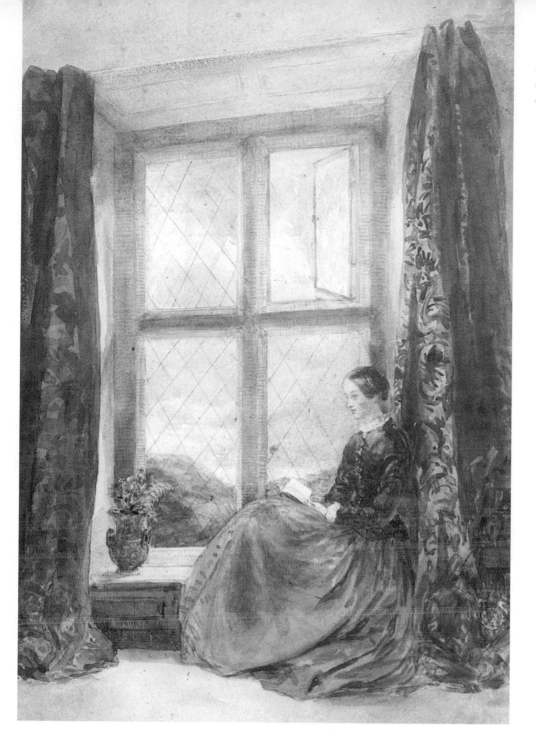

Florence reading at Lea Hurst c. 1852, in a watercolor by cousin Hilary

home aggravated Parthe's "monomania" (fixation) toward her that finally led Florence to realize that she could no longer wait for her family's support — that she herself must leave home to break this impasse in the family. After accompanying Parthe back to Lea Hurst, she wrote to Rev. Manning detailing her sister's condition:

> *… The opinion given is that imbecility or permanent aberration is the inevitable consequence, unless my sister is removed from home & placed under a firm & wise hand. My poor mother can be brought neither to see nor to understand. They go on ordering their winter clothes & arranging their autumn parties, as if this horrible fate were not hanging over them. They are like children playing … The medical men are decidedly of opinion that my presence at home aggravates the disease. I have therefore said that Sir James Clark having given this awful*

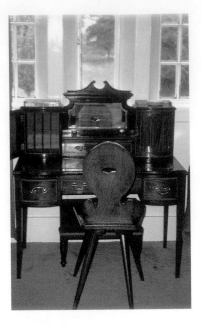

The writing desk and chair at Lea Hurst where Florence penned much of her Suggestions for Thought *in the early 1850s*

warning, I cannot think it right to take a part in a way of going on which he has said will have such consequences ... You asked me whether I had anticipated this [Parthe's breakdown]. Oh! for such long, long weary years have I been expecting it that it is almost a relief it has come at last ... Hardly any body has any idea of the true state of the case, excepting the medical men, for with the cunning of monomania, every thing is smooth ... Under these circumstances, I have but one course to pursue. No one will act but me ... I shall go ... to the duty nearest at hand — to nurse a sick aunt — & wait to see what I can find out to be God's work for me.[45]

After accompanying her father once again to Umberslade for a water cure, Florence returned to Derbyshire to nurse Aunt Evans during her final illness in the fall of 1852 and then went to Tapton to comfort the remaining sister, Grandmother Shore.

At the end of 1852, she wrote in her diary: "I have remodeled my whole religious belief from beginning to end. I have learned to know God. I have recast my social belief. Have them both ready written for use [early drafts of *Suggestions for Thought*], when my hour is come."[46]

Florence made another visit to Paris, where she stayed with Mary Clarke and Julius Mohl. There she visited major hospitals, met with influential doctors, collected hospital and nursing organizational reports, and tabulated this data for further reference. Once again, she made plans to study nursing with the Sisters of Charity — but this time her Grandmother Shore fell ill, and Florence returned home to nurse her. Throughout her life, Florence referred to the sacredness of being with loved ones while they were dying.

After Grandmother Shore died on March 25, 1853, W.E.N. wrote of Florence's last hours with her: "Great has been the occasion for her usefulness, great the comfort she has administered — her hands in hers till the last of her moments on earth. Judge of the sensation of Love in the mind of a dying sufferer."[47]

The compassionate, knowledgeable, and now professional care with which W.E.N. saw his daughter comfort his mother, and which he had also experienced in the two visits to Umberslade, changed something inside him that had long been ready. Florence's compassion for the sick, which had been so conspicuous throughout her life and had led her to the bedsides of innumerable relatives, friends, and villagers, was now about to move to a higher level. For, on the heels of Grandmother Shore's release from the world came Florence's opportunity for release from her own circumscribed world. Humanity beckoned, and Florence Nightingale was ready to heed the call.

Chapter 4

Harley Street

Should I be unable to effect the good which I have in view, I shall wish to feel at liberty to retire at the end of a twelvemonth.

— Florence Nightingale to Lady Charlotte Canning, April 29, 1853[1]

After the lingering illness and death of Grandmother Shore in the fall of 1852, Florence's father experienced a change of heart and mind regarding his younger daughter's role in the world. The veil of convention and habit lifted from his eyes after he witnessed Florence so efficient, helpful, and professional from her training at Kaiserswerth and such a spiritual comfort at the bedside of his dying mother.

His sister (Aunt Mai) and his brother-in-law (Uncle Sam) as well as other close friends had told him he ought to give Florence her freedom. He did so in a manner that counted — he agreed in 1853 to provide her with £500 a year (about £26,000 and US$43,000 in today's values[2]) to be paid quarterly in advance. Here at last was Florence's chance to move out of the family home and pursue her dreams. Because his wife and older daughter remained intractable on the subject of Florence's independence, W.E.N. advised her: "Better write to me at the Athenaeum [his private club] so as not to excite inquiry."[3] There was a similar open-mindedness, rare in English society, in the branch of the family that Florence was forbidden to see. Uncle Benjamin Smith had provided his eldest daughter, Barbara Leigh Smith (later Bodichon), an annuity of £300 on her 21st birthday 4 years earlier; like her cousin, she was at the beginning of her activist career.

Opportunity presents

One of Florence's friends, Lady Charlotte Canning, was on the governing committee of a charitable institution for sick gentlewomen on Chandos Street that was being reorganized. Lady Canning and Elizabeth Herbert suggested Florence for the position of Superintendent. Florence wrote to her friend Mary Clarke on April 8 describing the hospital: "It is a Sanatorium for sick governesses, managed by a Committee of fine ladies. But there are no surgeon-students nor improper patients there at all, which is, of course, a great recommendation in the eyes of the Proper."[4] Florence, in concert with the commit-

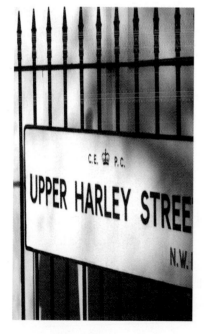

Street sign for Upper Harley Street in London, where the Institution for the Care of Sick Gentlewomen was located

Page 1   Page 2

tee, had looked at several sites for a new location. The existing building just off Cavendish Square was rundown and inadequate, and all had agreed upon her choice of No. 1
Upper Harley Street, only a few blocks away.

In keeping with the social protocols of the time, which dictated that a lady of
Florence's class could perform only charitable or philanthropic work, Florence was to
receive no salary as superintendent and would also be responsible for her own expenses
as well as those of the housekeeper (Mrs. Clarke) she would bring with her from home.

There was only one exception to this social convention. In the rigid class structure
of Victorian society, the only work that a lady of "gentle birth" could perform for pay
was that of governess, a woman entrusted with the care of children, usually in a private
household. In the hard economic times of the late 1830s and early 1840s, the number of
women seeking such positions had grown to the tens of thousands; yet in 1851, only
24,770 positions were available. The 1851 census had termed these unmarried ladies —
365,159 of them — "excess women."[5] Because of the huge surplus of "excess women"
throughout England, salaries remained at subsistence level for a job that often turned
out to be virtual slavery. One newspaper advertisement of the day gives an idea of the
duties expected of a governess:

> *Wanted, a young lady who has had advantages, for a situation as governess. To sleep in a room
> with three beds, for herself, four children, and a maid. To give the children their baths, dress
> them and be ready for breakfast at a quarter to eight. School 9-12 and half-past 2-4, with two
> hours' music lessons in addition. To spend the evenings in doing needlework for her mistress.*

Page 3

Page 4

To have the baby on her knee while teaching, and to put all the children to bed. Salary £10 a year and to pay her own washing.[6]

It was from thinly disguised workhouse conditions such as these that many of the physically and emotionally debilitated ladies came to the small, charitable institution for gentlewomen, their only haven.

In her formal letter of acceptance to Lady Canning on April 29, 1853, Florence looked ahead to what she wanted to accomplish in her first year. The thoughts she had been developing since her first attempt at nursing training in 1845 with Dr. Fowler at Salisbury Hospital had become clarified from her experience at Kaiserswerth and her observations of Catholic nursing orders and hospitals. She requested that the "Committee will take into their consideration on what terms volunteer Nursing Sisters shall be received into the Institution, should any such offer themselves."[7]

Before starting her new position, Florence returned to Paris in May to finish her nurses' training with the Sisters of Charity, which had been cut short by the death of Grandmother Shore. The sisters operated a hospital and an orphanage, and within a 10-minute walk were another children's hospital as well as a general hospital where she also could gain experience. However, her training was cut short once again when she contracted measles. Florence stayed in the home of the Mohls while recovering; Julius Mohl presciently wrote: "Her gentle manner covers such a depth and strength of mind and thought, that I am afraid of nothing for her, but that her health should fail her."[8]

Turning a vision into action

On August 12, 1853, Florence Nightingale, at last breaking free of her gender and class shackles at age 33, began her professional career as superintendent of the Institution for the Care of Sick Gentlewomen in Distressed Circumstances at No. 1 Upper Harley Street, London. It was the vocation for which she had been born. From her first day at Harley Street, Florence unleashed her original, clear, precise vision of how hospitals and institutions should be designed and managed to provide compassionate, patient-centered care in the most efficient manner possible. She led with the savvy and command of a born executive.

Florence's genius lay in her ability to create administrative systems through which her compassionate mission to carry out God's will could take shape. Her concept of management was all-encompassing. She was thrilled to be able to finally apply the ideas that swirled in her mind; she needed very little, if any, orientation. Since the age of 6, she had known that nursing was her vocation; since the age of 16, she had seen it as her Divine Call. Now all of the extensive self-education that had begun in her teens — the family nursing and cottage visiting where she had first trained herself; the observations and copious note-taking in hospitals and charitable institutions throughout the British Isles, Europe, and Egypt; the conversations with doctors and nursing Sisters whenever the opportunity presented itself; the endless reading; and the seed of Kaiserswerth — came together in her seamless, visionary design and plan for the hospital on Harley Street.

In this early stage of her nursing career, Florence was already exhibiting the superb organizational, intellectual, and administrative skills that enabled her to grasp the big picture of what needed to be done for these former governesses, many of whom were old and infirm or without work or family. Almost all of the problems that she would later encounter in her Crimean mission on a staggeringly larger scale she worked out in this small, three-floor, 27-bed hospital.

The many letters, notes, and lists she wrote during this period reflect her in-depth knowledge of hospitals as well as her sense of humor, which was invaluable in dealing with the disparity between her intuitive vision and the world she sought to change. Her four quarterly reports to the governing committee of the institution reveal her understanding of the principles of sanitation and their commonsense application, her skills in managing day-to-day operations and containing costs, as well as her uncanny psychological and spiritual insights into the lives of her patients.

It was here, at Harley Street, that Florence Nightingale first implemented her innovative ideas about sickness, health, and healing — what she referred to as "the art and science of nursing" — which addressed such matters as the harmful effects of noise, and the importance of proper ventilation and warmth, adequate light, variety, taking food, bed and bedding, cleanliness of rooms and walls, personal cleanliness, advising patients, observation of the sick, and much more. These were the ideas that she would later apply in the Crimean War and expound in her ground-breaking book, *Notes on Nursing,* in 1860.

First weeks on the job

Florence's first item of business was to redesign the physical plant and architectural layout so that nurses would be able to focus on caring for the patients rather than wasting time and footsteps in needless activity. She had inherited a talent for creating architectural plans and drawings from her father; as a child and young girl, she was at his side as he designed Lea Hurst, planned the remodeling of Embley, and designed the huge carriage in which they had toured Europe. Harley Street was her first opportunity to integrate structural planning into her vision of modern health care.

Among her administrative abilities was an aptitude for what are now called time and motion studies as well as a total command of detail, whether it be plumbing, kitchen placement, communications, or use of a dumbwaiter (the windlass), as reflected in the following letter written to Lady Canning in June 1853:

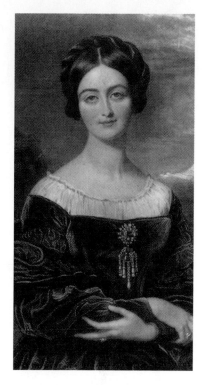

Lady Charlotte Canning (1817-1861), who recommended Florence for her first nursing position at the Institution for the Care of Sick Gentlewomen on Harley Street

> *The indispensable condition of a house for the purpose we require is 1st that the nurse should never be obliged to quit her "floor," except for her own dinner & supper, & her patients' dinner & supper — (& even the latter might be avoided by the windlass we have talked about).*
>
> *Without a system of this kind, the nurse is converted into a pair of legs for running up & down stairs. She ought to have hot & cold water upon her own floor, she ought to sleep upon her own floor — in her own bed-room, she ought to have the requisites for making poultices, barley water, warming all her medicines, dressings &c&c, (&, I should say, for making her patients' breakfasts & teas, & her own) so that she should never have occasion to leave the floor confided to her. Her bed-room & little kitchen (which may be one & the same) ... are therefore indispensably on the same floor as her patients. At Chandos St. & other places, where the nurses sleep all together on the ground floor, they might just as well sleep out of the house.*
>
> *2nd, the bells of the patients should all ring in the passage outside the nurse's own door, on that story, & should have a valve, which flies open when its bell rings, & remains open, in order that the nurse may see who has rung. If a nurse must go down into the kitchen for every thing, she has (if she has 3 patients,) 6 journies for their breakfasts, as many for everything they want &c, besides the waiting in the kitchen, because the cook cannot let her boil their eggs, or make their chocolate, or cut their bread & butter at that moment.*
>
> *Should it be impossible to spare one small room on each floor for the purpose mentioned, there ought to be one large room set apart on the 2nd floor, where everything for the nurses' use is ready & where all the nurses go to fetch what they want & to warm & to mess for their patients.*
>
> *The carrying of hot water all over the house is desirable. The cheapest way of doing it is, I believe, to have a boiler at the top of the house with a small fire to heat it (the boiler replenishing itself) & pipes bringing the hot water to each story ...*
>
> *Each nurse ought to have one or two Sub-nurses or Probationers [nurse-trainees] under her, according to the number of patients she has. Where the rooms are properly distributed & all the above precautions observed, I have seen one nurse & two probationers take the care of twelve patients (all in separate rooms), excepting in cases where a patient required a nurse to herself. But, if a nurse has one patient at the top of the house & another at the bottom, besides journeys to the kitchen & to her own bed-room, of course this is impossible ...[9]*

Florence closed this letter by suggesting that the committee might want to define the hospital's exact purpose and scope of treatment and decide whether it would also establish a training program for nurses, one of her chief objectives.

The early weeks at Harley Street were hectic; when Florence arrived for her first day on the job, the building was empty and little preparation or remodeling had been done. Not only had the committee been remiss in beginning the work outlined above, but it had also frustrated its new superintendent with its petty religious factionalism. Florence dashed off a note to her friend Mary Clarke ("Clarkey") Mohl that revealed both humor and exasperation:

> *My Committee refused me to take in Catholic patients — whereupon I wished them good-morning, unless I might take in Jews and their Rabbis to attend them. So now it is settled, and in print, that we are to take in all denominations whatever, and allow them to be visited by their respective priests and Muftis, provided I will receive (in any case whatsoever that is not of the Church of England) the obnoxious animal at the door, take him upstairs myself, remain while he is conferring with his patient, make myself responsible that he does not speak to, or look at, any one else, and bring him downstairs again in a noose, and out into the street. And to this I have agreed! And this is in print!*
>
> *Amen. From Committees, charity, and Schism — from the Church of England and all other deadly sin — from philanthropy and all the deceits of the Devil, Good Lord, deliver us.[10]*

In another letter to Clarkey, Florence reaffirmed her decision to leave home and live at Harley Street despite Fanny and Parthe's protests:

> *I have not taken this step, Clarkey dear, without years of anxious consideration. It is the result of the experience of years and of the fullest and deepest thought; it has not been done without advice, and it is a step, which, being the growth of so long, is not likely to be repented of or reconsidered. I mean the step of leaving them. I do not wish to talk about it — and this is the last time I ever shall do so, but as you ask me a plain question, Clarkey dear, I will give you a plain answer. I have talked matters over ("made a clean breast," as you express it) with Parthe, not once but thousands of times. Years and years have been spent in doing so. It has been, therefore, with the deepest consideration and with the fullest advice that I have taken the step of leaving home, and it is a fait accompli.[11]*

Because the committee had overspent its small budget, Florence had everything useable from Chandos Street brought to the new location. The condition of many of the items reflected the sad state of hospitals and the poor understanding of hygiene at the time. Florence's insistence on cleanliness reflected her exhaustive attention to theory-based procedures that were then considered state-of-the-art. In a straightforward report to the institution's governors, she described the situation facing her:

> *… On the removal of the Institution to Harley St., the linen & furniture were found to be in a most dirty & neglected condition. The table cloths, kitchen cloths, towels, &c, were ragged. There appeared no trace of any mending or darning having been made for many months. The sheets were good. Everything else was rat-eaten. The counterpanes [quilts] were ragged, & have all been since patched & darned. The towels, though nearly new, had large holes in them. The dusters & the kitchen-cloths were if possible, in a worse condition. The blinds were unfit for use, but have been applied to the purpose of lining chair covers. The furniture-covers were*

unwashed, & the color, in many cases, could hardly be distinguished for dirt ... Many nearly new blankets, mattresses & pillows were spoiled, even to rotting, by large stains ... Vermin ran about tame in all directions.[12]

In the midst of all the start-up difficulties, with patients already admitted and carpenters, plumbers, and other tradesmen working away, the always curious W.E.N. paid a visit to the lively scene and got a stiff dose of the realities of hospital reform in progress. Florence wrote on August 30 that her father "was almost suffocated with gas which went off with a series of partial explosions. Added to this we had 5 patients dying in the house, the foreman got drunk, and there was a fight between workmen in the drawing room."[13]

Yet after only a month, Florence was able to write to Lady Canning on September 13 a cheerful and informal progress report whose first words were about the patients, always her central focus: "Mrs. Parez bore the moving like a hero, & was decidedly the better for it! Now however she is failing, & sometimes, I think, cannot live through the night ... " She then went straight to personnel matters: "I have parted with the under-housemaid, & I have been obliged to give poor Nurse Bellamy warning, though I had no fault to find with her, farther than that she had nothing of a nurse but the name and the wages."[14]

An eye for detail

With an eye always on economy, cost, and proper accounting, Florence found no detail too small to comment upon:

Your [Lady Canning's] furniture from Mr. Fisher's has not yet all arrived. That which has come we like exceedingly. The curtains for the great ward are all made, & look very gay — but they are not yet all up, owing to 3 doz. of Gutta Percha rings being still wanting. I have been to the place in Bond St about them twice. They will not let us have them for less than 2/6 per doz. (but they say the price to other customers is 3/9) ... The arm chairs you ordered from Mr. Fisher's have been the delight of the Patients & are all in use.[15]

Replying to a question from Lady Canning about her personal feelings, Florence revealed the practicing mystic's characteristic self-denial and devotion to service:

With regard to my own share in the business, I have been so busy for the last fortnight that I really had never asked myself the question till your letter came. Now I ask myself, in obedience to your desire, how do I like it? And I can truly say that, as far as the Patients are concerned, my business is full of joy & consolation. They are much easier to manage than I expected, & they are always to be cheered, tho' not always cheerful. Indeed I think we are most fortunate in our Patients — & we are going to lose one on Thursday, who is going home to die, because Dr. Farre can do nothing for her, whose loss I shall regret as if it were my own sister.[16]

Although Florence's mother had forcefully resisted her younger daughter's decision to devote herself to nursing, she sent Florence flowers, food and game, old clothes, and other items that were put to good use at the hospital. Among these items were some books based on originals printed by William Caxton, who had established the first printing press in England in 1477. Florence's letter thanking her mother reveals her early awareness of the mind-body connection, her belief in treating the whole person, an almost unheard-of approach to patient care at this time: "[The] Caxtons are being read aloud in the common room at this moment ... only one of the patients can read aloud & she has only half a lung. The Cs. are much admired."[17] In encouraging her patients to read, Florence revealed an implicit understanding of the salutary effect that reading and other relaxing activities could have on a sick person. She would clearly articulate these values in her reports and correspondence over the next few years as well as in *Notes on Nursing* in the sections "Noise" and "Variety."

Quarterly reports & committee politics

Florence's four quarterly reports to the governing committee show that her talent for managing others for the purpose of delivering improved patient care was equal to her passion for bedside caregiving. She sought ways to improve working conditions, wages, and hours for nurses and made plans to develop formal training for them. She changed the medication purchasing system, the content of diets, and the physical design of the hospital kitchen. She began requiring accountability for all supplies. She revised individual task assignments and wrote job descriptions for all workers. She also rejected the inefficient and counterproductive practice of appointing hospital personnel based on their connections rather than on the skills they brought to the job.

First quarterly report

The first quarterly report, dated November 14, 1853, contained characteristically detailed reports of inventory and improvements, beginning with a description of everything that had been brought from Chandos Street and an itemized list of basic necessities. With an eye for economy and efficiency, Florence noted that old carpets recovered from Chandos Street were cleaned and "not a square inch remains unused."

She knew exactly the qualities she wanted in personnel and was never reluctant to hire and fire. When she found people with good attitudes, she was ready to patiently train them but never minced words on the reality of the situation: "The house has not now the advantage of efficient cleaning — the housemaids being two inexperienced girls, who, though willing and anxious to do all in their power, are unequal to their work without constant superintendence — and therefore more has fallen upon Mrs. Clarke [the housekeeper Florence had brought from home]." There were now three nurses on staff "with whom I am perfectly satisfied," one to each floor.

Her comments on shortages of kitchen and household implements unknowingly foreshadowed a time soon to come when a dearth of supplies would be a matter of life and death for British soldiers and would help rouse England to reform. For now, she merely noted that the "kitchen-utensils were deficient, no preserving-pan, no saucepan for steaming potatos, no dust-pan, no brushes, no brooms."

The report shows that Florence Nightingale, granddaughter of a successful banker on her father's side, completely changed the way purveying was done at Harley Street:

I have thought it, also, desirable to change some of the Trades people — it having been the cus-
tom, as may be seen by the books, to have in articles by the oz. & the half oz — the Grocer's
man frequently coming to the house as many as three times a day ... I now lay in groceries
monthly from Fortnum & Mason's, flour by the sack from Rymer's ... candles by the
4 doz lbs from Davie's ... thereby making the saving between wholesale & retail prices.

Florence didn't hesitate to use her own money to enhance the patients' comfort when she thought it appropriate. She concluded her first report with the observation that "Finding a little more light-reading desired by the patients, I take in the 'Times,' & subscribe to Mudie's [Britain's largest circulating library] for them, but not at the expence of the Institution."

In a postscript, she summarized the number of patients admitted in the first quarter (18), how many remained (13), and how many had been discharged (5):

Of these five, 1 considerably benefited (the Case being an incurable one), is now wishing to
return (Internal Tumour), 1 discharged as unfit for the Institution (Chronic Rheumatism),
1 benefited (Central Amaurosis), 1 completely cured by an Operation (Cancer of the breast),
1 completely cured by the prospect of New Zealand (Weakness) ...[18]

Although some committee members were threatened by the extensive changes their new superintendent was initiating or proposing, Florence, who had been around politics all her life, handled her opposition skillfully; she simply implemented the needed changes while creating the appearance that the ideas came from the governing board. A letter she wrote to her father after she had been at Harley Street for nearly 4 months reveals her talent for administrative politics, her ability to read people, and her enjoyment of the responsibilities of leadership:

You ask for my observations upon my Time of statesmanship. I have been so very busy that I
have scarcely made any Resume in my mind, but upon doing so now for your benefit, I per-
ceive ... when I entered into service here, I determined that, happen what would, I never would
intrigue among the com'tee. Now I perceive that I do all my business by intrigue. I propose in
private to A, B, or C the resolution I think A, B, or C most capable of carrying in Com'tee &
then leave it to them — & I always win.

I am now in the hey-day of my power. At the last Gen'l Com'tee, they proposed & carried
(without my knowing anything about it) a Resolution that I should have £50 per month to
spend for the House & wrote to the Treasurer to advance it me — whereupon I wrote to the
Treasurer to refuse it me. Ly [Lady] Cranworth, who was my greatest enemy, is now, I under-
stand, trumpeting my fame thro' London. and all because I have reduced their expenditure
from 1/10 (1s. 10d.) per head per day to 1/ (1s).

The opinions of others concerning you depends not at all, or very little, upon what you are
but upon what they are. Praise & blame are alike indifferent to me, as constituting an indica-
tion of what my-self is, tho' very precious as the indication of the other's feeling ... My popular-
ity is too great to last. At present I find my Com'tee only too easy to manage. But if they could
be so taken in by my predecessor?

She then went on to list a series of proposals that she had presented to the committee as having come from the "medical men" — including having the house surgeon dispense medications instead of the druggist (to save money) — and then shown to the "medical men" without telling them that the proposals had already been passed in committee.

> *It was a bold stroke, but success is said to make an insurrection into a revolution. The Medical Men have had two meetings upon them, & approved them all, nem. con. [unanimously] — & thought they were their own. And I came off with flying colours, no one suspecting my intrigue, which, of course, would ruin me, were it known, as there is as much jealously of the Com'tee of one another & of the Medical Men of one another, as ever Napoleon had of Wellington ... And so much for the earth-quakes in this little mole-hill of ours.[19]*

A letter written to Aunt Hannah Nicholson in January 1854 reflected the type of spiritual dialogue that the two women had shared for a decade:

> *Our vocation is a difficult one, as you, I am sure, know — & though there are many conso-lations & very high ones, the disappointments are so numerous that we require all our faith & trust. But that is enough. I have never repented nor looked back, not for one moment. And I begin the New Year with more true feeling of a happy New Year than ever I had in my life.[20]*

Second quarterly report

In her second quarterly report, dated February 20, 1854, Florence recorded details about patient admissions, fees paid, types of cases and outcomes of treatment, surgery, discharge information, and care of the dying. The report revealed her concern that many women with no serious health problems were using the hospital as a temporary refuge simple because they had no place else to go:

> *A Hospital is good for the seriously ill alone — otherwise it becomes a lodging-house where the nervous become more nervous, the foolish more foolish, the idle & selfish more selfish & idle. For two of the elements essential to a Hospital are want of occupation & directing the atten-tion to bodily health ... There is not a trick in the whole legerdemain of Hysteria which has not been played in this house.*
>
> *On Sundays & Thursdays, patients prepare themselves for the Ladies' Committee & the Medical Men — exactly as Roman Catholic women do for confession — by getting up a case. It is dull to be always saying the same thing. Therefore some patients leave off their flannels on Sunday in order to have a cough for Monday. I have known a patient, so hungry as to steal another patient's meal, who yet left all her own meals untasted (in order to prove her want of appetite) & ate them in the night ...*
>
> *Conclusion — that, if the Medical Certificate be not strictly enforced, this will become, not a Hospital for the Sick, but a Hospital for incompatible tempers & for hysterical fancies ...*

To prevent this, Florence proposed that the Ladies Committee restrict admission to seriously ill women or accept other cases "on approval" for a week or two and allow the doctors to determine whether medical care would benefit them; limit the hospital stay to 2 months; and help discharged patients find occupations.[21]

Third quarterly report

The third quarterly report, dated May 15, 1854, contained observations, comments, and conclusions that were similar to those in the first two reports but also included some interesting major administrative issues and patient situations, including one woman "cured of self-mismanagement":

> ... She came to us, having been confined to her bed for 3 years, & believing herself incapable of taking solid food or anything but Port Wine & cream. She left us, (in two months) restored to the use of her feet & senses, eating meat & taking long walks like other people. But this could only have been done by isolating her from other patients & all influences which would have strengthened her illusions. She was cured, almost without a grain of medicine ...

Florence realized that comfort and compassion were as important in healing as medical treatment. She wrote: "The benefits which this Institution ought to afford to the sick are perhaps best seen when we are enabled to give comfort in the time of danger & to lessen the agony of death ..." She informed the board that she intended to be present at all doctor's visits to patients in order to avoid having their directions misunderstood. To do otherwise would be "incompatible with the good order of the house & [her] duty to the Institution."

She also called the committee's attention to the fact that, because of a decline in the average number of patients in the preceding 2 months, she was having trouble maintaining her previous low expenses of about 1 shilling per patient per day. "The fact of the deficiency of Patients calls for immediate attention. Otherwise, this institution will degenerate into a luxurious piece of charity, not worth burthening [sic] the public with. The expenses now amount to £1500 pr an — the Receipts, including Subscriptions & Patients' Payments, to less than £1000 pr an." She added a final word on personnel matters: "I have changed one housemaid, on account of her love of dirt and inexperience, & one nurse, on account of her love of Opium & intimidation."[22]

Ready for the next challenge

As her year at Harley Street came to an end, Florence's primary goal of training nurses seemed improbable, and her friend Selina Bracebridge and others advised her to leave the hospital because she was wasting her talents. Florence concluded her final quarterly report, dated August 7, 1854, as follows:

> The year having now expired, for which I undertook the office of Sup^t of this Institution, the Ladies' Committee will naturally expect that I should give some notice to them of my views as to our success. I would wish therefore to express that I consider my work is now done, & that the Institution has been brought into as good a state as its capabilities admit.
>
> I have not effected anything toward the object of training nurses — my primary idea in devoting my life to Hospital work for, owing to the small number of applications, the committee have not been able to select, in all cases, proper objects for Medical & Surgical treatment — and accordingly the result has not been satisfactory to me. In every other respect, viz. as to good order, good nursing, moral influence & economy, the result has been to me most satisfactory.

I therefore wish, at the close of the year for which I promised my services, to intimate that, — having, as I believe, done the work as far as it can be done, — it is probable that I may retire, if, in pursuance of my design & the allegiance which I hold to it, I meet with a sphere which is more analogous to the formation of a Nursing School. I would wish to give a notice of three months, to be extended, if possible, to six months ...[23]

By now Florence Nightingale's reputation had spread throughout medical circles in London and beyond. Her friend Louisa Twining, daughter of the tea company family, began negotiations for Florence to become the new superintendent of nurses at the re-organized King's College Hospital, where Dr. William Bowman, the leading ophthalmic surgeon of the day, practiced. Florence had assisted Bowman in surgery while at Harley Street, and he was highly impressed with her abilities. He urged her to accept the position.

Florence was considering the move for the fall and had plans to enroll farmers' daughters into a nurse training program based on the Kaiserswerth model. She seemed poised to take the next step in her nursing career. Aunt Mai wrote to her: "If you will but be ready for *it*, something is getting ready for you, and you will be sure to turn up in time."[24]

At the forefront of medical science

As a nurse assisting with surgical procedures in which chloroform was used as an anesthetic — both at Kaiserswerth and Harley Street — Florence was participating in one of the greatest medical advances of the 19th century. Antiseptic surgery and conclusive evidence of the germ theory were still unknown. It was not until 1867 that Joseph Lister presented his landmark paper on antiseptic surgical procedures, and 1879 that Robert Koch's paper, "The Etiology of Traumatic Infectious Diseases," finally proved the germ theory of infection.

Chloroform: A salvation

The development of anesthesia for pain-free surgery and childbirth had been a slow, sporadic process. Although ether and nitrous oxide had been known before the turn of the century and chloroform had been discovered independently in the early 1830s in France, Germany, and the United States, there had been no systematic medical applications. Several factors contributed to the slow spread of knowledge: A unified medical profession didn't exist; there were no common or universally accepted procedures for scientific inquiry and validation; and the technical language hadn't developed the precision necessary to convey clear and unambiguous meaning to all readers. Finally, the personalities, politics, and social status of the players often far outweighed — for good or bad — their discoveries or theories.

Sir James Young Simpson (1811-1870), an obstetrician and surgeon, discovered the use of chloroform as a practical anesthetic in November 1847. Simpson was Professor of Midwifery at the University of Edinburgh and one of the towering medical figures of his time. In addition to obstetric and gynecologic topics, he wrote widely on pathology,

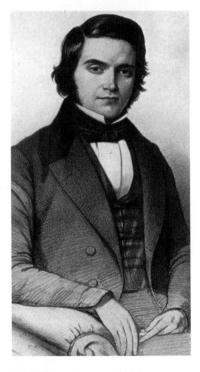

Dr. William Bowman (1816-1892), eminent ophthalmic surgeon, who recommended Florence for superintendent of nurses at King's College in London before the Crimean War intervened

homeopathy, mortality, and many other subjects. The first British doctor to support women in medicine, he would accept Dr. Emily Blackwell, Elizabeth's sister, as a pupil and assistant in 1854 and, in the early 1860s, Elizabeth Garrett, the first woman on the British Medical Registry, when the establishment had closed the medical college doors to women in the aftermath of Elizabeth Blackwell's success.

At a time when many doctors seemed to adhere to a stuffy orthodoxy, Simpson's boundless curiosity and concern for the well-being of his patients led him to explore any technique or procedure that would reduce pain and promote healing. Before using chloroform in surgery, he experimented for almost a year with ether, which a few forward-thinking surgeons had just begun to test. Simpson used ether successfully in childbirth throughout 1847 but became increasingly aware of its shortcomings. In an era of gaslights, candles, and coal fires, ether was dangerously flammable; it could cause vomiting and irritate the eyes and lungs; it had a noxious odor; and, in cases of prolonged labor, the sheer quantity of ether was a consideration due to lack of knowledge about appropriate dosages over long periods and the practical consideration of carrying heavy containers of the liquid up flights of stairs for home deliveries.

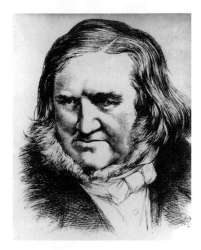

Dr. James Young Simpson (1811-1870), pioneer in the use of chloroform as an anesthetic in obstetric and gynecologic procedures

Undertaking his own research, Simpson personally inhaled the vapors from a wide variety of substances prepared by chemist friends until, on November 4, 1847, he found that chloroform worked amazingly well. Within 2 weeks, he had used it "with perfect success, in tooth-drawing, opening abscesses, for annulling the pain of dysmenorrhoea and of neuralgia ... and ... also in obstetric practice"[25] and had written a pamphlet extolling its advantages over ether. Chloroform, he said, required less chemical to achieve anesthesia, worked faster and lasted longer, was more pleasant for the patient, and was easier and safer to handle. The pamphlet sold 1,500 copies within 2 weeks.[26]

Over the next 5 years, Simpson received support from two other influential men: Dr. John Snow of London, who would soon prove that cholera was essentially a waterborne disease, and Dr. James Syme, the eminent Edinburgh surgeon. Both used chloroform in thousands of cases without a single fatality. They expanded on Simpson's work by emphasizing specific protocols for its use: The chloroform must be chemically pure, correctly stored, and correctly and consistently administered, and indicators for each patient must be carefully observed. Their published work, refinement of procedures, and statistical evidence provided a near-unassailable base for Simpson's broader arguments.

A third source of support was indispensable. On April 8, 1853, under Snow's supervision, Queen Victoria, in her eighth confinement, was anesthetized with "that blessed chloroform," gave birth painlessly, and proclaimed the experience "soothing, quieting & delightful beyond measure."[27] Despite opposition to the use of chloroform by the most conservative elements of the medical establishment, the royal example carried immense weight, and chloroform rapidly became the anesthetic of choice throughout Europe and America.

The use of chloroform, which Nightingale supported, made possible the development of modern surgical procedures, an advance that would require greater knowledge and training of nurses.

A deadly outbreak of cholera

Florence was in the thick of the action when the worst attack of cholera in the history of London broke out in late August 1854, not far from Harley Street. In 10 days, some 500 people in the neighborhood died of the disease; the mortality would have been even greater had it not been for the wholesale flight of the inhabitants. Within 6 days of the outbreak, three-fourths of the homeowners, lodgers, and tradesmen in the neighborhood had fled for their lives.

Florence took a temporary leave of absence from the Harley Street hospital on August 31 to take over as superintendent of cholera patients at Middlesex Hospital, on the north edge of Soho. A constant stream of cholera patients poured in, day and night.

> *The prostitutes come in perpetually — poor creatures staggering off their beat! It took worse hold of them than of any. One poor girl, loathsomely filthy, came in, and was dead in four hours. I held her in my arms and I heard her saying something. I bent down to hear. "Pray God, that you may never be in the despair I am in at this time." I said, "Oh, my girl, are you not now more merciful than the God you think you are going to? Yet the real God is far more merciful than any human creature ever was, or can ever imagine."*[28]

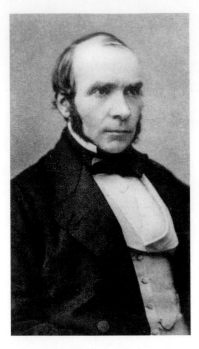

Dr. John Snow (1813-1858), renowned medical scientist who first linked cholera to contaminated water supplies

The same Dr. John Snow who had administered chloroform to Queen Victoria was assigned to investigate the cholera outbreak in Soho. Snow had been investigating the causes of cholera since the disease first broke out in the coal pits of Tyneside over two decades earlier. During the second epidemic in 1849, he had become certain that the disease was water-borne, but lacked convincing proof. The third wave of cholera that swept through England in 1854 produced a distribution pattern in London that provided Snow with the conclusive evidence he needed.

Snow determined that the acute Soho epidemic had broken out on August 31, the same day that Florence had gone to help at Middlesex Hospital. His inquiries in the neighborhood immediately led him to suspect the Broad Street water pump as the source of contamination. After obtaining a list of deaths in the area from the General Register Office, he found that 89 persons had died in the week ending September 2 and that "nearly all the deaths had taken place within a short distance of the pump."[29]

When Snow reported his findings to neighborhood officials on September 7, they asked him what could be done to stop the epidemic. He replied: "Take the handle off the Broad Street Pump."[30] The handle was removed the following morning, and the outbreak immediately began to subside. Snow's map of the outbreak, showing the location of the pump and the individual deaths nearby, wasn't the first of its kind but, because it provided decisive evidence of the water-borne nature of cholera, it became a classic in the field of medical cartography.

After the cholera onslaught subsided, Florence took a 2-week holiday at Lea Hurst, where one of the most popular authors of the day, Elizabeth Gaskell, was visiting. A writer of warm and humorous vignettes of village life and novels that reflected the plight of women, the workers, and the poor, Gaskell shared the same political and social views as Florence as well as an appreciation of the supernatural.

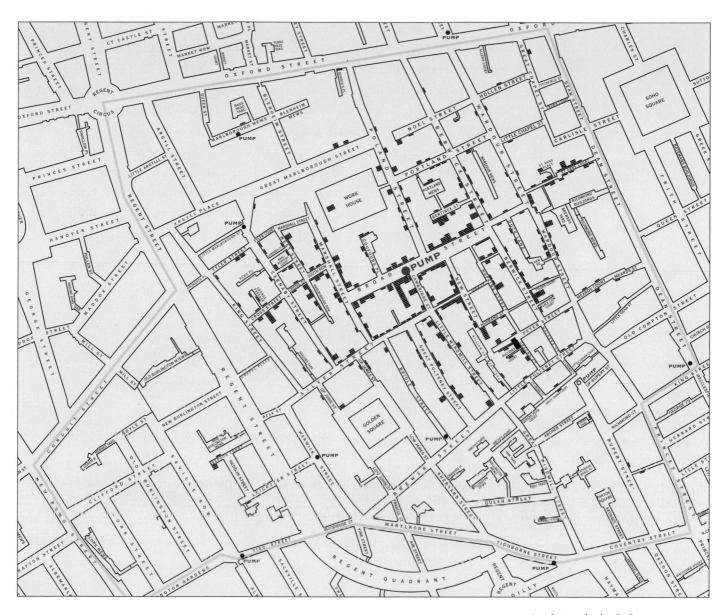

By plotting the deaths from cholera on this street map during the epidemic of 1854, Dr. John Snow linked the outbreak to the Broad Street pump (red dot in center of map) and ultimately helped establish that cholera was a water-borne disease.

Gaskell was impressed by Florence's single-minded sense of purpose and selflessness in ministering to the sick; she wrote that she had never seen such intellect in a woman and only twice among men. She was captivated by Florence's struggle to break free from the family and to obtain nursing training and secure a professional career:

> *Is it not like St. Elizabeth of Hungary? The effort of her family to interest her in other occupations by allowing her to travel, etc. — but the clinging to one object! ... She must be a creature of another race, so high and mighty and angelic, doing things by impulse or some divine inspiration — not by effort and struggle of will. But she seems almost too holy to be talked about as a mere wonder.*
>
> *Mrs. Nightingale says, with tears in her eyes (alluding to Andersen's Fairy Tales), that they are ducks, and have hatched a wild swan. She seems as completely led by God as Joan of Arc. I never heard of any one like her. It makes me feel the livingness of God more than ever to think how straight He is sending His Spirit down into her as into the prophets and saints of old.[31]*

While Florence was at Lea Hurst, the first British troops to fight a major war since Waterloo in 1815 had steamed across the Black Sea and disembarked on the beaches of the Crimean Peninsula. England, along with France and Turkey, had declared war on Russia the previous spring. News of the first battle success was quickly overshadowed by alarming reports of an ensuing debacle in caring for the sick and wounded. The country exploded in a fury of indignation and rage.

Florence returned to London, where her decision to become a superintendent of nurses gathered speed, but it would not be at King's College Hospital as Louisa Twining and Dr. Bowman were urging. As Aunt Mai had said, "Something is getting ready for you."[32] Among the British forces in the Crimea there were no women nurses, and there was only one woman in all of England fit for the task of leading such a group.

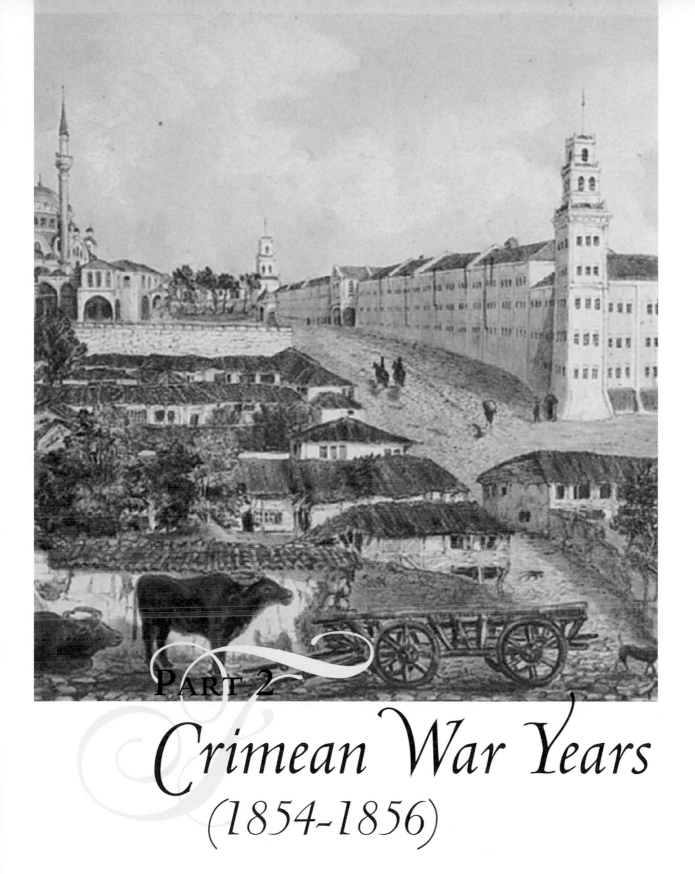

PART 2
Crimean War Years
(1854-1856)

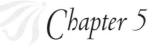

Chapter 5

Departure for the East

*T**here is but one person in England that I know of who would be capable of organizing and superintending such a scheme; and I have been several times on the point of asking you hypothetically if ... you would undertake to direct it.*

— *Sidney Herbert to Florence Nightingale, October 15, 1854*[1]

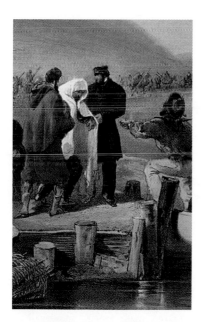

"Embarkation of the sick at Balaclava" (detail of painting on page 108)

The Crimean War, which catapulted Florence Nightingale to fame, was rooted in Czarist Russia's expansion southward toward the Mediterranean and the Middle East. Britain and France opposed this Russian drive in order to maintain the balance of power and to protect their spheres of influence in the area. English policy aimed to maintain naval control of the eastern Mediterranean and thereby protect the overland trade routes to India and other parts of the British Empire. By the 1850s, with the Turkish Ottoman empire in decline, Russia took renewed interest in Persia and neighboring European lands that formed its own back door — the western coast of the Black Sea and the lands of the Balkan peninsula. Aside from these geopolitical considerations, both France and Russia claimed rights of protection for Christians in the Holy Land. France claimed guardianship of Roman Catholics, while Russia stood for the Greek Orthodox church, of which the reigning Czar Nicholas I was *ex officio* head.

The flash point came in the summer of 1853 when Roman Catholic monks in Jerusalem attempted to place a silver star over the manger in the Church of the Nativity. Orthodox monks intervened, a fight broke out, and several Orthodox monks were killed. The Russians, furious at Turkish authorities for not keeping order, used the incident as a pretext to move troops into Wallachia. After futile negotiations, the Turks declared war on Russia in October 1853. On November 30, the Russian Black Sea fleet destroyed the Turkish naval force at Sinope harbor and massacred the sailors in the water, an act that inflamed European public opinion. With Turkey now defenseless on her Black Sea coast, the English and French demanded that the Russians withdraw from the Balkans. When they refused, France and Britain declared war at the end of March 1854.

Both countries immediately dispatched troops to Turkey and entered the war as allies of Turkey, primarily to block Russia from gaining control of the Bosporus and the

Dardanelles. In June 1854, the Russian troops, decimated by cholera, met stiff resistance from the Turks along the Danube and retreated homeward, thus ending the threat to Constantinople. The Allies then shifted their strategic attention to the Russian naval base at Sebastopol, on the Crimean peninsula.

The British were commanded by Lord Raglan, who had lost an arm at Waterloo (and for whom the "raglan sleeve" was named). Raglan had served as the Duke of Wellington's military secretary for 42 years and, upon Wellington's death, became Master General of the Ordnance, a bureaucratic position. He was an honorable gentleman who spoke perfect French, but at age 67, he had never even commanded a company. He was a bureaucrat, not a general.

Military operations on both sides were to be marked by great stubbornness and gallantry by the rank and file, but the British were hampered by Raglan's incompetence. Raglan wasn't the only problem. In the 40 years since Waterloo, the British army hadn't been involved in a major war. At a time when modern administrative practices were slowly developing in business and some areas of government, the army organization remained an outmoded bastion of aristocratic privilege. Organization was one area where Florence Nightingale would soon make a major contribution.

Seven different departments supported the army in the field, and administrative procedures were a hodge-podge of accumulated practice and overlapping duties. There was no system for organizing and transporting supplies; even adequate maps of the rugged Crimean terrain weren't available.

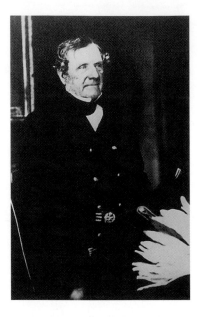

Lord Raglan (1788-1855), Commander-in-Chief of the British army during the Crimean War

RIGHT: *Routes taken by Florence Nightingale and British troops to Turkey and the Crimea (close-up of this map appears on page 106)*

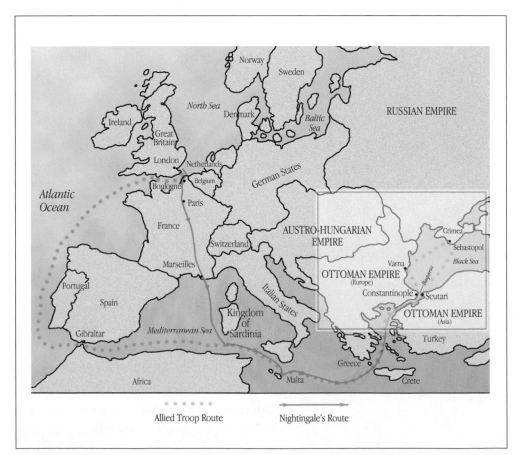

Allied Troop Route Nightingale's Route

DEPARTURE FOR THE EAST

The medical service suffered from the same problems as the other army departments and, like the civilian sector, from the slow advance of medical science in general. In February 1854, Dr. Andrew Smith, Director-General of the army's Medical Department in England, sent a team of three doctors to Varna, a small Bulgarian port on the Black Sea, to find suitable locations for hospitals and facilities for troops. They found that the existing buildings were infested with rodents and other vermin and that the nearby countryside was low and swampy, but their negative reports were virtually ignored by the government.

In June 1854, Dr. John Hall, a 42-year veteran of the army's Medical Department, was appointed Inspector-General of Hospitals for the Crimean campaign at age 63. Reassigned from Bombay, Hall stopped briefly in Constantinople, where he made preliminary recommendations on area hospitals before proceeding to the Crimea.

In early June, 27,000 British troops and some 25,000 French troops arrived at Varna. Most Turkish troops were camped farther north along the Danube river. The soldiers soon felt the effects of summer heat, poor sanitation, and the unhealthy, swampy location. Between June and August, 20% of the entire expeditionary force were hospitalized with cholera, diarrhea, dysentery, and other serious enteric disorders; nearly 1,000 lives were lost before a shot had been fired.[2] Over 600 British troops died in one night from cholera; the Russian army, decimated by the same disease, retreated and didn't attack the base at Varna.

To deter any further Russian aggression, the British and French decided they must remove the threat of the Russian naval base at Sebastopol. In early September, Allied troops, still weakened by cholera and other diseases, took 2 days to march the 10 miles from the encampment near Varna to the ships bound for the Crimea. Two weeks later, the fleet of 600 ships anchored at Calamita Bay, 35 miles north of Sebastopol. The French and Turkish troops made camp and unfurled their tents upon arriving at the beach; the British had only what each man could carry, but no tents. A wind-driven rainstorm lashed the exposed British troops the entire night. It was later calculated that the addition of only two more ships to the existing fleet would have provided all the supplies the British needed.

This was just part of the medical, competency, and logistical nightmare that was soon to face Florence Nightingale.

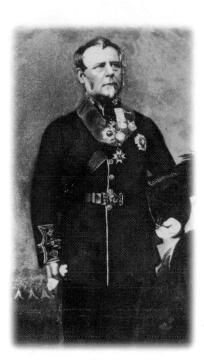

Dr. John Hall (1795-1866), Inspector-General of Hospitals and Nightingale's nemesis during the Crimean campaign

Crimean battles & Turkish hospitals

On September 20, 1854, the British and French routed the Russians at the Battle of the Alma river just above Sebastopol, but losses were heavy and compounded by sickness among troops who had fought with inadequate food, water, and supplies. The Allies failed to exploit their victory to take Sebastopol while the Russians were in disorganized retreat. Instead, they marched around Sebastopol, encamped outside the British supply port of Balaclava, and made preparations for a siege.

At dawn on October 25, a Russian force of 25,000 attacked the Allied positions around Balaclava but was driven off in separate engagements by Major-General Colin Campbell and his "thin red line" of the 93rd Highlanders and Sir James Scarlett's Heavy

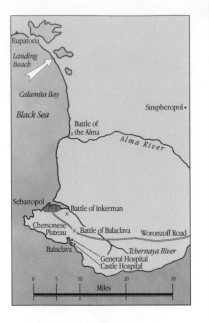

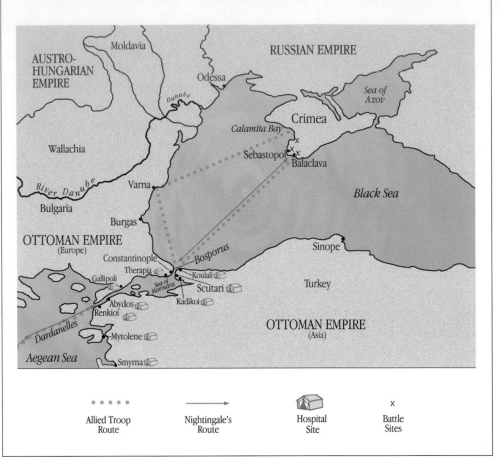

ABOVE: *Southwest portion of the Crimea, showing the locations of major battles*

RIGHT: *Important routes, hospitals, and battle sites during the Crimean War*

Cavalry Brigade. The low point of the day was the ill-fated Charge of the Light Brigade, a disaster later immortalized in Tennyson's poem of the same name. Because of an ambiguous order, Lord Cardigan foolishly led an unsupported cavalry charge of 670 men across a mile and a half of open ground in the face of enemy artillery and riflemen on three sides. Nearly 40% of Cardigan's force and almost 75% of the horses were quickly lost; swift action by French cavalrymen helped save the survivors in their retreat. Despite this infamous debacle, the Allies held the field and secured the British supply base at Balaclava, which left the Russians on the defensive for the remainder of the conflict.

The bloody battle of Inkerman followed on November 5, but the Allies managed to beat off this Russian attempt to lift the siege despite poor weather and even worse generalship. The battle followed by a day Florence Nightingale's arrival in Turkey, and she would lose no time in beginning to make a difference to the fighting men. On November 14, a severe hurricane sank the British supply ship *Prince,* laden with winter clothes, supplies, food, and ammunition, and severely damaged other ships in the harbor, producing additional material losses and a further test of Nightingale's ingenuity.

Balaclava, while secure, was hardly suitable for supplying a huge field army. The only supply road from this tiny port rose 600′ (183 m) up to the plateau above Sebastopol where the siege positions lay. Transporting supplies and casualties over this dirt track was difficult in good weather and nearly impossible in rain, sleet, and ice.

For the sick and wounded, the situation was a nightmare because they had to be carried by other soldiers on foot or transported down to the harbor strapped to mules or slung into ox-drawn Turkish carts. Then they were either lifted aboard steamships at wharfside or rowed out into the harbor in small boats to be lifted onto the ships. Here they waited days or weeks without any care, lying on the hard wooden deck or on straw pallets, surrounded by filth, until the ships were full and ready to sail. They then faced the ordeal of an exhausting voyage lasting 2 days to 1 week (depending on the weather and type of ship used) across the Black Sea to the Turkish hospitals with no medical or surgical care. On arrival at the dilapidated Scutari docks, they often had to lie for hours in pain, half-naked and in squalid conditions, before being unloaded once more into small boats, taken to the docks, and then assisted on foot, strapped to mules, or loaded in carts for the last agonizing journey to the military hospitals. The medical officers, doctors, and orderlies weren't trained to handle so many casualties and lacked medicines, bandages, surgical supplies, tables, and other hospital equipment. Even basic supplies for the soldiers, such as beds, tables, chairs, kitchen equipment, plates, cups, utensils, bath tubs, brushes, combs, and soap, weren't available.

When the Allied troops first arrived at Gallipoli in May 1854, the French, far more practiced in logistics from their land campaigns under Napoleon I and colonial wars in Algeria, had already settled into the choicest sites on the European side of the Bosporus near the Grand Bazaar. With no other space available, the British army moved its troops and hospitals to Scutari, directly across on the Asian side.

Lithograph by William Simpson of the ill-fated "Charge of the Light Brigade" at Balaclava, October 25, 1854

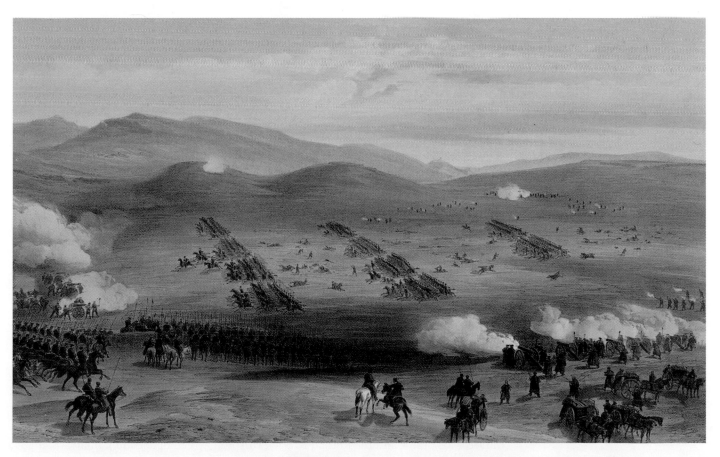

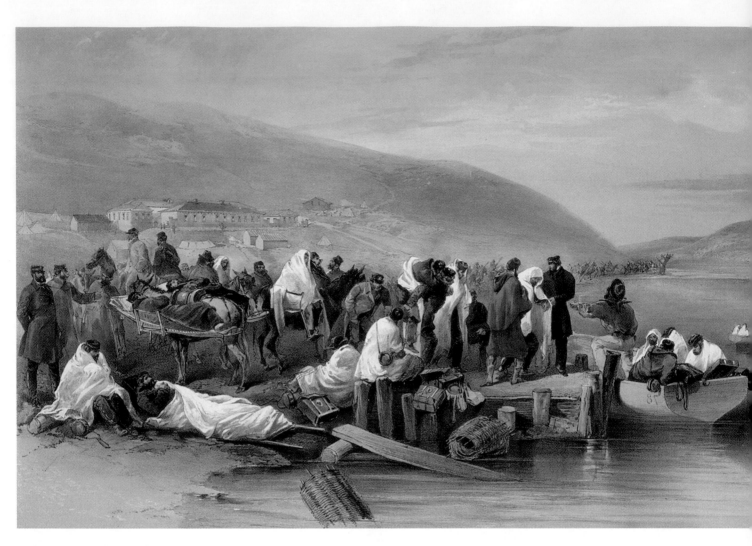

"Embarkation of the sick at Balaclava," William Simpson's lithograph of the wounded being evacuated to Scutari hospitals

The Turkish Hospital on the Asian shore of the Bosporus, loaned to the British army, was the first hospital established by the British during the war; it became known as the General Hospital. Originally designed as a hospital for 1,000 patients, it was in only fair condition and remained that way until the end of the war.

Situated a half-hour's walk from the General Hospital was the Selimiye Barracks, built between 1794 and 1799. After the Battle of the Alma, the Turkish authorities turned the Selimiye Barracks over to the British for use as a second large hospital, which became known as the Barrack Hospital. Dominating the high hill north of the General Hospital, this enormous, three-floor rectangular building was built around a huge interior courtyard for training and parades, with imposing square towers at each corner. During the Crimean War, the Barrack Hospital held an average of 2,000 patients in a space that was designed for 1,200. Off the long corridors were individual wards where more than 72 patients were placed in a space with the capacity for 30.[3]

South of the General Hospital was the officers' facility at Kadikoi, known as the Palace Hospital. This facility, which was part of the Sultan's Summer Palace, was occupied as a hospital until January 1855. Five miles north of Scutari on the Asian side of the Bosporus, were two hospitals at Koulali: the Koulali General Hospital, which opened in December 1854, and the Koulali Barrack Hospital, which opened in January 1855.

To relieve the pressure at Scutari, additional military hospitals run by a civilian medical staff were established in 1855 at Renkioi and Smyrna. There was also a naval hospital at Therapia as well as hospitals at Abydos, Gallipoli, and Varna, none of which had female nurses.

News reports & public outrage

In early October 1854, Dr. Hall had inspected the Barrack Hospital at Scutari before the wounded and sick arrived from the battles of Balaclava and Inkerman. He issued a perfunctory report claiming that preparations were satisfactory and passed the word to Lord Stratford de Redcliffe, the British ambassador at Constantinople. The ambassador, who rarely ventured outside his own diplomatic and social circles, took Hall's report at face value and sent it on to the Secretary at War, Sidney Herbert, in London.

An opposite picture soon reached the public. The scandalous treatment of the soldiers and the terrible incompetence of the army organization and general staff were exposed by the first modern war correspondent, William Howard Russell of the *Times*, who accompanied the troops to Turkey. He was ably assisted by Thomas Chenery, the diplomatic correspondent in Constantinople. Russell's descriptions of soldiers being left without medical care were to have a major impact on the war and the future course of the British army. Russell himself had been wounded in 1850 while covering a territorial dispute between Denmark and Prussia. Although the wound was slight, this experience left him acutely sensitive to the plight of the wounded and sick. A large and genial Irishman, he wrote from an outsider's perspective and forever demolished the idea of war as a gentleman's game.

The newspaper reports infuriated the British officers and doctors because they made them appear inept. However, their most important effect was in shaping public opinion. In previous wars, news had been circulated only by official dispatches, sometimes a month or more after the events described. The Crimean War was the first in which independent reporters, vigorously supported by their publishers, submitted critical first-person accounts of action in the field. Steam-driven printing presses and fast railroads allowed newspapers to reach a large public within hours of printing. The detailed coverage and immediacy of the news from the Crimea shattered the facade of a competent army high command and ignited a storm of outrage. Reformers at all levels seized the opportunity to initiate change.

Russell had seen evidence of military mismanagement at Malta and at Gallipoli before arriving in the Crimea in the spring of 1854. He privately reported to his editor in London:

> The management is infamous, and the contrast offered by our proceedings to the conduct of the French most painful. Could you believe it — the sick have not a bed to lie upon? They are landed and thrown into a ricketty house without a chair or table in it. The French with their ambulances, excellent commissariat staff ... in every respect are immeasurably our superiors.[4]

On October 12, three weeks after the Battle of the Alma, the *Times* carried the first of many horrifying reports about the conditions at the Barrack Hospital — this one by

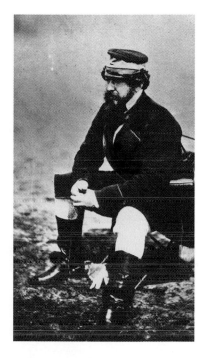

William Howard Russell of the Times, *the first modern war correspondent, whose reports from the front exposed the terrible conditions of the British soldiers*

Chenery, who echoed Russell's earlier observations. Chenery's account of the arrival of the wounded at Scutari was a far cry from Hall's confident report of a few days earlier:

> *It is with feelings of surprise and anger that the public will learn that no sufficient preparations have been made for the cure of the wounded. Not only are there not sufficient surgeons ... not only are there no dressers and nurses ... but ... there is not even linen to make bandages for the wounded ...*
>
> *Can it be said that the battle of Alma has been an event to take the world by surprise? Has not the expedition to the Crimea been the talk of the last four months? And when the Turks gave up to our use the vast barracks to form a hospital and depot, was it not on the ground that the loss of the English troops was sure to be considerable when engaged in so dangerous an enterprise? And yet, after the troops have been six months in the country, there is no preparation for the commonest surgical operation!*
>
> *Not only are men kept, in some cases for a week, without the hand of a medical man coming near their wounds; not only are they left to expire in agony, unheeded and shaken off, though catching desperately at the surgeon whenever he makes his rounds through the fetid ship; but now, when they are placed in the spacious building, where we are led to believe that everything was ready which could ease their pain or facilitate their recovery, it is found that the commonest appliances of a workhouse sick-ward are wanting, and that the men must die through the medical staff of the British Army having forgotten that old rags are necessary for the dressings of the wound. If Parliament were sitting, some notice would probably be taken of these facts, which are notorious and have excited much concern; as it is, it rests with the Government to make inquiries into the conduct of those who have so greatly neglected their duty.[5]*

The next day another Chenery dispatch spelled out the superiority of the French medical arrangements:

> *... The worn-out [British] pensioners who were brought as an ambulance corps are totally useless, and not only are surgeons not to be had, but there are no dressers or nurses to carry out the surgeon's directions, and to attend on the sick during the intervals between his visits. Here the French are greatly our superiors. Their arrangements are extremely good, their surgeons more numerous, and they have also the help of the Sisters of Charity, who have accompanied the expedition in incredible numbers [actually 50 were sent out]. Those devoted women are excellent nurses.[6]*

Nightingale summoned

Nightingale, who yearned for a larger mission in caring for the sick and suffering, was stirred by the newspaper reports from the front. Within 2 days of reading the articles in the *Times,* she was asked to lead a volunteer group to Scutari. Understanding political protocol, she contacted Dr. Andrew Smith, Director-General of the army's Medical Department; Lord Clarendon, the former Secretary of Foreign Affairs; Lord Palmerston, her friend and neighbor at Embley, now Home Secretary; and the Duke of Newcastle, the Secretary for War in Prime Minister Aberdeen's government.

She also wrote to her friend Elizabeth Herbert, wife of Sidney Herbert, about these plans. Because she was still under a contractual agreement at Harley Street, she asked

Mrs. Herbert to request that the Ladies' Committee release her for this mission. In her letter of October 14, 1854, she also asked for her feedback and assistance on several other matters:

> *My Dearest ... A small private expedition of nurses has been organized for Scutari, and I have been asked to command it. I take myself out and one nurse. Lady Maria Forester [a wealthy widow] has given £200 to take out three others. We feed and lodge ourselves there, and are to be no expense what ever to the country. Lord Clarendon has been asked by Lord Palmerston to write to Lord Stratford [British ambassador at Constantinople] for us, and has consented. Dr. Andrew Smith of the Army Medical Board, whom I have seen, authorized us, and gives us letters to the Chief Medical Officer at Scutari. I do not mean to say that I believe the Times accounts, but I do believe that we may be of use to the wounded wretches ...*
>
> *Now to business.*
>
> *(1) Unless my Ladies' Committee feel that this is a thing which appeals to the sympathies of all, and urge me, rather than barely consent, I cannot honorably break my engagement here. And I write to you as one of my mistresses.*
>
> *(2) What does Mr. Herbert say to the scheme itself? Does he think it will be objected to by the authorities? Would he give us any advice or letters of recommendation? And are there any stores for the Hospital he would advise us to take out? Dr. Smith says that nothing is needed ... We start on Tuesday if we go, to catch the Marseilles boat of the 21st for Constantinople, where I leave my nurses, thinking the medical Staff at Scutari will be more frightened than amused at being bombarded by a parcel of women, and I cross over to Scutari with some one from the Embassy to present my credentials from Dr. Smith, and put ourselves at the disposal of the Drs.*
>
> *(3) Would you or some one of my Committee write to Lady Stratford [wife of the British Ambassador at Constantinople] to say, 'This is not a lady but a real Hospital Nurse,' of me? 'And she has had experience ...'*[7]

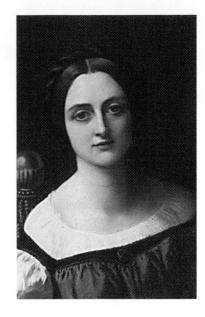

Elizabeth Herbert, wife of Sidney Herbert, who helped Florence prepare for her nursing mission to Turkey (detail of painting on page 61)

The next day, Nightingale wrote a similar letter to her friend Selina Bracebridge about her planned expedition. She indicated that Smith, who like many thought the war would be over in a matter of weeks, had told her that the party might be too late; it would be 3 weeks since the wounded arrived at Scutari and any soldiers with gangrene or hemorrhage would be either dead or well. Smith would support a small party of nurses initially, to be followed by another small group in 10 days. He was opposed to a larger party because he felt the troops might be moved from Scutari, and he couldn't envision a group of British women following the troops around as the Sisters of Charity followed the French troops.

Aware that a Kaiserswerth establishment existed at Constantinople, Nightingale wrote to them about housing. Her own housekeeper, Mrs. Clarke, volunteered to go with her, and Nightingale also considered taking a few more nurses from Harley Street.

The notion of using women nurses at English military hospitals had previously arisen on several occasions, but resistance to change had always scuttled the idea. In 1847, Sir Edward Parry, Captain-Superintendent of Haslar (naval) Hospital, had suggested a training program based on the Kaiserswerth model for nurses at his institution, but he was ignored.[8] At the outbreak of the Crimean War, officials at the War

Office had discussed using women nurses, but this idea was, in the words of an 1855 inquiry, "mooted at a very early stage (before, in fact, the army left this country), and the general opinion of military men was adverse to their employment."[9]

However, the huge public outcry that followed the reports in the *Times*, and the realization by officials that it was their "duty to remedy such a state of things,"[10] paved the way for Sidney Herbert's breakthrough initiative. The two remaining obstacles to such a plan were quickly overcome. First, the military men were mollified because the contingent of nurses would be assigned to a rear-area hospital, Scutari, and not to the battlefield. Second, the difficulty of finding "any lady who was competent to undertake so great a task"[11] was solved by Herbert's suggestion that Nightingale, an acquaintance of the Duke of Newcastle, should lead the party. The whole process was facilitated by the fact that Newcastle and Herbert were more than colleagues; they had been good friends since their days together at Oxford.

Sidney Herbert's letter

Mrs. Herbert didn't receive Nightingale's letter immediately because she and her husband had already left town for a weekend at Bournemouth on the English Channel. On October 15, 1854, a day after Nightingale wrote to Mrs. Herbert about her planned private expedition, Sidney Herbert wrote to Nightingale from Bournemouth, formally inviting her to go to Scutari and supervise a group of female nurses on behalf of the government. The two letters crossed in the mail; Herbert was apparently unaware that Lady Forester, whom he mentions, had already contacted Nightingale:

> *Dear Miss Nightingale,*
>
> *You will have seen in the papers that there is a great deficiency of nurses at the Hospital at Scutari. The other alleged deficiencies, namely of medical men, lint [bandages], sheets, etc., must, if they have really ever existed, have been remedied ere this, as the number of medical officers with the Army amounted to one to every 95 men in the whole force, being nearly double what we have ever had before, and 30 more surgeons went out 3 weeks ago, and would by this time, therefore, be at Constantinople. A further supply went on Thursday, and a fresh batch sail next week. As to medical stores, they have been sent out in profusion; lint by the ton weight, 15,000 pairs of sheets, medicine, wine, arrowroot in the same proportions; and the only way of accounting for the deficiency at Scutari, if it exists, is that the mass of stores went to Varna, and was not sent back when the army left for the Crimea; but four days would have remedied this. In the meanwhile fresh stores are arriving.*
>
> *But the deficiency of female nurses is undoubted, none but male nurses having ever been admitted to military hospitals. It would be impossible to carry about a large staff of female nurses with the army in the field. But at Scutari, having now a fixed hospital, no military reason exists against their introduction, and I am confident that they might be introduced with great benefit, for hospital orderlies must be very rough hands, and most of them, on such an occasion as this, very inexperienced ones. I receive numbers of offers from ladies to go out, but they are ladies who have no conception of what a hospital is, nor of the nature of its duties; and they would, when the time came, either recoil from the work or be entirely*

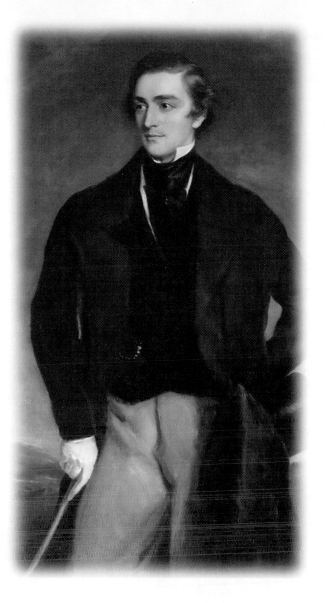

*useless, and consequently — what is worse — entirely in the way. Nor would these ladies
probably ever understand the necessity, especially in a military hospital, of strict obedience
to rule.*

*Lady Maria Forester (Lord Roden's daughter) has made some proposal to Dr. Smith, the
head of the Army Medical Department, either to go with or to send out trained nurses ...*

*But ... Lady M. Forester probably has not tested the willingness of the trained nurses to go,
and is incapable of directing or ruling them. There is but one person in England that I know of
who would be capable of organizing and superintending such a scheme; and I have been several times on the point of asking you hypothetically if, supposing the attempt were made, you
would undertake to direct it. The selection of the rank and file of nurses will be difficult; no one
knows it better than yourself. The difficulty of finding women equal to a task after all, full of
horrors, and requiring, besides knowledge and goodwill, great energy and great courage, will
be great. The task of ruling them and introducing system among them, great; and not the least
will be the difficulty of making the whole work smoothly with the medical and military authorities out there. This it is which makes it so important that the experiment should be carried out
by one with a capacity for administration and experience.*

My question simply is, Would you listen to the request to go and superintend the whole thing? You would of course have plenary authority over all the nurses, and I think I could secure you the fullest assistance and co-operation from the medical staff, and you would also have an unlimited power of drawing on the Government for whatever you thought requisite for the success of your mission ... I do not say one word to press you ... but I must not conceal from you that I think upon your decision will depend the ultimate success or failure of the plan. Your own personal qualities, your knowledge and your power of administration, and among greater things your rank and position in society give you advantages in such a work which no other person possesses.

If this succeeds, an enormous amount of good will be done now, and to persons deserving everything at our hands; and a prejudice will have been broken through, and a precedent established, which will multiply the good to all time ... I am certain the Bracebridges would go with you and give you all the comfort you would require ... I have written very long, for the subject is very near my heart. Liz [Mrs. Herbert] is writing to Mrs. Bracebridge to tell her what I am doing ...

There is one point which I have hardly a right to touch upon, but I know you will pardon me. If you were inclined to undertake this great work, would Mr. and Mrs. Nightingale give their consent? The work would be so national, and the request made to you proceeding from the Government who represent the nation comes at such a moment, that I do not despair of their consent. Deriving your authority from the Government, your position would secure the respect and consideration of every one, especially in a service where official rank carries so much weight. This would secure to you every attention and comfort on your way and there, together with a complete submission to your orders.

I know these things are a matter of indifference to you except so far as they may further the great objects you have in view; but they are of importance in themselves, and of every importance to those who have a right to take an interest in your personal position and comfort. I know you will come to a wise decision. God grant it may be in accordance with my hopes! Believe me, dear Miss Nightingale, ever yours, Sidney Herbert.[12]

Mrs. Herbert wrote Nightingale on the same day urging her to accept the challenge. Nightingale immediately accepted, becoming the Superintendent of the Female Nursing Establishment in the English General Military Hospitals in Turkey. However, in the haste of the moment (and because no one expected the war to last long), the hospitals at Scutari were the only ones specifically designated in her mission; the regimental hospitals in the Crimea weren't included in her official orders. Neither Mr. Herbert nor Nightingale noticed this flaw in wording, which set the stage for later problems when she tried to assert her authority in the hospitals in the Crimea, some 300 miles across the Black Sea from Scutari.

When Sidney Herbert officially met with Nightingale on October 16 to discuss plans for her departure, she said with confidence that she could be ready to leave in 5 days. Herbert agreed to send no more nurses to the East unless Nightingale asked for them. She felt the initial number of nurses shouldn't exceed 20; Herbert, however, pushed for 40. In the end, only 38 could be found who satisfied the minimum qualifications. It's important to remember that this venture was without precedent. Never before had female nurses been used in British military hospitals, which argued for keeping the contingent small.

Controversy over Catholic nuns

On October 17, the Herberts' town house at 49 Belgrave Square, London, became the headquarters for the nurse selection committee members — Nightingale, Mrs. Brace-bridge, Mrs. Herbert, and Mary Stanley (whom Florence had met in Rome in late 1847). Nightingale was fully occupied in getting ready to depart, so she delegated Mrs. Brace-bridge and the others to interview candidates. The selection committee sought not only to recruit qualified women, which was difficult enough, but also to maintain a balance between the various religious factions in the country.

Sidney Herbert realized that for the nursing mission to succeed, it would have to include Catholic nurses, not only for the nearly 10,000 Irish soldiers, who constituted one-third of the troops at the front, but also to maintain political harmony among the more prominent religious factions at home. In the last few decades of reform, English society and even high political and Anglican circles had grudgingly begun to acknowledge that the Catholic Church and other non-Anglican congregations must be accommodated under the law.

One underlying reason was the swelling stream of Irish immigrants, nearly all Catholic, that had flooded England and provided the cheap labor that helped build the tunnels and railways and man the looms and factories of the industrialized North. The other was the political need for friendly relations with a Vatican hierarchy that was more liberal than in previous years. As a result of these and many other issues, the Church of Rome in 1850 established 10 bishoprics in England for the first time since Henry VIII broke with the Pope three centuries earlier. Although England had always been deeply religious, the country had also been anticlerical and this sentiment reached a new high at midcentury, especially among the more fervent Evangelicals, who cried "No Popery!" at the establishment of the 10 bishoprics, railing against all things Catholic, including nuns.

Catholic Bishop Thomas Grant of Southwark quickly saw an opportunity for the Catholic sisters to be of service to the army while performing a valuable public relations role. Acting on his own, he contacted the Convent of Mercy in Bermondsey (a part of London south of the Thames), an order of the Sisters of Mercy and the first Catholic religious house to be erected in England since the Reformation. Under the leadership of Reverend Mother Mary Clare Moore, this convent's capable nuns had nursed patients during several cholera epidemics and ministered well to the poor in their neighborhood. Five of them prepared to go. Bishop Grant proclaimed: "Let the nuns who are so fiercely assailed [on the home front] proceed at once to the battlefield. There their daily life, seen by the whole world, and their devotedness to the cause of charity, will be the best answer to the vile calumnies uttered against them."[13]

Because Catholic circles offered the most spontaneous support for nurses, the government agreed to increase their number to 10, one-quarter of the total being recruited. Bishop Grant appealed to the Sisters of the Faithful Virgin of Norwood, who managed a home and shelter for orphans. Although they knew nothing about nursing, five Norwood sisters offered their services, and Bishop Grant had his quota.

Meanwhile, Herbert and Nightingale met on October 17 to make a final decision on the selection of nurses. Nightingale intentionally engaged no volunteers of high social standing in her original party because she believed that their position in society failed to prepare them for the work ahead. The 38 nurses who were finally selected included:

• 10 Roman Catholic Sisters: 5 Bermondsey nuns, who would become the most valuable members of this party, and 5 Norwood nuns, who were affable but inexperienced

• 14 Anglican Sisters: 8 Sellonites (named after their founder, Priscilla Lydia Sellon), who had little experience other than treating cholera patients (also known as the Sisters of Mercy); and 6 from St. John's House, a High Church group

• 14 unaffiliated nurses from various English hospitals who were, as Nightingale's friend Mary Clarke tartly remarked, "of no particular religion, unless the worship of Bacchus should be revived."[14] (Clarke's remark reflected the fact that heavy drinking was common among the working class at the time.)

The rules that Herbert and Nightingale developed were simple and straightforward. All the nurses (including Catholic) were to follow Nightingale's orders about work hours, duties, and responsibilities. They were also to do their work without reference to religious creed and weren't to try to influence the religious opinions of the patients. Nightingale would report directly to the Principal Medical Officer at Scutari, the first of whom was Dr. Edward Menzies. All expenses and wages were to be paid by the Purveyor, acting through the Chief Medical Officer of the hospital.

Following the final selection, Herbert met with the nurses and told them that they were under Nightingale's supervision. The nurses would be required to wear a uniform, a cap, and a hospital badge embroidered with the words "Scutari Hospital." They weren't allowed to go out unless there were at least three in a group or they were accompanied by Mrs. Clarke, Nightingale's housekeeper.

Still acting on his own, Bishop Grant dispatched Mother Moore and four of her Sisters of Mercy to Paris on October 17 with still-incomplete plans for their Crimean mission. The next morning they received a telegram from Bishop Grant, who had been contacted by the government, telling them to wait in Paris until further notice. The nuns had already stated that they were on a mission of charity and, therefore, expected no remuneration from the government for their services. However, they learned that the War Office had agreed to pay their expenses from Paris to the Crimea.

They soon learned more. Bishop Grant's departure orders to the Sisters had stipulated that they were free to have their devotional exercises and to introduce religious topics, although only to Catholic soldiers. However, Bishop Grant, practical and realistic, quickly agreed with the government that the Catholic Sisters would be under the hospital authority of Nightingale. When Nightingale visited the Sisters at their hotel in Paris, they were surprised to hear that they were to take their orders from her and not from their Mother Superior. However, Mother Moore gracefully accepted the change in mission, which marked the beginning of a lifelong friendship with Nightingale.

When Bishop Grant's agreement with the government became known, Catholics were appalled to learn that nuns were to be placed under the direction of a Protestant lady who had the power to select, distribute, or dismiss. To place a Mother Superior under secular authority was unacceptable and a risky precedent. A Vatican staff member wrote to Bishop Grant that the Pope said "Such a thing ought not to be,"[15] whereupon it was decided that if a second party of nuns was sent to the Crimea, they would go under a different agreement.

"Who is Mrs. Nightingale?"

The entire October 15th letter from Mr. Herbert to Nightingale found its way to the pages of the *Daily News* on October 19, which caused protests that the government was selecting too many Catholic and High Anglican nurses. That issue of the *Times* also incorrectly reported that a "Mrs." Nightingale was to head the party of nurses bound for the Crimean campaign. Although she was well known in the upper echelons of English society, she was unknown to the general public. In fact, a headline in the *Examiner* on October 28 read, "Who is Mrs. Nightingale?"

Days later the *Times* discovered its error, and so did the public. The fact that the head of the nursing expedition was not a matron, but a graceful and rich young lady, *Miss* Florence Nightingale, added to the popularity and public support of the venture. From the very beginning, "Miss Nightingale" captured the imagination of the people.

That month, as a response to the alarming war news in the *Times,* Sir Robert Peel, son of the former prime minister, started a national fund to help purchase supplies for the sick and wounded in the Crimean campaign. The *Times* Fund, as it came to be known, started on October 13 with a £200 contribution from Peel and quickly began to receive public donations. The English people were inspired by the idea of an expedition of female nurses headed by Nightingale, and within a short time the fund raised £7,000. The *Times* appointed Bence Macdonald to administer the Fund and to cooperate with Nightingale in meeting her needs. Nightingale herself donated her £500 annual allowance to the *Times* Fund.

The *Times* also announced that any nonmonetary gifts would be given to the soldiers. At this time, the Nightingale family took a house in Cavendish Square that became the headquarters for the public's donated gifts. The *Times* Fund money and gifts, to which Nightingale had immediate access, would later evoke a great deal of hostility and jealousy from the military toward her because, when supplies were lacking, she was still able to get what she needed.

Ironically, Nightingale's family, especially Fanny and Parthe, who had been so adamantly opposed to her plans for a nursing career, now took great pleasure in her growing fame. They were also proud of her ability to remain calm and composed under the tremendous pressure of decision making. However, the frenzied activity preceding her departure produced one small casualty: The family forgot to feed her pet owl, Athena, and the little bird died on the eve of her departure. The family quickly had it embalmed and mounted, and presented it to her before she left. Parthe remarked that the only tears her sister shed during the exhausting week of preparations were "when I put the little body into her hands." Nightingale commented through her tears, "Poor little beastie, it was odd how much I loved you."[16] Athena was returned to her family for safekeeping and remains on view today at Lea Hurst.

In the flurry of activity that preceded her departure for the Crimea, Nightingale found time to save a few important letters of support from among the many she received. At her death 56 years later, a small notebook containing those letters was discovered. One was from her mother:

> *Monday morning. God speed you on your errand of mercy, my own dearest child. I know He will, for He had given you such loving friends [the Bracebridges who accompanied her] and they will be always at your side to help you in all your difficulties. They came just when I felt that you must fail for want of strength, and more mercies will come in your hour of need. They are so wise and good, they will be to you what no one else could. They will write to us, and save you in that and in all ways. They are to us an earnest of blessings to come. I do not ask you to spare yourself for your own sake, but for the sake of the cause.— Ever Thine.[17]*

Another letter she kept was from Henry Manning, now a Catholic priest, with whom she had corresponded on religious and philanthropic matters:

> *God will keep you. And my prayer for you will be that your one object of Worship, Pattern of Imitation, and Source of consolation and strength may be the Sacred Heart of our Divine Lord. Always yours for our Lord's sake.[18]*

A third letter, written on October 18, 1854, was from her old suitor, Richard

Ball at Guildhall in aid of the Patriotic Fund, which was established to care for soldiers' widows and children

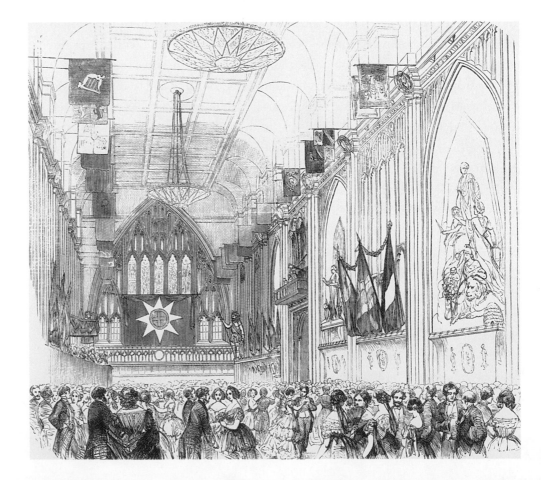

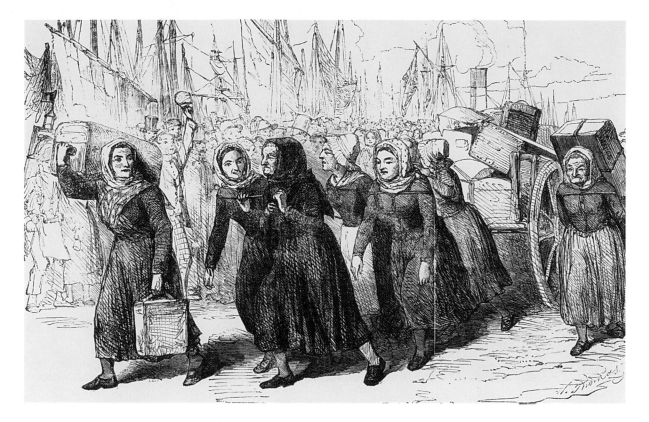

French fisherwomen in Boulogne carrying the luggage of Florence Nightingale and the nurses on their journey to Scutari

Monckton Milnes, whose friendship she still treasured:

> *My Dear Friend, I hear you are going to the East. I am happy it is so, for the good you will do there, and the hope that you may find some satisfaction in it yourself. I cannot forget how you went to the East once before, and here am I writing quietly to you about what you are going to do now. You can undertake that, when you could not undertake me. God bless you, dear friend, wherever you go.* [19]

Departure at last

Three days later, on October 21, the 34-year-old Nightingale, along with Mr. and Mrs. Bracebridge, her contingent of nurses, and her Uncle Sam Smith, who would accompany the party as far as Marseilles, departed London and crossed the English Channel to France. News of Nightingale's destination and purpose had preceded them, and the reception was exuberant. Arthur Clough, now married to cousin Blanche Smith, accompanied the party to Boulogne, where fisherwomen, many with sons or brothers in the French expeditionary army, met them at the docks and carried their luggage to the hotel. The landlord refused to let them pay for the meals and accommodations. The next night they were greeted by cheering crowds in Paris, where Julius Mohl (Clarkey's husband) had arranged lodging.

Despite the official government line that supplies were abundant at Scutari, Nightingale's intuition told her otherwise. At Marseilles, she had a strong hunch that she should independently procure a wide array of items for her nursing party. Her Uncle Sam helped her interview shopkeepers and merchants, from whom she bought miscella-

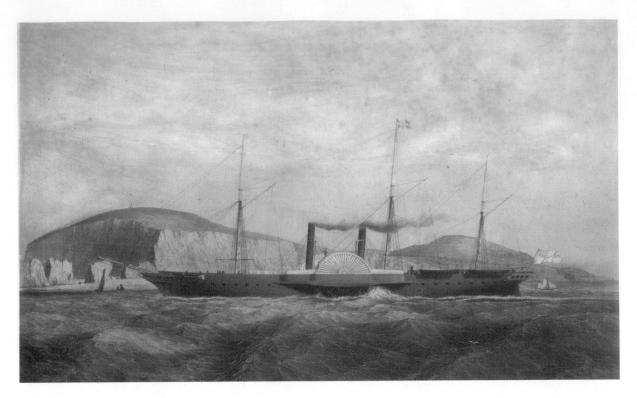

The paddle steamer Vectis, *which carried Florence Nightingale and the nurses from Marseilles to Scutari in October 1854*

neous provisions. When the party eventually arrived in Turkey, these last-minute supplies proved indispensable to the group's initial survival and success.

Throughout the trip, Nightingale made every effort to look after the nurses, even arranging separate sleeping quarters for the different religious sects. The women commented that they had never received such kind treatment, and certainly not from a lady.

The party left Marseilles on October 27 on the paddle steamer *Vectis*, built for speed to carry the mail. The ship was notorious for its tendency to roll in high seas, and the government had difficulty in gathering a crew. On its second day in the Mediterranean, the ship was buffeted by gales; the stewards' cabin and the galley were washed overboard, and the cannon had to be jettisoned. When the group finally reached Malta, Nightingale was too weak from days of seasickness to go ashore. The days of hardship had begun.

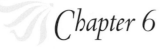
"The Whole Army is Coming"

I have not a moment. The whole army is coming into the hospitals. The task will be gigantic. Alas, how will it all end? We are in the hands of God. Pray for us. We have at the moment five thousand sick and wounded. My only comfort is, God sees it, God knows it, God loves us. Remember us to my sisters.

— *Florence Nightingale to Caroline Fliedner, December 1854[1]*

After a 9-day voyage from Marseilles via Malta, the weary and seasick Nightingale party anchored at Constantinople on November 4, 1854, in a pouring rain. Lord Napier, the envoy of British Ambassador Lord Stratford de Redcliffe, came aboard to greet them. Later that day, Nightingale wrote a quick note home to her family describing the last day of the voyage and news of the Battle of Balaclava:

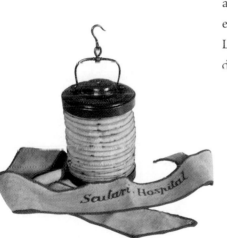

"Scutari Hospital" sash worn by the Nightingale nurses and the actual Turkish lantern Nightingale used when making evening rounds at the Barrack Hospital at Scutari

> *At six o'clock yesterday morn I staggered on deck to look at the plains of Troy, the tomb of Achilles, the mouths of the Scamander, the little harbor of Tenedos, between which and the mainshore our Vectris [the Nightingale party's ship], with steward's cabins and galley torn away, blustering, creaking, shrieking, storming, rushed on her way. It was in a dense mist that the ghosts of the Trojans answered my cordial hail ...*
>
> *We ... reached Constantinople this morn in a thick and heavy rain, through which the Sophia, Sulieman, the Seven Towers, the walls, and the Golden Horn looked like a bad daguerreotype washed out. We have not yet heard what the Embassy or Military Hospital have done for us, nor received our orders.*
>
> *Bad news from Balaclava. You will hear the awful wreck of our poor Cavalry, 400 wounded, arriving at this moment for us to nurse — the bad conduct of the Turkish commanders — cowardice in one — the other shot. Our two ships damaged, Arethusa and Albion. But Lord Raglan says he shall take Sebastopol. We have just built another hospital at the Dardanelles. It is quite true that a sortie of 8000 Russians was repulsed by 1500 of ours. One man killed 14 Russians with his own hands ...*
>
> *Just starting for Scutari. We are to be housed in the Hospital this very afternoon. Everybody very kind. The first wounded I believe to be placed under our care. They are landing them now.[2]*

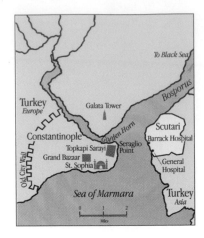

Map showing Constantinople, with its Grand Bazaar, and Scutari, the site of the Barrack Hospital, where Nightingale served as superintendent of nurses throughout the war

BELOW: *19th-century skyline of Constantinople, showing the mosques and minarets visible from the port*

In the afternoon the nurses were lowered from the ship into small boats and rowed across to Scutari, which lay directly across the Bosporus. They were housed in the Barrack Hospital, on the second and third floors of the northwest tower, which soon became known as the "Sisters' tower." Their windows overlooked the Sea of Marmara and the Princes' Islands on one side, and Constantinople on the other.

Nightingale's sketch of the tower floor plan shows the party's six rooms on the second floor in a space that formerly lodged three medical officers and their servants. There was a large kitchen or storeroom, and from it other doors opened to smaller rooms. The Bracebridges slept in one small room that shared a common sitting room with Nightingale. One larger room was allocated to the 14 lay nurses. Another room was given to the 10 Catholic nuns whom Nightingale labeled "black and white" for the colors of their habits. The Anglican nurses took the three remaining small rooms directly overhead.

The nurses' quarters were abysmal: The cramped rooms were infested with rodents and vermin; the roof leaked; and the windows were often torn off during storms. In one room, the dead body of a Russian general was discovered. Washing facilities, privies, and water supplies were inadequate; the party had to take turns bathing in a single basin. There were no drying facilities for clothes; anyone who got wet in harsh weather had to stay in bed for several hours while her soaked garments dried in front of a kitchen fire. Although supplies for cleaning were scarce, Nightingale obtained wash basins and scrub brushes to clean the area as well as raised platforms to keep the mattresses off the floor.

Proper food was also scarce; milkless tea, sour bread, and tainted meat were often the only rations available. Fasting became a common practice.

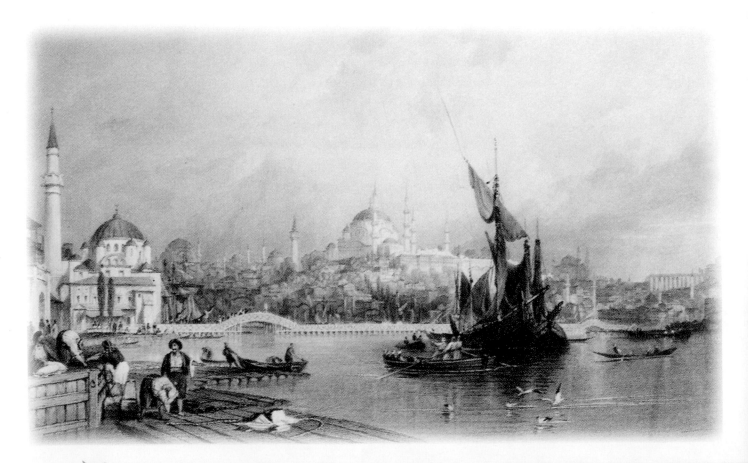

"THE WHOLE ARMY IS COMING"

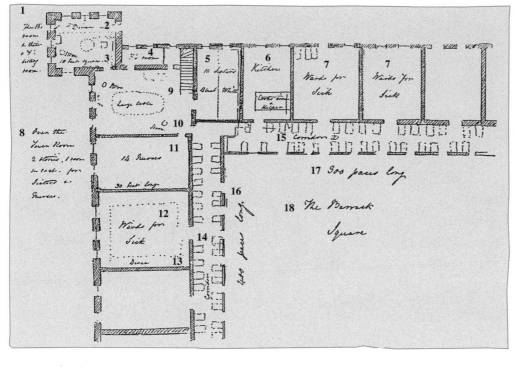

Nightingale's hand-drawn floor plan of the nurses' tower at the Barrack Hospital, showing where she and her party of nurses lived:
1. The Bracebridges' room and the joint sitting room
2. Divan
3. Stove
4. Nightingale's room
5. 10 Sisters "black and white" [referring to the orders of nuns]
6. Kitchen, cook's room
7. Wards for sick
8. Over the tower room, 2 stories, for Sisters and nurses
9. Large room
10. Stove
11. 14 nurses (30 feet long)
12. Wards for sick
13. Divan
14 & 15. Corridor
16. 400 paces long
17. 300 paces long
18. The Barrack Square

Early challenges

As soon as the nursing party was settled in their quarters, Nightingale approached the medical officers and offered her services, according to her orders. The medical officers on the scene saw Nightingale's group as meddling outsiders and declined their services. It had never occurred to Secretary at War Sidney Herbert or Nightingale that the nurses might be rejected. The fact that no General Orders had been issued describing the nurses' mission turned out to be a critical flaw.

When Dr. John Hall, Inspector-General of Hospitals, learned that the government was sending female nurses led by Nightingale to Scutari, he was less than enthusiastic. To Hall, Nightingale was merely a wealthy woman seeking adventure and was exploiting her class and connections to further her scheme. For her part, Nightingale saw Hall as an antagonist — a large cogwheel in the military machinery. The two were almost bound to clash, given the ambiguity of Nightingale's instructions from the War Office, which authorized her dominion over nurses in *Turkey* but which Hall interpreted as giving her no authority in the *Crimea,* which was 300 miles away.

In addition to being antagonistic toward the nursing party, Hall was also woefully behind the times in medical science, specifically in his opposition to the use of anesthesia in surgery. Seven years after Sir James Simpson had published his pamphlet on the successful use of chloroform and a year after Queen Victoria had used the anesthetic in childbirth, Hall was still cautioning his medical officers against its use during treatment of serious gunshot wounds. He believed few would survive its use, saying: "The smart of a knife is a powerful stimulant, and it is much better to hear a man bawl lustily than to see him sink into the grave."[3] Fortunately, Hall never issued a clear directive on the matter, so many surgeons used chloroform whenever it was available.

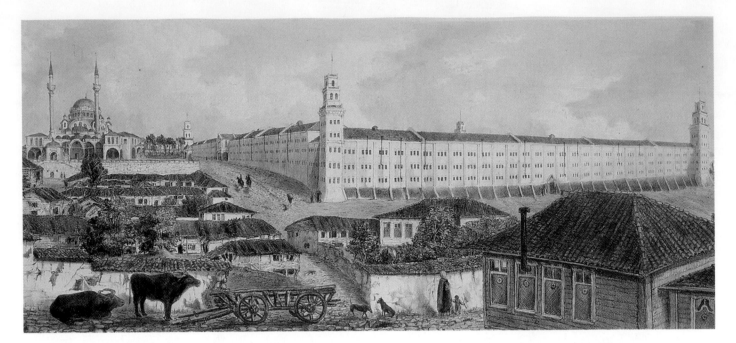

A painting of the Barrack Hospital at Scutari, Nightingale's headquarters during the Crimean War. The "Sisters' tower" is in the rear, near the mosque.

A few doctors at Scutari did welcome Nightingale's arrival. Dr. Alexander Mc-Grigor, a surgeon, worked closely with her to introduce basic reform following her arrival. Unfortunately, he died of cholera in the fall of 1855. Senior Medical Officer Dr. William Cruikshanks also recognized the nurses' value and told Nightingale that her best nurse, Mrs. Eliza Roberts, dressed wounds and fractures more skillfully than any of the dressers or assistant surgeons. Dr. William Linton, who became one of the Senior Medical Officers at Scutari in 1855, also provided valuable assistance in the many reports Nightingale wrote during and after her Crimean mission. Lord William Paulet, Commandant at Scutari, was a disappointment to her, but General Henry Storks, who succeeded Paulet in 1855, was a greater supporter.

Despite her initially cool reception by the military medical hierarchy, Nightingale immediately began keeping detailed daily records of wounds, diseases, and deaths; contaminated food and water; lack of supplies; and major organizational problems with the army's Medical Department. She set the nurses to work making mattresses, stump pillows, and shirts for the soldiers from the miscellaneous supplies she had purchased in Marseilles.

To gain the confidence of the medical officers and surgeons on the scene, Nightingale gave strict orders that no nurses were to enter the hospital wards until they had received an official request from the medical officer on duty. This was upsetting to many of the nurses, who were unaware of the ambiguous orders and the administrative parrying that followed; they were eager to help the soldiers who were in agony and dying all around them. However, Nightingale, who was task-oriented and capable of driving herself mercilessly, didn't pause to adequately explain her motives and management strategy to her staff. As a result, a few nurses interpreted her actions as arbitrary and unsympathetic and failed to support her.

The Anglican Sisters and lay nurses weren't accustomed to the rigorous discipline that Nightingale insisted on and soon became discontent. While some nurses chafed under the discipline, others complained about the ill-fitting uniforms. Hastily designed and fabricated in England, these consisted of a loose-fitting gray tweed dress, or "wrapper," worsted jacket, cap, and short woolen cloak, and a brown sash on which were embroidered in red script the words "Scutari Hospital." Mrs. Rebecca Lawfield, one of the six St. John's House nurses, told Nightingale:

> I came out, Ma'am, prepared to submit to everything — to be put upon in every way — but there are some things, Ma'am, one can't submit to — There is caps, Ma'am, that suits one face, and some that suits anothers, and if I'd known, Ma'am, about the caps, great as was my desire to come out to nurse at Scutari, I wouldn't have come, Ma'am.[4]

Nightingale did, however, have some key supporters; among these, Mother Mary Clare Moore of Bermondsey understood from the beginning the need for unit discipline and insisted that her nuns follow Nightingale's orders. Mother Moore was to become one of Nightingale's most trusted and respected friends during the war and after.

"Four miles of beds"

The medical officers, exhausted and overworked, quickly changed their attitude toward the nurses on November 9, when the sick and wounded from the Battle of Balaclava streamed into the already overcrowded hospitals. Still more casualties from the Battle of Inkerman followed shortly. There were already 1,715 Crimean casualties at the Barrack Hospital and 650 severely wounded in the General Hospital, when word was received to prepare for 570 more. At Inkerman, 1,859 were wounded and 480 killed. Unable to cope with the flood of new casualties, the military staff turned to Nightingale for help. On November 14, Nightingale wrote to Dr. William Bowman, her friend and colleague from Harley Street, describing the scene:

> I have no doubt that Providence is quite right and that the Kingdom of Hell is the best beginning for the Kingdom of Heaven, but that this is the Kingdom of Hell no one can doubt. We are very lucky in our Medical Heads — two of them are brutes, and four of them are angels — for this is a work which makes either angels or devils of men, and of women too. As for the Assistants, they are all cubs, and will, while a man is breathing his last breath under the knife, lament the "arrogance of being called up from their dinners by such a fresh influx of wounded." But wicked cubs grow up into good old bears, tho' I don't know how — for certain it is, the old bears are good.
>
> We have now four miles of beds — and not eighteen inches apart. We have our quarters in one Tower of the Barrack — and all this fresh influx has been laid down between us and the Main Guard in two corridors with a line of beds down each side, just room for one man to step between, and four wards ... I take rank in the army as Brigadier-General, because 40 British females [38 nurses, Mrs. Clarke, and Mrs. Bracebridge], whom I have with me, are more difficult to manage than 4000 men ... These poor fellows have not had a clean shirt nor been washed for two months before they came here, and the state in which they arrive from the transport is literally crawling. I hope in a few days we shall establish a little cleanliness. But we have not a basin nor a towel nor a bit of soap nor a broom — I have ordered 300 scrubbing brushes ... But one half the Barrack is so sadly out of repair that it is impossible to use a drop of

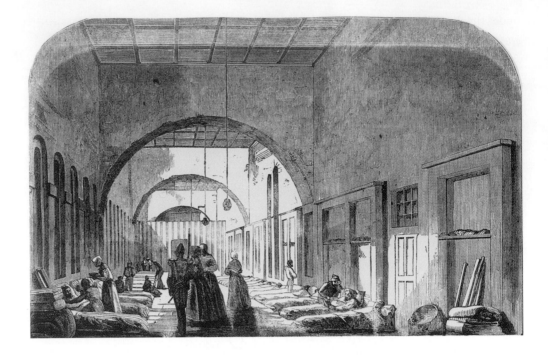

water on the stone floors, which are all laid upon rotten wood, and would give our men fever in no time ... I am getting a screen now for the Amputations, for when one poor fellow who is to be amputated tomorrow, sees his comrade today die under the knife it makes impression — and diminishes his chances. We have Erysipelas Fever and Gangrene ...[5]

Nightingale placed 10 nurses in the General Hospital and 28 in the Barrack Hospital. She rotated the nurses from time to time, sending the most trustworthy to other hospitals and keeping the least disciplined under her watchful eye. Three were dismissed for drunkenness in the first few weeks. Of the first 38 nurses who served, Nightingale considered 16 very efficient and 5 or 6 excellent. One of the best was Mrs. Elvira Roberts, from St. Thomas's Hospital in London.

Appalling conditions

The vermin-infested wards were as bad as the worst slums of London. Overflow casualties were laid on both sides of the long corridors. Sick and wounded soldiers insisted on keeping their own blankets, no matter how filthy or tattered, because the hospital blankets were made of coarse canvas.

The Barrack Hospital sat over a network of cesspools, but sewer lines were blocked and privies overflowed into the hallways. Windows were closed against the cold, wind, and rain, trapping the stench from the sewers together with smoke from the stoves. The water supply was visibly contaminated with organic matter. Not surprisingly, cholera, typhoid, and typhus added to the roll of illness and death.

One of the army's most serious oversights was its failure to establish a central warehouse in which to receive supplies sent from England. Consequently, goods unloaded from merchant ships were detained by the Turkish Customs House. Long delays in processing and rampant pilferage caused Nightingale to call the Customs House "a bottomless pit whence nothing ever issued of all that was thrown in."[6] Supplies coming by government ships were often delayed by being transported to Balaclava and back again, if at all. Sometimes supplies were left on the ships for lack of storage space ashore. To solve this problem, Nightingale agitated for a government storehouse on the Scutari side of the Bosporus, which was eventually established.

Ironically, a three-member commission of inquiry, appointed by Sidney Herbert to investigate the appalling conditions of the soldiers and the lack of supplies, had arrived in Scutari with the Nightingale party. Although the three men — two doctors and a barrister — were empowered to draft a report, they had no authority to make recommendations or changes. The group's work was further hampered when one of its members drowned in the sinking of a supply ship in the hurricane of November 14.

One of the first nonmilitary people to see firsthand the difficulties Nightingale faced was the clergyman and journalist Reverend Sydney Godolphin Osborne, who wrote for the *Times* under the initials "S.G.O." Osborne, who arrived at Scutari 2 days before Nightingale, described her as having "the tact and diplomacy of a Palmerston" and commented on her other qualities:

> ... *Her manner and countenance are prepossessing, and this without great self-possession of positive beauty; it is a face not easily forgotten, pleasing in its smile, with an eye betokening great self-possession, and giving, when she wishes, a quiet look of firm determination to every feature. Her general demeanor is quiet and rather reserved; still I am much mistaken if she is not gifted with a very lively sense of the ridiculous. In conversation, she speaks on matters of business with a grave earnestness one would not expect from her appearance. She has evidently a mind disciplined to restrain under the principles of the action of the moment every feeling which would interfere with it. She has trained herself to command, and learned the value of conciliation towards others and constraint over herself. I can conceive her to be a strict disciplinarian; she throws herself into a work as its head. As such she knows well how much success must depend upon literal obedience to her every order...*
>
> *Every day [at Scutari] brought some new complication of misery to be somehow unraveled. Each day had its peculiar trial to one who had taken such a load of responsibility, in an untried field, and with a staff of her own sex, all new to it ... and in my opinion, [she] is the one individual who in this whole unhappy war had shown more than any other what real energy guided by good sense can do to meet the calls of sudden emergency.*[7]

The bureaucratic maze

Obtaining supplies was one of Nightingale's ongoing nightmares; she had to deal with at least three departments to obtain anything. The Medical Department provided doctors and other staff, supplied drugs and equipment, and oversaw the management of the hospitals; the Commissariat was responsible for food, fuel, and transport; and the Purveyor's Department, under Mr. Wreford, was responsible for preparing and serving the food for men too sick to eat their normal rations. Yet the Purveyor didn't control his own food purchases; he depended on the Commissariat for raw foodstuffs.

Nightingale enlisted three able men to help her obtain the needed supplies: Bence Macdonald, the *Times* Fund administrator; Osborne, the *Times* journalist; and Augustus

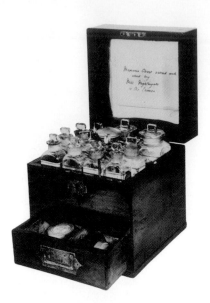

Nightingale's medicine chest that she took with her to Scutari, which contained such medications as Powered Rhubarb, Carbonate of Magnesia, Quinine, Carbonate of Potassium, Carbonate of Soda, Ipecacuanha Wine, Paregoric Elixir, Citric Acid, Essence of Ginger, Carbonate of Zinc, tonic pills, and cough pills

Stafford, a member of Parliament who had come to see conditions for himself. Drawing on the *Times* Fund and Nightingale's private monies, the reformers bypassed the Purveyor's Department and bought supplies in Constantinople's Grand Bazaar, the world's largest marketplace, then stored them in Nightingale's own storeroom. Soon people knew that if they needed supplies or had to get something done, they should see Nightingale. However, she never released supplies without official medical authorization and only after an inquiry had first been made to the Purveyor's Department for the goods. She became the *de facto* source for such things as stump pillows, arm slings, splints and padding, flannel, calico, medicinal wine, and basic washing supplies.

Food preparation was primitive; at the Barrack Hospital, cooking was done in 13 huge copper pots, which also were used to make tea. Orderlies detailed as "cooks" identified their assigned chunks of meat with nails, buttons, or any other handy marker, and dropped them into the pots, often pulling the meat out again before the water had begun to boil. Some servings were nearly all bone and no meat; when Nightingale requested that only boned meat be used, she was told this was impossible because it would require a new army regulation.

Despite the presence of the nearby bazaar, vegetables were rarely served; one day Nightingale saw thousands of cabbages dumped into the sea because no one was authorized to receive the shipment. Although scurvy was rampant, no one would authorize the distribution of existing stocks of lime juice. To improve this situation, Nightingale opened two extra kitchens in different parts of the building and installed three supplementary boilers for preparing tea as well as arrowroot and sago, two easily digestible plant starches.

The Barrack Hospital had no laundry facilities, which meant no clean clothes, bed sheets, or blankets. The original boiler had broken down, and no official could decide who should authorize its repair. When the newly arrived soldiers realized this, they wouldn't give up their filthy garments because they preferred sleeping with their own lice rather than the lice of others. When Nightingale's request for new boilers was denied, she obtained boilers from the Army Engineer's Office, paid for them out of the *Times* Fund, and had them installed in a nearby building, which became the washing house. The arrival of a drying closet, designed by philanthropist Lady Angela Burdett-Coutts, also helped to improve the laundry situation.

Nightingale soon discovered that some 200 women who had followed their husbands or lovers from the encampment at Varna to Scutari were living in squalor beneath the hospital — some with babies and small children. When the Reverend Dr. J. S. Blackwood arrived for duty as chaplain, his wife, Lady Alicia, asked Nightingale how she could help. Nightingale promptly assigned Lady Alicia the responsibility of helping with the poor women and children. As the health of the women improved, they were put to work doing laundry in the newly equipped washing house, fulfilling hospital requisitions, and making linens.

On top of all this, Nightingale and her nurses found time to write letters home for soldiers who were illiterate or too ill to lift a pen. She made sure that letters of sympathy were always sent to mothers, wives, and families of dead soldiers, telling of their last moments and words. Many of these letters were circulated and printed in the local newspapers throughout England, providing a balm to the communities as well as winning hearts and minds to the cause of women as nurses.

Making progress

Nightingale worked sometimes 20 hours each day. Soon even the most hardened officers noticed the effects of her commanding authority and healing presence. She had an utter disregard of contagion and spent hours over men who were dying of cholera or other fevers. On one occasion, surgeons laid five soldiers aside to die, deeming their condition hopeless. Nightingale and a few nurses got permission to care for these men through the night, and by morning they were fit for surgery. When doctors would say "we can't," her response was "we must." However, some officers continued to show their contempt by calling her "the Bird"; when faced with an unpleasant task, they would excuse themselves by saying "It's the Bird's duty."

For her part, Nightingale remained self-assured amid the tension and jealousy. To her family she wrote: "Praise, good God! He knows what a situation He had put upon me. For his sake I bear it willingly, but not for the sake of Praise. The cup which my Father hath given me shall I not drink? But how few can sympathize with such a position!"[8]

Within a few weeks, Nightingale had made tremendous progress in obtaining supplies with the help of her three "assistants" — Macdonald, Osborne, and Stafford. By the end of November, she wrote to Herbert that she was "Barrack Mistress, Purveyor, and

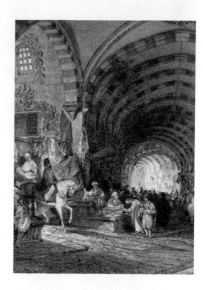

The Grand Bazaar in Constantinople, where Nightingale sent her assistants to buy supplies that she could not obtain from the Purveyor's Department

BELOW: *Drying closet designed by Lady Burdett-Coutts and sent to Nightingale for use at the Barrack Hospital*

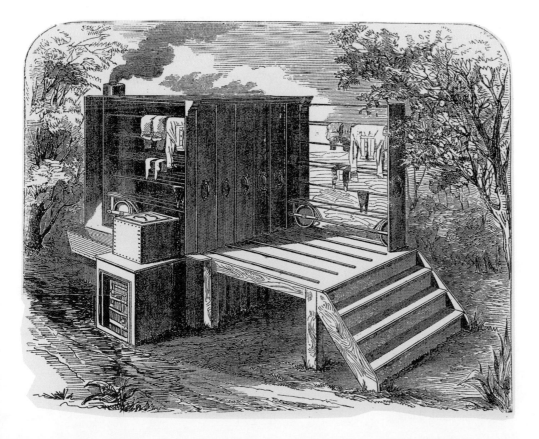

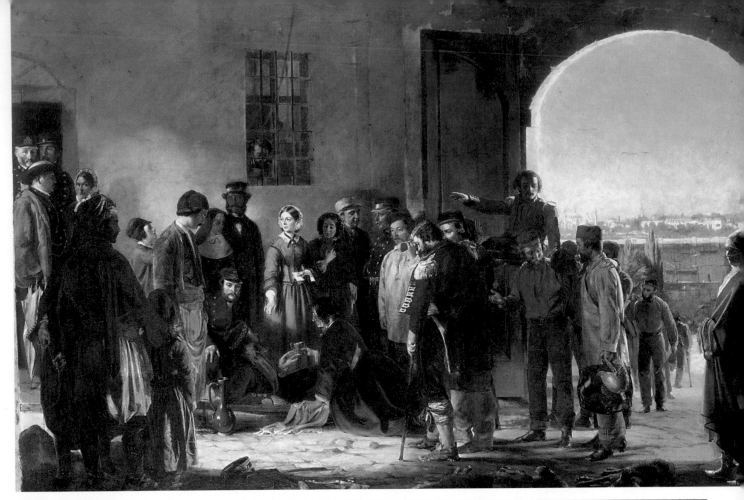

"*The Mission of Mercy: Florence Nightingale Receiving the Sick and Wounded at Scutari,*" painted in 1857 by Jerry Barrett, showing Nightingale, paper and pen in hand, with her colleagues at Scutari

RIGHT: *study diagram showing the following people:*
1. *Florence Nightingale*
2. *Mrs. Eliza Roberts*
3. *Selina Bracebridge*
4. *Charles Bracebridge*
5. *Lord William Paulet*
6. *Colonel Charles Sillery (military commandant at Scutari, 1853-54)*
7. *Dr. William Cruikshanks*
8. *Reverend Mother Mary Clare Moore*
9. *Robert Robinson*
10. *Miss Harriet Tebbutt (Mary Stanley party)*
11. *Alexis Soyer*
12. *General Henry Storks*
13. *Dr. William Linton*
14. *Jerry Barrett (artist)*

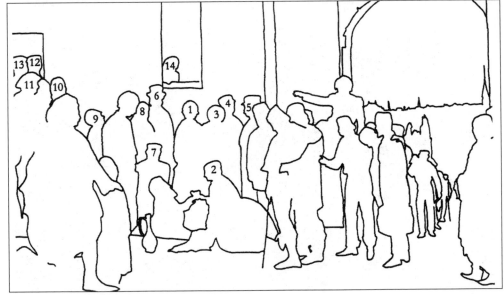

Clothier of the British Army" and a "General Dealer" in 6,000 shirts, 2,000 socks, 500 pairs of drawers, nightcaps, slippers, knives, forks, wooden spoons, trays, tables, forms, clocks, operating room tables, scrubbers, towels, soap, screens, spoons, tin baths, combs, precipitate for destroying lice, scissors, bedpans, and stump pillows.

The letters Herbert received from Nightingale as well as other friends and colleagues provided him with an eye-opening account of the army's administrative bungling and enabled the government to begin planning remedial action:

... When we came here, there was neither basin, towel nor soap in the Wards, nor any means of personal cleanliness for the Wounded except the following. Thirty were bathed every night by Dr. McGrigor's orders in slipper-baths, but this does not do more than include a washing once in eighty days for 2300 men. The consequences of all this are Fever, Cholera, Gangrene, Lice, Bugs, Fleas — & maybe Erisypelas — from the using of one sponge among many wounds ... The fault here is, not with the Medical Officers, but in the separation of the department which affords every necessary supply, except medicines, to them — & in the insufficient supply of minor officers in the Purveying Department under Mr. Wreford, the Purv'r Genl, — as well as in the inevitable delay in obtaining supplies, occasioned by the existence of one single Interpreter only, who is generally seen booted ...[9]

In a small sitting room in the Sisters' tower, Nightingale held meetings at which the military officers and surgeons gave orders for the regulation of the female nurses in the wards. She also received assorted ladies, nuns, orderlies, Turks, Greeks, French, Italians, and others, all speaking their own languages, who were waiting with requisitions for supplies. The nurses referred to her quarters as their "Tower of Babel."

Support from the queen

In early December 1854, word came from Lord Raglan, Commander-in-Chief of the British army, that the Barrack Hospital should soon expect up to 800 more casualties. Because there was no more floor space, Nightingale turned her attention to renovating a run-down wing of the hospital that was previously uninhabitable. With McGrigor's support, she got permission from Lady Stratford de Redcliffe, wife of the British ambassador to Turkey, who instructed the engineering staff to begin the necessary repairs. The first group of 125 workmen soon went on strike, whereupon Lord Stratford withdrew his support. Not to be deterred, Nightingale hired 200 new workmen to complete the job and paid them from her private funds.

On January 19, 1855, 800 sick and wounded soldiers arrived at Scutari from their grueling trip across the Black Sea to a clean hospital wing, warm clothes, and palatable food. Not everyone was impressed with this display of "the Nightingale power," as indicated by the derisive comment of a Colonel Sterling: "Miss Nightingale coolly draws a cheque. Is this the way to manage the finances of a great nation?"[10] Indeed, it was the only way at Scutari. Despite these sentiments, the War Office subsequently approved Nightingale's ward reconstruction and reimbursed her for it.

Thanks to the efforts of Secretary at War Sidney Herbert, support for the nursing mission was growing among government officials. Even more important, Queen Victoria began to take a personal interest in Nightingale's efforts. In a letter to Herbert written on December 6, 1854, the queen complained that she wasn't getting enough information about the condition of her soldiers:

Would you tell Mrs. Herbert that I beg she would let me see frequently the accounts she receives from Miss Nightingale or Mrs. Bracebridge, as I hear no details of the wounded, though I see so many from officers, etc., about the battle field, and naturally the former must interest me more than any one. Let Mrs. Herbert also know that I wish Miss Nightingale and the ladies would tell

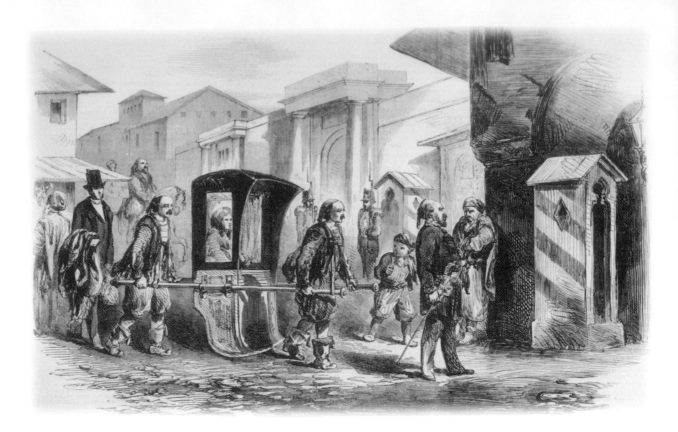

Lady Stratford de Redcliffe,
wife of the British Ambassador
to Turkey, on her way to visit
Nightingale at the Barrack
Hospital

*these poor, noble wounded and sick men that no one takes a warmer interest or feels more for
their sufferings or admires their courage and heroism more than their Queen. Day and night she
thinks of her beloved troops. So does the Prince. Beg Mrs. Herbert to communicate these my
words to those ladies, as I know that our sympathy is much valued by these noble fellows.[11]*

From this time forward, the queen received copies of Nightingale's letters on a
wide variety of reform issues as well as reports on the care of troops. When Nightingale
received the queen's message, she had the chaplain read it to the men in the wards and
posted copies on the walls of several of the hospitals. She wrote Herbert that "the men
were touched" by the queen's message. The soldiers' comments showed the sense of duty
and loyalty that English soldiers in the 19th century felt toward their sovereign:

*"It is a very feeling letter," they said. "She thinks of us" (said with tears). "Each man of us
ought to have a copy which we will keep till our dying day." "To think of her thinking of us,"
said another; "I only wish I could go and fight for her again."[12]*

Soon, Nightingale received a letter from the Keeper of the Queen's Purse announcing that she would soon receive gifts of warm scarves for the soldiers and the nurses,
which Nightingale was to distribute at her own discretion. Such gifts and direct communication from the queen were an indicator not only of her heartfelt concern for the
soldiers and nurses, but also of her personal support of Nightingale and her mission:

*Windsor Castle, December 14 [1854]. Madam — I have received the commands of Her
Majesty the Queen to forward by the ship* Eagle *some packages containing some comforts and
useful articles which Her Majesty wishes to be placed in your hands for distribution, as you
may think fit, amongst the wounded and sick at Scutari.*

Her Majesty has wished to mark by some private contribution from herself her deep personal sympathy for the sufferings of these noble soldiers, and her admiration of the patience and fortitude with which they have suffered both wounds and hardships.

The Queen has directed me to ask you to undertake the distribution and application of these articles, partly because Her Majesty wished you to be made aware that your goodness and self-devotion in giving yourself up to the soothing attendance upon these wounded and sick soldiers had been observed by the Queen with sentiments of the highest approval and admiration; and partly because, as the articles sent did not come within the description of Medical or Government stores, usually furnished, they could not be better trusted than to one who, by constant personal observation, would form a correct judgment where they would be most usefully employed. [13]

Around this time, Nightingale wrote to Herbert that she was pleased with the progress she was making in many areas. Cleaning supplies had arrived and been distributed, 2,000 shirts had arrived, an extra kitchen had been established, and a maternity hospital had been started. Most important, the administrative machinery and personnel relations in the hospital were improving, the most competent nurses were able to spend more time in dressing compound fractures, and the renovation of the hospital wing was nearing completion.

Then, within days of sending this sunny report, Nightingale discovered to her surprise, through a letter from Herbert's wife to Mrs. Bracebridge, that a second party of nurses — unsolicited by her — was en route.

Mary Stanley & the Kinsale nuns

After Nightingale's departure for Scutari, Elizabeth Herbert and Mary Stanley continued to interview women in case more nurses might be needed. Sidney Herbert had originally agreed not to send any more nurses to the East unless Nightingale specifically requested them. Now, however, facing a growing mass of logistical and administrative problems, Herbert hastily misinterpreted a letter from Mr. Bracebridge to mean that Nightingale would welcome more help and he rashly allowed a second group of nurses to be organized in the fall of 1854.

At the same time, Herbert's friend Rev. Henry Manning, a former Anglican archdeacon who had converted to Catholicism in 1851 and was now a priest in London, had been quietly promoting the dispatch of a second group of nurses composed mainly of an order of Irish nuns known as the Sisters of Mercy. The politically astute Manning saw a chance to strengthen the position of the Catholic Church as well as provide additional nurses, mainly to minister to the Irish Catholic soldiers. He urged Mary Stanley, a mutual friend of the Herberts and Nightingale (and a member of the nurse selection committee) to head the delegation. Stanley, a Protestant, would quietly convert to Catholicism within the year.

Although Bishop Thomas Grant and Mother Mary Clare Moore had agreed that the Bermondsey nuns would work under Nightingale's direct supervision, this time Manning and the Vatican establishment balked at conceding any supervisory authority,

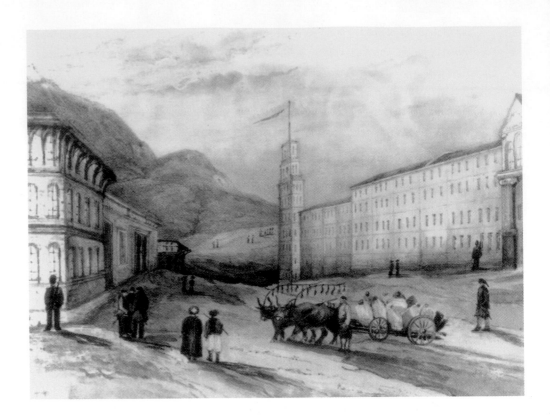

beyond the minimum necessary, to a Protestant nursing superintendent. For this second group, Manning set down new conditions he thought would guarantee the nuns' religious autonomy:

> *i. That the Sisters proceeding to the hospitals in the East shall be under their own Superior in all matters out of the wards of the hospitals.*
>
> *ii. That they shall, within the wards of the hospitals, be under the Medical Officers and the Superintendent of the nurses in all matters of hospital regulations.*
>
> *iii. That in all matters (except the details of nursing by the bedside of the sick where direct communication may be necessary) the Superintendent shall communicate with the Sisters only through their own Superior...*
>
> *vi. I have, further, a written promise from those to whom the direction of all the household details is committed, to the effect that the Sisters shall form a separate community under their own superior, in a house of their own, or a distinct quarter of any larger building.[14]*

Herbert and other Protestant government officials were not aware that, in the minds of Manning and the Catholic hierarchy, "from first to last the mission of the Sisters was not from the Government, but from their own Ecclesiastical and Religious Superiors."[15] To secure as much independence as possible, Manning raised a sum of £160, to which he added £60 from his own personal account, to pay for the nuns' incidental expenses.

The woman chosen as religious leader of the second contingent of nuns was Reverend Mother Mary Francis Bridgeman of Kinsale. Manning had noted in one of his early meetings with Mother Bridgeman that she was "an ardent, high-tempered and, at first, somewhat difficult person — but truly good, devoted and trustworthy."[15] Although the Irish nuns came from many different convents, they became known as the "nuns of

Kinsale" after their leader's home convent. Mother Bridgeman had at first suggested that the Sisters be placed under the supervision of Mother Mary Clare Moore of Bermondsey, who was already working under Nightingale. However, the mothers superior at the other Irish convents were adamant that Mother Bridgeman retain full authority and responsibility for the Irish Sisters, to which she agreed. She also agreed, as the Bermondsey nuns had, that her Sisters wouldn't try to convert Protestant soldiers but would be free to minister to Catholic soldiers.

To maintain a balance of Catholic and Anglican nurses, the government recruited 33 Protestant women to accompany the Sisters of Mercy. When the entire second party — 15 Sisters of Mercy, plus 9 ladies and 24 other nurses — gathered at Herbert's residence before their departure, Herbert advised them of the necessity of obeying their superiors, that as hospital nurses they were all on the same footing, and that no one was to consider herself better than her companions. Mother Bridgeman wrote in her diary that "it did not need much foresight to conclude how ineffectual this experiment would prove, and what the result was likely to be."[17]

On December 2, the whole party gathered at the London Bridge Station with Mary Stanley in overall command and Mother Bridgeman in charge of the Irish nuns. Even in their attire, the 15 nuns stood apart from their colleagues. While the 33 ladies and nurses all wore the same Scutari Hospital uniforms, the Sisters of Mercy were permitted to wear their black serge habits, white coifs and guimpes, and long, flowing veils.

"A cloud of locusts"

By the time the ship carrying the Stanley party anchored off Constantinople on December 15, 1854, Mother Bridgeman had won the hearts of all the Sisters, the volunteer ladies, and many of the lay nurses for her ability to bring calm after many days of suffering, anxiety, and fear during the rough sea voyage. However, this rough voyage was only a prelude to the turmoil ahead.

Neither Nightingale nor any of the senior medical officers were expecting the new contingent of nurses. When the ship arrived, Charles Bracebridge came aboard and advised the group that there was no room for them at Scutari — 40 people were already living in a space originally allocated for three people. Both Dr. Alexander Cumming, the Principal Medical Officer at Scutari, and Nightingale refused to accept responsibility for the new nurses. Nightingale was angry because her original agreement with Herbert specified that she would formally request additional help if she needed it. Now a second party of 46 nurses (plus Stanley and Mother Bridgeman) had arrived when no authorities at Scutari had requested them and none were prepared to accept them.

As Bracebridge exclaimed, "The 46 have fallen on us like a cloud of locusts. Where to house them, feed them, place them is difficult; how to care for them, not to be imagined."[18] Until arrangements could be worked out, the British ambassador lodged everyone in a house owned by the Embassy in Therapia. On December 15, Nightingale composed an anguished letter to Herbert, summarizing her present plight:

> *When I came out here as your Sup't. it was with the distinct understanding (expressed both in your own handwriting & in the printed announcement which you put in the Morn[ing]*

Chron[icle] which is here in every one's hands) that nurses were to be sent out at my requisition only, which was to be made only with the approbation of the Medical Officers here.

You came to me in your distress, & told me that you were unable for the moment to find any other person for the office, & that, if I failed you, the scheme would fail. I sacrificed my own judgment, & went out with forty females, well knowing that half that number would be both more efficient & less trouble — & that the difficulty of inducing forty untrained women, in so extraordinary a position as this, (turned loose among 3000 men) to observe any order or even any of the directions of the Medical Men, would be Herculean. Experience has justified my foreboding. But I have toiled my way into the confidence of the Medical Men. I have, by incessant vigilance, day & night, introduced something like system into the disorderly operations of these women. And the plan may be said to have succeeded in some measure, as it stands. But the Medical Officers, (under whose orders my written instructions & my own judgment equally concur in placing me) have, while expressing themselves satisfied with things as they are, repeatedly given their opinion that more women cannot be usefully employed nor properly governed. And in this opinion I entirely agree.

To have women scampering about the wards of a Military Hospl. all day long, which they would do, did an increased number relax the discipline & increase their leisure, would be as improper as absurd. At this point of affairs arrives, at no one's requisition, a fresh batch of women, raising our number to eighty-four. You have sacrificed the cause so near my heart; you have sacrificed me, a matter of small importance now. You have sacrificed your own written word to a popular cry.

I will not say anything of the cruel injustice to me. The Medical Men are disgusted, & decline absolutely to employ more, or to make any change in existing arrangements ... You must feel that I ought to resign, where conditions are imposed upon me which render the object for which I am employed unattainable — & I only remain at my post until I have provided in some measure for these poor wanderers ...[19]

When this letter reached Herbert on December 24, he quickly apologized, refused to accept Nightingale's resignation, and authorized her to send the entire party back to England if she so chose. While this round of correspondence was in the mail, Nightingale and the other authorities turned to the immediate task of resolving the problem. Lord Napier, Lord Stratford's envoy, astutely pointed out that sending the nuns home might cause a near rebellion in Ireland and returning the others to England would be a major setback for the cause of women nurses in the military.

During the delicate negotiations to resolve the problem, Nightingale and all the hospital staff were stretched to their limits with an overwhelming workload. An even greater number of sick and wounded were flowing in from the Crimea. The terrible winter had set in and 4,000 casualties, many suffering from exposure, arrived at Scutari between December 17 and January 3.

On December 24, Nightingale worked out a temporary solution for the Irish nuns. Dr. Cumming agreed to raise the total number of nurses at Scutari to 50; Mother Bridgeman and four of her Sisters would work temporarily in the Barrack Hospital, pending confirmation from their superiors in Ireland. To make room for them, five of the Sisters from the original contingent, who had little nursing experience, would be sent home.

Although Mary Stanley had planned to return to England as soon as her group was settled, she now felt responsible for the women placed in her charge and decided to remain with them for several months. During this period, Stanley's inexperience in supervisory matters, combined with her reluctance to relinquish her accidental authority, frustrated Nightingale, and the two women soon came to view each other as adversaries.

Nightingale, still feeling betrayed by Herbert, wrote to him on Christmas Day with news of the actions she had taken to resolve the situation:

> You have not stood by me, but I have stood by you. In this new situation, I have taken your written instructions as my guide, &, carrying them out with the best discretion which God has given me, I have endeavored to establish — in circumstances however perplexing & anomalous — a consistent action. Had I not done this, we should have been turned out of the Hospitals in a month, & the War Office would have borne the blame of swamping the experiment ...
>
> The [essence] of my instructions appears to me to be this —
>
> (1) Establish no separate action from the Medical Men but be their lieutenant & purveyor to carry out their intentions.
>
> (2) Control among your charge all these different sects & views so as to prevent these Hospitals from becoming a "polemical arena" — I quote your own words.
>
> The ... proposition which the Superior of the new Nuns (who is obviously come out with a religious view — not to serve the sick, but to found a convent, completely mistaking the purpose of our mission) makes is that the whole of the 15 nuns should come in or none — they cannot separate & they cannot separate from her — Why? [B]ecause it would be "uncanonical." ... [B]y this word, she has brought herself against the barrier of the War Office Instructions...
>
> (And, I assure you that, in the midst of my own overwhelming troubles, my heart bleeds for you that you, the centre of the parliamentary row, should have to attend to these miseries, tho' you have betrayed me.)
>
> ... I believe it may be proved as a logical proposition that it is impossible for me to ride through all these difficulties ... None the less shall I do what I believe to be your first will & that of Common Sense.[20]

Nightingale and Mother Bridgeman, whose roles had been predetermined by religious politics and the force of their personalities, continued to clash over the placement of the Irish Sisters at the Barrack Hospital — Nightingale, maintaining administrative authority according to her original instructions and wanting to avoid a "polemical arena," and Mother Bridgeman, carrying out the rules and wishes of the Catholic hierarchy. Finally, on January 5, 1855, Mother Bridgeman and four of her Irish Sisters agreed to temporarily serve under Mother Mary Clare Moore at the Barrack Hospital, pending clarification of their orders from their religious superiors. Gradually, the other nurses were placed: Stanley and some of her party went in January 1855 to staff the new hospital at Koulali, 5 miles north of Scutari; 11 volunteers were sent to Balaclava; and several women who had nursing experience chose to work at Barrack Hospital. Ten nuns who couldn't be placed, along with the other ladies and nurses, temporarily remained at the embassy house in Therapia and at a Sisters of Charity establishment in Galata.

Later that month, there was an outbreak of cholera in which four surgeons and three nurses died. The Kinsale Sisters proved excellent nurses, relieving the pain and suffering of the soldiers, distributing food and wine, and thoroughly cleaning the wards. The Irish soldiers were elated at the sight of their own nuns: "Sure, and it's our own Sisters, glory be to God!"[21]

Religious friction emerges

Within weeks, the first religious controversies in the hospital wards surfaced, as Nightingale and Herbert had feared. The senior Protestant chaplain at Scutari informed Nightingale that the Irish Sisters were trying to convert Protestant soldiers, an act clearly forbidden by their orders. Nightingale described the situation to her friend Lady Charlotte Canning in London:

> The second party of nuns who came out now wander over the whole hospital out of nursing hours, not confining themselves to their own wards but "instructing" (it is their own word) groups of orderlies and convalescents on the corridors, doing the work of ten chaplains and bringing ridicule on the whole thing while they quote the words of the War Office.[22]

The arrival of letters from Herbert to Nightingale and Mother Bridgeman helped rectify the situation. The letter to Nightingale was his reply to her letter of December 15th, in which he admitted his error in sending the second party and authorized her to return the group to England, an action that Nightingale realized was "morally impossible" and no longer necessary.

In the letter to Mother Bridgeman, which Nightingale seems not to have been aware of, Herbert explained that he "acted under a misconception of Miss Nightingale's wants and wishes" in sending out the second party to Scutari and that "under these circumstances, Miss Nightingale has been advised by me to select such of the Sisters and nurses as she considered the most efficient for the work in which she was engaged, and to send back the remainder." In a postscript, he added, "I am informed here that your kind services may very possibly be required in Galata, which, if it relieve you from your present difficulties, I should be glad to hear had been the case."[23]

Although Herbert seemed to be specifically restating that Nightingale was to superintend all the nurses, Mother Bridgeman interpreted the postscript to mean that he was allowing her group to serve in other hospitals without Nightingale's supervision.

The arrival of Father Ronan, the nuns' chaplain, in Scutari on January 21 helped resolve the awkward problem of the Kinsale nuns. He soon drafted a new agreement consisting of the following main points:

• The 15 Sisters of Mercy would serve under Mother Bridgeman "for she is their duly appointed Superior and cannot transfer her authority to any other."

• Ten of the 15 would be sent to the hospital at Koulali and the remaining 5 would be employed at either the General or Barrack Hospital at Scutari; those at the Barrack Hospital would form a separate community under Mother Bridgeman.

• The Sisters would be allowed to tend to the spiritual needs of their Catholic patients, especially when requested by the patients themselves or by the Catholic chaplains.

• The Sisters would pledge not to interfere with the religious concerns of the Protestants, "to give undistinguishing relief to the corporal sufferings of all, and to promote amongst them all respect for the hospital authorities."[24]

Ronan incorrectly assumed that his chaplaincy and guardianship extended to the Bermondsey nuns, but Mother Moore, always a firm ally of Nightingale, objected to this, and he limited his attentions to the Kinsale nuns. This occasion signaled a widening breach between Mother Moore and Mother Bridgeman.

The situation was settled for the time being: Mother Bridgeman and 10 of her Sisters went off to Koulali Hospital, where Stanley and others of the second party also were placed; 5 of the Irish Sisters were assigned to the General Hospital, with Nightingale approving of Mother Bridgeman's right to visit. At the request of Lord Raglan, Nightingale sent 8 of Stanley's group to Balaclava to assist the army surgeons. One of these women, Lady Jane Shaw Stewart, served over the next 15 months as superintendent of three Crimean hospitals — the General, Castle, and Land Transport Corps Hospitals — and later provided much help to Nightingale in writing her reports. Two other members of Stanley's group were sent home — one for ill health, the other for intoxication. Nightingale agreed to have the remaining Kinsale nuns replace some of her original group who had been sent home for intoxication or other disciplinary problems.

News of the conflict stemming from the Kinsale nuns' arrival began to appear in the *Times* and other newspapers:

> *When the batch of sisters and nurses brought out by Miss Stanley arrived here very considerable difficulty was experienced by Miss Nightingale in turning the services of even a portion of*

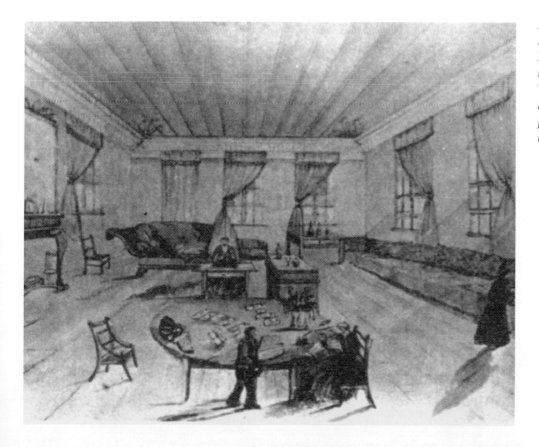

Nightingale reading, Mrs. Smith writing, and Mrs. Roberts getting a paper from the divan in a drawing by Ann Ward Morton, one of many she did in the spring of 1856, when pressure in the Barrack Hospital had eased

them to useful account. Having proved herself a vigorous reformer of hospital misrule, she was at that moment contending against the tacit opposition of nearly all the principal medical officers; her nurses were sparingly resorted to even in the Barrack Hospital, and in the General Hospital, Dr. Menzies' headquarters, she held a very insecure footing.[25]

To protect the tenuous support she had gained from some of the medical officers, Nightingale battled fiercely for administrative control of all the nurses. Allowing personnel problems and religious rivalries to develop outside her control would risk ridicule and ruin of the entire nursing enterprise. As she wrote to Herbert:

> *I never look at the* Times, *but they tell me there is a religious war about poor me there, & that Mrs. Herbert has generously defended me. I do not know what I have done to be so dragged before the Public. But I am so glad that my God is not the God of the High Church or of the Low — that He is not a Romanist or an Anglican — or an Unitarian. I don't believe He is even a Russian — tho' His events go strangely against us ... A Greek once said to me on Salamis, I do believe God Almighty is an Englishman.*[26]

Establishing standards of care

The standards of care and personal and ethical qualities routinely demanded of today's nurses were virtually unknown in the 19th century. Nightingale had to create not only a structure, but also a culture to support that structure. It was her mission to establish the concept of women nurses in the military — women with excellent clinical skills as well as high moral character and a selfless desire to serve others. She also tried to introduce the role of nurse superintendent, to follow all the rules and procedures set forth by the Medical Department, and to develop consistent, measurable patient outcomes.

In recruiting potential nursing candidates, Nightingale always applied a particular test: Was she a good woman and did she know her business? It wasn't sufficient to be merely good or religious. She meant for nurses to nurse, not to flirt with the soldiers or try to save their souls. (Her concerns were well-founded; one day, six of her best nurses, accompanied by six soldiers, came to her declaring that they wished to be married.) Because of her high standards, Nightingale always had difficulty finding qualified nurses.

Reforming the corrupt, inefficient army system of hospital care and troop supply was now becoming another major goal. Writing to her mother in early February 1855, Nightingale laid out her future course and added a few words about Mary Stanley's support of Mother Bridgeman:

> *Pray tell Aunt Mai that ... I often think of what we said together — of the great reformers who have died of disappointment — & I find our principles hold good in time of trial, the anchor is firm. I say "I expected this — I will not die of disgust & disappointment." I have often thought in early life (how little I then expected Scutari) that I should throw my body in the breach, that I bridge the chasm to reform, — that there must be an Originator, a Promulgator, An Executor to each Reformation. Christ said, I am the way and the truth and the life — in general, there is the way, (the thinker), the truth, (the speaker), the life, (the actor), separate persons to each great step — the originator perishes without credit & without success, the promulgator is ruined*

in pocket, the third succeeds. I remember thinking, So perish those who pioneer the way for Mankind. But they may perish, but I shall endure.

I shall not break my heart of disappointment, though even mine own familiar friend [referring to Mary Stanley] turns against me. No, dearest Mother, I shall do nothing, the originator never does, but greater things than these shall others do — the Army shall be reformed, the Army Medical Board, the Military Hospitals — those three sinks of jobbery & official vice — & I have done all I hoped by representing these things.[27]

The bleak winter of 1855

The greatest foe the British faced in the war was the severe Crimean winter. Czar Nicholas boasted that "Generals January and February" would be his best allies during the bleak winter of 1855, and he was very nearly proved right. Europe was unseasonably cold that year, and in the Crimea the temperature dropped to 13° F (–10° C). Inkwells froze, toothbrushes had to be thawed before use, and icicles 4″ (10 cm) long and as thick as a man's little finger formed on mustaches. The knitted helmets with openings for the nose and eyes that the troops wore to cover the head and neck — called "balaclavas" — were little protection against the frigid wind, rain, ice, and snow.

The few tents that made it to the field were flimsy, lacked floors, and were of little use against the winds howling over the steppes. Most of the troops made do with wet blankets in the mud. Trenches were filled with water and ice; boots froze to the soldiers' feet and had to be boiled off, the skin coming off in huge patches. Because there were not enough mule litters and no ambulance vans, the Turks had to carry disabled soldiers on their backs to the harbor at Balaclava for evacuation to hospitals in Scutari.

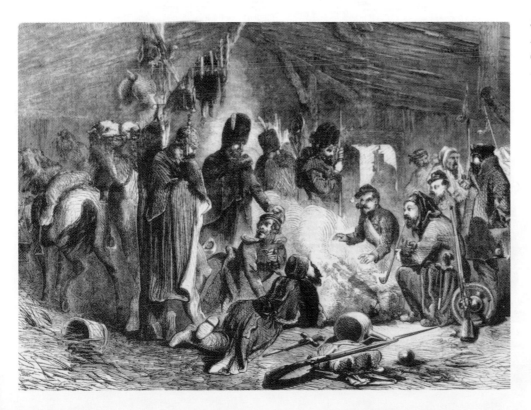

Soldiers crowded into Lord Raglan's stable with their horses during the winter storms of 1855

William Howard Russell, war correspondent for the *Times*, continued to send graphic reports from Balaclava of the casualties arriving from the encampment above Sebastopol. In late January 1855, he wrote of one column bound for the hospitals:

> ... *[They] formed one of the most ghastly processions that ever poet imagined. Many of these men were all but dead. With closed eyes, open mouths and ghastly attenuated faces, they were borne along two by two, the thin stream of breath visible in the frosty air, alone showing they were alive. One figure was a horror — a corpse, stone dead, strapped upright in its seat ... the head and body nodding with frightful mockery of life at each stride of the mule over the broken road. No doubt the man had died on his way down to the harbor. As the apparition passed, the only remarks the soldiers made were such as this, "There's one poor fellow out of pain anyway." Another man I saw with the raw flesh hanging from his fingers, the naked bones of which protruded in to the cold air, undressed and uncovered. This was a case of frostbite ... All the sick on the mules' litters seem alike on the verge of the grave.[28]*

It wasn't just Russell's vivid reporting that fueled public indignation against the army and the government; it was the full weight of the *Times* itself. With ten times the circulation of its nearest competitor, the London daily served the rising business and middle classes now coming to power in England. Its editor, John Thadeus Delane, was considered the greatest newspaperman of his era and had enormous influence. Outraged by Russell's detailed accounts, Delane thundered against the entrenched "aristocracy," which he accused of:

Turks carrying the British sick and wounded to Balaclava in January 1855, one of the main ways of transporting soldiers down the mountain to the ships bound for Scutari hospitals

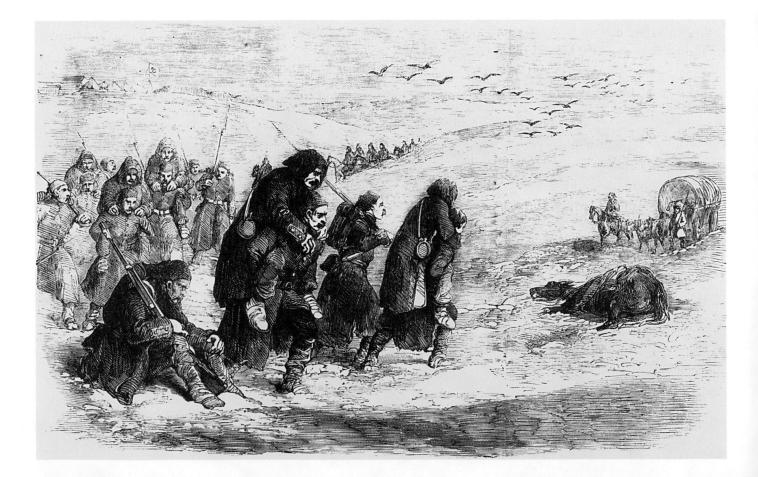

... trifling with the safety of the army in the Crimea ... Incompetency, lethargy, aristocratic hauteur, official indifference, favour, routine, perverseness and stupidity reign, revel and riot in the Camp before Sebastopol ... We say it with extreme reluctance, no-one sees or hears anything of the Commander-in-Chief [Raglan].[29]

Echoed now by other newspapers, the *Times* publicized the same terrible realities that Nightingale and others had been describing privately to Sidney Herbert. The public demanded sweeping reforms. On January 26, 1855, John Roebuck, the Radical member of Parliament from Sheffield, introduced a motion to convene a committee "to inquire into the condition of our Army before Sebastopol, and into the conduct of those departments of the government whose duty it has been to minister to the wants of that Army."[30] The motion passed after a stormy debate. As a result of the uproar, Lord Aberdeen's government fell, and Herbert was forced to resign as Secretary at War.

The country now turned to a man who could get things done, the Nightingales' old friend and neighbor, Lord Palmerston. After 48 years in government, Palmerston became Prime Minister and got to work immediately. He combined the posts of Secretary for War and Secretary at War and appointed Lord Panmure to the new position — Secretary of State for War. Panmure had served as Secretary at War from 1846 to 1852.

Sidney Herbert accepted Palmerston's invitation to become Colonial Secretary. However, when the Roebuck committee began its inquiry, Herbert resigned from the cabinet as a matter of conscience, although it was understood by all that the failures in the Crimea weren't his fault and that he had labored diligently to improve conditions. Although he was out of the cabinet, Herbert remained a member of Parliament; he urged Nightingale to continue her correspondence with him so that he could continue to fight for army reform at home.

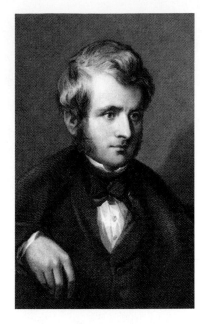

Hon. John A. Roebuck, head of the Roebuck Committee in the House of Commons, which investigated the Crimean War muddle and concluded that "the state of the hospitals was disgraceful"

An "unparalleled" calamity

As the winter weather intensified, the Scutari hospitals were deluged with severe cases of frostbite, gangrene, dysentery, and other illnesses. On January 4, the census showed 2,500 men in the Barrack Hospital, 1,122 men in the General Hospital, and 250 convalescents in the Sultan's Serail, another facility behind the Barrack Hospital. Then another 1,200 sick troops arrived from Balaclava, primarily suffering from dysentery, fever, and frostbite. There were more men in all the hospitals combined than in the camps above Sebastopol. Nightingale, having calculated the peak mortality rate in January at 1,000 per 1,174 men, described the situation as "... a calamity, unparalleled in the history of calamity."[31]

To cope with the flood of casualties, the army's Medical Department opened two more emergency hospitals at Smyrna and Renkioi in February 1855. These hospitals used civilian doctors and nurses because of the shortage of military personnel. Forty additional volunteer ladies and nurses were sent out by the War Office to staff them. These hospitals were independent of Nightingale, although she was consulted many times about their operation.

Under Palmerston's leadership, practical improvements soon began to appear. Construction of a railroad to run from the port of Balaclava up the incline to the troops on the plateau at Sebastopol was begun in January and completed in March 1855. A new harbormaster was appointed at Balaclava and, as spring brought milder weather, supplies began to move steadily to the soldiers in the field for the first time.

The push for reform

Nightingale believed that the Barrack Hospital could be made into a model facility — the best in the world — with a proper restructuring of operations and division of labor. She insisted that the Purveyor's Department should have adequate stores so the staff and patients wouldn't have to live "from hand to mouth" each day. She also insisted on the importance of careful record-keeping: of exactly how many beds were in all the hospitals, how many were ready for use, how many patients were arriving, and the regular inspection of patients' diets, kitchens, laundry, and cleaning. Above all, she wanted a patient to become a patient the minute he entered the hospital and to cease being a soldier. Up to this time, soldiers had been expected to care for themselves.

However, Nightingale was as concerned with overall reform of the army departmental systems as she was about hospital operations. As she wrote to Herbert:

> There is a far greater question to be agitated before the country than that of these eighty-four miserable women — eighty-five including me. This is whether the system or no-system which is found adequate in time of peace but wholly inadequate to meet the exigencies of a time of war is to be left as it is, — or patched up temporarily, as you give a beggar halfpence, — or made equal to the wants, not diminishing but increasing, of a time of awful pressure ...
>
> I am afraid to get back today to my immense first question how this Hospt. is to be purveyed — how, instead of living from hand to mouth, — we pouring in stores which are to be renewed again every 4 or 5 weeks, the men having left with all the stores on their backs — we ought to know (1) exactly how many beds there are in the Hospital ... ready for use, (2) how many vacant, (3) how many patients to come in,— each ward ought to have its own complement of shirts, socks, bedding, utensils, etc. etc. etc.— the new sick succeeding to the old sick's things — instead of keeping a Caravanserai [Turkish desert encampment where people and animals sleep together] as we do ... I will send you a picture of my Caravanserai, into which beasts come in & out. Indeed the vermin might, if they had but "unity of purpose," carry off the four miles of beds on their backs, & march with them into the War Office.[32]

War supplies were often stolen, held up by the Turks, or shipped to the wrong destinations. Nightingale proposed a government storehouse where goods could be unloaded and registered on a ship-to-storekeeper's receipt. She devised practical strategies to circumvent the labyrinthine Purveyor's system. As soon as she got word that a ship had docked, she would petition the military authorities to intercept the supplies bound for the hospital stores, knowing that if the supplies wound up under the Purveyor's control, she might never see them. She still had to search in the Purveyor's store almost daily to get what she needed — often to find the necessary supplies lacking. By this time, the Purveyor's Department appeared to have totally broken down. Taking matters into her own hands, Nightingale continued to send her assistants to the Grand Bazaar to purchase supplies or to order them from Marseilles.

Administrative proposals

In her letters to Herbert, Nightingale clearly articulated the root cause of the lack of leadership in the Purveyor's Department and among the medical officers. Because these officers belonged to the *civil* department of the army, they had no power to command the soldiers. This meant that a hospital medical officer could instruct an orderly to do something but couldn't discipline the orderly for failure to carry out the order. Official orders had to come from a line officer, who instructed the wardmaster or hospital sergeant, who could then take action.

When Bence Macdonald, administrator of the *Times* Fund, returned to England in February 1855, Nightingale urged Herbert to meet with him to learn about the continuing logistical problems, which she described to Herbert in a letter about the administrative tangle:

> *A great deal has been said of our "self-sacrifice," "heroism," so forth. The real humiliation, the real hardship of this place, dear Mr. Herbert, is that we have to do with men who are neither gentlemen, nor men of education, nor even men of business, nor men of feeling, whose only object is to keep themselves out of blame, who will neither make use of others, nor can be made use of ... I am so glad you are out of office, though VERY sorry for our country, because I can now have no shame in telling you sincerely ... of the dirt of this nest of official vice. And of course, you will be listened to at home as much as if you were in office.[33]*

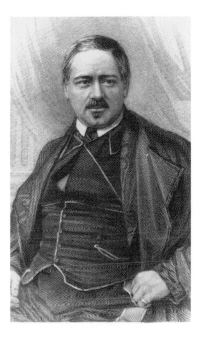

Alexis Benoit Soyer, the famous French chef of London's Reform Club, who went to Scutari at his own expense in 1855. His improvements in the hospital kitchens and training of chefs dramatically improved the soldiers' diet.

Nightingale proposed reforming the hospital administration according to three specific job functions — to provide food, to supply hospital furniture and clothing, and to establish an orderly daily routine. Although these three functions technically existed in the Purveyor's Department already, they weren't being carried out as they should.

To improve the soldiers' meals, she wanted a Commissariat Officer to reside at the Barrack Hospital so he could make a complete list of full diets, half diets, and spoon diets (the three levels of rationing specified by the army) and the number of each that was required. She suggested a system of bed-tickets, which would enable orderlies to pass through the wards and easily track the meals that needed to be served.

Alexis Benoit Soyer, the famous chef of the Reform Club in London, came to Scutari at his own expense in March 1855 to correct deficiencies in the hospital kitchens. At Nightingale's request, he recruited men and trained them as proper cooks, dramatically improving the soldiers' diets. Each kitchen was provided with a large teapot as well as supplies of sugar, tea, arrowroot, and beef tea so that each wardmaster could use these items as needed.

Feeding men on the battlefield was another major problem. Soldiers not only had to fight the battles, but also find their own wood and cook their own meals. This meant they often didn't eat because they lacked the strength necessary to search for firewood, which was virtually nonexistent after the first weeks of winter. To remedy this, Nightingale developed recommendations for feeding the men on the front lines — a system that later came to be known as *rationing* — yet her idea was ignored at the time because it would require a new army regulation.

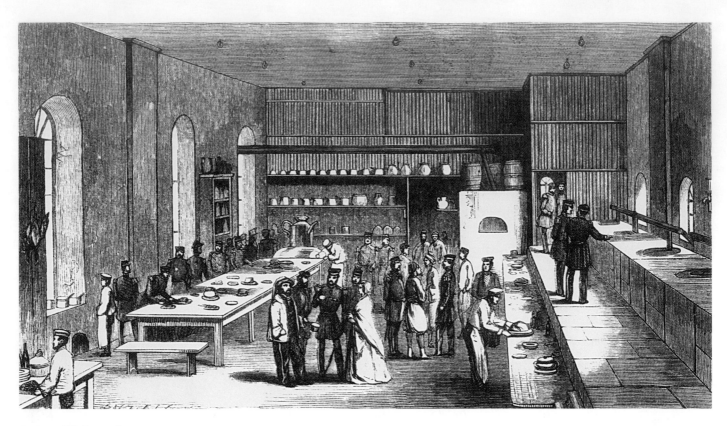

Improved kitchen at the Barrack Hospital after Alexis Soyer's culinary campaign

In addition to reporting her problems with Mr. Wreford of the Purveyor's Department, Nightingale complained bitterly to Herbert about the lack of initiative shown by the British ambassador, Lord Stratford de Redcliffe:

> *I think it matters little whether a vain, silly swearing old man, like Wreford, is kept "in" or "out." But it matters much whether ... our Embassy at Constantinople is to continue to be the laughing-stock of Europe, & the principle consecrated (in the person of Lord Stratford) of making diplomacy — not the protection of his country men, not correlative assistance to the war — the business of his Ambassador-ship. Here has that old man been four months with the British Army perishing within sight of his windows. He has been over once for 1½ hours during those four months when I forced him into the wards ...*
>
> *What have the French been doing? They now have ten Hospitals in Constantinople, while the British position is nil. Within the last week they, the French, have taken the last available building, (a large building in the neighborhood of St. Sophia) for 3,000,000 fr ... We have nothing. I will send you a plan of their position on the other side. What is an Ambassador for? Is not this trifling with the sufferings of the British Army?[34]*

Proposals poured from Nightingale's pen. To facilitate the delivery of furniture and clothing, she wanted the Purveyor's Department to supply the hospital completely, all at once, as it should be — 2,000 beds, totally outfitted. Thereafter, this allotment would remain fixed. She wanted the wardmaster to keep an inventory on the door of each ward, listing all items and the quantity of each. She developed a list of supplies needed for each bed and each patient. She felt the soldiers must be taught to respect their supplies, which many didn't. When they lost or broke an item, she wanted the replacement cost deducted from their pay. Each morning, the soldiers were to remove their dirty clothes and be given clean ones. When they left again for the battlefields or went to another hospital to convalesce, they should leave all their hospital supplies (blankets, pillows, utensils, and so on), not take them along. The quartermaster was to inspect the rooms to be sure this procedure was done. By the end of February 1855, Nightingale had secured approval to have locked supply cupboards placed in some of the wards.

More reform proposals

Not content with reforming the army medical bureaucracy, Nightingale focused on still other ways to help the soldiers. She was disturbed by the disparity in pay between sick and wounded soldiers. Prior to 1854, if a soldier had a disease or injury that wasn't contracted in the line of duty, most of his daily wage was docked for the length of his hospital stay. This policy, known as "hospital stoppage," was aimed primarily at men who had contracted preventable disorders such as venereal disease. Nightingale felt that if a soldier became ill while on duty, his pay should be the same as for a wounded soldier. Thanks to her repeated requests to both Herbert and the queen, sick and wounded soldiers began receiving the same pay in February 1855.

That same month she proposed to Herbert that a military medical school be established at Scutari. She had already found a building in front of the Barrack Hospital that could be purchased for £300 to £400. The medical school was authorized shortly thereafter; it included a dissection room, microscopes, instruments, chemical apparatus, and other needed supplies. Nightingale believed the young English surgeons at Scutari were first-rate anatomists, but miserable pathologists. In April, Dr. Peter Pincoffs came to Scutari and started conducting pathology lectures and dissections, but the medical

A watercolor sketch by Ann Ward Morton of men dining in Barrack Hospital

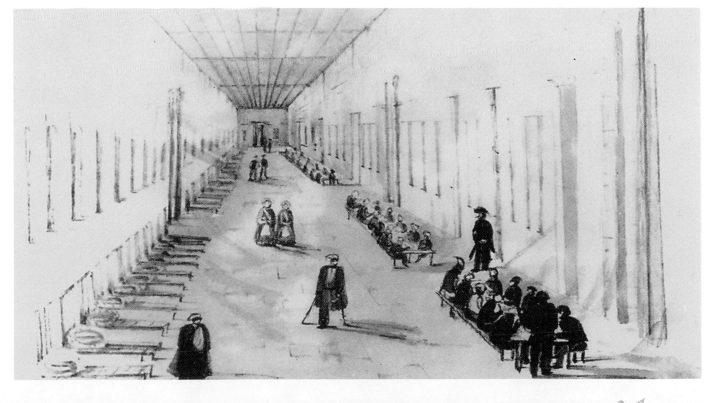

school program, like so many others, was unable to go forward because of professional jealousies among the medical officers. This project, however, eventually led to the formation of the Army Medical School at Chatham, England, in 1860, a major reform of the army's Medical Department after the war.

Another of Nightingale's radical proposals was to form a corps of orderlies in each hospital, composed of 10 specially trained men chosen for their good character. They would remain at each hospital and not be returned to the battle front, as was the current practice. Pointing out that this policy worked well for the French, she recommended that the orderlies be well paid, well fed, and well housed, and be supplied a uniform that could be easily recognized. Eventually, she was able to get 40 orderlies assigned to regular duty at the Barrack Hospital, but it wasn't until the colonial wars of the 1880s that training of orderlies was clearly established.

Nightingale also believed that the daily routine of the hospital could be improved if a house steward was appointed to direct the washing, cooking, cleaning, and coordination of the orderlies. She also wanted a governor (administrator) appointed to each military hospital. Most of all, she wanted the medical officers to come in, prescribe, and then leave, as they did in English hospitals back home. She felt that they weren't capable of attending to patients and running the wards.

By June 1855, many of her suggestions had been implemented and a royal warrant was issued for delivering better care of the sick and wounded. Two years later the Medical Staff Corps was reorganized and replaced by the Army Hospital Corps.

All in all, Nightingale's tedious and laborious work in dissecting problems and developing extensive documentation was the beginning of her far-reaching influence in eventually reforming the army medical administration. Her letters to Herbert provided factual ammunition for the needed reforms and were essential in developing the seminal *Royal Commission Report on the Sanitary Condition of the Army*, which finally appeared in 1858.

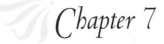
Commissions, Illness, & Accolades

*P*oor old Flo steaming up the Bosphorus & across the Black Sea with four Nurses, two Cooks & a boy ... in the Robert Lowe or Robert Slow (for an uncommon slow coach she is) taking back 420 of her Patients, a draught of convalescents returning to their Regiments to be shot at again. A "Mother in Israel," old Fliedner called me — a Mother in the Coldstreams [Coldstream Guards, the famous British army unit] is the more appropriate appellation. What suggestions do the above ideas make to you in Embley drawing room? Stranger ones perhaps than to me — who, on the 5th May, year of disgrace 1855, year of my age 35, having been at Scutari this day six months, am, in sympathy with God, fulfilling the purpose I came into the world for ...

— Florence Nightingale to the Nightingales, May 5, 1855[1]

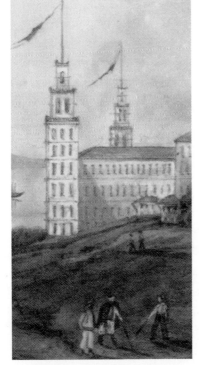

View of the Bosporus and the Barrack Hospital towers from the road into the British cemetery, by Ann Ward Morton

The new government, headed by the Nightingales' long-time friend and neighbor Lord Palmerston, was as close to Florence Nightingale as Broadlands (Palmerston's home) was to Embley. Nightingale's father and uncle, as leaders of the reform committee in Hampshire two decades before, had helped to secure a parliamentary seat for Palmerston in the first election after passage of the Great Reform Bill of 1832.

Palmerston was one of the first English politicians to understand the emerging power of public opinion that came with the widening of the electoral franchise and the growth of newspapers. He clearly understood his mandate to remedy, as one member of Parliament put it (echoing Nightingale's private words), the catastrophe that had "occurred without a parallel in history; that an army three times victorious has been left to perish — to be utterly destroyed — by the incompetence of those whose duty it was to have supported it."[2]

Palmerston's nearly half-century experience as Secretary at War, Foreign Secretary, and then Home Secretary, combined with his shrewd political instincts and intellect, provided him with great administrative abilities and, just as important, with a broad personal knowledge of the men involved at all levels of government. Within a week of taking office, he held a cabinet meeting in which seven measures were resolved "to establish a better order of things in the Crimea:

1. A Land Transport Corps to be formed.

2. A Corps of Scavengers [garbage collectors] to be procured.

3. A Sanitary Commission to be sent out.

4. A Commission, of which Sir John McNeill is to be the head, to be sent out to inquire into the working of the Commissariat in all its branches of supply and issue, and every other detail.

5. Civil medical men to be sent out, and a hospital at Smyrna formed.

6. Major-General Simpson to proceed to the Crimea as Chief of the Staff, etc.

7. A Sea Transport Board to be formed at the Admiralty.[3]

Creation of the two commissions brought Nightingale into close contact with new networks of reformers, one of whom she already knew well. It was Lord Shaftesbury (formerly Lord Ashley), Palmerston's son-in-law, who had first suggested to the young Florence some 15 years earlier that she study the Blue Books, the government inquiries into social problems. Shaftesbury had been a board member on the first national General Board of Health (1848 to 1854), along with Lord Morpeth and Edwin Chadwick, a leading advocate of sanitary reform.

Sanitary Commission

The Sanitary Commission, third on Palmerston's list of reforms, was a response to the Crimean emergency, but it was also an outgrowth of the steady stream of public health reform that had been developing in Britain over the past 30 years. The commission was composed of three men: Dr. John Sutherland, the head, who had been one of two chief medical inspectors on the first General Board of Health; Dr. Hector Gavin, a former government official who had combated cholera in the West Indies; and an engineer, Robert Rawlinson.

The details for the Sanitary Commission were largely drawn up by Shaftesbury, based on an idea of Gavin's. Shaftesbury urged Lord Panmure, Secretary of State for War, to proceed at once with the plan "to purify the hospitals, ventilate the ships, and exert all that science can do to save life where thousands are dying, not of their wounds, but of dysentery and diarrhoea, the result of foul air and preventable mischiefs."[4]

The Sanitary Commission arrived at Scutari on March 6, 1855, and Gavin wrote to Shaftesbury of his first impressions: "There is not that energy and decision at work which should characterize Englishmen. Your Lordship would wonder how men in their sober senses could do the absurd things which seem to be common here."[5] Unfortunately, his further counsel was lost as, 6 weeks later, Gavin was mortally wounded by accident when handing a revolver to his brother.

From the time that she first arrived in Scutari, Nightingale recognized the poor sanitation, but she didn't have the power to correct the problems that she identified.[6] Her first 4 months of work had focused on organizing the nurses and improving hospital supplies, general cleanliness, and the soldiers' welfare. Sutherland and the other commissioners quickly went to work to remedy the appalling conditions.

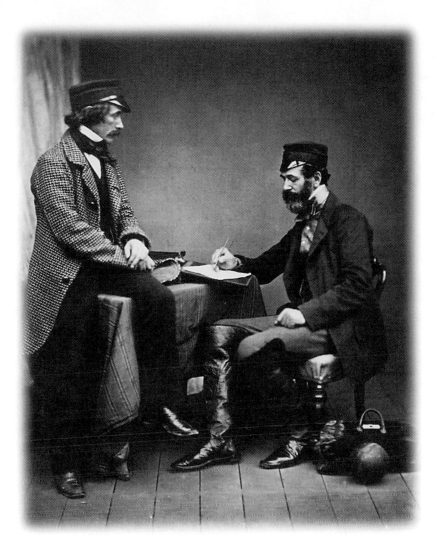

The commission discovered that the water source for the hospital was being contaminated by open privies that couldn't be flushed and had never been cleaned out. A horse carcass was even found in the fresh water supply. Beneath the Barrack Hospital were clogged sewers; the hospital literally sat atop a huge cesspool. Dead animals and hundreds of cartloads of rubbish were removed from under the hospital, and a system was installed to flush out the sewers. Openings were made in the roof to improve air circulation. Rotten shelves and floors were torn out, eliminating breeding places for rats and mice. The inside walls and floors were painted with disinfectant. The courtyards around the building were paved and rubbish was removed. The double rows of mattresses were decreased to one, and orderlies were assigned to empty waste containers and debris from the wards and corridors on a daily basis. Aided by the improving weather and the lack of major fighting, these sanitary improvements had a striking effect: By June — only 3 months later — the mortality rate at Scutari had fallen from 42.7 deaths per 1,000 to 2 per 1,000.

Although Nightingale didn't conceive the idea for the commission, her letters to former Secretary at War Sidney Herbert, along with the personal correspondence of many others to those in government and the newspaper reports, helped create the

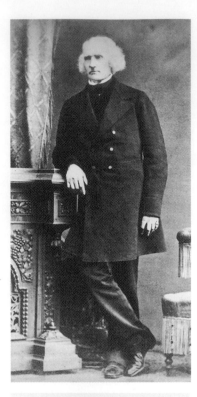

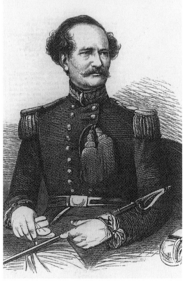

Sir John McNeill, (1795-1883), top, and Colonel Alexander Tulloch (1801-1864), who were sent to the Crimea in 1855 by the government to report on the management of the Commissarial system

momentum that eventually led to its creation. Nightingale stated in 1857 that it was the Sanitary Commission that had saved the British army. The Commission's head, Dr. Sutherland, became one of Nightingale's staunchest supporters as well as her personal physician. After the Crimea, he worked with her almost daily on army and sanitary reform until his retirement in 1888. Rawlinson, the third Commission member, also remained good friends with Nightingale after the war.

Commissariat Commission

The Commissariat Commission was to investigate the status of supplies, food, and clothing for the British army in the Crimea. The two members of the commission were Sir John McNeill and Colonel (later Major General) Alexander Tulloch.

Born in Scotland, McNeill joined the East India Company as an assistant-surgeon in Bombay in 1816 and rose rapidly through the ranks. He served in several positions in the Foreign Service and was appointed minister plenipotentiary to Persia in 1836. Since 1845, he had served in his native Scotland as Chairman of the Poor Law Board, where his skillful management greatly mitigated the effects of the potato famine, which devastated Scotland as it had Ireland. McNeill had also been a friend and colleague of Lord Palmerston since the 1830s and was known as an authority on Russian and Middle Eastern affairs.

Tulloch was an army internal affairs investigator who had trained in the law. While serving with the army in India, he took up reform issues, such as improved diets for soldiers, better salary policies, and improved canteen services, and collected data on troop sickness and mortality, which he published privately in 1835. This report led to an assignment to investigate mortality in the entire army. He also uncovered fraud in pensioners' payments, which led to the creation of a pensioner corps. Tulloch also put his experience with field bakeries to good use in the Crimea, arranging for the baking of fresh bread; many soldiers whose teeth were rotting from scurvy craved a morsel of soft bread because they couldn't eat the hard rolls.

At Scutari, the problems involving supplies, food, and equipment that McNeill and Tulloch identified were precisely those that Nightingale had been writing about to Herbert since her arrival. Although Tulloch wanted to assign personal blame for the blunders and incompetence that the team found, McNeill, who was older and more politically astute, calmed his colleague and made sure that their reports were careful and free of personal recriminations. Because of his many years in Persia, McNeill was familiar with the countries bordering the Black Sea and personally knew many of the British diplomats. He immediately began obtaining and delivering fresh beef and poultry, vegetables, forage, and fuel to the army in the Crimea.

The two commissioners mandated a new system of inventory and release of supplies by the Purveyor's Department. Their report, known as the McNeill-Tulloch Report, published in January 1856, created a long-running controversy in England between the reform politicians and the obstructionists in the War Office. Both McNeill and Tulloch would remain close colleagues of Nightingale's after the war.

A rare healing presence

Nightingale's compassion and care elicited the appreciation and admiration of the soldiers. Whenever a new group of sick and wounded soldiers arrived, she was often up for 20 hours at a stretch, dressing wounds and tending to dying patients without stopping. She was especially attentive to the severest cases, often asking to take care of them. When she walked the wards at night with her lantern, the soldiers saluted her. Nightingale's midnight vigils in the wards were made famous by descriptions such as this one in the *Times*:

> *Wherever there is disease in its most dangerous form and the hand of the despoiler distressingly nigh, there is that incomparable woman sure to be seen. Her benignant presence is an influence for good comfort, even amid the struggles of expiring nature. She is a "ministering angel" without any exaggeration in these hospitals, and as her slender form glides quietly along each corridor, every poor fellow's face softens with gratitude at the sight of her. When all medical officers have retired for the night and silence and darkness have settled down upon those miles of prostrate sick, she may be observed alone, with a little lamp in her hand, making her solitary rounds.[7]*

She talked to the soldiers and cheered them with her calm voice, warm smile, and gentle touch, and they hung on her every word. She often wrote personal, caring letters to the mothers or wives of soldiers who died, such as the following:

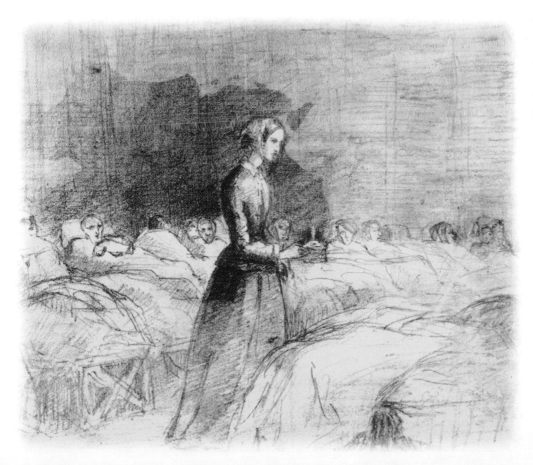

A sketch that appeared in the Illustrated London News in 1855 of Nightingale making rounds in one of the wards, carrying the lamp later immortalized in Longfellow's poem "Santa Filomena"

The first time I saw your son was in going round the wards in the General Hospital at Bala-clava. He had been brought in, in the morning ... He was always conscious, and remained so till the very last. He prayed aloud so beautifully that, as the Nurse in charge said, "It was like a sermon to hear him." He asked "to see Miss Nightingale." He knew me, and expressed himself to me as entirely resigned to die. He pressed my hand when he could not speak. He died in the night ... He was decently interred in a burial-ground we have about a mile from Balaclava. One of my own Sisters lies in the same ground, to whom I have erected a monument. Should you wish anything similar to be done over the grave of your lost son, I will endeavour to gratify you, if you will inform me of your wishes. With true sympathy for your loss, I remain, dear Madam, yours sincerely, Florence Nightingale.[8]

The soldiers she so caringly ministered to and many of the medical officers and surgeons she worked with sang Nightingale's praises in letters to families and friends, which were then circulated to others. Soon, Florence Nightingale became a household name in all the villages, cottages, and factories of England. One soldier wrote home: "What a comfort it was to see her pass even. She would speak to one and nod and smile to as many more; but she could not do it to all, you know. We lay there by hundreds; but we could kiss her shadow as it fell, and lay our heads on the pillow again, content." Another wrote: "Before she came there was cussin' and swearin', but after that it was holy as a church."[9]

By all accounts, Nightingale had a rare healing presence among the soldiers, conveying hope in a way that helped them endure pain and suffering. Member of Parliament Augustus Stafford, who had assisted Nightingale at Scutari, told Richard Monckton Milnes, her former suitor, that "Florence in the hospital makes intelligible to him the Saints of the Middle Ages. If the soldiers were told that the roof had opened, and she had gone up palpably to Heaven, they would not be the least surprised. They quite believe she is in several places at once."[10] Some soldiers even likened her to Joan of Arc. Her obvious leadership qualities led many at the hospital to say, "If she were at their head, they would be in Sebastopol in a week."[11]

More improvements

With sanitary conditions much improved at the Barrack Hospital, Nightingale now began to focus on other ways of helping her patients. She found the soldiers eager for education — they weren't the "scum of the earth," as some officers called them. She hired two schoolmasters to teach the men how to read and write, and she provided books, stationery and stamps for writing letters home, maps, newspapers, and games. She also established the "Inkerman Cafe," an alternative to the canteen, in a small house midway between the two main hospitals in Scutari. Some of the officers viewed her initiatives with disdain and told her to quit spoiling the "brutes." Instead she increased her efforts, setting up a second school in a hut between the two large hospitals.

No smooth mechanism existed for the soldiers to send money home when they were paid. Continuing the work of Rev. Sydney G. Osborne, who had since left Scutari, Nightingale established a temporary Money Order Office, where on four afternoons

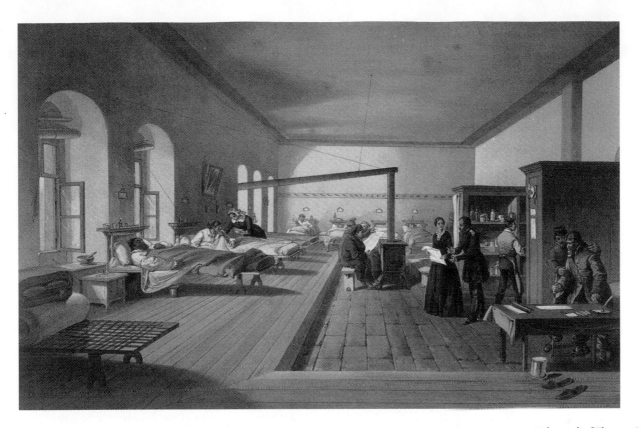

Lithograph of Florence Nightingale speaking with a British officer in the Barrack Hospital, c. 1855

each month she would receive soldiers' money and send it to her Uncle Sam Smith back in England. He in turn would obtain English money orders, which he'd then forward to the soldiers' families. At first, around £1,000 was collected each month, but word soon spread and the soldiers in the Crimea wanted the plan extended to them. Nightingale's proposal to accommodate their wishes was accepted by the war's end.

Religious friction continues

Although the nurses eventually won the respect of many of the doctors at Scutari for their caregiving skills, there was ongoing mistrust between Nightingale and the Kinsale nuns, primarily over the issue of "proselytizing." Some of the friction arose from their different perceptions of what constituted appropriate "ministering" to their patients. Nightingale felt that Mother Bridgeman and the Kinsale nuns were taking advantage of their situation and sometimes doing the work of priests.[12] To Mother Bridgeman, however, the nuns weren't preaching doctrine or administering the sacraments, they were simply sympathizing with and caring for the soldiers as a good mother might.

Above all, Nightingale wanted to avoid having the proselytizing controversy spread back to England, where it could cause difficulty for the government and possibly derail her sacred mission of saving lives and establishing a military nursing system. However, word did filter back to England, to Catholic circles in Ireland, and even to the Vatican. Mother Bridgeman received a blessing from the Pope with instructions to "hold your ground until you shall be sent away by force, but do not let your enemies frighten you away."[13]

The agreement with the government that Henry Manning had originally crafted, with its loophole of autonomy for the Kinsale nuns, guaranteed that religious friction would continue until the end of the war. However, the intent of Herbert, now out of office, and the government was always clear, as he wrote to Nightingale in March 1855:

There is no doubt that the unwelcome batch of nurses were meant to be under your authority ... As regards the agreement with the R.C. sisters, if they have represented that it was not binding on them they have deceived you, as they were bound by it in the same way and to the same extent as those who went out with you.[14]

Doctrinal disputes aside, Mother Bridgeman made many improvements at the Koulali hospitals and the General Hospital in Balaclava. She taught the orderlies in the General Hospital about cleanliness and job responsibility. After she took over the delivery of stimulants to the patients, the orderlies became more sober and useful on the wards. She soon won the respect and admiration of soldiers, doctors, and orderlies alike.

Mary Stanley, who had led the second group of nurses to Scutari, found herself unsuited to the rigors of hospital work and returned to England in March 1855. Several more contingents of nurses arrived after the Stanley party. By April, 125 ladies, nuns, and lay nurses were working in the various British military hospitals. Although Nightingale, through administrative bungling at the beginning of her mission, didn't supervise the women working outside of Scutari, she was responsible for keeping records on them.

Memorial for the dead

Nightingale witnessed 3,000 deaths in January and February 1855 and was saddened by the sight of the many graves near the Barrack Hospital. She often saw the Turkish workers who buried the British dead kneel toward Mecca and pray when they heard the call to prayer from the minarets of the nearby mosques. Around this time, at the request of Queen Victoria, the Sultan of Turkey granted permission to establish an official British cemetery at Scutari.

When the queen asked Nightingale if she might do anything else to assist her, Nightingale requested that an obelisk be erected as a memorial to the dead in a lovely spot overlooking the Sea of Marmara, between the General Hospital and the Barrack Hospital. It was a spot that Nightingale described in a letter to her family, early in March 1855:

... I was walking home late from the Gen'l Hospt'l round the cliff, my favorite way, & looking, I really believe for the first time, at the view — the sea glassy calm & of the purest sapphire blue — the sky dark deep blue — one solitary bright star rising above Constantinople — our whole fleet standing with sails idly spread to catch the breeze which was none ... the domes & minarets of Constantinople sharply standing out against the bright gold of the sunset — the transparent opal of the distant hills, (a color one never sees but in the East) which stretch below Olympus always snowy & on the other side the Sea of Marmara ...[15]

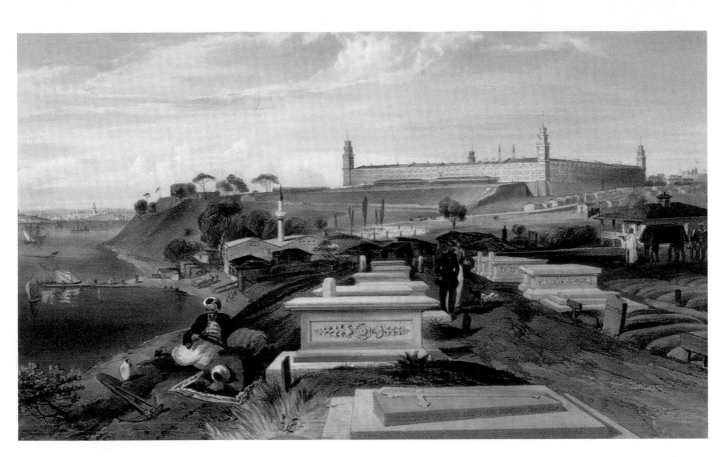

An 1856 lithograph of the British military cemetery in Scutari, with a Turkish gravedigger kneeling on his prayer rug, and the Barrack Hospital in the background

The queen sent the Sultan an official request to allow a memorial to be built in the British cemetery. The Sultan granted approval and, in March, Nightingale began planning the memorial. In a letter enlisting her sister's help in obtaining a design for the monument and determining its cost, Nightingale also reflected on her own role and that of her fellow Englishmen:

My dearest, I hope you are doing something about the Monument. The people here want to have a Cross — they do not see that immediately will arise the question, Greek or Latin Cross — that we cannot have our Cross in a country where all [Christians] are Greek — still less can we have the Greek Cross — besides the ill grace of our setting up a Cross at all who are fighting for the Crescent. But these people cannot be made to see this ...

The whole of the gigantic misfortune has been like a Greek tragedy — it has been like the fates pursuing us. Every thing that has been done [the entire Crimean campaign] has been a failure & nobody knows the reason why — the Gods have punished with blindness some past sin & visited the innocent with the consequences ...

... first [ascertain] ... whether [the] Queen wishes to interfere. If she has no commands, set to work at once. I should like "Wingless Victory" for Chapel — one single solitary column for monument to greet first our ships coming up the Sea of Marmara. It is such a position — high o'er the cliffs we shall save in vain ...

... Let us live at least in our dead. Five thousand & odd brave hearts sleep there — three thousand, alas! dead in Jan. & Feb. alone — here ... I wish to keep their remembrance on earth — for we have been the Thermopylae of this desperate struggle, when Raglan & cold & famine have been the Persians, our own destroyers. We have endured in brave Grecian silence

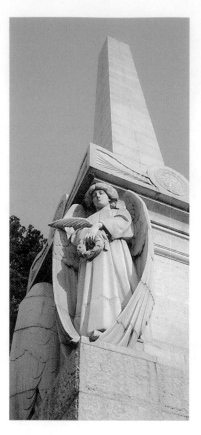

Closeup of the British Soldiers Memorial, erected at Nightingale's request at the British military cemetery, today known as the Haydarpasa Cemetery, Üsküdar, Turkey

...We have folded our mantles about our faces & died in silence without complaining. No one can say we have complained.

And as for myself, I have done my duty. I have identified my fate with that of the heroic dead, & whatever lies these sordid exploiteurs of human misery spread about us these officials, there is a right & a God to fight for & our fight has been worth fighting. I do not despair — nor complain — It has been a great cause.[16]

Parthe began recruiting help for the memorial, and individual grave markers began to be placed at the request of families. The finished monument, erected in 1857, carried the inscription: "To the memory of the British soldiers and sailors, who during the years 1854 and 1855 died far from their country in defence of the liberties of Europe. This monument is erected by the gratitude of Queen Victoria and her people. 1857."

By April 1855, Nightingale was physically exhausted and overcome with a sense of failure because of the slow pace of army reform and her continuing administrative and religious problems with the diverse group of ladies and nuns serving as nurses. In May, summing up the chaos of the first 6 months, Nightingale said:

The horrors of the war were not wounds, blood, fever, dysentery, and famine, but intoxication, drunken brutality, demoralization, and disorder on the part of the inferior; jealousies, meanness, indifference, selfish brutality on the part of the superior.[17]

First trip to the Crimea

After the physical improvements had been made at the Barrack Hospital and the number of casualties began to level off, Nightingale obtained approval from the War Office in the spring of 1855 to make her first trip to the Crimea to inspect the hospitals there.

In addition to the regimental hospitals in the Crimea, there were four general hospitals. The General Hospital at Balaclava was established shortly after the arrival of troops in September 1854. In April 1855, after Palmerston's reforms had began to produce improvements, the Castle Hospital, built of prefabricated huts and capable of accommodating 2,500 patients, opened on the hillside above Balaclava. The Hospital of St. George Monastery also consisted of huts for convalescents and ophthalmic patients, as did the hospitals of the Land Transport Corps near Karani. All of these hospitals had female nurses, although the Monastery Hospital had none until December 1855 and the Land Transport Hospitals not until 1856. By spring of 1855, the nurses at the General Hospital and the Castle Hospital had their own superintendents, assigned by the medical officers.

On May 2, 1855, 10 days before her 35th birthday, Nightingale began the 300-mile journey by ship from Scutari across the Black Sea to the Crimea. She was accompanied by Charles Bracebridge; four nurses, one of whom one was her favorite, Mrs. Roberts; Alexis Soyer, the London chef who had made major improvements in the hospital kitchens, and his manservant; a 12-year-old drummer boy named Thomas, who called himself "Miss Nightingale's man"; an invalid soldier from the 68th Light Infantry, whom Bracebridge had hired as a messenger; and 420 soldiers returning to the trenches.

The party arrived in Balaclava on May 5, with Nightingale feeling healthy, but tired. Word had spread that she was coming to visit, and the vantage points along the small harbor and on the decks of ships were packed with people eager for a glimpse of the already famous Lady Superintendent.

One of her first duties was to pay a formal visit to the headquarters of Lord Raglan, the Commander-in-Chief of the British army in the Crimea, but he was away from camp. Being a good horsewoman, Nightingale was mounted "upon a very pretty mare, which, by its gambols and caracoling, seemed proud to carry its noble charge, and our cavalcade produced an extraordinary effect upon the motley crowd of all nations assembled at Balaclava, who were astonished at seeing a lady so well escorted."[18] She was taken to a mortar battery, and along the way the troops cheered for her:

> *The brave 39th, whose Regimental Hospitals are the best I have ever seen, turned out & gave Florence Nightingale three times three, as I rode away. There was nothing empty in the cheer nor in the heart which received it. I took it as a true expression of true sympathy — the sweetest I have ever had. I took it as a full reward of all I have gone through. I promised my God that I would not die of disgust or disappointment, if he would let me go through this. In all that has been said against me & for me, no one soul has appreciated what I was really doing, none but the honest cheer of the brave 39th ...[19]*

One day, Nightingale, Bracebridge, and their party rode on horseback to survey Sebastopol from the heights, not far from the British camp just beyond the Russian artillery range. She wrote to Parthe of the experience:

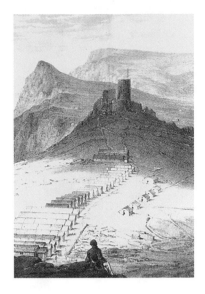

The Castle Hospital huts that were built near Balaclava in April 1855 with contributions by British citizens

BELOW: *Nightingale, en route to the Crimea, tending to a soldier on deck*

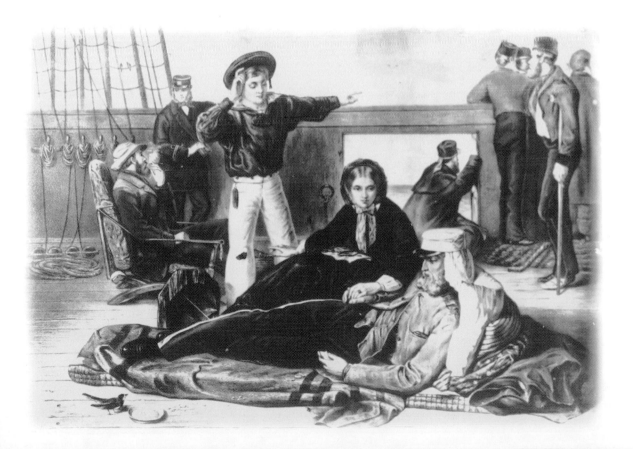

It was a wonderful sight looking down upon Sebastopol — the shells whizzing right & left. I send you ... some little flowers. For this is the most flowery place you can imagine — a beautiful red Tormentilla which I don't know, yellow jasmine & every kind of low flowering shrub. A sergeant of the 97th picked me a nosegay. I once saved Serjt.'s life by finding him at 12 o'clock at night lying — wounds undressed — in our Hospl. with a bullet in his eye & a fractured skull. And I pulled a stray Surgeon out of bed to take the bullet out ...[20]

Nightingale wrote about the striking 20-square-mile scene of huts and tents at the main encampment on the heights above Sebastopol. Troop reinforcements had begun to arrive in the spring, and she was inspired by the panorama of some 150,000 troops working for a single purpose.

During her stay in the Crimea, Nightingale actively investigated the hospitals and regiments and attended to business matters in connection with the various nursing groups. She received Sir John McNeill and Colonel Alexander Tulloch, who had worked wonders with the Commissariat Commission. She discussed the building of new huts and improved kitchens with Soyer, the chef who had accompanied her. She and her party toured the General Hospital and the Castle Hospital, and she wrote about the conditions she found:

Nothing which the "Times" has said has been exaggerated of Hardship. Sir John McNeill is the man I like the best of all who have come out. He has dragged [sic] Commissary General out of the mud. He has done wonders. Every body now has their fresh meat 3 times a week, their fresh bread from Constantinople about as often.[21]

Nightingale had interpreted her orders as an authorization to consult the Principal Medical Officer and inspect the nursing establishment at each hospital. However, her original orders, issued with the understanding that she was to be supervisor of all

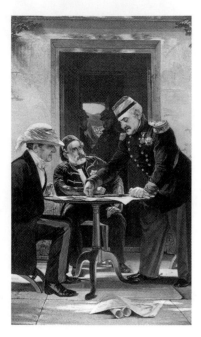

Lord Raglan, British Commander (left), Omar Pasha, Ottoman Turkish Commander (center), and General Pelissier, French Commander (right), meeting during the siege of Sebastopol

RIGHT: *Lord Raglan's headquarters*

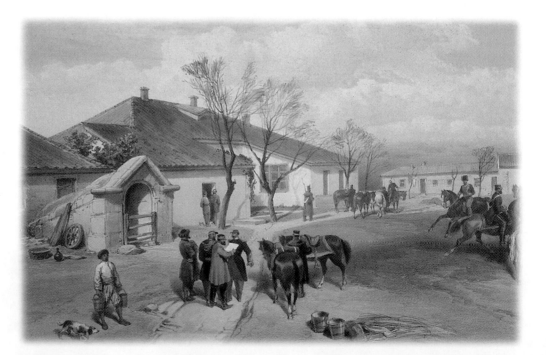

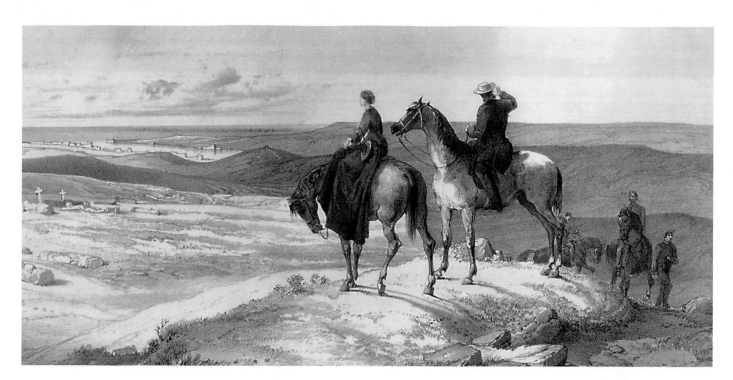

Florence Nightingale and Charles Bracebridge surveying Sebastopol in May 1855 in a drawing by Nightingale's sister, Parthe

nurses, had been issued when the government had anticipated that the war would be over in a matter of weeks and that only a limited number of nurses would be used at a few hospitals near Constantinople. Moreover, Nightingale's trip to the Crimea exposed the flaw that named her superintendent of nurses only in Turkey, not in the Crimea.

Dr. John Hall, Inspector-General of Hospitals for the Crimean campaign, was only too happy to interpret her orders by the letter and the word. She referred to him in her private notes as a "fossil of the pure Red Sandstone."[22] Although Hall and David Fitzgerald, the Chief Purveyor in the Crimea, were cordial to her face, both men continually blocked her suggestions and requests for supplies.

Felled by illness

Fearless in the face of contagion, Nightingale attended to patients stricken with fever. When Alexis Soyer expressed distress over the length of time she spent with one infectious soldier, Nightingale said that she had seen too many cases to dread the experience of infection.[23]

Nevertheless, on May 12, 1855, Nightingale fell ill, complaining of tremendous fatigue. She sent for Dr. Arthur Anderson, the Principal Medical Officer at Balaclava, who believed that she was suffering from a severe case of Crimean fever and advised her to leave the ship on which she was staying. Although it was only a 5-minute walk to the Castle Hospital, Nightingale was carried on a stretcher by four guardsmen and was placed in a private hut behind those of the wounded soldiers.

During the next 2 weeks, Nightingale's condition fluctuated between satisfactory and critical, with sudden relapses in the morning, followed by recovery and then another relapse in the evening. Her long hair was cropped short, probably to increase her comfort. Although she was advised to rest, then the only treatment known, Nightingale

The strangers in whom she most delighted were Mr & Mrs Bracebridge, both well acquainted with her birthplace, & who always addressed her in Greek, and she spent a great part of every day investigating the shelves in the library, hours indeed she used to remain at the back of the largest quartos. Her toilette (as is supposed to be the case sometimes with literary ladies) suffered much from these excursions, and by the end of the winter she generally had not a feather left in her tail. Her French attendant used to be exceedingly unhappy on such occasions, & remark that company was coming, & that "Monsieur Iuir" as Athena was occasionally called) was "tout rond et pas beau du tout, & what a pity it was, & could nothing be done?

tip & finger to receive her one daily meal, opening her wings wide as she swallowed each piece of meat at her hand.

The following year she took a second journey into Germany, the waters of Karlsbad having been thought good for her health. She seemed to enjoy her travels & the respect that was paid to her exceedingly, tho objecting to the universal 'Kalbfleisch' as much as others

Two drawings of Nightingale's pet owl, Athena, from the book Parthe created to amuse her sister during her convalescence from Crimean fever

was not without her pen and paper. Writings during this time reveal that her mind wandered and she was unable to concentrate. Soyer recorded in his diary that Anderson said that she "suffered from as bad an attack of fever as I have seen."[24] Nursed by Mrs. Roberts, Nightingale was extremely weak for several more weeks and was unable to feed herself or to speak above a whisper.

One day when a soldier arrived to see her, Roberts refused him entry, until he said that he had ridden a long way to see her and that she knew him well. It was Lord Raglan, who had come to pay his respects. On May 24, Raglan telegraphed back to London that Nightingale was out of danger, and all of England rejoiced. A month later Raglan himself became sick and died within a few days.

Although Nightingale was advised to return to England to recover fully, she was determined to stay in the East until the last soldier had returned to England. In July 1855, Lord Stratford, the British ambassador, arranged for Nightingale to recuperate at his summer residence at Therapia, a few miles west of Constantinople. She was reported to look much older than her age because she was emaciated, weak, and pale.

During her recovery, Nightingale was showered with gifts. Sidney Herbert sent her a terrier, and the troops gave her a baby owl to replace her departed pet, Athena. Parthe wrote and illustrated a charming little book called *Life and Death of Athena, an Owlet from the Parthenon,* and sent it to her. Selina Bracebridge read it aloud while they both laughed and cried. Sutherland announced that Nightingale's fever had saved her life because it forced her to rest.

Near the end of July, Nightingale resumed her letter writing and began to take long evening walks on the shore of the Sea of Marmara. In a letter to Parthe, she commented on the praise being showered on her at home:

> I do not affect indifference towards real sympathy — but I have felt painfully, the more painfully since I have had time to hear of it, the éclat which has been given to this adventure. The small still beginning, the simple hardship, the silent & gradual struggle upwards — these are the climate in which an enterprise really thrives & grows — time has not altered our Saviour's lesson on that point — which has been learnt successively by all reformers, down to Fliedner [pastor at Kaiserswerth], from their own experience ...[25]

Return to the Crimea

By August, Nightingale was back at work. The Bracebridges had returned to England in late July, and her devoted Aunt Mai came to Scutari to assist her. In several letters that Aunt Mai wrote to family and friends, she described firsthand Nightingale's toil behind the scenes:

> ... Hers is perplexing brainwork ... She habitually writes till 1 or 2, sometimes 3 or 4 (AM); has in the last pressure given up 3 whole nights to it ... Such questions as food, rest, temperature never interfere with her during her work ... She is extremely quick and clear ... She has attained a most wonderful calm and presence of mind ...[26]

Nightingale continued to document the organizational chaos and logistical blunders of the British army, generating an enormous correspondence to doctors, both in the East and back in England, and to various government officials. She recognized the political problems and personal jealousies amid the bureaucratic tangles, but she was

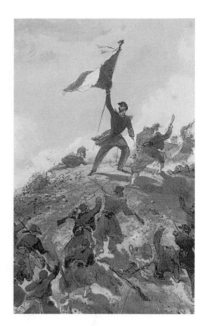

French attack on the Malakoff Fort before the final surrender of the Russians at Sebastopol

LEFT: British officers at Christmas dinner in the camp above Sebastopol. The banner in the rear spells out recent British victories at the Alma River and at Inkerman.

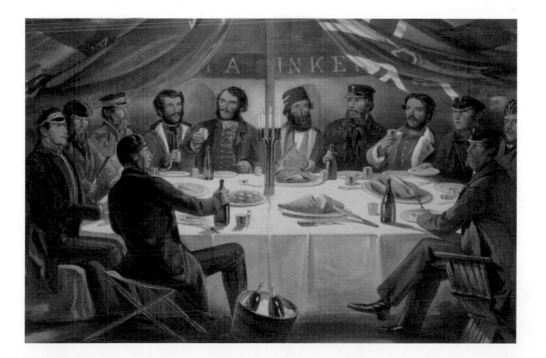

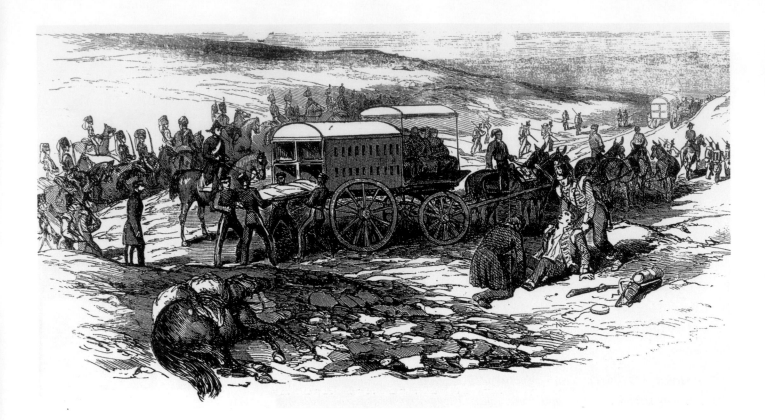

The British army's new ambulance wagon, first used in the later stages of the siege of Sebastopol to transport the wounded

also very aware of her own political strength. She said at one point, "There is not an official who would not burn me like Joan of Arc if he could, but they know that the War Office cannot turn me out because the country is with me."[27]

Ongoing power struggle

On September 9, 1855, after a siege of almost a year, the Russians began to evacuate Sebastopol, and the end of the war was in sight. However, because Secretary of State for War Lord Panmure still hadn't clarified her orders, Nightingale was unable to assert her authority in the Crimea. There was much confusion and resentment between Nightingale, Mother Bridgeman, and the ladies who had been in charge of various hospitals since their arrival in January 1855.

After the fall of Sebastopol, Mother Bridgeman realized that the Sisters' services were no longer needed in Koulali, where they were stationed. She knew that they were needed at Scutari, but she refused to return there to work under Nightingale. Instead, she offered her services to Hall, who accepted. On October 2, she notified Nightingale:

> ... As it seems to me our services should be more needed in the Crimea than elsewhere during the winter, I offer them to Dr. Hall, who has accepted them. I shall therefore, be obliged to withdraw the Sisters from the General Hospital, Scutari. I trust my doing so shall cause no inconvenience. We hope to sail for the Crimea at the beginning of next week. We only got Dr. Hall's reply by last night's post.[28]

Nightingale was aghast that Mother Bridgeman and her Sisters could go to Balaclava in this manner, but she had no recourse to stop them. She and her ally, General

Storks, decided that Nightingale should accompany the women to maintain an appearance of authority. The entire party left for the Crimea on the same ship. Both women were cordial to each other, but shortly after their departure both became seasick and stayed in their cabins until land was sighted. Mother Bridgeman was quickly confirmed as Superintendent of the General Hospital, and Nightingale now pushed harder for clarification of her orders to extend to the Crimea.

As she had foreseen, personnel problems proliferated among the various contingents of ladies, nuns, and nurses — sent without her approval, yet ultimately, she believed, her responsibility — with their differing religious affiliations, political loyalties, social status, and levels of training. Her relationship with Hall worsened, and Mother Bridgeman continued to follow Hall's orders and not Nightingale's.

At the beginning of October, Nightingale had to be admitted to the General Hospital in Balaclava for severe sciatica, symptoms related to her bout of Crimean fever 5 months earlier. By the end of November, she would also be suffering from earaches, chronic laryngitis, dysentery, rheumatism, and insomnia.[29]

To further complicate her work, on October 16, the *Times* reported on a lecture given by Charles Bracebridge that severely criticized the medical and military handling of the war. Although Bracebridge tried to backtrack, saying his comments had been misrepresented, Hall and others believed that Nightingale was behind the attack and this further strained their relationship. Nightingale wrote to Bracebridge urging him to be an "active friend" rather than a "disagreeable enemy," and to avoid such "mere irresponsibility of opposition."[30]

With all of these persistent problems and frustrations facing her, Nightingale became plagued by periodic feelings of despair. Stymied by the bureaucrats' refusal to grant her supervisory authority over all the nurses, she felt that her mission to standardize patient care at all the military hospitals had failed and that she too was a failure.

Nightingale Fund, the Sultan, & the Queen

As word spread throughout England that Nightingale was determined to stay in the East until the last soldier returned home, Sidney Herbert and other leaders saw an opportunity to create something positive out of the Crimean experience. On November 5, 1855, a provisional committee of some 70 distinguished individuals, including the Lord Chief Justice, the Speaker of the House, and Secretary of State for War Lord Panmure, met in London to discuss the creation of a new national fund, to be called the Nightingale Fund, that would be used to promote nurse's training in England as a tribute to Nightingale. A few days later, the following resolution was drafted:

1. The noble exertions of Miss Nightingale in the hospitals of the East demand the grateful recognition of the British people.
2. That while it is known that Miss Nightingale would decline any such recognition merely personal to herself it is understood that she will accept it in a form that may enable her, on her

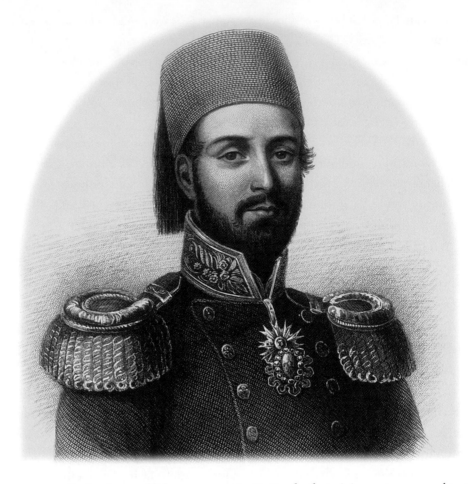

*return to England, to establish a permanent institution for the training, sustenance and protec-
tion of nurses and to arrange for their proper instruction and employment in ... hospitals.*

*3. That to accomplish this object on a scale worthy of the nation and honorable to Miss Night-
ingale herself, a public subscription be opened to which all classes be invited to contribute and
application be made for the "red" [high-ranking] of the clergy, the mayors of corporate towns
and other available sources of assistance.*

*4. That the sums thus collected be applied to these objects according to the discretion of Miss
Nightingale and under regulations formed by herself, the subscribers have entire confidence in
her tried energy and judgement.[31]*

This resolution was amended the following week to state that in the meantime, the
trustees would be considered "protectors of the Fund."

On November 29, the committee held a public meeting chaired by the Duke of
Cambridge, the queen's cousin and head of the army, and an ardent supporter of Nightingale. According to the *Times,* the hall was filled to bursting and the meeting was
"brilliant, enthusiastic, and harmonious."[32] A few blocks away at the Burlington Hotel,
the Nightingale family, too nervous to attend, waited for news of the meeting. They
were gratified to hear of the speeches by Herbert, the Duke of Argyll, Richard Monckton
Milnes, Lord Stanley, and others. W.E.N. wrote to his sister, Aunt Mai, of "our joy at the
universal oneness of the meeting which has honoured Flo with its absolute fiat of 'Well
Done' and well to do."[33] The idea of a training school for nurses, which Florence had
conceived of a decade earlier, was headed toward reality.

Fanny, enjoying her greatest social moment as the elite of England gathered to honor her daughter, later wrote to Nightingale:

It is very late, my child, but I cannot go to bed without telling you that your meeting has been a glorious one. I believe that you will be more indifferent than any of us to fame, but be glad that we feel that this is a proud day for us ...[34]

Nightingale replied:

If my name and my having done what I could for God and mankind has given you pleasure, that is real pleasure to me. My reputation has not been a boon to me in my work: but if you have been pleased, that is enough. I shall love my name now, and I shall feel that it is the greatest return that you can find satisfaction in hearing your child named, and in feeling that her work draws sympathies together some return for what you have done for me. Life is sweet after all.[35]

In the next month, nearly 20,000 circulars about the Nightingale Fund were sent to mayors and prominent clergymen around the country. Pledges totaling £7,000 were soon received, the first installment in a bold venture that would open a new path for women and for nursing.

Rulers' thanks

As a token of his appreciation, the Sultan of Turkey presented Nightingale with a diamond and carnelian bracelet and a sum of money for the nurses, both of which Queen Victoria permitted her to accept. The diamond link-chain bracelet had a deep red-orange carnelian agate medallion, surrounded by diamonds, with a Turkish inscription that translates as "The color of the agate resembles the ruby, and the brilliance of the sunlike diamond [referring to Nightingale] who had a heart like the brilliant sun that radiated love and care. 1855."[36]

About the same time, Nightingale received a letter from the queen:

You are, I know, well aware of the high sense I entertain of the Christian devotion which you have displayed during this great and bloody war, and I need hardly repeat to you how warm my admiration is for your services, which are fully equal to those of my dear and brave soldiers, whose sufferings you have had the privilege of alleviating in so merciful a manner. I am, however, anxious of marking my feelings in a manner which I trust will be agreeable to you, and therefore send you with this letter a brooch, the form and emblems of which commemorate your great and blessed work, and which, I hope, you will wear as a mark of the high approbation of your Sovereign!

It will be a very great satisfaction to me, when you return at last to these shores, to make the acquaintance of one who has set so bright an example to our sex. And with every prayer for the preservation of your valuable health, believe me, always, yours sincerely, Victoria R.[37]

In November, Nightingale received Queen Victoria's gift, which had been designed by Prince Albert. The words "Blessed are the merciful" encircle the badge, which also bears the word "Crimea," with a St. George's cross in red enamel and the royal cypher surmounted by a crown of diamonds. The inscription on the reverse side reads, "To

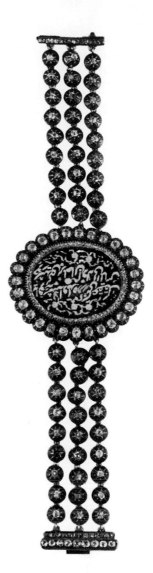

Diamond and carnelian bracelet presented to Nightingale in 1855 by the Sultan of Turkey as a token of appreciation

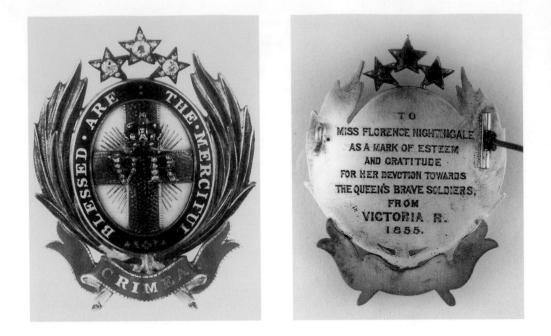

Front and back of the brooch designed by Prince Albert and given to Nightingale by Queen Victoria in 1855

Miss Florence Nightingale, as a mark of esteem and gratitude for her devotion towards the Queen's brave soldiers, From Victoria R. 1855." The queen's gift was publicly announced in the *Morning Post* on December 20.

When Nightingale attended festivities at the British Embassy in Constantinople on Christmas Day, she wore the queen's brooch on a plain black dress with a high collar. She reportedly appeared frail and slight of height, with penetrating eyes, and short hair covered with a white cap and and a lace kerchief. She was too weak to play games but she sat on a sofa and was seen laughing until tears came to her eyes.

Nightingale wrote to thank Queen Victoria for the brooch on December 21. Knowing that her letter would be read to other influential people and not one to miss an opportunity, she also laid out her plan for soldiers to send money home. The Queen sent the letter to Prime Minister Palmerston and Lord Clarendon, the Foreign Secretary, both of whom thought it was a good idea. Despite the reservations of some officials, who doubted that British soldiers would send any money home, the government established post offices for money orders at Constantinople, Scutari, and Balaclava. By the end of the war, the soldiers had sent £71,000 back to England — money that otherwise would most likely have been spent in local taverns.

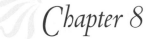
Achieving Command & Control

> *The War Office gives me tinsel & plenty of empty praise which I do not want — and does not give me the real business-like efficient standing which I do want ...*
>
> Florence Nightingale to Sidney Herbert, February 21, 1856[1]

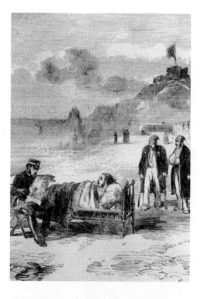

Soldiers convalescing by the Black Sea at their Castle Hospital huts overlooking Balaclava

Notwithstanding her rising fame at the battlefront and at home and the many improvements she had made at Scutari, Nightingale continued to struggle for overall control of her visionary Crimean nursing mission. She was frustrated by the ambiguity of her general orders, which failed to explicitly give her control over the nursing staff in all military hospitals, and by the ongoing administrative conflict with Mother Bridgeman, the head of the Kinsale nuns, who refused to take orders from Nightingale, a Protestant layperson. On top of all this, in January 1855 the Deputy Purveyor, David Fitzgerald, wrote a specious "confidential report" praising Mother Bridgeman and blasting Nightingale. This report was circulated in antireform circles by Dr. John Hall, Inspector-General of Hospitals in the Crimea. After a year in the East, Nightingale felt as if she were fighting for the very existence of her work.

Help was on the way, however. In early October 1855, Colonel John Henry Lefroy, the Confidential Advisor in Scientific Matters to Lord Panmure, Secretary of State for War, arrived in Scutari to draft a secret report for Panmure on the true state of the military hospitals. Nightingale told him of her political and bureaucratic struggles stemming from her ambiguous general orders and of her ongoing clashes with Mother Bridgeman, Dr. Hall, and Fitzgerald, who was one of Hall's allies. After hearing Nightingale's side of the story, Lefroy went on to the Crimea with admiration for her work, insight about her mission, and an understanding of the jurisdictional problems created by the ambiguity of her original orders regarding Turkey and the Crimea.

When he arrived in Balaclava in January 1856, Lefroy met with Mother Bridgeman, observed the Sisters at work (and was impressed by them), and asked about her prob-

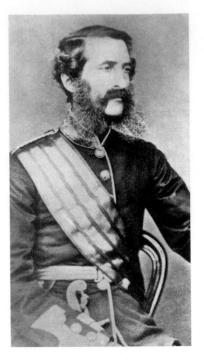

Colonel John Henry Lefroy, whose confidential report to the Secretary of State for War resulted in Nightingale's finally receiving official orders as General Superintendent of the Female Nursing Establishment of the Military Hospitals of the Army

RIGHT: *Florence Nightingale, c. 1856, making her rounds between the Crimean hospitals in her buggy, which was provided by the army*

lems with Nightingale. While conducting his investigation, he also asked Fitzgerald to draft a confidential report on the Crimean nursing contingent since its introduction in January 1855. Fitzgerald's report praised Mother Bridgeman and her Sisters highly and criticized Nightingale and the nurses who worked under her at Scutari. It also opposed the idea of appointing Nightingale superintendent of all nurses in the Crimea. Despite Fitzgerald's conclusions, when Lefroy returned to London in February he strongly recommended to Panmure that the entire nursing staff should be centralized under one superintendent — Florence Nightingale.

That same month, Nightingale realized she must firmly fight for her cause with the Medical Department and the War Office. To her, it seemed that Fitzgerald's negative report had undermined all her work, and she wrote to her friend Sidney Herbert, former Secretary at War, pressing him to do everything he could to convince Lord Panmure to clarify her orders. To strengthen her position, she enclosed a letter from her friend and advisor, Dr. John Sutherland of the Sanitary Commission, which urged Nightingale to obtain a formal mandate extending her authority to all hospitals north of the Bosporus and giving her the final approval on the transfer of nurses to different hospitals. He felt that these points were imperative to her mission and must be written into the general orders, particularly if the war in the East continued.

Nightingale's ascendancy complete

After studying Lefroy's report, Panmure decided at last that a strong, centralized nursing authority was the best way to maintain the health of the troops in the field and, on February 25, 1856, he finally put in writing the authority Nightingale had requested. On March 16, the day she set sail for her third trip to the Crimea, Nightingale's clarified role was officially placed in the general orders. Nightingale had achieved a major objective

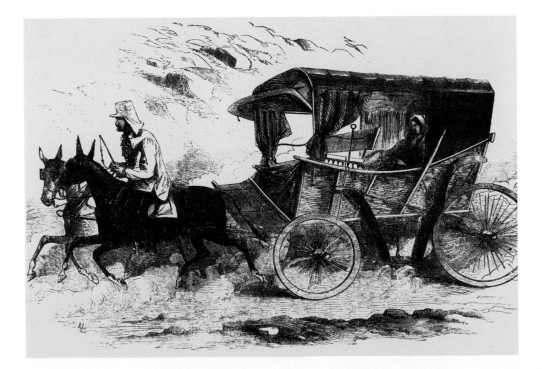

that would be followed in all future wars: All nurses in the military would henceforth be accountable to one superintendent.

Nightingale considered her last trip to the Crimea the third great period of her service during the war — the first being her initial work at the Barrack Hospital in Scutari through the difficult winter of 1855, and the second, caring for the wounded at Balaclava during the fall of 1855 and winter of 1856. On this last Crimean journey she was able to consolidate her authority, travelling long distances between scattered hospitals to set up programs for recuperating soldiers, such as recreation and reading rooms, and arranging for them to send money home.

When Nightingale met with Mother Bridgeman at the General Hospital on March 25 to inform her of her new official status, Mother Bridgeman still refused to submit to her authority. To avoid further difficulty with Nightingale and the possibility that the Sisters of Mercy might eventually be sent home like the Norwood nuns, Hall and Fitzgerald advised Mother Bridgeman to resign "before Miss Nightingale could humble or mortify her with the only alternative."[2]

Sisters of Mercy return home

Despite all her differences with Mother Bridgeman, Nightingale didn't want the Sisters to resign because she felt such an action would "make [them] martyrs."[3] However, Mother Bridgeman refused to reconsider. On April 12, 1856, the Sisters of Mercy boarded a steamship and left Turkey — much more quietly than they had come. They arrived in London on May 8 and were accommodated at the Convent of Mercy in Blandford Square in Chelsea.

It's a sad fact in the history of the Crimean War and of nursing in general that the Sisters of Mercy were never recognized by the English government in the way that Nightingale was and that the memory of their dedicated service was allowed to fade. The War Office never sent them any decorations, offered them eulogies, or even recorded the names of those who had served. Because they had volunteered their services, they weren't even reimbursed for their travel expenses back to their different convents.

They were, however, offered a gift of £230 from the Sultan of Turkey as a token of appreciation for their services. Because they feared that they would offend the Sultan if they refused it, the sisters asked their superiors how best to handle the gift. They were told to distribute the money among the poor and keep none for themselves. Each of the Convents of Mercy received its pro rata share of the money according to the number of Sisters from each establishment who served in the war.

When the Irish Sisters returned to their respective convents later in May, they tried to arrive without fanfare but word spread rapidly and the countryside was ablaze with bonfires and tar barrels at special vantage points to welcome them home. Hundreds of townspeople in Kinsale showed their affection for Mother Bridgeman by attending a solemn Mass of Thanksgiving in her honor. Soon after, she was appointed Mistress of Novices at the convent, a position in which she assisted the young nuns in developing their talents. She was later reappointed Mother Superior, a position that she held until her death 30 years later. Today Mother Bridgeman is remembered in her convent and in the annals of the Sisters of Mercy as a great nun and a woman of prayer, kindness, and gentleness. Her community continues to view her assertiveness in the Crimea as a virtue, not as rebellion, as seen by Nightingale and other officials.

Controversy over the Nightingale Fund

As the Crimean War drew to a close, support was building back in England for the Nightingale Fund's plan to establish the first secular nursing school based on Nightingale's principles. Nightingale herself, however, had mixed feelings about the Fund. Although she appreciated the sympathy and confidence in her that the Fund implied, she doubted whether her health would allow her to take on the burden of administering it. She suggested that the collected monies be entrusted to Sidney Herbert, Charles Bracebridge, and a few others she recommended, who could then decide on the appropriate use.[4] She confided to Bracebridge on January 31, 1856:

> 1. The people of England say to me by this Subscription — "We trust you — we wish you to do us a service." No love or confidence can be shown to a human being greater than this — and as such I accept it gratefully and hopefully. I hope I shall never decline any work God — & the people of England offer me. But 2. I have no plan at all ... and no fear presents itself more strongly to my mind, no certainty of failure more complete — than accompany the idea of beginning anything of the nature proposed to me ...
>
> ... If I have a plan in me ... it would be simply this — to take the poorest & least organized Hospital in London, & putting myself in there — see what I could do — not touching the "Fund" perhaps for years — not till experience had shown how the Fund might be best available ...
>
> At the same time — would I could say (which I cannot) how much I feel the love & confidence of the people of England — in whose service as I have lived — so I shall die.[5]

Religious rivalries began almost as soon as the Fund was announced. Although Nightingale, an Anglican, had envisioned a secular training program, some Catholics soon began expressing suspicions that the fund was intended to honor Nightingale personally or to establish a Protestant charity. A letter to the Catholic journal *The Table* on February 29, 1856, revealed some of these concerns:

> You are aware ... that a large sum of money is being collected for what is called the "Nightingale Fund." When asking the contribution of the poor Catholic soldiers, the expression used by the collectors is "Your subscription is expected for Miss Nightingale and the Sisters of Mercy"... Now Sir, will you in your journal ... inform the Catholic soldiers whether the Sisters of Mercy or Charity will have any part in this collection? And you will oblige me, and perhaps check a fraudulent scheme, by informing the public whether the fund is for the purpose of personally complimenting Miss Nightingale or for the establishment of a Protestant charitable institution? If for either object, the present manner of collecting the Fund is a swindle — an obtaining of money under false pretenses.[6]

Some Protestants, on the other hand, wrote articles attacking Herbert and Nightingale about their beliefs, suggesting that Nightingale was almost a Roman Catholic. It was difficult for many people to conceive of a nurse training program outside the framework of the Catholic or Anglican Church. For her part, Nightingale didn't have a clear idea of how the money would be used — other than that it would be for some sort of secular training program — or when she would be able to begin the program.

The Fund's committee members distributed leaflets in railway stations and gave public speeches to raise money, and the *Times* published articles about meetings, reports, and subscribers. The people of New Zealand sent a contribution of £1,000. Sir William Codrington, who had succeeded Raglan as Commander-in-Chief of the British Army in the East, recommended that each soldier donate a day's pay. Only three doctors contributed, but the troops gave enthusiastically. In the end, the army donated £9,000 to the Fund, and the Navy and the Coast Guard also donated.

The largest individual donations came from the upper class, the highest being £300. Many £25 gifts came from unmarried women for whom Nightingale and her work held a special meaning. Even people who donated just a few shillings had their names placed on the subscribers list. A March concert in London by Jenny Lind, the famous soprano known as "the Swedish nightingale," brought in nearly £2,000.

In the end, the Nightingale Fund raised about £44,000 (approximately £2,036,100 or US$3,380,000 in today's values) as of June 20, 1856.[7] A Deed of Trust was drawn up stating that Nightingale would direct the investment of the funds and could use the money at a date yet to be determined. The nurses training program was eventually established in 1860 using a portion of the money from the Nightingale Fund.

Last months in the Crimea

In March 1855, Czar Nicholas I of Russia died, and his successor, Alexander II, made peace overtures to the Allies. In September, after the French had seized a key position, the Russian army evacuated Sebastopol. Leaving nothing of valve, they set fire to the town and ships in the harbor, and blew up the forts behind them. The Crimean War ended on March 30, 1856, with the signing of the Treaty of Paris.

Nightingale remained in Balaclava with four Sisters of Bermondsey to tend to the dwindling number of convalescing soldiers. She spent much of her time during this period writing her final reports. When her loyal supporter Mother Mary Clare Moore was forced to leave because of ill health in April, Nightingale wrote her a farewell letter:

> *Your going home is the greatest blow I have had yet ... I do not presume to express praise or gratitude to you, Rev'd Mother, because it would look as if I thought you had done the work not unto God but unto me. You were far above me in fitness for the General Superintendency, both in worldly talent of administration, & far more in the spiritual qualifications which God values in a Superior. My being placed over you in our unenviable reign of the East was my misfortune & not my fault ... I will ask you to forgive me for everything and anything which I may unintentionally have done, which can ever have given you pain, remembering only that I have always felt what I have just expressed — & that it has given me more pain to reign over you than to you to serve under me ...[8]*

Nightingale and her four assistants lived under harsh conditions for the remainder of their stay in the Crimea. In the meantime, as donations to the *Times* Fund continued

Profile of the 10 parties of women (totaling 229) sent to serve as nurses in British military hospitals in Turkey during the Crimean War, most of whom Nightingale never had the opportunity to supervise

British Nursing Parties in Turkey

Party	Number of women	Superintendent	Date of arrival	Destination
1	39	Florence Nightingale	Nov. 4, 1854	Scutari
2	47	Mary Stanley	Dec. 15, 1854	Scutari
3	43	Mrs. Holme Coote	Unknown	Smyrna
4	7	Not identified	Unknown	Scutari
5	27	E. Hutton	Apr. 9, 1855	Koulali
6	14	Not identified	Apr. 21, 1855	Koulali
7	6	Mrs. C. Willoughby Moore	Unknown	Officers
8	26	Mrs. Newman	July 23, 1855	Renkioi
9	3	Rev. Mr. Sabin	Unknown	Scutari
10	3	Sr. Mary Ellis	Jan. 22, 1856	Scutari

Adapted with permission by Irene Sabelberg Palmer. Florence Nightingale and the First Organized Delivery of Nursing Services. *Washington, D.C.: American Association of Colleges of Nursing, 1983.*

to grow, and as the Purveyor's Department became more efficient, Nightingale was actually able to offer aid to the other Allied armies. When typhus broke out among the French in the spring of 1856, she sent them medical supplies, wine, and arrowroot. She also provided assistance to the Turks and Greeks and gave medical supplies to the Sardinian Sisters of Mercy when one of their supply ships was destroyed in a fire.

Final reports on the nurses

Nightingale's work in the Crimea represented the first organized delivery of British nursing services in wartime with female nurses under a woman superintendent. During her 20 months in the East, 229 nurses were sent to serve in the British hospitals; 11 died there of typhus, cholera, and other diseases.[9] Only 17 served for the duration of the war.

Although Nightingale emerged as the central figure in the Crimean drama, the heroic work of all these women demonstrated to the British military that women could make a vital contribution to the army in wartime. In addition, the nurses' efforts were politically important because they set the stage for later expansion of nursing in many areas and provided a valuable impetus to the women's movement.

The range of nursing tasks carried out under extreme conditions during the Crimean War showed that direct patient care and support services were necessary to recovery. Simple nursing activities included moistening parched lips, adjusting blankets, and assisting with bathing, dressing, feeding, and positioning. Nursing care for more serious cases involved applying hot and cold compresses, linseed meal poultices for frostbite, and simple and wet dressings; washing wounds; and dressing amputations. Some of the nurses also accompanied the doctors on their rounds and took directions from them.

The nurses were responsible for administering medications and controlling the dispensation of wine, which was used as a treatment for sick and wounded soldiers and was a staple in the diet of patients and nurses. They often maintained night watch in the wards or hospital corridors, especially to prevent delirious patients from pulling off dressings or endangering themselves. The women also saturated handkerchiefs with eau de cologne to counteract foul-smelling odors from wounds and dressings.

Compassion was an important aspect of the care administered; the nurses' healing words and presence often helped to soothe patients suffering from depression or insanity. The ladies and some of the nurses wrote letters for the soldiers to their families and also wrote to the families of soldiers who had died. They also kept the soldiers' valuables because the orderlies and fellow soldiers couldn't be trusted.

Other recognized tasks included housekeeping and the preparation and serving of meals. Before the medical staff even accepted the nurses' services, Nightingale set the women to work making shirts, stump pillows, slings, and straw-filled mattresses; up to then, soldiers were usually left lying on the dirt or stone floors. Nightingale established workable laundries and recruited some of the soldiers' wives to do the washing. She also saw that adequate sewage and drainage facilities were maintained, as ordered by the Sanitary Commission. Nightingale established her own kitchens to supplement the army rations for the sick and wounded because many were starving, either because they couldn't feed themselves, or because food was scarce or inedible.

Although Nightingale's orders weren't clarified soon enough to establish her superintendency over all 229 nurses who served in Turkey and the Crimea, she nevertheless kept detailed records on all of them and on the care they delivered. In her official reports, Nightingale provided a character sketch of each nurse who served, along with a résumé of skills, knowing that some of the women would be seeking work when they returned home. She wrote glowing reports on three of her finest nurses: Mother Mary Clare Moore; Mrs. Roberts, who had nursed her during her illness; and Lady Jane Shaw Stewart, whom she had designated as her successor in the event of her death.

Preparing to go home

In her private notes and letters from the Crimea after the war had ended, Nightingale expressed relief and excitement about going home. On April 22, 1856, she sent her sister, Parthe, a humorous skit describing the conditions under which she was living:

> *Would not you like to see me hunting rats like a terrier-dog? Me!*
> *Scene in a Crimean Hut*
> *Time midnight*
> *Dramatis Personae -*
> *Sick Nun in fever perfectly deaf, me the only occupant of the hut except rat sitting on rafter over sick nun's head & rats scrambling about.*
> *Enter me, with a lantern in one hand & a broom-stick in the other (in the Crimea, terrier dogs hunt with lanterns in one paw & broom-sticks) me, commonly called "Pope" by the Nuns, make ye furious Balaclava charge, i.e. the light cavalry come on & I am the Russian gun ...*
> *Broom-stick descends — enemy dead — "Pope" executes savage war dance in triumph, to the unspeakable terror of Nun ... Slain cast out of hut unburied ... If there is anything I "abaw," it is a Rooshan & a rat.[10]*

Status of British Women Sent to Turkey	
Members of Religious Communities	
Protestant	
Deaconess — unpaid	1
Sellonites (Sisters of Mercy) — unpaid	8
Sisters of St. John's House — paid	20
Roman Catholic — unpaid	
Sisters of the Faithful Virgin	5
Sisters of Mercy, Convents in Ireland	
Carlow	2
Charlesville	2
Cork	2
Dublin	2
Kinsale	3
Sisters of Mercy, Convents in England	
Bermondsey	8
Chelsea	3
Liverpool	1
Laywomen	
Ladies — unpaid	40
Hospital nurses — paid	117
Servants — paid	15
TOTAL	**229**

Disposition of Women after Arrival in Turkey	
Died	
April 1, 1855 to February 23, 1856	11
Discharged	
Incompetence or unsuitability for the work	
November 6, 1854 to December 10, 1856	12
Intoxication	
November 6, 1854 to January 29, 1856	18
Left or abandoned job	
April 22, 1855 to June 1856	2
Misconduct	
December 21, 1854 to January 29, 1856	17
Invalided home	
December 21, 1854 to April 27, 1856	37
Resigned	
November 1854 to March 28, 1856	40
Returned home after peace treaty	
May 16 to July 28, 1856	92
TOTAL	**229**

Adapted with permission by Irene Sabelberg Palmer. Florence Nightingale and the First Organized Delivery of Nursing Services. *Washington, D.C.: American Association of Colleges of Nursing, 1983.*

Religious and lay status of the 229 women in the British nursing parties in Turkey (left) and their disposition between November 4, 1854, and January 22, 1856 (right)

On July 7, she wrote another letter to Mother Moore, who was back in England:

... I am now winding up accounts as fast as I can. I do not yet know when I shall come home. But when I do, I shall come as quietly as possible, see no one in London but you, dear Revd. Mother, and go straight into the country to my father's house, whence I shall report myself to the War Department.

Dearest Revd. Mother, I am sure that no one, even of your own children, values you, loves you and reverences you more than I do. Take care of your precious health, do. In closing this work, I can never sufficiently express how much I feel all that you and your Sisters have been to it. It is beyond expression.[11]

In spite of the magnitude of her pioneering accomplishments and the heroic status she had achieved around the world, Nightingale left the Crimea with a sense of failure. At the end of her 21-month-long mission, she felt the army Medical Department was still where it had been at the beginning of the war; only the flow of supplies had improved significantly. The primary force that had sustained her during all her difficulties was her certainty that she was doing God's chosen work. Now, as she prepared to return to England in July 1856, she saw her achievements in the Crimea as only the starting point for her future work.

DIAGRAM OF THE CAUSES OF MORTALITY
IN THE ARMY IN THE EAST.

APRIL 185[...]

AUGUST SEPTEMBER OCTOBER N[...]

APRIL 1854 MAY JUNE BULGARIA JUL[...]

MARCH 1855.

FEBRUARY

JANUARY 1855

...edges are each measured from
...re of the circle represent area
...or Mitigable Zymotic diseases; the
...e the deaths from wounds; & the
...tre the deaths from all other causes.
...i Nov.r 1854 marks the boundary
...ring the month.
...area coincides with the red;
...lue coincides with [...]

Part 3
Post-War Years
(1856-1861)

Chapter 9

"At the Altar of the Murdered Men"

*I*f we are permitted to finish the work He gave us to do, it matters little how much we suffer in doing it. In fact, the suffering is part of the work ... But surely it is also part of that work to tell the world what we have suffered & how we have been hindered, in order that the world may be able to spare others. To act otherwise is to treat the world as an incorrigible child which cannot listen or a criminal which will not listen to right.

— *Florence Nightingale, Private Note, 1857*[1]

Nightingale returned to England in 1856 in a solemn state. In the Crimea, she had looked death in the face; the surreal chaos and horror of war were forever etched in her mind. She had been soiled with soldiers' blood and had seen the fearful and suffering faces of thousands of sick and dying, the "dear children" for whom she felt responsible. Yet she had also seen that war could imbue in people a profusion of virtues — love, compassion, heroism, and devotion.

The daily crises of war she had faced for almost 2 years had unleashed her own warrior spirit and united her with the soldiers in a common cause — that of reforming the entire army's Medical Department. The intensity with which she would now devote her life to service was heightened and inspired by her idea of "Mankind creating Mankind," the concept that man must discover the organization by which he can live in harmony with God's purpose. Having seen the worst, she was now determined to devote her life to ameliorating human suffering in both war and peace.

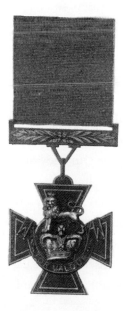

The Victoria Cross, which the queen presented personally to men who had served with distinction in the Crimean War

A quiet homecoming

Anxious to avoid a gala homecoming in England, Nightingale was silent about her travel plans, even to her family. The government offered to bring her home on a man-of-war, but she refused. Instead, she and Aunt Mai left Constantinople on July 28, 1856, travel-

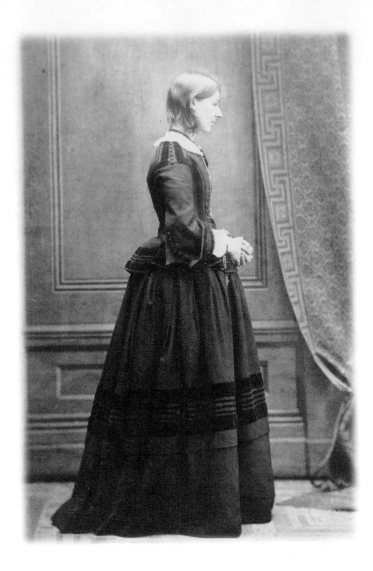

A rare photograph of Florence Nightingale c. 1858 without her scarf, showing her hair that was first cropped following her bout of Crimean fever in May 1855

ing incognito as "Mrs. and Miss Smith." With a queen's messenger in attendance to help them with their passports, they sailed on a French steamer to Athens, Messina, and Marseilles. At Paris, where she and Aunt Mai separated, Nightingale spent the night at the Mohls', then continued on and arrived in London on August 6.

Nightingale's first stop the next morning was the Convent of Our Lady of Mercy at Bermondsey to visit with Mother Mary Clare Moore and the nuns. It was the first day of their annual retreat, and she spent a few hours with them in prayer. She then took the train north to Derbyshire, getting off at a small country station 1½ miles from home. In the summer twilight, she walked across the fields to her beloved Lea Hurst, arriving without advance notice on August 7, 1856, after nearly 2 years' absence in the East. Parthe wrote that "a little tinkle of the small church bell on the hills, and a thanksgiving prayer at the little chapel next day, were all the innocent greeting."[2]

Nightingale now needed a period of seclusion to recuperate from the 21 months of anxiety, strain, and hardship she had endured as well as time to weep for the brave soldiers whom she had come to regard as her "children." She felt that the fierce emotions she had brought back home required no explanation to anyone, least of all to those who had experienced war for themselves. She would face her great sadness alone and in silence, relying only on her own inner strength and the conviction that she was doing God's will. Her healing would come by recalling the sacrifices of the soldiers, remembering what she had endured, and envisioning what she might do better in the future. In a private note at the end of 1856, she wrote:

> *Oh my poor men who endured so patiently. I feel I have been such a bad mother to you to come home & leave you lying in your Crimean grave. 73 percent in eight regiments during six months from disease alone — who thinks of that now? But if I could carry any one point which would prevent any part of the recurrence of this colossal calamity ... then I should have been true to the cause of those brave dead.[3]*

Nightingale's somber mood was apparent to her family, who often found her deep in profound reflection. She was physically and mentally exhausted and still suffering from chronic insomnia, anorexia, and nausea at the sight of food — the aftereffects of her initial bout of Crimean fever in 1855. Parthe wrote to Elizabeth Herbert from Lea Hurst on August 13:

> *Our dear one is home at last. They came back as quietly & as rapidly as they could, to avoid the receptions & greetings with which she was threatened, & which you know are little to her taste. Lord Lyons wished to send her in the Caradoc [warship] to any port she pleased, but she cannot bear giving trouble, besides this would have "published" her, so they came in the French steamer ...*
>
> *We had to put an extinguisher on the race of Mayors, & had stopped all proposals here to drag her home in triumph &c &c, so poor dear quietly she came in at her own door & quietly to her own people. She looks well in the face & seems well for a few hours in the morning, then she sinks down quite wearied out for the rest of the day — we are most anxious to give her the breathing time which alone can restore her to a chance of work for the future. We see how little she feels equal to anything of the kind at present. She feels quite worn out at heart & absolute quiet is all that she desires. A great deal of necessary business she must have, but we shall strive to ward off everything else, even her best & kindest friends ... She says "I find I cannot do work for more than half an hour at a time." We cannot but feel very uneasy about the extreme exhaustion which she shews. She sends her very best love to you ...[4]*

Before returning to England, Nightingale had sent home three orphaned boys she called her "Crimean treasures"; they were William Jones, a one-legged sailor boy, who had been with Nightingale for 10 months in Scutari and for whom she later found employment; Thomas, a 12-year-old drummer boy who called himself "Miss Nightingale's man" and vowed to devote his civil and military career to her; and Peter Grillage, a Russian boy who had been taken prisoner and brought to the hospital, where Nightingale had taken charge of him. When asked by one of the nurses where, as a good boy, he would go when he died, he answered "to Miss Nightingale." He later became a footman at Embley and married a longtime maid at the estate.

On their trip to England, these boys were accompanied by Robert Robinson, an invalid from the 68th Light Infantry, who had been Nightingale's messenger in the Crimea. She later sent Robinson to agriculture school, gave him funds for a short period, and then got him a job on an estate in Scotland. Also sent home was a puppy named

Rousch, "soldier" in Russian, who had been found near Balaclava and given to Nightingale by the soldiers.

There were few material things from the Crimea that Nightingale treasured, but two favorites were a bunch of grass that she had picked out of the ground "watered by our men's blood at Inkerman" and a cross made either during or after the war out of musket balls and a piece of shrapnel.

A few weeks after Nightingale's return, Parthe wrote another letter to Elizabeth Herbert, describing her sister's continued ill health and increasingly beatific state:

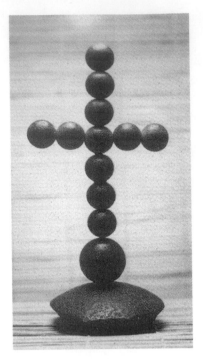

One of Florence Nightingale's few keepsakes from the Crimea, a cross made for her out of shrapnel and musket balls

I am sorry to say that F does not make so much progress as we hoped & there comes in so much business that she does not get the rest so needful to her — such heaps of letters, & among the business ones such queer ones, begging of course, one from a Clergyman in Queen's Bench asking for 70£, the next from a Costermonger asking for a donkey "by return of post" ... addressed "Miss N on her return from the Crimea" or "Miss N at her home England" & amongst this rubbish such beautiful little tributes, 1800 workmen in some iron works in Newcastle on Tyne to say how glad they are to hear that she is come home ... a big clasped Bible with a beautiful address from "the female tenantry" down to the smallest cottages of an estate of Papa's where we hardly ever go — & little tokens of the affection & confidence of the people such as touch her to the heart.

I must say I cannot conceive anything more beautiful than her state of mind, she is so calm, so <u>holy</u> — I can use no other word. In telling of all the horrors she has gone through (& I don't think you have any idea of what they have been, <u>we</u> did not know how much) it is as if she dwelt in another atmosphere of peace & trust in God where nothing wicked can touch her. The physical horrors we cannot get her to tell us of, & she speaks of the mental ones, which are so far worse to bear, the indifference, ignorance, bigotry & cruelty as one fancies they must be looked upon in Heaven, sadly & compassionately, without a personal feeling, about them — I could not have conceived such an entire abnegation de soi [of self] possible in this world — she always had it, but it has increased very much — Her whole soul is in her work & in her strong desire to see it make progress ... As for her perfect indifference to praise it is something almost incredible, I cannot get her to hear the things in the papers ...

God must prosper work in such hands, which are so truly striving to do all for Him & through Him — nothing else could have held her up under the superhuman fatigues of the last 22 months, night & day — & this Crimean 3 months which I think have been the worst of all — But it has seriously undermined her & I cannot believe that she will live long, I see she does not think so herself, not that she ever says so, but I know what certain signs mean — Well, long or short we bless God & are content: that our darling has been permitted & enabled to do so much for Him & for mankind ...[5]

During her first month at home, Nightingale worked with her Uncle Sam Smith to balance accounts and different claims with the nurses and to distribute to them the Sultan's monetary gift that the queen had allowed her to accept. She herself took no money, but the queen had allowed her to keep the carnelian and diamond bracelet given to her by the Sultan. Nightingale wrote letters to each of the nurses who had served with her, enclosing a copy of a letter of thanks she had received from Lord Panmure, Secretary of State for War. The following letter was sent to Mother Moore and the Bermondsey Sisters:

"AT THE ALTAR OF THE MURDERED MEN"

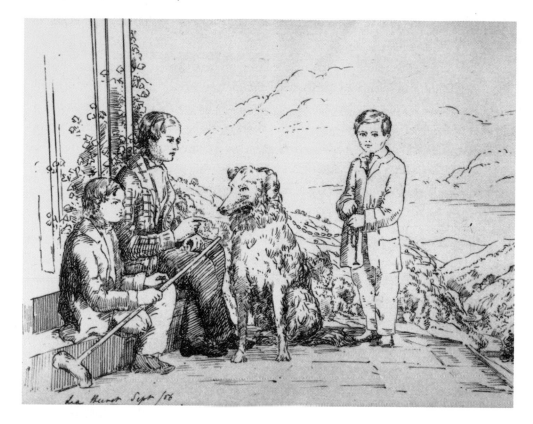

LEFT: *A sketch drawn by Parthe in September 1856 of her sister's "Crimean treasures," the three homeless boys whom Florence sent home from the Crimea: William Jones, a one-legged sailor; Thomas, a 12-year-old drummer boy; and Peter Grillage, a Russian orphan who later became a footman at Embley, with "Rousch," a captured Russian puppy given to Nightingale by some soldiers*

BELOW: *Wood engraving of the Crimean War army medal for valor, The Victoria Cross, and scenes of bravery in battle by six medal recipients, including two privates*

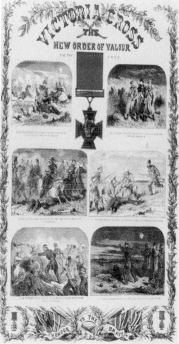

It is with the sincerest pleasure that I enclose to each of those who rendered such valuable service in the British War Hospitals of the East, the tribute paid by the War Secretary to their services. I rejoice that this as well as the Sultan's offering have testified how great was the appreciation of their labors.

I may here humbly add my own most grateful acknowledgments for all the assistance which I have received in this work. The devotion to it which I have witnessed both in Catholic and Protestant can never be forgotten by me. It is a remembrance to make glad the memory even of those scenes of suffering, which must also remain with us while life endures. With every fervent prayer that love can offer for my fellow workers, I remain their grateful and affectionate friend, Florence Nightingale.[6]

Heroes of the war: Soldier & nurse

Two groups of people emerged from the Crimean War as heroes — soldiers and nurses. The change in the British soldier's status was dramatic: Previously, an enlisted man was looked down upon as a drunk, a criminal, or a man who was simply too incompetent to find work elsewhere. After the newspaper reports of heroism on the battlefield and stoic dignity in the hospitals, the soldier was considered a prized member of society and the epitome of loyalty and courage.

Throughout the late spring and summer of 1856, British troops had been returning from the Crimea and Turkey, and national awareness of their homecoming was at a peak. Newspaper reports described Queen Victoria personally receiving "her dear soldiers." The queen commissioned a special medal to honor those who had served in the

Crimea with conspicuous bravery, both officers and ordinary soldiers. The coveted Victoria Cross, bearing the simple inscription "For Valour," was first presented by the queen herself on May 21, 1856, a day marked by parades and ceremonies; it was the first time that common soldiers had met the queen in person.

Thanks to Nightingale and her colleagues, the image of the nurse was also completely transformed: She was now seen as an angel of mercy with a high calling. By proving that women could successfully serve as nurses in military hospitals, Nightingale had almost single-handedly awakened England to the idea that women did indeed have a capacity for purposeful work and could make major contributions to society.

Caroline Bathurst, a family friend, wrote to Parthe:

> A movement has been begun ... I believe the movement is of God — & that the true & the good in it will prevail. Florence's whole influence will have been thrown exclusively into the scale of "grace & truth." What a veiled & silent wonder she has always been — manifesting her womanhood in deeds, not in words, but the fulfilment of duties, not by the assertion of rights ..."[7]

"Lady with a lamp"

From the beginning of the war, Nightingale's popularity with the British public had been enormous because of the letters that the soldiers wrote to family and friends about her and the articles in the *Times* that described her tireless work on behalf of the sick and wounded. As word of her accomplishments spread, she became a kind of national heroine-cum-saint in Britain and beyond. Newspapers and other publications were full of her biography as well as articles, poems, and columns about her Christian devotion in the Crimea. In 1857, these tales inspired the American poet Henry Wadsworth Longfellow to write one of his best-known poems, "Santa Filomena," from which came the famous image of Nightingale as the "lady with a lamp":

Queen Victoria distributing medals to soldiers who had served in the Crimean War, c. 1856

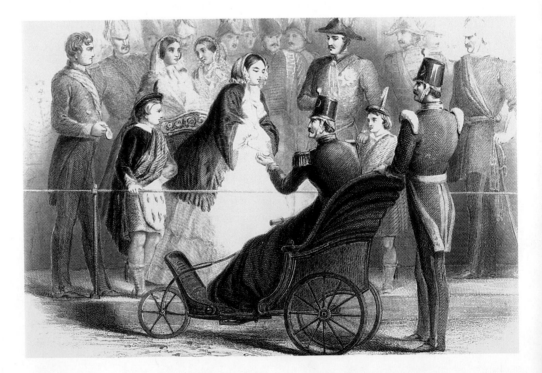

"AT THE ALTAR OF THE MURDERED MEN"

... The wounded from the battle-plain,
In dreary hospitals of pain,
The cheerless corridors,
The cold and stony floors.

Lo! in that house of misery
A lady with a lamp I see
Pass through the glimmering gloom,
And flit from room to room.

And slow, as in a dream of bliss,
The speechless sufferer turns to kiss
Her shadow, as it falls
Upon the darkening walls ...

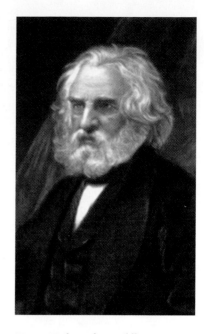

Printers produced woodcuts of the "Lady with the Lamp," and artisans created portraits, statuettes, Staffordshire china figurines, and sketches of her, which were sold in shops and on the street.

Henry Wadsworth Longfellow, the American poet whose poem "Santa Filomena," published in the first issue of the Atlantic Monthly *in November 1857, fixed the image of Nightingale and her lamp firmly in the public mind*

LEFT: *Florence Nightingale sheet music, c. 1856*

"Florence" became one of the most popular names for baby girls; even ships and racehorses were named after her. Cities and towns created "Fairground Exhibitions of Miss Florence Nightingale Administering to the Sick and Wounded." She was honored in songs with such titles as "Angels with Sweet Approving Smiles" and "The Star of the East" and even with an anagram in which the letters of her name were transposed as "Flit on, cheering angel."

Nightingale's wartime work and experiences continued to be the talk of all the parties and social gatherings, and she was flooded with letters and invitations for speeches, receptions, and parades. Her mother and sister pushed her to attend private and public gatherings, but Nightingale, concerned only with following her inward spiritual path and in recovering her health in preparation for the work to come, refused all appearances except a few personal engagements. Fanny and Parthe were especially disappointed when she refused to attend an elaborate garden party at Chatsworth, the home of the Duke and Duchess of Devonshire, a few miles from Lea Hurst. The Duke, a great admirer of Nightingale, had compiled a collection of newspaper clippings about her, which he later presented to the Derby Free Library. He also later presented her with a silver owl in recognition of her wisdom and in memory of her pet owl, Athena.

A mission of reform

During her initial period of recuperation, Nightingale was haunted by the memories of the thousands of soldiers who had died because of the glaring deficiencies and unpreparedness of the army's Medical Department. Of the 97,800 soldiers who had fought in the Crimean War, 4,500 had died of battle-related causes, but nearly four times as many — 17,600 — had died of disease and exposure.[8] She also began to realize that the lack of clear-cut army policies for the British soldier wasn't confined to the battlefield; horrible sanitation problems, poor nutrition, lack of job descriptions, and lax organizational structure dogged the army in peacetime as well.

Nightingale now embarked on a new mission: to ensure that the devastating experiences she had witnessed in the Crimea would never happen again. She believed that God had presented her with a unique opportunity to combine her mystical vision with social action. She was resolved to be "a savior" — a term she used to refer to all those who save from error — and to press home every defect she had witnessed and every lesson she had learned in the East. A private note she wrote in August 1856 summarized her feelings: "I stand at the altar of the murdered men, and while I live I fight their cause."[9]

Working tirelessly, she began to spearhead the major reforms for the army's Medical Department that she had begun formulating while at Scutari and in the Crimea. Knowing that her facts and figures would be the cornerstone for reform, she compiled extensive statistics to back up her ideas. She also began to correspond with some of her former political allies in the Crimea to begin developing a strategy: Dr. John Sutherland and Sir Robert Rawlinson, of the Sanitary Commission; Sir John McNeill and Colonel Alexander Tulloch, members of the Commissariat Commission; and Colonel John Lefroy, who had investigated the hospital situation on behalf of Lord Panmure. The

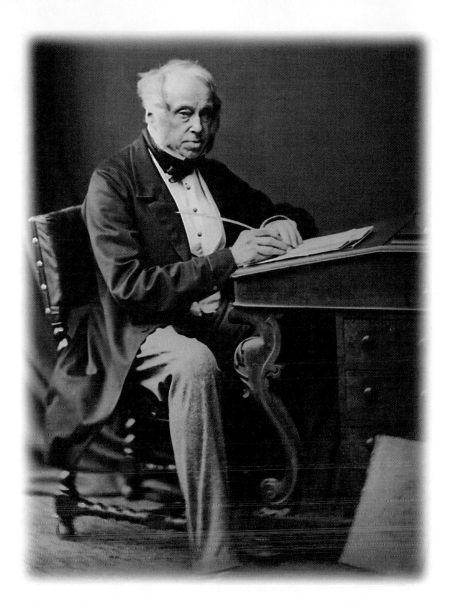

leader of this unofficial group would be her dear friend the incorruptible Sidney Herbert, politically astute member of Parliament as well as another staunch supporter of reform.

The reformers' task was formidable because the army bureaucracy, staffed by the old system of aristocratic patronage, had been virtually untouched by reform and was skilled at obstructionism. In April 1856, the government appointed a Board of Enquiry (known as the Chelsea Board because it met at the Chelsea Military Hospital) to investigate the wartime supply debacle revealed by the McNeill-Tulloch Report. First published in 1856, this report described the army's gross inefficiency in supplying the troops and mandated a new system of inventory and release of supplies. However, the Chelsea Board's final report assigned no personal blame for the supply fiascos, stating that the cause of the muddle was the failure of the Treasury to send out, at the proper time, a particular consignment of hay.

The Chelsea Board's report, which the *Times* lambasted as a "gross farce,"[10] triggered a huge public outcry; most of the country was infuriated with what it rightfully believed was a whitewash. However, it was quietly accepted by the Prime Minister, Lord

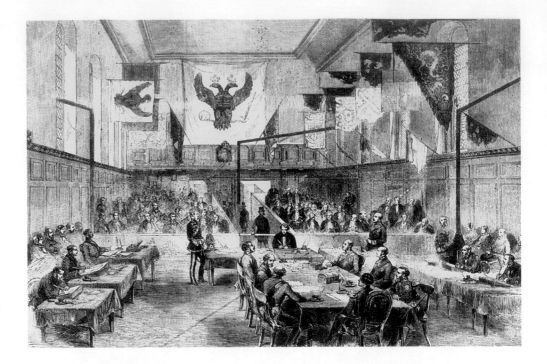

Palmerston, who was liberal in many areas but still believed that the army should be led by the landed aristocracy. By the following March, however, when Herbert rose in the House of Commons to ask that the queen recognize the efforts of McNeill and Tulloch — and thereby send a strong political signal favoring reform — Palmerston sensed the mood of the House and the country and didn't oppose the motion, which passed.

The vote that approved the findings of the McNeill-Tulloch Report reflected the complex web of political interests and obstruction that the reformers faced. Although Palmerston's government had sent McNeill and Tulloch to the Crimea to solve the Commissariat problems — which they clearly did — their report revealed such deep faults in the army structure that it created a political liability for the very government that had sent them. Nightingale understood Palmerston's reasons for wanting to downplay the report but she also realized the implications of the victory in the House when she later wrote to McNeill, "Silently, all over the country, no doubt this is sapping the country's trust in the Aristocracy more than any thing else could have done."[11] In the end, the McNeill-Tulloch Report, and the reaction to it, consolidated the political base for continuing reform.

Invitation to Balmoral

A few weeks after Nightingale's return home, Sir James Clark, doctor and friend of Queen Victoria and the Nightingales, invited Nightingale to visit his home in Scotland, where she had gone in 1852 to accompany Parthe home. Queen Victoria, staying nearby at the royal residence of Balmoral Castle, wished to meet her. Excited by this unique opportunity to personally report to the queen and Prince Albert on her experiences in the Crimea and her ideas about reform, Nightingale immediately began preparing for this historic meeting. Although she had already formulated some basic ideas, she also wanted advice from those who were experienced in dealing with the queen.

Nightingale immediately turned to the men she had come to trust during her 21 months in the Crimea, all reformers in their own right. Sidney Herbert advised her to talk openly and to illustrate her points with facts, details, and statistics. Colonel Lefroy, who had met Nightingale in Scutari during his confidential mission for Lord Panmure in October 1855 and had the highest regard for her, offered valuable insights. Currently posted at the War Office, he fully understood the personalities involved as well as the obstructionist tendencies of the government departments. Lefroy wrote that he had met on several occasions with Prince Albert:

> The Prince exhibited such a remarkable knowledge of the subjects he was enquiring about, so strong and clear and business-like a capacity that you will, I think, find it both expedient and necessary ... to enter into a full and unreserved communication of your observations, and be tempted irresistibly to let fall such suggestions as are most likely to germinate in that high latitude. If I am correct in this impression, a similar frankness with Lord Panmure follows.
>
> I was once amused by the Prince (Albert) remarking on a point of military education, "I have urged it over and over again; they do not mind what I say," showing that even he cannot always overcome the vis inertiae of Department indifference or prevail on people. It may be so in any question of medical reform. Lord Panmure hates detail, and does not appreciate system. He can reform but not organize. It is organization we want, but which arouses every instinct of resistance in the British bosom, and it is this which can be least influenced by H.M.'s personal interest. Like a rickety clumsy machine, with a pin loose here and a tooth broken there ... so is our Executive, with the Treasury, the Horse Guards, the War Department, the Medical Department all out of gear ... He will be stronger than Hercules, who gets out of it the movement we require ...
>
> In some form or other we have almost a right to ask at your hands an account of the trials you have gone through, the difficulties you have encountered, and the evils you have observed — not only because no other person ever was or can be in such a position to give it, but because, permit me to say, no one else is so gifted. It will be no ordinary task; and no ordinary power of reasoning, illustrating, grouping facts will be requisite. Another might repeat what you told him, but the burning conviction, the vis viva of the soul cannot be imparted ...[12]

On her way to Clark's home in September, Nightingale stopped in Edinburgh to consult with McNeill and Tulloch; she also inspected the barracks and hospitals at Edinburgh to gather more data that might be useful later. McNeill and Tulloch urged her to tell the whole truth and to fortify her descriptions with facts, just as Herbert had suggested. They advised her to proceed slowly, first giving her personal accounts and observations, and then, if encouraged, to provide general suggestions. If the meeting went as desired, she would then offer to write a formal report of her observations.

Nightingale decided to follow their advice. She would give the queen an honest account of her experiences and offer to submit a written report of her observations. Although some of her friends thought it would be appropriate to request a position as Superintendent of Nurses in all the military hospitals, she planned to ask nothing for herself, only reform for the soldiers. To this end, she would also propose that a Royal Commission be established to inquire into the condition of barracks, hospitals, and the army's Medical Department.

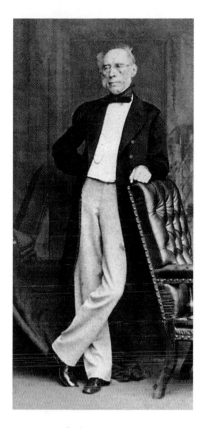

Sir James Clark (1788-1870), c. 1867, personal physician to Queen Victoria and in earlier years to the Nightingales, who arranged for Nightingale to report her Crimean War experiences to the queen after her return from the East and who supported her work for many years

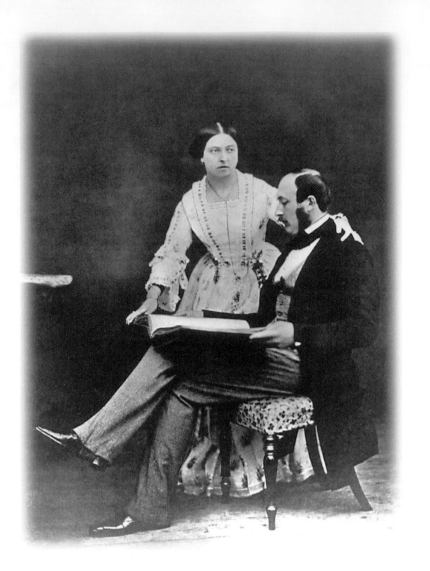

Queen Victoria (1819-1901) and her husband, Prince Albert (1819-1861), who were profoundly impressed with Florence Nightingale after their meeting with her at Balmoral

The meeting with the queen would set in motion 5 years of complex, arduous, and continuous work. Joining Nightingale would be influential politicians and leading sanitation experts who could provide leadership and support in Parliament, persuade cabinet ministers to appoint commissions to address and enforce reform, draft official reports for the government and then privately print condensed versions for a larger audience, and persuade influential journalists to print timely articles on reform issues.

On September 21, Clark introduced Nightingale to Queen Victoria and Prince Albert at Balmoral. In an informal meeting, Nightingale communicated her keen perceptions calmly and clearly. The queen, the prince, and Sir George Grey, the queen's private secretary, all asked penetrating questions in joint as well as separate meetings. Nightingale had already formulated in her mind 5 specific army reforms and 12 points that were a mixture of army and medical reform.

Five proposals for army reform

The proposals for reform of the army included the following:
• In all army units, soldiers must be taught to take care of themselves both in war and peace: to bake their own bread, kill their own cattle, build their own huts, repair shoes,

tailor clothes, fix drains, and in all matters be self-sufficient instead of relying on civilian contracts.

• The Commissariat Department should be put on the same footing as the East Indian Commissariat, the supply arm of the army in India, which had worked well for many years.

• A summary of the items in the Quartermaster General's warehouses must be periodically reported to officers in the field, who then would know exactly where to obtain the supplies they needed. For instance, many soldiers in the Crimea had suffered from scurvy (lack of vitamin C) when the known cure — lime juice — sat unused in the storehouse at Balaclava, only a few miles away. Troops also suffered needlessly from exposure while those same warehouses bulged with winter coats, blankets, and even rugs.

• In time of war, the transport of supplies must be under military command and control. During the Crimean War, supplies had arrived on civilian ships and some naval vessels, and there was no command structure in place that could recruit available civilian or naval crews to move the supplies the last few miles from the Balaclava port to the army camps.

• A sanitary officer must be assigned to every Quartermaster General's office to advise on proper encampment sites, diet, clothing, placement of huts, transport of the sick, and similar matters. One example Nightingale gave was of a fever-stricken unit at Balaclava that was camped in an area so damp that the huts were covered with green algae. After much needless delay, the huts were moved 20 yards to higher ground without altering the military position, and the fever abated.

Other proposals for reform

Nightingale's 12 recommendations for combined army and medical reform included:

• The management of general hospitals must be consolidated under one department. In Turkey and the Crimea, the hospitals had been run by eight departments, and the officers were all appointed by different authorities. This patchwork system led to delays, inefficiency, and irresponsibility; for instance, a requisition to mend a broken pane of glass had to pass through six departments.

• In hospitals, a new standard of cleanliness and hygiene should be developed for the wards and all other areas; floors, walls, ceilings, furniture, storage closets, staircases, and all other surfaces and fixtures should be kept clean.

• The army's Medical Department should be restructured and modernized, specifically in the following areas: clearly defined job descriptions, policies, and procedures for administrative and professional personnel; uniform pay and promotion policies; staff education and training; and creation of an army medical school that would train all medical personnel in the military aspects of disease prevention, hygiene, pathology, and surgical practice.

• Each hospital should be self-sufficient and maintain a complete inventory of supplies necessary for patients, such as gowns, robes, slippers, bedding, and eating utensils.

• Cooks should be trained and assigned to their kitchens; menus should be planned to provide proper nutrition; and kitchens and prepared food should be inspected daily.

- Policies for washing should be established, with separate facilities for three categories: bedding, personal linen, and surgical cloths and wrappings.
- Canteens (recreation rooms) for soldiers should be established at all barracks and camps, and should include libraries and reading rooms, facilities for letter writing, coffee-rooms, indoor and outdoor games, lectures, and other educational and recreational opportunities that would provide an alternative to taverns.
- Hospital facilities and medical services should be provided for soldiers' wives and children.
- Both male and female nurses should be used in military hospitals, under appropriate regulations, after comprehensive training.
- A new policy should govern stoppage of a soldier's pay. At the time, a soldier's pay was reduced by different amounts depending on whether he was sick in the field, on board ship, in hospital with wounds, or in hospital with an illness. Nightingale felt that a soldier who became ill while on duty should receive the same pay as one wounded in action to avoid damaging morale.
- All hospitals should be engineered to provide the best conditions for lighting (especially direct sunlight), adequate sewerage and drainage, ventilation, heating and cooling, water supply, ample cubic space per patient, and similar considerations.

Balmoral Castle, Aberdeenshire, the Scottish country residence of Queen Victoria and Prince Albert

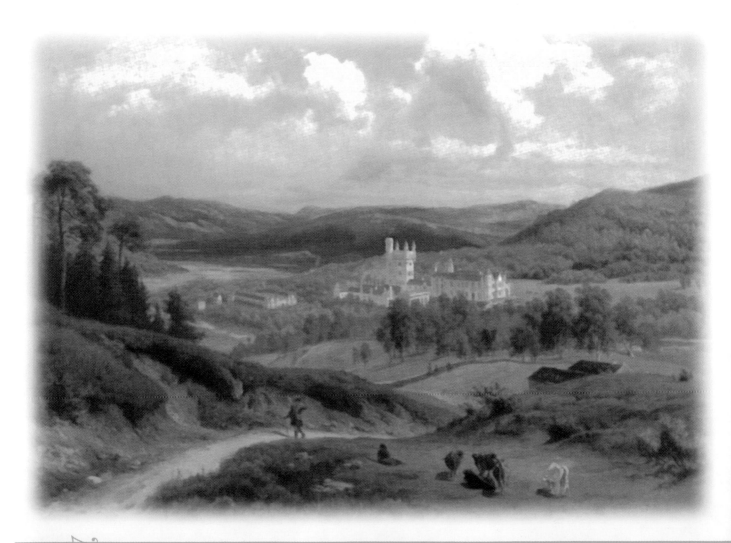

"AT THE ALTAR OF THE MURDERED MEN"

• Army hospitals should maintain a uniform system of meaningful statistics that would provide information on mortality; types and frequency of diseases, injuries, and operations; and duration of cases. This data would allow analysis of hospital sanitation as well as the efficacy of treatments and surgical procedures.

"We are much pleased with her . . ."

Nightingale's first 2-hour meeting with the queen and prince made a favorable impression on them. Prince Albert later wrote in his diary: "She put before us all the defects of our present military hospital system and the reforms that are needed. We are much pleased with her; she is extremely modest." Several days later, the queen called at Clark's home, where she and Nightingale had "tea and a great talk." In a letter to her cousin, the Duke of Cambridge, Queen Victoria wrote: "I wish that we had her at the War Office."[13]

Nightingale made yet another visit to Balmoral and, on October 6, accompanied the queen to church and later to a ball, where she sat with the royal family. This afforded her another chance to tell the prince about the army problems and also to talk with him about metaphysics and religion, subjects that were of considerable interest to him. Parthe wrote to Nightingale that Lord Clarendon, the Foreign Secretary, had said that "the queen was enchanted with her."

The royal couple enthusiastically supported Nightingale's ideas, but under the British Constitution the power to initiate action lay not with the Crown, but with the appropriate government ministers. The queen could only persuade the Secretary of State for War, Lord Panmure, of the need for army reform. Panmure was scheduled to visit Balmoral the next week, and Queen Victoria asked Nightingale to extend her visit and meet with him at Balmoral. In order to define their grounds for discussion, Nightingale wrote the queen a letter with her reform recommendations, and the queen provided a copy to Panmure, noting that she had accepted the original.

When Panmure reached Balmoral, he met with a composed, reserved, yet intensely focused Nightingale. The burly Scotsman heard the same precise observations and specific proposals for army and medical reform that Nightingale had presented to the queen. In a second visit to Nightingale at Clark's home, Panmure agreed that Nightingale should write a formal report describing her experiences in the war along with suggestions for necessary army reforms. He agreed in principle to the establishment of a royal commission of inquiry as well as an army medical school. He then volunteered another item for her consideration: He asked her to review and comment on plans for the first general military hospital at Netley, for which Queen Victoria had laid the foundation stone a few months earlier.

News of the success of the Highland meetings invigorated the reformers. On her way home, Nightingale stopped to confer again with Sir John McNeill in Edinburgh. She reached Lea Hurst on October 15, and from there began making arrangements for further strategy sessions with her colleagues. In November, Nightingale and her family departed for London to take up residence at the family's favorite hotel, the Burlington. Here she would be close to the government offices and homes of her colleagues for the long campaign ahead.

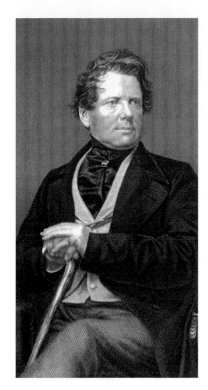

Lord Panmure (1801-1874), Secretary of State for War from 1855 to 1858

The "Little War Office"

Long before they received a royal warrant authorizing the creation of a Royal Commission of Inquiry, Nightingale and her "cabinet" set to work at her residence in the Burlington, which soon became known unofficially as the "Little War Office." Over the next 5 years, this "band of brothers," as they referred to themselves, met at the Burlington or at Sidney Herbert's Belgrave Square residence almost daily. If they didn't meet in person, they communicated with each other through messengers or the mail, which was delivered two to three times daily. They not only collaborated professionally, but also became good friends, sharing jokes, emotional outbursts and tempers, secrets, prayers, greetings, condolences, anniversaries, birthdays, and gifts.

Nightingale and Herbert: A meeting of the minds

Florence Nightingale and Sidney Herbert were allies, devoted friends, and colleagues who brought out the best in each other. Their relationship was the blending of two minds in a common cause. They referred to their Burlington group as "our cabal," "our mess," or "our cabinet." Their ceaseless work together was to have far-reaching effects — more than either could have ever imagined — in the years to come. Nightingale worked in the background, providing Herbert with the facts, arguments, and refutations that he needed to gain support for the proposed reforms. Herbert, in turn, served as her public voice, becoming the chief spokesman in Parliament for army reform.

With over two decades of parliamentary and governmental experience, Herbert was ideally suited to make the case for reform. He had championed various reform issues in his long career, was an astute reader of men, and had an impeccable sense of political timing. Perhaps most important, he was held in the highest personal and professional esteem by his colleagues. Even though he had been Secretary at War when the Crimean War broke out, he received no personal blame for the debacle that developed; his reputation remained untarnished.

Herbert and Nightingale spent huge amounts of time working together during their 5-year collaboration. Between meetings, they constantly exchanged notes: "What do you think?" "What am I to do?" "Give me your notes on this," "Your report is excellent," "I am at a stand still until I see you." Elizabeth Herbert fully supported her husband in his endeavors. Ever since the two women had met in Rome in 1847, they had been great friends and colleagues. They remained friends even after Herbert's death in 1861, but their contact lessened when Elizabeth converted to Roman Catholicism in 1865.

Dr. John Sutherland: Staunch ally

Another key member of the reform team was Dr. John Sutherland, who had become Nightingale's close friend and supporter since leading the Sanitary Commission to Scutari. Sutherland was one of the most knowledgeable men in England on sanitation practices and had served as one of two chief medical inspectors on the nation's first General Board of Health (1848-54). This short-lived board was an unprecedented experiment in government that laid the foundations for modern public health in England.

Born in Edinburgh in 1808, Sutherland received a medical degree from the Royal College of Surgeons of Edinburgh in 1831. After briefly practicing medicine in Liverpool, he served as editor of *The Liverpool Health of Towns' Advocate* in 1846 and the *Journal of Public Health and Monthly Record of Sanitary Improvement* from 1847 to 1848. As a chief medical inspector for the General Board of Health, one of Sutherland's main responsibilities was to provide technical assistance to local boards for the removal of cesspools and construction of sewers for the drainage of houses, towns, lands, and roads, using newly developed glazed earthenware piping. Other duties included framing bylaws that guided local boards; developing policies on water supply, slum clearance, lodging houses, and burials; and responding to outbreaks of disease, especially the two cholera epidemics of 1848-1849 and 1853-1854. At a Paris conference on quarantine law in 1852, Emperor Louis Napoleon presented Sutherland with a gold medal in honor of his work. Sutherland also helped to implement new burial laws to deal with the abysmal graveyard conditions that had developed as England's population doubled from 9 million to 18 million in the first half of the century.

After his important work on the wartime Sanitary Commission, which exposed the unsanitary conditions of the army hospitals in Scutari, Sutherland returned to England in August 1855. Queen Victoria summoned him to Balmoral to report his findings and make recommendations on ways to improve conditions for the British troops.

Sutherland was later to serve on almost every commission that Nightingale became involved in until his retirement in 1888. Even when his name didn't appear on the official list, Nightingale usually included him in some capacity. He became her private consultant and secretary for official matters and would often write the first draft of her reports.

Sutherland played an active role, with Nightingale and Herbert, in preparing the *Report of the Royal Commission on the Health of the British Army*, published in 1858. This report led to the formation of the Barrack and Hospital Improvements Commission, whose members included Sutherland and Herbert. This Commission inspected every barrack and hospital in England, and its reports ultimately resulted in vast improvements in the health of British soldiers.

Dr. William Farr: Expert on statistics

At a dinner at the home of Colonel Alexander Tulloch in the fall of 1856, Nightingale met Dr. William Farr, the leading medical statistician in England. Farr served as the first Compiler of Abstracts in the General Register Office, from 1838 until his retirement in 1879. His 1837 article on "Vital Statistics" in MacCulloch's *Account of the British Empire* was pivotal in establishing statistics as a social science, and his annual letter on death statistics and related questions, which began in 1841, opened a new field of medical literature in England. He made the number of deaths per thousand of population a standard measure in the field.

Farr became Nightingale's valuable ally, placing at her disposal his expertise and two decades of official statistical and actuarial data on death and disease in England. It was from him that she conceived the idea of comparing the morbidity and mortality rates in Scutari to those of the peacetime army as well as the civilian population.

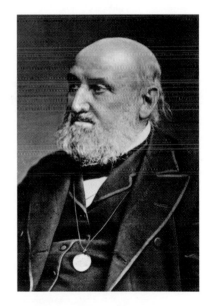

Dr. William Farr (1807-1883), physician and pioneering medical statistician who helped Nightingale with her statistical work on the Crimean War

Farr, an 1832 licentiate of the Apothecaries' Society, made many contributions in the field of public health. Before the germ theory of disease was conclusively proved by Koch in 1879, Farr proposed his own "zymotic" theory of disease, which synthesized the most practical aspects of the two major theories of the day — the contagion and miasma theories. According to Farr, the "pathologic transformations" that occurred during an epidemic, an endemic, or a contagious disease were of a "chemical nature ... analogous to fermentation."[14] He believed that disease could be caused by both person-to-person contact and "emanations" or "effluvia" from dung heaps or dead matter, and that zymotic diseases were more prevalent in filthy and crowded environments, such as the hospitals at Scutari and in the Crimea.

In addition, he developed "Farr's Law," which stated that the curve of an epidemic ascends rapidly at first, inclines slowly to a peak, and then falls more rapidly than it mounted. He first plotted this curve based on the spread of the 1840 smallpox epidemic. (The epidemic curves later developed by Brownlee, Ross, and others are usually of the bell-shaped Farr type, called the Pearson's class iv.)[15] Farr also served on the census commission and was an active member of the Statistical Society for more than 30 years.

Setting up the Royal Commission

In spite of her limited physical reserve and the lingering effects of Crimean fever, Nightingale drew up ideas for the Royal Commission as well as a list of potential members, including Dr. John Sutherland, Dr. William Farr, Colonel John Lefroy, and Sidney Herbert as chairman. Hopes ran high when her fellow reformers received her recommendations along with an account of her meeting with the queen and Lord Panmure. Sutherland's humorous letter of acceptance on November 12 showed his mild surprise at the great progress Nightingale had made so far:

> I have just received your letter and am led to believe that there must be a foundation of truth under the old myth about the Amazon women somewhere to the East of Scutari. All I can say is that if you had been queen of that respectable body in old days, Alexander the Great would have had rather a bad chance. Your project has developed itself far better than I expected, and I think I see a way of doing good and therefore I shall serve on the Commission ...[16]

Although not all of her original nominees were selected, Nightingale was pleased for the most part with the final 10 members appointed to the Royal Commission: Sidney Herbert (chairman), Sir James Clark, Dr. John Sutherland, Dr. Graham Balfour (secretary), Dr. J. Ranald Martin, General Henry Storks, Dr. Andrew Smith, Sir T. Phillips, Dr. Thomas Alexander, and Augustus Stafford, a member of Parliament.

Balfour, one of Nightingale's recommendations, had served in the statistical branch of the army and would later become Surgeon General (1873) and President of the Royal Statistical Society (1889-90). Martin, a 64-year-old surgeon and a good friend of Herbert's, had served in India and was a supporter of sanitation. Smith, Director General of the army's Medical Department, was the only commission member from the old army regime, which many people blamed for the major problems that had occurred in the Crimean War. Phillips was a lawyer and another friend of Herbert's. Storks had been Chief Commander at Scutari in 1855 and had supported Nightingale's efforts to set up reading rooms and other diversional activities for convalescing soldiers. Stafford had visited the Crimea in 1854 and later gave an eyewitness account to the House of Commons. Although William Farr wasn't appointed to the Commission, he worked behind the scenes with Nightingale.

Nightingale's vision of a commission to reform the army's Medical Department arose out of the mystic's view of "possibility":

> Mystics want to heal the disharmony between the actual and the real: and since, in the white-hot radiance of that faith, hope, and charity which burns in them, they discern such a reconciliation to be possible, they are able to work for it with a singleness of purpose and an invincible optimism denied to other men ... it was this instinct which drove St. Catherine of Siena from contemplation to politics; Joan of Arc to the salvation of France; St. Teresa to the formation of an ideal religious family ... [and] Florence Nightingale to battle with officials, vermin, dirt, and disease in the soldiers' hospitals.[17]

Nightingale's lessons on English history and government in her father's library, her own self-education, and her family's political history had helped provide her with the determination and political savvy she would need for the task at hand. Her plans covered all political bases: She had started at the top with the queen and vowed to "eat straight through England" and, if necessary, go directly to the people to achieve her goals.[18]

A catalyst for reform

While waiting for the royal warrant for the Royal Commission to be signed in the fall of 1856, Nightingale visited civil and military hospitals, interviewed doctors and chaplains, inspected barracks, and continued to compile data and statistics on sickness and mortality in the Crimean War as well as in England and abroad. She interviewed reformers and politicians in the fields of sanitation, prison reform, and all areas that impacted the quality of life of the British soldier.

These visits to public and military institutions in the months after her return from the Crimea produced catalytic effects. Many officials with whom she had no previous relationships began contributing advice or sharing their ideas on needed reform. One such person was Sir John Liddell, Director-General of the navy's Medical Department, who asked her to take an interest in the sailors and to help him introduce female nurses into the naval hospitals. She inspected Haslar Hospital, a naval facility, in January 1857 and consulted with Liddell on another naval hospital. She provided Liddell with some of her works in progress for his private use and he, in turn, provided her with information on naval stores, dietary matters, and statistics. He also accompanied her on an inspection of Chatham, a military and naval station.

Nightingale also wrote a number of reports during this period. At Lord Panmure's request, she prepared a memorandum titled *Female Nurses in Military Hospitals*. With Charles Bracebridge's assistance, she also wrote *Statements Exhibiting the Voluntary Contributions Received by Miss Nightingale for the Use of the British War Hospitals in the East, with the*

Mode of their Distribution in 1854, 1855, and 1856. This detailed document listed all of the gifts sent by contributors to Turkey and the Crimea, their quantity, and their final distribution among the various hospitals. She submitted both these reports to Lord Panmure in 1857.

Nightingale kept in regular touch with her friends from the Crimea. From General Henry Storks, she received drafts of proposed new army regulations, and from Colonel Lefroy, a draft of the plan for a School of Military Medicine and Surgery, which Panmure had approved. Lefroy also helped in another matter of great importance to her. He got permission for Nightingale to contribute, as a private citizen, to the establishment of a reading room and canteen at Aldershot, an army training base where her friend Mr. Sabin, the former principal chaplain at Scutari, was now stationed. The facility opened on July 17, 1857.

Despite all this activity, by early December 1856, Nightingale had grown tired and discouraged. Panmure, who took months to accomplish the most basic of tasks, was still dragging his heels on officially sanctioning the Royal Commission. Even Sidney Herbert, she feared, didn't share her sense of urgency about reform.

Dispute over Netley Hospital

As a response to lessons learned in the Crimea, the government had begun construction of England's first general military hospital in the small Hampshire town of Netley, below Southampton, sited directly on the waterfront. Thinking Nightingale would be pleased, Lord Panmure sent her the plans for the hospital in December 1856, but he soon regretted it. With construction already advanced, Nightingale warned Panmure that the plans were based on the outdated corridor system and consequently would concentrate too many patients in too small a space as well as be inconvenient for nurses. She advocated the pavilion system for hospital construction based on Lariboisiere Hospital in Paris. Nightingale was so convinced of the defects in the Netley plan that she paid a special visit to her neighbor, Lord Palmerston, the Prime Minister, during Christmas vacation at Embley to discuss the matter. Convinced by her misgivings, Palmerston wrote to Panmure in January 1857:

> *It seems to me that at Netley all consideration of what would best tend to comfort and recovery of the patients has been sacrificed to the vanity of the architect, whose sole object has been to make a building which should cut a dash when looked at from the Southampton River ... Pray, therefore, for the present stop all further progress in the work till the matter can be duly considered.*[19]

Panmure protested strongly, saying he couldn't justify wasting the £70,000 (approximately £3,236,400 or US$5,372,500 in today's values)[20] that had already been spent on construction. Palmerston finally allowed hospital construction to continue, but Nightingale suggested ways to correct some of the defects, which resulted in more open corridors, improved ventilation, more windows for the wards, and elimination of unnecessary corners. When finished in 1863, the Royal Victoria Hospital at Netley had 1,000 beds and a dock on the water to allow direct unloading of hospital ships from all points of the Empire.

Although she was defeated on the Netley matter, Nightingale didn't stop campaigning for the use of the pavilion plan in all future military hospitals. In her private report that was later included in the formal Royal Commission report, she proposed that all hospital construction plans be submitted first to competent sanitation authorities and that all new hospitals be constructed with separate pavilions to enhance ventilation and to avoid crowding a large number of sick people under one roof.

Report on her Crimean experience

Nearly 6 months after first meeting Nightingale at Balmoral, Lord Panmure, "who seldom did to-day what could be put off till to-morrow"[21] formally requested Nightingale to submit a report on the medical care and treatment of the sick and wounded in the Crimea as well as her observations on the sanitary requirements of the army in general.

Working continuously for the next 6 months, she wrote an 830-page report entitled *Notes on Matters Affecting the Health, Efficiency, and Hospital Administration of the British Army*. This remarkable document, completed in August 1857, became the cornerstone of the reform efforts. The introductory chapter was devoted to a history of the health of the British armies in previous wars. The next three sections addressed the organizational structure of regimental and general hospitals. The remaining pages discussed in depth the scope of her practice, observations, and various changes made during the Crimean War. Among the topics addressed were the need for sanitation officials and a statistics department in the army, soldiers' pay, cooking and dietary matters, washing and canteens, soldiers' wives, the construction of army hospitals, the mortality of armies in peace and war, and the education, employment, and promotion of medical officers.

Shortly after requesting her official report on her experience, Panmure asked Nightingale to write another report on nurses. She later expanded this 1857 report, called *Female Nurses in Military Hospitals*, into *Subsidiary Notes as to the Introduction of Female Nursing into Military Hospitals in Peace and in War*. In this report, Nightingale described her specific ideas about nursing: what it was and what it wasn't, organization and administration, job descriptions and task allocations, wages, and the best criteria for selecting nurses. Much of this work used military terms that are still used in nursing today, such as "on duty," "off duty," "absent or on sick leave," and "has left the service." These two landmark reports on army health and military nursing were submitted to Panmure but never released to the public.

Although Panmure and the government had agreed in principle on the formation of a Royal Commission and on its members, a Royal Warrant still hadn't been issued by February 1857 to begin work. Nightingale despaired at Panmure's inertia. Sidney Herbert wrote that Panmure was sometimes afflicted by gout "in the hands." She replied that "his gout is always handy," but reminded herself that "the Bison [Panmure] himself is bullyable, remember that."[22] Frustrated by Panmure's delays, she threatened to use her power publicly and wrote to Herbert on February 12, 1857, "Three months from this day I publish my experience of the Crimean Campaign and my suggestions for improvement, unless there has been a fair and tangible pledge by that time for reform."[23]

As Nightingale continued to compile data, it became clear to her that the same conditions that had existed in the Crimea existed in varying degrees in the army posts at home. On March 1, 1857, she wrote to Sir John McNeill:

With our present amount of sanitary knowledge it is as criminal to have a mortality of 17, 19, and 20 per 1000 in the Line, Artillery, and Guards in England, when that of Civil life is only 11 per 1000, as it would be to take 1100 men per annum out upon Salisbury Plain and shoot them — no body of men being so much under control, none so dependent upon their employers for health, life, and mortality as the Army.[24]

On March 28, she wrote again to McNeill:

This disgraceful state of our Chatham Hospitals, which I have been visiting lately, is only one more symptom of a system which, in the Crimea, put to death 16,000 men — the finest experiment modern history has seen upon a large scale, viz. as to what given number may be put to death at will by the sole agency of bad food and bad air.[25]

No matter how conscientious or how neglectful the individuals in the bureaucracy might be, the fault was one of system and organization. Nightingale was determined to alter both.

Chapter 10

The Drive for Army Reform

W*e have much more information on the sanitary history of the Crimean Campaign than we have on any other. It is a complete example — history does not afford its equal — of an army, after a great disaster arising from neglects, having been brought into the highest state of health and efficiency. It is the whole experiment on a colossal scale ...*

— Florence Nightingale, Report of the Royal Commission, 1859[1]

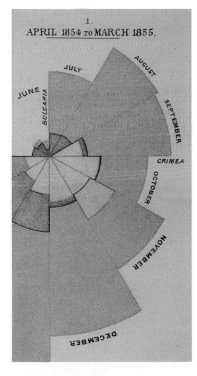

Detail of Nightingale's famous wedge diagram showing the different causes of death of British soldiers during the Crimean War

On May 5, 1857, Lord Panmure issued the Royal Warrant for the Royal Commission on the Health of the Army. The commission's task was to investigate the sanitary conditions of the army, the organization of military hospitals, and the treatment of the sick and wounded. Although Nightingale couldn't sit on the commission, her "Little War Office" supplied its members over the next 3 months with facts, tables, and statistics from Nightingale's voluminous materials. From this information, the reformers and commission members developed questions to ask the commission's witnesses.

The reformers' initial efforts had already yielded results. That spring, a British expeditionary force had been dispatched to China to resolve a dispute in Canton. Sir James Clark, personal physician to the queen and the Nightingale family in earlier years, persuaded the War Office to implement measures to improve ventilation on the ships, the troops' diet, and other matters relating to health and sanitation. As a result of these measures, the mortality rate of the forces in China was little more than 6% per year, compared to 50% for the troops in the early stages of the Crimean War and 17.5 per 1,000 each year for soldiers in the barracks at home (whom the reformers hadn't yet reached).

Throughout May 1857, Nightingale prepared briefs for the examination and cross-examination of all commission witnesses. She made a special effort not to put the men she had clashed with in the Crimea on the defensive. Of her old nemesis, Sir John Hall, former Inspector-General of Hospitals in the Crimea, she wrote that she didn't wish "to badger the old man in his examination, which would do us no good and him harm."[2]

Royal Commission proceedings

By June 1857 the Royal Commission was underway. Nightingale coached Commission Chairman Sidney Herbert on how to present the data and what questions to ask. As the reformers' spokesman in Parliament, Herbert depended on Nightingale and Dr. John Sutherland, former head of the Sanitary Commission in the Crimea, for their firsthand knowledge of events in Scutari and the Crimea.

The reformers decided that Nightingale should *not* appear in person before the commission because of her poor physical condition and because her testimony might place Herbert in an unnecessary and delicate political situation. The fact that he had received inside information from Nightingale in numerous letters while he was Secretary at War and during the entire Crimean conflict might have been considered "bad form" because they were operating outside official channels. However, the risks of *not* calling Nightingale as a witness were equally great: Her absence might compromise the credibility of the commission's final report and raise rumors about why she hadn't been called.

In the end, the "Little War Office" decided that the best solution was to have the commissioners submit written questions to Nightingale and let her respond in the same way. This strategy enabled her to answer in detail a wide range of questions about her background as a hospital expert, her experiences in the Crimea, her statistical methods, and topics related to the Purveyor's Department, medical officers, and hospital supplies and organization. Nightingale's report to Lord Panmure, *Notes on Matters Affecting the Health, Efficiency, and Hospital Administration of the British Army,* formed the basis of her written answers to the questions of the Royal Commission.

Continuing to disregard her health, Nightingale worked almost every day, sometimes 20 hours at a time. She took no holidays, ate and slept poorly, lost weight, and became more demanding and irritable. At the end of July, she submitted to Herbert her final recommendations to be included in the Royal Commission report.

Four subcommissions created

In August, just 3 months after the Royal Warrant was issued, the Royal Commission concluded its work. It recommended that four subcommissions be set up to initiate the following reforms:
- put the army barracks in a sanitary order
- establish a statistical department for the army
- institute an army medical school
- restructure the army medical department, revise the hospital regulations, and draw up a warrant for the promotion of medical officers.

The degree to which Herbert relied on Nightingale during this period was expressed in a note he wrote her on August 7, 1857, "I never intend to tell you how much I owe you for all your help during the last three months, for I should never be able to make you understand how helpless my ignorance would have been among the Medical Philistines. God bless you!"[3]

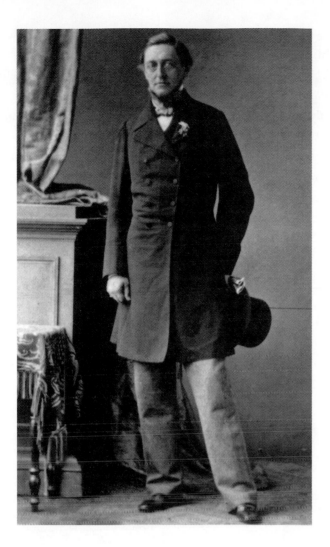

Nightingale, in turn, admired Herbert for never personalizing the conflict and always keeping attention focused on the reformers' ultimate goals. She later wrote of him:

> *He was a man of the quickest and most accurate perception that I have ever known. Also he was the most sympathetic. His very manner engaged the most sulky and the most recalcitrant of witnesses. He never made an enemy or a quarrel in the Commission. He used to say, "There takes two to be a quarrel, and I won't be one."[4]*

Having recommended the four subcommissions as well as the prospective members months earlier, Nightingale was anxious to see them approved and had already threatened to release her report to the public — at the risk of embarrassing the government — if immediate action wasn't taken. Although Panmure quickly agreed to form the subcommissions, which would be chaired by Herbert, they weren't appointed until October 1857. In the meantime, they received an interim grant to begin work and were given executive power to order any changes needed to improve the health of the army.

Herbert recruited Commission Secretary Dr. Graham Balfour to head the Statistics Subcommission and Captain Douglas Galton (who was married to Nightingale's cousin Marianne Nicholson) to head the Barracks Subcommission. Nightingale also brought in her old friend from the Crimea, the noted chef Alexis Soyer, to improve the kitchens.

Herbert began writing the official report of the Royal Commission with data supplied to him by Nightingale as well as data from commission witnesses.

Although Nightingale's *Notes* had been finished for months, the reformers decided that all of the data in it, along with all the data in the Royal Commission Report, should be carefully analyzed by medical statistician Dr. William Farr before being released. Nightingale consulted with Farr many times in 1857 while preparing her statistical tables and diagrams. He reviewed her syntheses and conclusions, comparing them to a "light shining in a dark corner."[5] He also made suggestions for improvement, such as dividing the material into chapters and providing explanations for readers unfamiliar with statistical methods.

Nightingale did write an explanatory memorandum, entitled *Mortality of the British Army at Home and Abroad, and during the Russian War, as Compared with the Mortality of the Civil Population in England,* and convinced Herbert to use it as an appendix to the Royal Commission Report. She realized that she could later distribute the memorandum anonymously with the legend "Reprinted from the Report of the Royal Commission" to give it added impact. In a letter to Nightingale in November 1857, Farr called her memorandum "the best [thing] that ever was written on statistical 'Diagrams' or on the

Nightingale's diagrams illustrating the causes of mortality of the British army in the Crimean War with different colored wedges that compared deaths from "Preventible or Mitigable Zymotic diseases" (blue), from wounds (red), and from all other causes (black)

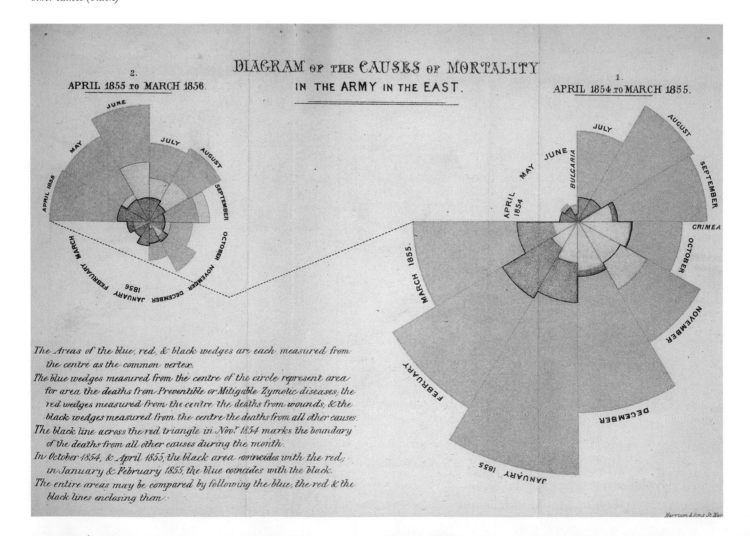

THE DRIVE FOR ARMY REFORM

ADDRESSED TO MISS NIGHTINGALE BY THE COMMISSIONERS
APPOINTED TO INQUIRE INTO THE

Regulations affecting the Sanitary Condition of the Army,

Reprinted (with some alterations) from the Report of the Royal Commission.

I.—SANITARY STATE OF THE ARMY AND HOSPITALS.

HAVE you, for several years, devoted attention to the organization of civil and military hospitals?

Yes, for thirteen years.

What British and foreign hospitals have you visited?

I have visited all the hospitals in London, Dublin, and Edinburgh, many county hospitals, some of the naval and military hospitals in England; all the hospitals in Paris, and studied with the 'sœurs de charité;' the Institution of protestant deaconesses at Kaiserswerth, on the Rhine, where I was twice in training as a nurse; the hospitals at Berlin, and many others in Germany, at Lyons, Rome, Alexandria, Constantinople, Brussels; also the war hospitals of the French and Sardinians.

When were you sent out to the British war hospitals at Constantinople?

We arrived at Constantinople on November 4, 1854, the eve of the Battle of Inkermann.

What hospitals did you find occupied there by the British?

Two large buildings on the Asiatic side, near Scutari, viz., a Turkish barrack and a Turkish military general hospital, both of which had been given over by the Turkish government for the use of the British troops.

How many patients did they contain at that date?

The Barrack contained 1500, the General hospital 800 patients, total 2300.

By how many nurses and ladies were you accompanied?

By 20 nurses, 8 Anglican 'sisters,' 10 nuns, and 1 other lady.

Where did you take up your residence?

We were quartered the same evening in the Barrack hospital, and two months afterwards, a reinforcement of 47 nurses and ladies having been received from England, we had additional quarters assigned us in the general hospital, and later at Koulali.

To what do you mainly ascribe the mortality in the hospitals?

To sanitary defects.

Will you now state what the rate of mortality was? And how you have calculated it?

I have calculated it, (1.) on the cases treated; (2.) on the sick population of the hospitals.

I beg to put in a Table.

Average of Weekly States of Sick and Wounded, from October 1st to January 31st, deduced from those given by R. W. Lawson, Deputy Inspector-General, Principal Medical Officer, Scutari.

Date.	No. of Days.	Sick Population of the Hospitals (mean of weekly numbers remaining)	Cases treated (mean of admissions and discharges including Deaths.)	Deaths.	Mortality.	
					Annual rate per cent. per annum on the sick population	Per cent. on cases treated.
1854.						
Oct. 1st to Oct. 14th . .	14	1,993	590	113	148	19·2
Oct. 15th to Nov. 11th . .	28	2,229	2,043	173	101	8·5
Nov. 12th to Dec. 9th . .	28	3,258	1,944	301	121	15·5
Dec. 10th to Jan. 6th (1855)	28	3,701	3,194	572	202	17·9
1855.						
Jan. 7th to Jan. 31st . .	25	4,520	3,072	986	319	32·1
	123	3,140	10,843	2,145	203	19·8

February, 1855 *

Hospitals.	Sick Population.	Cases treated.	Deaths.	Rate of Mortality per cent.	
				Annually on sick Population.	On cases treated.
Scutari and Koulali	4,178	3,112	1,329	415	42·7
Koulali alone . .	648	581	302	608	52·0

* This mortality is considerably understated. If to the Adjutant's Head Roll of Burials for Scutari, page 26, which is probably the correct return, had been added the Medical Officer's Return of Deaths for Koulali, here given, which is the only one we have, the total deaths would have been, not 1329, but 1453; and the rate of deaths on cases treated, not 42·7, but 46·7 per cent.

Army."[6] A year later, Nightingale became the first female member of the Statistical Society of London, based on Farr's recommendation.

Nightingale's conclusions about the causes of mortality in the Crimean War, developed with Farr's assistance, were frightful: She concluded that most of the deaths — both wound- and disease-related — were due to overcrowding, poor sanitation, and improper ventilation, *not* to inadequate food and supplies, as she had initially believed. She used original wedge diagrams, a novel method of presentation at the time, to compare data both cross-sectionally and over time.

On Christmas Day, 1857, Nightingale wrote Herbert that she had had 2,000 copies of her memorandum on *Mortality of the British Army* privately printed and planned to have copies sent to the queen and Prince Albert, Lord Palmerston, Lord Panmure, Dr. Andrew Smith (former Director-General of the army's Medical Department), all the Crowned Heads in Europe (through their ambassadors or ministers), all the commanding officers in the Army, all army surgeons and medical officers at home and abroad, and all the newspapers, reviews, and magazines in the country.

She also wrote that when the changes in the army Medical Department went into effect, she planned to "frame & glaze Proofs of all the Diagrams, & have them hung up at the 1. Army Medl. Board, 2. Horse Guards, [and] 3. War Department. For these are the facts they will have to work upon. This is what they do not know & did ought to!"[7]

Two pages of the Royal Commission Report showing Florence Nightingale's answers to written questions submitted to her

Official Report of the Royal Commission

The Royal Commission's final report — officially called the *Report of the Commission Appointed to Inquire into the Sanitary Condition of the Army, the Organization of Military Hospitals, and the Treatment of the Sick and Wounded* — wasn't released until February 1858, after Dr. William Farr had made a final check of the politically explosive data. Although Nightingale was not an official member of the commission, most members of Parliament and many others who read the report were aware that it contained her observations and theories.

Nightingale's statistical data conclusively demonstrated the causes of the high mortality rate during the Crimean War as well as the precarious situation of British troops in peacetime, whose mortality rate was double that of the civilian population. Overall, the report received excellent reviews in the nation's dailies, monthlies, and quarterlies — publications which, at the time, carried great weight in forming public opinion. An army doctor, Dr. Andrew Combe, later praised her report in the *Edinburgh Medical Journal*:

> [Miss Nightingale] ... *reasons with a strong, acute, most logical, and, if we may say so, masculine intellect, that may well shame some of the other witnesses. They maunder through their subjects as if they had by no means made up their minds on any one point ... and they seem almost to think that two parallel roads may sometimes be made to meet, by dint of courtesy and good feeling, amiable motives that should never be trusted to in matter of duty.*
>
> *When you have to encounter uncouth, hydra-headed monsters of officialism and ineptitude, straight hitting is the best mode of attack. Miss Nightingale shows that she not only knows her subject, but feels it thoroughly. There is, in all that she says, a clearness, a logical coherence, a pungency and abruptness, a ring as of true metal, that is altogether admirable.*[8]

The ties that bind

Nightingale took up residence at the Burlington Hotel in London in November 1856 so that she could meet regularly with her "Little War Office" to work on the urgent reform issues that were now the focus of her life. Unfortunately, she was accompanied by her mother and sister, whose lives still revolved around social activities. Although Fanny and Parthe were immensely proud of her accomplishments, they totally failed to comprehend the nature and magnitude of her continuing work. This was made clear to Nightingale one evening when they commented that "she led an amusing life."[9]

Nightingale now reacted to Fanny and Parthe with understandable impatience, indifference, and extreme annoyance. She was annoyed and frustrated by their continuous interruptions of her work to discuss trivial matters that didn't interest her. She was also irritated by financial arrangements and complained to her father about having to share the costs of a common parlor that she never used as well as other expenses that her mother was charging to her account.

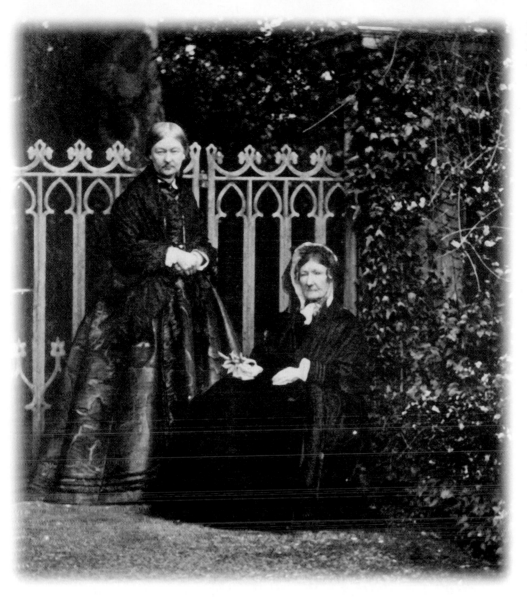

To Nightingale, women fell into two categories. In one group were women such as Queen Victoria and Mother Mary Clare Moore of Bermondsey, who devoted their lives to a serious purpose. In the other were idle women, such as her mother and sister, who cared only for frivolous social pursuits. In a painfully honest private note written in 1857, Nightingale reflected bitterly on the complex, strained relationship she had always had with Fanny and Parthe:

Moses said "Honour thy father & thy mother ..." Christ said "My mother & my brethren are those which hear the word of God & do it." How much farther advanced this was than that ...

What have my mother & sister ever done for me? They like my glory — they like my pretty things. Is there any thing else they like in me? I was the same person who went to Harley St. & who went to the Crimea. There was nothing different except my popularity. Yet the person who went to Harley St. was to be cursed & the other was to be blessed ... this false popularity, based on ignorance, has made all the difference in the feeling of my "family" towards me. There has been nothing really learnt by them from experience. But the world thinks of me differently — i.e. I have won, but by an accident ...

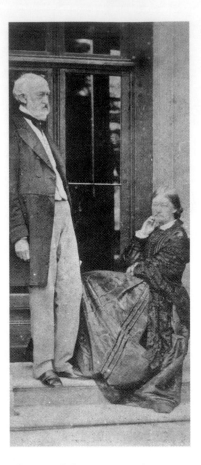

Florence's father, W.E.N., and sister, Parthe, at Embley, c. 1870

When we consider what a mother's feeling really is for her child, how flimsy, how unsubstantial it is, when compared with that of some "Virgin-Mothers" we see the truth. A pretty girl meets a rich man. And they are married. Is there any thought of the children? The children come without their consent even having been asked, because it can't be helped. Sometimes they are not wanted. Sometimes there is need of an heir. But, in reality, for every one of my 18,000 children, for every one of those poor tiresome Harley St. creatures, I have expended more motherly feeling & action in a week than my mother has expended for me in 37 years ...

We have seen what mothers do for their children — and what are children, at least daughters, expected to do in return? To be the property of their parents, till they become the property of their husbands. And I was expected to be not only the property of my parents, but the property of my sister. Because she had the world's opinion with her then. I had not.

Since I was 24 (probably long before, but certainly since then), there never was any vagueness in my plans & ideas as to what God's work was for me. I could have taken different kinds of work — education, Hospitals &c. But each was definitely mapped out in my mind after a plan. I cannot, after having had the largest Hospital experience man or woman has ever had, perceive that the plan I formed, at 24, for learning in Hospitals was imprudent or ill-advised ...

Upon what principle my "family" opposed this inexorably, overbearingly — I do not know — other than the "principle" of following the world's words & opinion. In fact, I know they take credit now for having promoted that which they called me unprincipled for proposing. (My mother even taxed me with having "an attachment I was ashamed of.")

When I was 30, I had an Adult Evening School for factory-girls, which was, on the whole, the most satisfactory thing I ever did. My sister went into hysterics because I attended this. And my mother requested me to abstain for 6 months from doing anything my sister disliked & to give up for that time entirely to her. To this I acceded ... When I went to Kaiserswerth the second time for 3 months, being then 31, my sister threw my bracelets, which I offered her to wear, in my face. And the scene which followed was so violent that I fainted ...

To Harley St., with which they now believe themselves to have "associations" dear to them, I was all but "taboo"ed for going. My sister said something to the effect that she could never pass the threshold. And though she did pass the threshold more than once, the first time she ever came was to go almost into hysterics. She hated the place — & treated me like a criminal for taking it. And I felt like one, then & all my life till within the last 4 years ...

Nightingale pointed out Fanny and Parthe's hypocrisy in now congratulating themselves on — and accepting society's praise for — having "given [her] up" to do God's work when they had actually hindered her in every way for so many years:

... I wish to shew how false & cruel it is to make success the test of right. While I was struggling through the very steps ... necessary to accomplish that for which I am now praised — for want of which same steps others have failed in the self-same thing — all men forsook me — & chiefly my own family. Now, because I have succeeded by an accident which never might have happened ... all men praise me. What is such praise worth?

But let me say whose support has been of "worth." 1. my spiritual mother's [Madre Santa Colomba] 2. that of one who has been a mother to me too in another way — Mrs. Bracebridge — & 3. singularly enough that of Mr. & Mrs. Herbert. They did not wait to send me to the Crimea in order to support me, as far as they could, in doing God's work ...

Undoubtedly thinking of her mother and sister, she concluded by pointing out how living an idle life could cause the human brain to become as delusional as the brain of people "who conceive themselves to be tea-pots, or to have 30,000 men fighting in their insides:"

... I have seen scenes among [the idle rich] quite worthy of Molière, where two people, in tolerable & perfect health, lying on the sofa all day long & doing absolutely nothing, have persuaded themselves & others that they are the victims of their self-devotion for an other who perhaps is really dying from over-work ... I believe these delusions, bred of idleness, to be absolutely incurable (in this world)...[10]

New symptoms of chronic illness

Since returning to England and immersing herself in the work of her "Little War Office," Nightingale had continually suffered from extreme fatigue, insomnia, lack of appetite, nausea at the sight of food, irritability, nervousness, and intermittent depression. In August 1857, the same month in which the Royal Commission ended its inquiry, she suffered a severe bout of palpitations and finally collapsed. Her doctors ordered her to go to Malvern for the popular "water cure."

Nightingale traveled in an invalid carriage from London to Malvern, a health resort in the west of England known for its medicinal waters. She begged Aunt Mai, who had moved to the Burlington to help with correspondence and manage her domestic affairs, not to tell anyone how ill she was. The doctors at Malvern diagnosed Nightingale as suffering from extreme exhaustion and recommended bed rest. Although her aunt and friends also blamed her ill health on overwork, Aunt Mai wrote to the Nightingales that "the intense desire to complete the work keeps her alive when nature otherwise decides."[11]

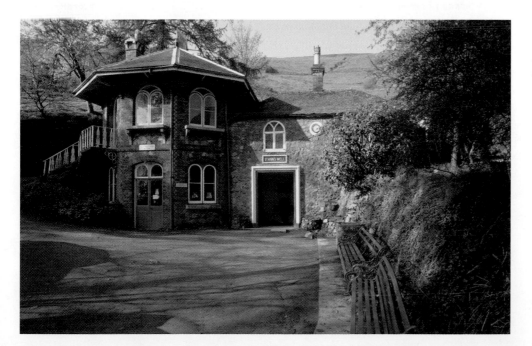

The building housing St. Anne's Well at Malvern, where Nightingale received hydrotherapy treatments in 1857

Dr. Sutherland wrote to implore her to think of herself and stop working. He advised her to eat at least 28 ounces of solid food per day and said she looked like all her blood needed "renewing." She responded to him:

And what shall I say in answer to your letter? Some one said once, He that would save his life shall lose it; and what shall it profit a man if he gain the whole world and lose his own soul? He meant, I suppose, that "life" is a means and not an end, and that "soul," or the object of life, is the end. Perhaps he was right. Now in what one respect could I have done other than I have done? or what exertion have I made that I could have left unmade?... Had I "lost" the Report, what would the health I should have saved have "profited" me? or what would ten years of life have advantaged me, exchanged for the ten weeks this summer? Yes, but, you say, you might have walked or driven or eaten meat ... Let me tell you, O Doctor, that after any walk or drive I sat up all night with palpitations. And the sight of animal food increased the sickness. The man here put me, as soon as I arrived, on a sofa and told me not to move and take no solid food at all till my pulse came down ...[12]

Her extreme frustration over the slow pace of army reform, combined with repeated bouts of severe, debilitating illness, made her feel as if she might die at any time without having accomplished any of her goals. While recuperating at Malvern, she wrote to Sutherland about a dream she had of old times in Egypt and the death of her pet owl, Athena:

I have been greatly harassed by seeing my poor owl lately, without her head, without her life, without her talons, lying in the cage of your canary (like the statue of Rameses II in the pool at Memphis), and the little villain pecking at her. Now that's me. I am lying without my head, without my claws, and you all peck at me.[13]

Sutherland's devoted friendship, understanding, and humor, as well as his confidence in their relationship, are evident in his response to her complaint:

What can I say, my dear friend, to your long scold of a letter? ...You are decidedly wrong in passing yourself off for a dead owl, and in thinking that I have joined with other equally charitable people in pecking at you. It is I that have got all the pecking, altho' I hope that I am neither an owl or dead; and your little beak is one of the sharpest. But like a good, live hero, I bear it all joyfully because it is got in doing my duty to you.

I want you to live, I want you to work. You want to work and die, and that is not at all fair. I admire your heroism and self-devotion with all my heart, but alas! I cannot forget that it is all within the compass of a weak, perishing body; and am I to encourage you to wear yourself in the vain attempt to beat not only men, but time? You little know what daily anxiety it has cost me to see you dying by inches in doing work fit only for the strongest constitution.[14]

Invalidism and premonitions of death

Nightingale's deteriorating physical state caused her family great concern. After she suffered another attack in September, Parthe wrote to longtime friend Mary Clarke Mohl in Paris:

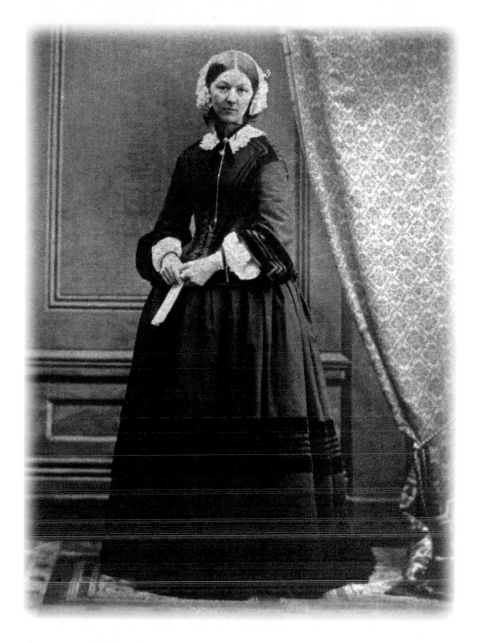

The accounts of F. have been very anxious. Aunt Mai says she does not sleep above two hours in the night and continues most feverish and feeble, and cannot eat. She never left that room where you saw her, was scarcely off her sofa for a month. Now she goes down for half an hour into a parlour, to do business with a Commissioner who has been there to see her. Aunt Mai says it throws her back more to put off work for "the cause" she lives for than to do a little every day — so we reconcile ourselves. Tuesday, she says, was a very uneasy day, and F. said she felt as she had done when recovering from the fever at Balaclava. Still both doctors say there is no disease, that it is only entire exhaustion of every organ from overwork, and that rest will alone restore her — rest for much longer than she will give herself, I fear.

She has two "packs" a day; this is all the water-curing; it seems to bring down her pulse, and she lives at that open window the chief part of the day, not reading or writing, only just still. She cannot be better anywhere, no one can get at her; Aunt Mai is a dragon, and the Commissioner is the only person who has seen her. Aunt M. says, "I cannot disguise to myself that she is in a very precarious state."[15]

Because of her chronic fatigue and severe symptoms, Nightingale declared herself an invalid in September 1857, at the age of 37. She took this drastic step in order to limit any demands on her time and health that were not relevant to her reform work, which was her sole mission. She realized that she had never been completely well since her first bout of Crimean fever and that her chronic weakness and palpitations were significant even though the doctors hadn't been able to provide a definitive diagnosis.[16]

On November 6, 1857, Nightingale wrote a letter to Sidney Herbert containing premonitions of her death and expressing confidence in his ability to carry on their army reform work. The envelope was marked "To be sent when I am dead. F. N."

1. I hope you will not regret the manner of my death. I know that you will be kind enough to regret the fact of it. You have sometimes said that you were sorry you had employed me. I assure you it had kept me alive. I am sorry not to stay alive to do the "Nurses" [nurse training school]. But I can't help it. "Lord, here I am, send me" has always been religion to me. I must be willing to go now as I was to go to the East. You know I always thought it the greatest of your kindnesses sending me there. Perhaps He wants a "Sanitary Officer" now for my Crimeans in some other world where they are gone.

2. I have no fears for the Army now. You have always been our "Cid" — the true chivalrous sort — which is to be the defender of what is weak & ugly & dirty & undefended, rather than of what is beautiful & artistic. You are so now more than ever for us. "Us" means, in my language, the troops & me.

3. I hope you will have no chivalrous ideas about what is "due" to my "memory." The only thing that can be "due" to me is what is good for the troops. I always thought thus while I was alive. And I am not likely to think otherwise now that I am dead ...[17]

Nightingale's family also felt that she was near death and gathered around her. The *Times* even composed her obituary. She drew up a will, which provided that any property she might be entitled to after the death of her parents be used to build a model barrack, with day and reading rooms as in Scutari and the Crimea. She designated Herbert, Sutherland, and Sir John McNeill as the men who should carry on her work. In a wave of emotion, she indicated that she wanted to be buried in the Crimea, "absurd as I know it to be. *For they* [the souls of the dead soldiers] *are not there.*"[18]

Back to work

In December 1857, Nightingale regained some of her strength and resumed her intense workload, conferring with Herbert for 3 hours in the morning, with Sutherland for 4 hours in the afternoon, and with Dr. Graham Balfour, Dr. William Farr, and Dr. Thomas Alexander as needed. Much work was now needed to implement the four subcommissions' recommendations for improving the health of the soldiers, not only in England but throughout the Empire.

From this period until the 1890s, Nightingale adopted a rigid routine of enforced invalidism, which allowed her to focus uninterruptedly on her work while conserving her limited physical strength. From her invalid-chair, bed, or couch, she would usually see only one visitor at a time, and no more than three or four a day. Nearly all visitors received a written invitation, with an appointment time specified to the half hour. When intensely engaged in her work, or if she were feeling ill, she might send the waiting visitor (even royalty) a note postponing the meeting. She ate her meals in solitude.

At this time she moved into the Burlington Hotel Annex because it was quieter. Although she hated publicity, her work kept her name in the papers as well as in social and political circles. Aunt Mai once again served as an intermediary between Nightingale and her mother and sister, who frequently dropped by from Embley, interrupting her work for trivial matters or the latest gossip. Aunt Mai soon convinced Fanny and Parthe that Nightingale must be left alone for the sake of her health. During this period, Nightingale's old friend, Mary Clarke Mohl, gave her a family of Persian cats, which provided Nightingale much pleasure over the years. She wrote many notes about their antics, and their paw prints were found on some of her papers.

Throughout 1858, Nightingale's health was precarious, and she continued to take hydrotherapy treatments at Malvern. Often after the strain of receiving visitors, Sutherland described her as "trembling all over" and would administer medical aid. Some visitors, finding her calm and looking well, wondered whether her symptoms were real or imagined. However, Nightingale realized that it was important for her to appear composed and confident to others, because in so doing she could articulate her reform ideas with more authority.

Change of government

A change in government in February 1858 saw the departure of some of Nightingale's closest allies. Lord Derby replaced Lord Palmerston as Prime Minister, and General Robert Peel replaced Lord Panmure as Secretary of State for War. Nightingale and Sidney Herbert managed to block the appointment of Sir John Hall, her old nemesis from the Crimea, as Director-General of the army Medical Department to succeed Dr. Andrew Smith, who was retiring, because they felt he would be disastrous for reform. In June, General Peel appointed Dr. Thomas Alexander to the top position, but this victory for the reformers was short-lived because Alexander died suddenly in 1860.

Captain Douglas Galton became an invaluable member of the Barracks Subcommission. Dr. John Sutherland served on both the Barracks and Sanitary Subcommissions. Lord Stanley, a great admirer of Nightingale, became the Colonial Secretary and agreed to send Nightingale's report out to his colonial governors and to suggest an inspection of the colonial barracks. Shortly thereafter, Lord Stanley became head of the India Office, where he would become instrumental in the India sanitary reform.

Nightingale's "Little War Office" colleagues continued their intense work for reform, often referring to her as their "commander-in-chief" or "lady-in-chief." Aunt Mai, her son-in-law Arthur Clough, and Nightingale's cousin Hilary Bonham Carter — who never married — had by now joined the cause and were assisting her with correspondence and the steady stream of visitors, including government officials, consultants, and dignitaries, such as the Queen of Holland and the Crown Princess of Prussia. Nightingale often asked her family to invite her guests for a visit to Lea Hurst or Embley, which delighted the Nightingales as well as the guests.

Marriage of Parthe

Sir Harry Verney, a 57-year-old member of Parliament and noted philanthropist, visited Nightingale at the Burlington in the fall of 1857, having promised his recently deceased wife that he would introduce his daughters to her. She granted him an interview because he was known in the House of Commons as an advocate for reform in such matters as rural health, sanitation, and education.

Some writers say that Verney wished to marry Nightingale, but she was only interested in discussing ideas about reform. However, she introduced Verney to her sister in the hope that he might become attracted to her. Her strategy worked: Verney and Parthe were married in June 1858. Nightingale's parents were predictably thrilled with Parthe's marriage. The Verneys divided their time between Claydon House, Verney's historic mansion in Buckinghamshire, and London during sessions of Parliament. Parthe, now Lady Verney, was well suited to the responsibilities of entertaining and running a large mansion. Nightingale commented on her sister's marriage in a note to Lady McNeill:

> She likes it, which is the main thing. And my father is very fond of Sir Harry Verney, which is the next best thing. He is old and rich, which is a disadvantage. He is active, has a will of his own and four children ready-made, which is an advantage. Unmarried life, at least in our class, takes everything and gives nothing back to this poor earth ... I think these reflections tend to approbation.[19]

After Parthe's marriage, Nightingale began to seek her brother-in-law's advice on a variety of political matters. In addition, W.E.N. now increased her annual allowance and paid for all her expenses, including lodging.

Throughout the spring and summer of 1858, Nightingale redecorated her new quarters in the Burlington. The apartment space was ideal for her: It contained an upper-level bedroom where she could surround herself with mounds of government Blue Books, official papers, and statistics; a dressing room; a maid's room; a spare bedroom; and an informal lower-floor living room. Fanny honored her daughter's desire for solitude and would send fresh food and flowers. Her father wrote that he was sending her things for her drawing room, but she indignantly replied that she had no drawing room [formal salon], a thing she saw as the "destruction of so many women's lives."[20]

Collaboration with Harriet Martineau

Fearing that the career bureaucrats in the War Office would quietly scuttle the Royal Commission report, Nightingale in November 1858 asked the well-known journalist Harriet Martineau to help push the government to action on army reform. Martineau was a columnist for the *Daily News* whose articles appeared several times per week. Her early work had focused on stories of injustice to workers and women as well as religious essays.

Martineau became a national literary figure in 1832 with the publication of *Illustrations of Political Economy,* a series of short stories that explained such topics as taxation,

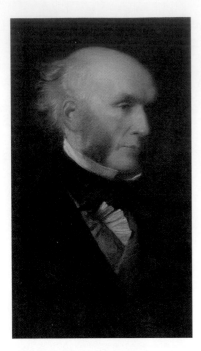

Sir Harry Verney (1801-1894), member of Parliament from Buckinghamshire who married Parthenope, Nightingale's sister, in June 1858

wages, and other economic issues. From 1834 to 1836, she traveled extensively in the United States and wrote *Society in America.* Her literary output was prodigious despite a lifetime of poor health. Among her better-known later works are *History of England during the Thirty Years' Peace* (1849) and *The Philosophy of Comte, Freely Translated and Condensed* (1853).

Nightingale had long been familiar with Martineau's life and work through Aunt Julia Smith, the writer's friend. In fact, during a serious illness in 1843, Martineau had once been "ministered" to by Nightingale, as she recalled in her autobiography: "... Still preserved and prized in my home are drawings sent me by the Miss Nightingales, and an envelope-case (in daily use) from the hands of the immortal Florence. I was one of the sick to whom she first ministered; and it happened through my friendship with some of her family."[21]

At this time in their lives, both women could sympathize with each other's health problems. Martineau, who had been deaf from an early age, was periodically bedridden for months at a time and sometimes so weak that she had to walk down the stairs backwards to maintain her balance.

Nightingale had sent a copy of her *Notes on Matters Affecting the Health, Efficiency, and Hospital Administration of the British Army* to Martineau, who immediately agreed to use the material to rouse public opinion. Both women agreed that Nightingale would review any articles for accuracy but that Martineau had full discretion thereafter for publication. As always, Nightingale preferred to remain in the background while supplying Martineau with any information she might need. When an unsigned pamphlet

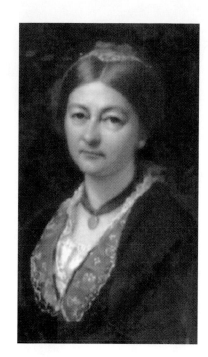

Nightingale's sister, Parthe, after her marriage to Sir Harry Verney

BELOW: *Claydon House, Sir Harry Verney's estate in Buckinghamshire, which Nightingale visited frequently in later years*

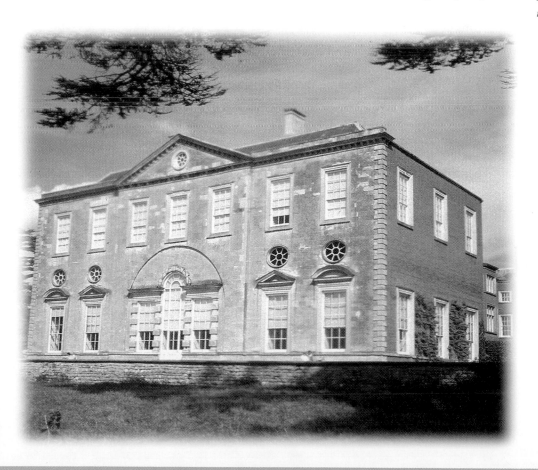

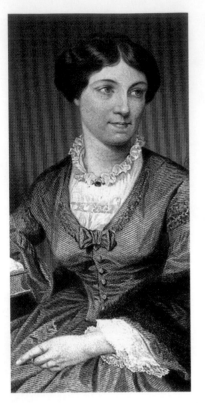

Harriet Martineau (1802-1876), famous journalist and author, who helped rouse public opinion in favor of army reform

appeared in 1859 attacking the Royal Commission report, Nightingale quickly penned one of her most effective pieces on this matter: a 16-page condensed version of her *Mortality of the British Army at Home and Abroad*, which contained her controversial statistical tables and diagrams. She had 150 copies of the piece, titled *A Contribution to the Sanitary History of the British Army in the Late War with Russia*, privately printed and immediately sent one to Martineau, asking her to make use of it "in the way you mentioned" without using Nightingale's name.[22]

In addition to circulating official documents, Nightingale sometimes wrote unsigned articles and essays for other journalists to use. In one such article, which Martineau used only for background purposes, she expressed her frustration with the government's inaction:

> Are the deliberate recommendations of a Royal Commission of "experts" to be adopted and future armies saved or has the whole plan so carefully considered and so intelligently framed been shelved by the genius of dullness and stupidity in the War Office to which Great Britain from time immemorial has committed the destinies of her soldiers, in peace and in war?
>
> Why all this delay? Or rather has not the time arrived when the nation should call for a Royal Commission of Inquiry into the manner in which the interests of the Army are neglected through the ignorance of a set of obscure paid officials who in all probability would never have been able to earn their salt in any other walk of life?[23]

Martineau wrote several articles in the *Daily News* that reviewed the commission's proposals for reform and the necessity of implementing them. She also wrote a book based on Nightingale's materials, entitled *England and Her Soldiers*, which appeared in 1859. This book explored Nightingale's premise that a whole new system of preventive measures was needed to improve the British soldier's health and quality of life, including good nutrition and sanitary measures to prevent disease and illness. To partially offset the expense of printing, Nightingale provided her with the printer's blocks so that they could be reused.[24] Displaying marketing savvy, she also advised Martineau to sell 5,000 copies at 2 shillings sixpence or 3 shillings, rather than 1,000 copies at 7 shillings, to make them more available.[25] Nightingale was pleased with the book and wanted each army regiment to have a copy, but the War Office refused to accept the books, fearing they would stir up discontent in the ranks. Undaunted, Nightingale paid a book distributor £20 to place copies in the soldiers' reading rooms across the country.

The beginnings of change

Ever since arriving at Scutari, Nightingale had been laying the foundation for reform of the British army's Medical Department. Her primary goal was the army's establishment of preventive measures that would keep British soldiers healthy — not merely tend to their wounds and sickness. From 1859 to 1861, through Nightingale's unrelenting work and leadership and the efforts of her fellow reformers, this vision slowly began to take form. In June 1859, political circumstances at last favored the initiation of real structural changes: Lord Palmerston returned as Prime Minister and appointed Sidney Herbert as Secretary of State for War. Herbert immediately wrote Nightingale:

I must send you a line to tell you that I have undertaken the Ministry of War. I have undertak-
en it because in certain branches of administration I believe that I can be of use, but I do not
disguise from myself the severity of the task nor the probability of my proving unequal to it.
But I know that you will be pleased to hear of my being there ... God bless you![26]

The subcommission reports

In April 1861, Sidney Herbert delivered to Parliament the reports of the four subcommissions, which had been appointed in 1857. These reports presented the progress that
had been made since that time in four key areas: sanitary conditions in barracks, establishment of an army Statistics Department, formation of an army medical school, and
the general restructuring of the army's Medical Department.

The report of the Barracks Subcommission reflected the tremendous reforms that
had taken place in hospital and barracks accommodations, including improvements in
ventilation, water supply, drainage, lighting, structure, and kitchen design. A School of
Practical Cookery and an official training program for orderlies had also been started.

The second subcommission report showed the reorganization of the army's
Medical Statistics Department. In the wake of these reforms, the British army's
Statistics Department became the best in Europe.

The third subcommission established the first Army Medical School after many
delays and near-defeat. Because of its precarious state, Nightingale had remained closely
connected with this particular project. The first medical students had arrived at Fort
Pitt, near Chatham, in September 1860. As Secretary of State for War, Herbert had appointed Nightingale and Sir James Clark to write the regulations for the medical school,
to nominate the professors, and to design the syllabus and lectures. Nightingale recruited several of her old Crimean friends for teaching positions, including Dr. E. A. Parkes
to chair the Department of Hygiene, Dr. William Aiken to head the Department of
Pathology, and Dr. Thomas Longmore to be Professor of Surgery.

In his introductory address at the school on October 2, 1860, Longmore noted
Nightingale's role in originating and establishing the school. Clark also wrote of
Nightingale's role in his introduction to Dr. Andrew Combe's *Management of Infancy*,
published in 1860:

> *In the Army Medical School just instituted hygiene will form the most important branch of the*
> *young medical officer's instruction. For originating this School we have to thank Miss*
> *Nightingale, who, had her long and persevering efforts effected no other improvement in the*
> *Army, would have conferred by this alone an inestimable boon upon the British soldier.*[27]

Nightingale called the fourth subcommission the "wiping commission" because it
took care of all the loose ends. Officially and primarily, it was responsible for the health
of the soldier. Newly enacted regulations and codes defined the responsibilities of the
Purveyor's Department; the distribution of all supplies to military hospitals; the operation of military and regimental hospitals in peace and war; and the duties of all officers
and personnel in the military hospitals, including the hospital governor (administrator), principal medical officers, captain of orderlies, orderlies, female nurses, and the

superintendent of nurses. A committee was also formed to address the moral health of the soldiers. Each barrack was considered up to standard if it had a library, reading room, recreation room, coffee shop, lecture room, outdoor recreation facility, and shops for learning different trades. These regulations were first instituted in 1861 at Woolwich General Military Hospital.

Seeing the fruits of their labors

Nightingale and her colleagues were blessed in a way that many reformers never experience: They saw change happen in their lifetime — and very quickly at that. In the first 3 years of reform, the fatality rate of soldiers stationed in England fell to less than one-half the number in earlier years, and the total mortality from all diseases dropped to less than the previous mortality from consumption (tuberculosis) and other respiratory diseases alone.

Even after these early victories, Nightingale continued to work unceasingly, energized by the results that were transforming her world and fired by her mystical vision to fight for "my country and my God."[28] If her contemporaries couldn't completely comprehend her inner motivations, they could at least see the outcomes of her labors. Sir John McNeill, writing to Nightingale from the perspective of a quarter-century of high government service, commented on the magnitude of what had been accomplished:

> It vexes me greatly to find that you are thwarted and annoyed by such things as you tell me of, but I am not in the least surprised. I did not expect you to accomplish so much in so short a time. Be assured that the progress from a worse to a better system is in almost every department of human affairs a progress slow and interrupted. Do not then be discouraged. If you have not done all that you desired — and who ever did? — you have done more than any one else ever did or could have done, and the good you have done will live after you, growing from generation to generation. I do not remember any instance in which new ideas have made more rapid progress.[29]

Chapter 11

Nurses Training &
Health Statistics

My principle has always been: that we should give the best training we could to any woman of any class, of any sect, "paid" or unpaid, who had the requisite qualifications, moral, intellectual & physical, for the vocation of a Nurse.

— Florence Nightingale to Dr. William Farr, October 13, 1866[1]

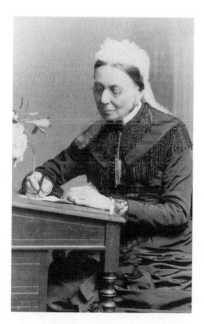

Sarah Elizabeth Wardroper, first matron of the Nightingale School of Nursing, which opened in 1860 at St. Thomas's Hospital in London

Fully occupied with army medical reform and struggling with her physical illness, Nightingale felt pressured by the additional responsibility of the Nightingale Fund. Since June 1856 when the Deed of Trust was drawn up between Nightingale and the fund trustees, the fund's investments had been managed by a council that included her friends and colleagues: Sidney Herbert as chairman, Charles Bracebridge, Sir James Clark, Dr. William Bowman, Sir John McNeill, and Dr. Henry Bence Jones.

In March 1858, Nightingale had asked Herbert to release her from any responsibility of organizing a formal training program for nurses because of her poor health, but he advised her against stepping down. She was too well known now: Nightingale *was* nursing. The fund council and the public wanted Nightingale herself to lead the effort.

In April 1859, McNeill suggested that the council form a governing subcommittee with a paid secretary in London to manage the fund's daily affairs. Herbert felt this would be a relief to Nightingale because of her fragile health and heavy workload. The subcommittee members included McNeill, Clark, Bowman, and Sir Joshua Jebb (Surveyor-General of Prisons). Arthur Hugh Clough, the husband of Nightingale's cousin Blanche Smith, was appointed Secretary of the Fund at £100 per year.

School for nurses takes shape

Nightingale felt that the most appropriate place to begin a new nurse training program would be St. Thomas's Hospital in London. She had met the matron (superintendent of nurses), Sarah Elizabeth Wardroper, while preparing to go to the Crimea and had seen her again after returning. Nightingale thought Wardroper, a 42-year-old mother of four, was the only person qualified to run a successful nurse training program. A gentlewoman and widow, Wardroper wasn't a nurse but had taught herself the role of matron, whose duties she assumed in 1854. Nightingale wrote about her to Herbert:

> I have discussed the matter with some of the authorities at St. Thomas's. The Matron of that hospital is the only one of any existing hospital I would recommend to form a School for nurses. It is not the best conceivable way of beginning. But it seems to me the best possible. It will be a beginning in a very humble way. But at all events it will not be beginning with a failure, i.e. the possibility of upsetting a large hospital — for she is a tried matron.[2]

Nightingale had written to Richard G. Whitfield, the current Resident Medical Officer of St. Thomas's, when she was at Balaclava in 1856 to thank him for sending to Scutari Mrs. Roberts, her favorite nurse who had nursed her while she was recovering from Crimean fever. She had also recommended to Whitfield Lady Jane Shaw Stewart, the former nursing superintendent at Balaclava, who wanted to come to St. Thomas's for surgical nurse training.

Whitfield was familiar with Nightingale's articles in the trade magazine *The Builder* in 1858, in which she advocated the pavilion plan of hospital construction using smaller wings, as opposed to the long corridor system used at Netley Hospital. Like Nightingale, Whitfield was a supporter of sanitary reformer Sir Edwin Chadwick and he sent her his booklet, *The Administration of Medical Relief to Outpatients at Hospitals,* which championed Chadwick's argument that it was false economy on the part of Poor Law (public welfare) authorities to provide medical care as cheaply as possible.

This developing relationship was to be of strategic importance. In 1859, St. Thomas's Hospital was in dire need of renovations and also happened to lie in the path of a projected railway line from London Bridge to Charing Cross. The hospital's governing board and staff members couldn't decide what to do. Some members wished to sell only part of the site to the railroad and maintain the existing buildings, while others, including Whitfield, wanted to sell the railroad the entire property, which would enable them to build a new hospital of the latest sanitary design in a healthier suburban area.

To break the impasse, Whitfield asked Nightingale to lend her support to his relocation plan. After studying the matter from all possible angles, she sided with Whitfield, wrote a report to Prince Albert (a member of the hospital's board), and enlisted the aid of her brother-in-law, Sir Harry Verney, and his friends in Parliament to convince the railroad to buy the entire hospital site.

Although the board agreed to relocate the hospital to a new suburban location, powerful interests led by Dr. John Simon, medical officer of the City of London, forced the board to rebuild in the heart of London. The new hospital finally opened in 1871 in its present-day location, across the Thames from the Houses of Parliament. In the interim, it was housed in temporary quarters in the old Surrey Gardens Music Hall.

After the relocation controversy was settled, Whitfield, Verney, and others put together an administrative agreement that called for St. Thomas's to provide facilities for the Nightingale Fund's nurse training program and for the fund to pay the cost. In

March 1860, Arthur Clough and the treasurer of St. Thomas's began assigning specific wards where the students, known as "nurse probationers," would train. In May, advertisements announcing the program were placed in the newspapers.

Nightingale's guidelines provided that the matron had the power to select as well as dismiss the probationers and to designate which Sisters (women with little nursing skill who did mostly housekeeping work) could give instructions to the probationers in certain areas. It was also agreed that some of the Sisters would be selected as probationers to receive further education and a certificate if they finished the training. Whitfield was to give lectures.

Even with these careful arrangements, the plan met opposition. The most antagonistic hospital doctor was John Flint South, a senior surgeon who felt that a training institution for Sisters and nurses was entirely unnecessary. In a pamphlet published in 1857, he wrote:

> As regards the nurses or ward-maids, these, as I have said, are much in the position of housemaids and require little teaching beyond that of poultice-making, which is easily acquired, and the enforcement of cleanliness and attention to the patients' wants. They need not be of the class of persons required for Sisters, not having such responsibility ... as a general rule the nurses do not stay in the same hospital or the same ward more than a year or two, being like many household servants, fond of a change.[3]

Despite South's objections, other doctors praised the plan and the nurse training and reform continued. R.H. Golden, another St. Thomas's doctor, wrote to Wardroper:

> ... I consider their [Nightingale's nurses] introduction a great advantage and blessing to the Hospital. The whole arrangement for the nursing since 1860 is most satisfactory and a great contrast to what it was before that time ... The advantage of training women for the special duties of nurses is so obvious to all persons, not only medical men, that I need hardly say that even some sacrifices should be made to do so ...[4]

Nightingale's training program launched

The Nightingale School of Nursing opened at St. Thomas's Hospital, then located on Borough High Street, on June 24, 1860. The first 11 nurse probationers arrived on July 9. Because of her chronic illness and the press of other work, Nightingale chose to work from behind the scenes on the details of managing the school. She and the Nightingale Fund Council made the following decisions about how the salaries were to be paid.

The council agreed to pay the hospital board £22 a year for the board and lodging of each nurse probationer. Wardroper, the first matron of the Nightingale School, was to be paid £100 per year in addition to her hospital salary of £150. Whitfield, the first appointed lecturer, would receive a stipend of £50 per year in addition to his existing income of £643. The ward Sisters would be paid £10 extra per year for instructing the nursing probationers on their wards.[5]

The nurse probationers, who had to sign a 4-year contract, were to be admitted free of charge and were to receive free room and board, their own tea and sugar, a washing allowance, and a wage of £10 for their first year. During their first year, they worked under the instruction of the Sisters on the wards. Unfortunately, no one had determined the competence of the Sisters to teach, and this aspect of the program remained a source of conflict for the next 10 years. Upon successfully finishing their first year's training, probationers were placed on the Nightingale Fund Register as "certificated" nurses. They then entered service as hospital nurses at St. Thomas's or other approved institutions for 3 years.

Nightingale clearly envisioned the nurse as one who delivered patient care — not one who merely did housekeeping work. In the beginning, she was reluctant to recruit "ladies" to train as nurses for fear that they wouldn't want to get their hands dirty. She hoped to recruit women who had received some education and were accustomed to earning a wage, such as the upper servant class consisting of the daughters of tradesmen and small farmers. Her aim was to gradually replace the existing St. Thomas's staff with trained nurses. As she wrote to Sir John McNeill, "the primary object is to be the establishment of a normal school for nurses with a view to elevation of that class to the position of a profession."[6]

Nightingale's vision was for trained nurses to go into hospital nursing and organized district nursing for the poor, not into private nursing in the homes of the wealthy. She also hoped that when enough nurses were trained, including some for leadership positions as matrons, teams of nurses would be sent out into the community to reform the existing practice of nursing and improve care. This eventually happened with the Liverpool Workhouse Infirmary in 1865.

According to the school application form, applicants were expected to be "sober, honest, truthful, trustworthy, punctual, quiet and orderly, clean and neat." And they were expected to become skillful in applying dressings and leeches; administering enemas; helping patients move, change position, and keep clean; making and applying bandages; understanding and maintaining adequate ventilation; and strictly observing the sick for secretions, expectoration, breathing, sleep, state of wounds, and effect of diet and medicines.[7] These basic skills are still learned in nursing fundamentals courses around the world today (minus the use of leeches, of course).

To assess the probationers' progress, Nightingale drew up her famous record sheet titled "Monthly State of Personal Character and Acquirements of Nurse During Her Period of Service." The probationers were also graded ("excellent," "moderate," or "0") on five personal characteristics: punctuality, quietness, trustworthiness, personal neatness and cleanliness, and ward management.

Postgraduate problems

From the outset, the major problem confronting the Nightingale School of Nursing was a shortage of qualified women to train as nurses and matrons. Another major problem was keeping the probationers in the program for the 3-year work period following the initial year of training. Because many of them viewed their contract as more like a servant's — even Nightingale thought the contract was terrible — very few of the original probationers were still in the program at the end of the first 4 years.

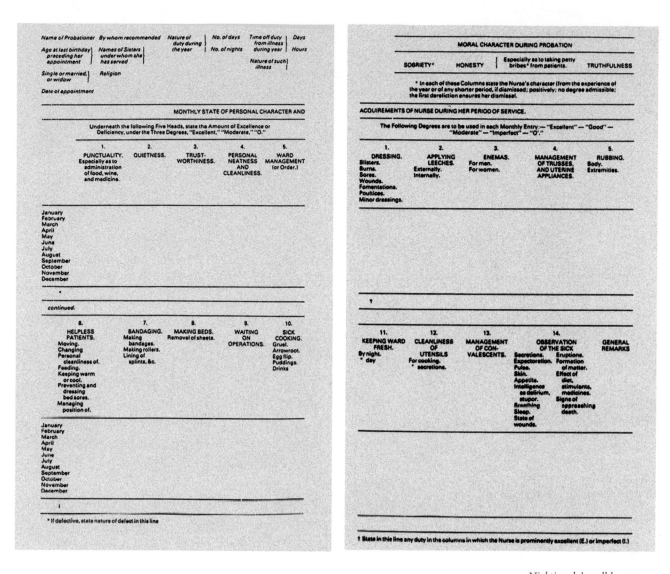

Nightingale's well-known record sheet, called "Monthly State of Personal Character and Acquirements of Nurse During Her Period of Service," which was used to assess students at the Nightingale School of Nursing

During the first year of the program, 3 of the 11 probationers were dismissed, 1 left because of poor health, and 2 were appointed as extra nurses at St. Thomas's Hospital. The 6 vacancies were filled by additional probationers. Thirteen probationers, including the 2 extra nurses at St. Thomas's, completed their year's course in June 1861 and were placed on the register as "certificated" nurses. However, only 4 out of this first group were still in nursing and able to collect their promised salary at the end of the second year. Of the others, 1 died of typhus and the others were dismissed for disobedience, drunkenness, or poor health.

Although the fund and trustees realized the many problems to be resolved, the first public report and the first council report were both favorable. The popular *St. James's Magazine* printed a glowing report on the Nightingale School in April 1861, describing the nurses in their brown dresses and snowy white caps and aprons moving noiselessly and cheerfully from bed to bed.[8]

Although there were other training programs in a few hospitals, they were all associated with religious orders. Nightingale's program was the first nurse training program with no religious affiliation. The more technical curriculum she developed was based on

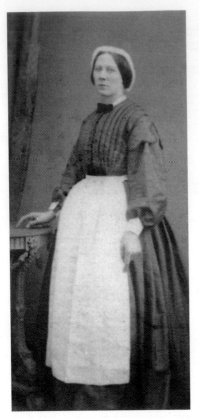

Mary Barker, a member of the first graduating class of the Nightingale School of Nursing in June 1861

the existing science of the day and stressed high moral character, the acquisition of 14 specific skills, and a basic understanding of anatomy and physiology.

As a result of her landmark training program, Nightingale became known as the founder of modern secular nursing. She began her system of nursing as a service and as an education for women, believing that nursing was a constructive way of providing work for women and freeing them from oppression. Other hospital boards and administrators, recognizing a new way to develop a trained nursing staff, began their own training programs based in whole or in part on Nightingale's model. These new programs soon competed with the Nightingale program for qualified applicants.

Revolutionizing hospital data collection

Having successfully initiated the reorganization of the army's Medical Statistics Department, Nightingale turned her attention to civilian hospitals in London, where she found similar problems in medical data collection. Hospitals in the mid-1800s had no scientific or standardized approach to gathering data on admissions and discharges, and each hospital followed its own system of disease nomenclature and classification.

Uniform hospital data

To remedy this situation, in 1859 Nightingale — with the help of medical statistician Dr. William Farr and others — designed a series of Model Hospital Forms that would ideally be used in all hospitals to provide uniform and consistent medical information about patients. These forms consisted of:

• the Admission and Discharge Form, which included such basic information as date of admission, date of recovery, date of death, state at discharge, number of days in hospital, and the patient's previous diseases — data that are taken for granted today but weren't routinely recorded in the mid-1800s

• the Disease Specification and Incidence Form, a standard list of classes and orders of diseases to replace the numerous systems of disease classification in use at the time (partly due to the ongoing debate between proponents of the miasma and contagion theories of disease)

• the Hospital Statistical Form, a huge sheet that contained 26 columns for entering the number of patients with specific conditions who were admitted, cured, dead, discharged incurable, or discharged at their own request as well as the number of days hospitalized per case.

The development of these forms was based on Nightingale's belief that proper analysis of accurate statistical data could help identify the best treatments for certain illnesses and the optimal number of days needed for treatment as well as mortality rates from various causes in different hospitals. In addition, analysis of complications and causes of death could reveal much about each hospital's sanitary conditions.

Nightingale had her Model Hospital Forms privately printed and circulated in various London hospitals that agreed to use them — St. Thomas's, St. Mary's, University College, Guy's Hospital, and St. Bartholomew's. With the help of these forms, Guy's

Hospital printed a statistical analysis of patients from 1854 to 1861, and St. Thomas's from 1857 to 1860; St. Bartholomew's printed a table of its cases for 1860 alone.

In addition, Nightingale had her Paris friend Julius Mohl circulate her model forms to doctors and hospitals in France. In October 1860, she enthusiastically wrote to Farr that the leading medical journals in Paris had published her article on the model forms.

Uniform surgical data

Having succeeded in developing standardized forms for specific diseases, in 1861 Nightingale started a campaign to promote uniform hospital surgical statistics with the help of Farr and her friend from St. Bartholomew's Hospital, Sir James Paget. She believed such records would help doctors ascertain the best surgical procedures for certain conditions and allow the comparison of sanitary conditions among hospitals and specific wards.[9]

Paget continued to help Nightingale refine her forms, which were still too vague and complicated. The revised forms included age, sex, accident, nature of operations, complications, and so forth. She had the new forms printed and supplied them to hospitals throughout England. In June 1861, delegates from eight London Hospitals — Guy's, St. Bartholomew's, St. Thomas's, London Hospital, St. George's, King's College, Middlesex, and St. Mary's — unanimously agreed that the metropolitan hospitals should adopt a standard system of patient registration, publish their statistics annually, and accept Nightingale's Model Hospital Forms.

Now that her Model Hospital Forms were launched, Nightingale printed and circulated her papers "Hospital Statistics" and "Proposal for a Uniform Plan of Hospital Statistics" among leading doctors, hospital officials, and other opinion leaders. She also sent a statistical paper to be read at the Social Science Congress in Dublin in August 1861. In September 1862, *The Journal of the Statistical Society* reported on the statistics of various hospitals that used her forms. The new forms and related statistics were pre-

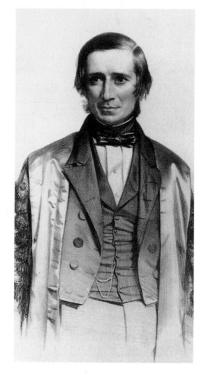

Sir James Paget, who helped Nightingale refine her Model Hospital Forms

BELOW: *Filled-in portion of Nightingale's Hospital Admission and Discharge Form, one of the Model Hospital Forms that she developed in 1859*

A.—HOSPITAL ADMISSION AND DISCHARGE BOOK.

No. of Case.	Date of Admission.	NAME.	AGE.	Sex. M. or F.	RESIDENCE, and Place where taken Ill or Injured.	TRADE or OCCUPATION.	DISEASE or ACCIDENT.	Date. Of ATTACK.	Of RECOVERY.	Of DEATH.	Of DISCHARGE (Relieved) or (Unrelieved,) or otherwise.	Of TRANSFER to other Division of Hospital.	DURATION OF CASE in Hospital, in Days and Quarters.	REMARKS. (Previous Diseases of Patients and of Parents.)
1					*Example of the Manner of filling up the Return.*									
2	May 17.	John Johnson...	35	M.	263, Strand.................. Run over by a cab on London Bridge.	Shoemaker...	Compound fracture of tibia and fibula. Amputation, May 20.	May 17	Aug. 18	—	Aug. 18	—	94 days	—
3	Aug. 5.	Maria Wood...	29	F.	28, Burrage Road, Plumstead.......... Attacked at her residence.	Laundress.....	Ague...............	Aug. 2	Aug. 28	—	Aug. 28	—	26 days	—
4	Nov. 3.	James Young...	14	M.	Workhouse. Attacked at workhouse school.	Son of a tailor	Smallpox, 12 days. Pneumonia, 3 days. (Not vaccinated.)	Nov. 3	—	Nov. 18	—	—	15 days	—

Portion of proposed Hospital Statistical Form, one of Nightingale's Model Hospital Forms developed in 1859 with detailed instructions provided on the right-hand side

sented at the International Statistical Congress in 1862 and 1863. In 1863, she had the forms incorporated into a new edition of her book *Notes on Hospitals*.

Nightingale takes on the census

Nightingale saw that it was but a short step from collecting disease and surgical data in hospitals to collecting health and illness data from the general population; she believed that such information could have far-reaching consequences in the improvement of public health. It seemed to her that adding a number of questions to the census form of 1860 (which was to be sent out in 1861) would be an excellent way of gathering such data. She specifically wanted information on the number of sick or infirm people living in each dwelling, which the Irish Census of 1851 had already included, and details on housing and sanitary conditions, which she considered directly linked to the health of the population.

Accordingly, she and Dr. Farr began redesigning the census form of 1860. In a letter to Farr, she wrote:

I feel so strongly about this Census bill that I cannot help writing to you of how much importance it would be, as bearing on all questions of the public health, to have a column in the enumeration paper in which should be entered the number of sick people in each house with the diseases. In this way we should have a return of the whole Sick and Diseases in the United Kingdom for one spring day, which would give a good average of the Sanitary state of all classes of the population.

The Mortuary Returns take no cognizance of a large amount of disease which rarely proves fatal, but which nevertheless represents a vast loss of efficiency in the population ... And, when taken with the Sick Returns of Hospitals, Asylums, Workhouses and so forth, they would afford insight into problems of great importance.[10]

Nightingale and Farr theorized that a complete census depended on the collection of consistent details. In a letter to him in April 1861, she described the comical way the census had been collected from her at the Burlington Hotel:

On Sunday morning (the 7th) a verbal message was sent up to me, not by the occupier of the Hotel but by his fac-totum (a kind of house-steward), desiring me to write my age (& my maid's) on a bit of paper — nothing more. This was the message, verbatim et literatim.

I swallowed the answer which rose to my lips — not thinking it worth while to have a war of words with this person — and, after ascertaining from his assertion that no Schedules had been left for the Families in this Hotel, I took one of the Specimen Forms you were so kind as to give me, & wrote the information fully & accurately therein concerning myself & maid ... & sent it down to him.

I leave you to think, if the message sent up to the other families occupying apartments in these 4 houses, were similar to that sent to me, of how dependable & valuable a nature is the information filled in by this person on his Sheet.

He appeared to consider the Census Act as an invention designed to afford him the amusement of asking people their ages — and of drawing upon his imagination for the rest of the information required.

As you know how much interested I am in the proper working of the Census & that I had rather the information required of us (as regards our health & houses) were more than less complete, I venture to suggest that all heads of families whether that family consist of one, two or more persons, wherever living, whether in hotels, lodgings ... should be required to fill up their own paper.[11]

Nightingale's proposals soon ran into opposition from the Census Bureau, the House of Commons, and the House of Lords, all of which felt that people shouldn't be asked so many questions. The government decided that the question of health or sickness was too indeterminate to ask each individual and that the answers would not be based on a uniform principle, thus providing inaccurate results. Nightingale attempted to answer their objections but, in the end, her proposals, too advanced for their time, were voted down in both Houses of Parliament.

A passion for statistics

Nightingale's development of the Model Hospital Forms and her efforts to expand the census form were both examples of her passionate belief that statistics could play a major role in improving public health and society in general. To her, statistics was the "most important science in the whole world, [because] upon it depends the practical application of every other science."[12] She believed that statistics could prove that the cost of crime, disease, and excessive mortality was greater than the cost of the sanitary improvements contained in her reform proposals. In addition, she showed how this type of information could be released to the press to shape public opinion and improve the health of the people.

International Statistical Congress of 1860

The statistical results obtained by the first hospitals to use Nightingale's Model Hospital Forms were so promising that she and Farr decided to introduce the forms at the International Statistical Congress in London in July 1860. Distressed by the lack of organization of the Congress's Sanitary Section, Nightingale worked with Farr, one of the General Secretaries, to design the format for this section. Although she didn't attend the Congress because of her chronic illness, she submitted a paper on "Hospital Statistics" and a detailed "Proposal for a Uniform Plan of Hospital Statistics."

In a letter to Lord Shaftesbury, who was head of the Sanitary Section, Nightingale pointed out that each of the governments attending the Congress had a vast amount of statistical information that could shed light on ways to prevent disease in its own country, and she asked all the delegates to share examples of successful cases of reduced mortality and disease. The delegates ultimately decided that all of the governments represented should adopt Nightingale's proposals for uniform hospital statistics.

Nightingale was keenly interested in the Congress's proceedings and, aided by her brother-in-law Sir Harry Verney and her cousin Hilary Bonham Carter, she entertained many of the international delegates at her residence at the Burlington Hotel. She wrote notes to Hilary about whom to invite, how to preside at breakfast meetings, and how to flatter the guests:

> ... *Put Dr. Balfour's big book back where he can see it when drinking his tea. Send me up one of my new copies. Please ask Quetelet to fix an hour & day (any hour) when he would come & see me, if he will be so good. Ask them to breakfast tomorrow. Let me see Sutherland before Chadwick goes. If Berg can stay now till twelve o'clock I will come down before that & see him. If Engel will come tomorrow, then ditto with him. If not, let them fix the hour.*[13]

Nightingale didn't attend these breakfasts herself, but afterward she invited selected guests to meet with her privately upstairs. One of these was Adolphe Quetelet, the Belgian statistician whose work on "moral statistics" was especially intriguing to Nightingale.

Visionary meets statistician

A statistician, astronomer, mathematician, and sociologist considered the founder of the modern science of social statistics, Quetelet was fascinated by numbers and collected an enormous amount of data from throughout Europe on human beings and their behavior. In addition to basic physical and social information, such as height, weight, age, educational level, occupation, and financial status (class), Quetelet collected data on crime, suicide, and marriage — which he called "moral statistics" because the individual had a choice of action in these areas. He believed that by correctly analyzing such data one could predict various types of behavior and events in society. For example, he showed that the number of crimes committed annually by persons in each age group was a constant.[14]

Quetelet astonished skeptics of his work when, in 1844, he predicted the extent of draft evasion among 100,000 Frenchmen. Based on the actual height distribution of those who answered the draft call, he predicted that 2,000 men had avoided the draft by pretending to be under the height requirement, an estimate that was found to be true. Using French statistics from 1826 to 1831, he also predicted the constancy with which crimes repeat themselves, including "how many would stain their hands with the blood of their fellow-creatures, how many would be forgers, and how many poisoners ..."[15]

Quetelet's theory was criticized by some people who construed it as denying men free will to choose between good and evil. However, Quetelet maintained that statistical analysis merely quantified the forces already operating in society and that this knowledge allowed societal conditions to be modified and peoples' lives to be improved. He organized people across Europe and America to gather census data that could serve as "moral statistics." He also organized an international forum at the Crystal Palace Exposition in London in 1851, which led to the First International Statistical Congress, held in Brussels in 1853.

Quetelet's moral statistics theory was a major influence on Nightingale's own concept of the social sciences as a system of laws and regulations that could be used to ascertain needed reforms for the improvement of public health. On a more personal level, she was especially fascinated by his law of the flowering of plants — the method he used to predict when a flower would bloom. According to this law, lilacs would bloom when the sum of the squares of the mean daily temperatures, counted from the end of the last frost date, equaled 4264° C. Using this theory, Nightingale for years sent her sister a lilac branch calculated to flower on April 19, Parthe's birthday.[16]

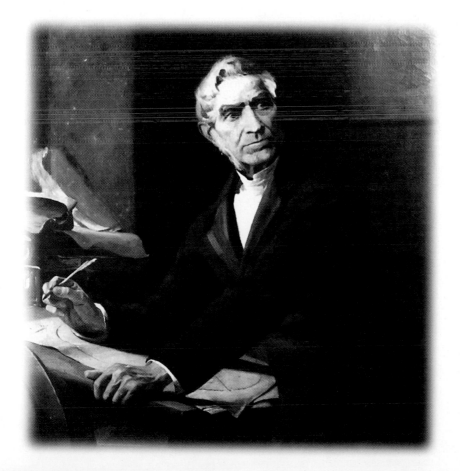

Adolphe Quetelet (1796-1874), Belgian statistician whose work on "moral statistics" was a major influence on Nightingale and who met Nightingale during the International Statistical Congress held in London in 1860

When Nightingale received from Quetelet his two-volume *Physique Sociale* in November 1872, she selectively annotated it and in 1873 wrote her own creed on the title page:

> *The sense of infinite power*
> *The assurances of solid Certainty*
> *The endless vista of Improvement*
> *from the Principles of*
> *PHYSIQUE SOCIALE*
> *If only found possible to apply on occasions when it is so much wanted* [17]

Nightingale's commitment to statistics was closely tied to her philosophical and spiritual beliefs. She considered Quetelet's *Essai de Physique Sociale* (1835; revised 1869) to be a religious work — a revelation of the will of God — and felt that his science was essential to all political and social administration. As she wrote in one of her annotations, the laws governing social phenomena were "God's laws, the laws of our moral progress:"

> *All Sciences of Observation depend upon Statistical methods — without these, are blind empiricism. Make your facts comparable before deducing causes. Incomplete, pell-mell observations arranged so as to support theory; insufficient number of observations; this is what one sees.* [18]

To Nightingale, politicians were untrained in the interpretation of statistics; as a result, legislation was "not progressive but see-saw-y," written by officials who "legislate without knowing what [they] are doing."[19] Her interest in the practical application of Quetelet's work came from her vast observation and experience of the world:

> *On my part this passionate study is not in the least based on a love of science, a love I would not pretend I possessed. It comes uniquely from the fact that I have seen so much of the misery and sufferings of humanity, of the irrelevance of laws and of Governments, of the stupidity, dare I say it? — of our political system, of the dark blindness of those who involve themselves in guiding our body social that ... frequently it comes to me as a flash of light across my spirit that the only study worthy of that name is that of which you have so firmly put forward the principles.* [20]

Chapter 12

Literary Fame & Personal Misfortune

I thank you sincerely & warmly for what you are kind enough to say about my "Notes on Nursing" — you do not know how, in the midst of much disappointment, such words cheer & strengthen us. The only possible merit of my little book is that there is not a word in it, written for the sake of writing, but only forced out of one by much experience in human suffering.

— Florence Nightingale to Harriet Martineau, July 29, 1860[1]

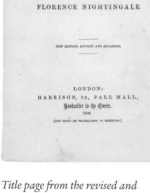

Title page from the revised and enlarged edition of Nightingale's Notes on Nursing, *published soon after the first edition in 1860*

At the end of the 1850s, Nightingale was busily organizing the world's first secular training school for nurses at St. Thomas's Hospital in London as well as preparing numerous statistical studies to support her work for army reform, with the help of her statistician friend Dr. William Farr. During this time, she developed a steady correspondence with many of the leading authorities on sanitary reform, one of whom was Edwin Chadwick, an outspoken leader of the sanitary movement in Britain. Their correspondence began in 1857 and continued for some 30 years until just before Chadwick died in 1890.[2]

Nightingale was familiar with Chadwick's work because he had served as a commissioner on the first General Board of Health from 1848 to 1854, the same board on which Dr. John Sutherland had served as one of two chief medical inspectors. Chadwick had also written or contributed to many of the government Blue Books on health and social issues that had raised Nightingale's — and the nation's — consciousness in the 1840s.

A friend of Jeremy Bentham and like him a staunch advocate of centralized government, Chadwick zealously advocated public control of the water supply and drainage business in the London metropolitan area. Private companies controlled this lucrative industry, and Chadwick aroused the opposition of powerful political interests. When the enabling legislation for the General Board of Health came up for renewal in Parliament in 1854, the opposition reorganized the board, removing Chadwick. However, he continued to be active in sanitary matters, the civil service, agricultural drainage, open spaces, and transportation issues.

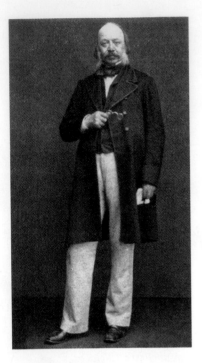

Sanitary reformer Edwin Chadwick (1800-1890), who encouraged Nightingale to write Notes on Hospitals *and* Notes on Nursing

Nightingale and Chadwick sometimes edited each other's papers for presentations at statistical meetings. Chadwick, adept at promoting and disseminating new ideas, realized that Nightingale's work needed to reach a wider audience. Confident that the public would respond to her advice, he suggested in December 1858 that she write a book on how improved sanitation in hospitals could help prevent disease. He further proposed that she write a nursing book for laymen that would teach them basic sanitary and caregiving measures that they could use to care for themselves and their families:

> *I do not feel equal to the task ... I am not in a position to be heard or should only be heard by hundreds — I am not a doctor, whereas you are the greatest national nurse, you would be heard by hundreds of thousands, and millions, who will give you a deep and a well deserved attention.[3]*

Nightingale had already assembled a vast "database" during her long campaign for army reform, and she now began to prepare her first two books, *Notes on Hospitals* and *Notes on Nursing,* with the idea of addressing a larger audience. (The word *Notes* in the title was her way of describing concise chapters of her works.) Chadwick was correct in foreseeing the large audience that Nightingale's publications might reach — her *Notes on Nursing* became a bestseller.

Notes on Hospitals

Even before she went to the Crimea, Nightingale was recognized in England as a leading authority on hospitals in Europe. Her *Notes on Hospitals,* published in 1859, raised the entire discussion to a higher level and had an immediate impact on hospital design and construction.

It's difficult for those living now to imagine the deplorably unsanitary conditions that existed in civilian hospitals in the mid-19th century. Sir Erich Erichsen, a surgeon of the day, wrote that one could find "the town free from infection [but] the hospital saturated by it, to such an extent as to induce its own surgeons to recommend their patients not to enter it, to compel them to refrain from operating."[4] Erichsen described most hospitals as:

> *... simply big houses, with basements containing kitchens, lavatories, cellars, and the ordinary offices ... with an operating-theatre and dead-house more or less closely connected with the main building, with every floor filled with sick and wounded people; on the ground floor, accidents and operating cases; on the first floor, probably medical patients; above, chronic, surgical and medical cases. Who can wonder at the development of pyaemia [blood poisoning] below, and erysipelas above? Who would live in an ordinary house thus filled? Who would expect to preserve his health if he ventured to inhabit it?[5]*

The first section of *Notes on Hospitals* focused on sanitary conditions of hospitals and hospital construction, and was based on two of Nightingale's papers that were presented at an October 1858 meeting of the National Association for the Promotion of Social Science in Liverpool. These papers included tables prepared by Farr from returns furnished to Nightingale from 15 metropolitan hospitals.

Nightingale listed four elements essential to the health of hospitals: fresh air, light, ample space, and subdivision of the sick into separate buildings, or pavilions. She also described specific problems in hospital construction and management that could promote ill health and provided measures to correct them:

• *Defective methods of ventilation and warming.* Sufficient fresh air (at least 2,500 cubic feet per bed per hour) should be provided to "keep wards perfectly sweet." Fireplaces should be located in the center of the ward rather than in a side wall, to distribute heat more evenly.

• *Defective height of wards.* To avoid accumulating foul air at the top of the ward, each ward of 30 beds should have ceilings about 16 to 17 feet high, with windows reaching to within 1 foot of ceilings.

• *Excessive width of wards between opposite windows.* To ensure adequate air exchange, the distance between opposite windows should be no more than 30 feet.

• *Beds arranged along a dead wall.* Placing beds along windowless walls deprives patients of fresh air and sunlight.

• *More than two rows of beds between opposite windows.* Double wards (with two rows of beds) are too wide for adequate ventilation, create a draft on the heads of the inner row of patients, and prevent the head nurse from seeing the entire ward at one time.

• *Windows on only one side of a ward or a closed corridor connecting the wards.* A "dead wall" or closed corridor on one side impairs the natural ventilation of the ward.

• *Use of absorbent materials for floors, walls, and ceilings of hospitals and washing rooms.* Floors, walls and ceilings should be made of pure white, polished, nonabsorbent cement to prevent the absorption of organic matter emitted from respirations.

• *Defective toilets and sinks.* Toilets and sinks should be properly constructed and ventilated, and set off from the wards to prevent outbreaks of fevers.

• *Defective ward furniture.* Beds should be of iron; all other furniture of oak. Mattresses should be of hair. For better cleanliness, all eating and drinking utensils and washing vessels should be of glass or earthenware instead of metal.

• *Inadequate accommodations for nursing and discipline.* Simplicity of construction allows for proper supervision and correct distribution of patients in a ward. A head nurse can supervise 32 patients per ward.

• *Defective hospital kitchens.* Adequate facilities are needed to prepare varied and nutritious meals for the sick.

• *Defective hospital laundries.* To lower the risk of fevers to washerwomen, laundries should have sufficient space and water for each washer, proper drainage and ventilation, and properly constructed drying and ironing rooms.

• *Erecting hospitals in towns.* Because land in cities is too expensive to allow correct hospital construction, hospitals should be located in suburban areas.

• *Defective drainage.* Sewers become cesspools if they are improperly sized or placed.

• *Construction of hospitals without free circulation of external air.* To encourage optimal ventilation, hospitals should not be surrounded by high walls or have enclosed courtyards. Even in a pavilion-style facility, the distance between the pavilions should be double the height of their walls to avoid interfering with light and air.

The second section of *Notes on Hospitals* contained the evidence that Nightingale had presented in the Royal Commission report. Recalling that she had been studying the organization of civilian and military hospitals for 13 years, she summarized the extent of her travels for hospital research:

> *I have visited all the hospitals in London, Dublin, and Edinburgh, many county hospitals, some of the naval hospitals in England; all the hospitals in Paris, and studied at the "Soeurs de Charité;" the Institution on the Rhine [Kaiserswerth], where I was twice in training as a nurse; the hospitals at Berlin, and many others in Germany, at Lyons, Rome, Alexandria, Constantinople, Brussels; also the war hospitals of the French and Sardinians.[6]*

The third section of the book contained her three articles on hospital design, first published in the *Builder* in August and September 1858, in which she advocated the "pavilion plan" of hospital construction rather than the commonly accepted corridor plan. The first and third sections of the book were intended to shape public opinion about hospital organization and design.

Nightingale believed that separate pavilions (wings) would prevent the spread of infection because infections would be limited to one wing rather than moving through corridors from one ward to another. She also espoused the use of windows on opposite sides of each wing to provide cross-ventilation and sunlight and to allow the nurses to

Nightingale's design for a hospital built according to the pavilion plan, which she believed was better for containing infection than the popular corridor plan

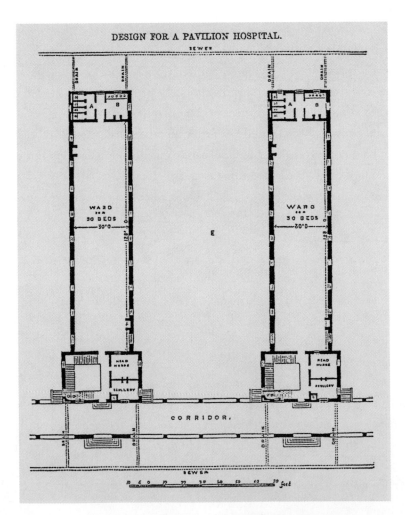

LITERARY FAME & PERSONAL MISFORTUNE

easily see the patients. The following excerpt on natural lighting is typical of Nightingale's notes:

> Now let us see how light is treated by some popular physicians and ignorant nurses. In nine cases out of ten a physician will draw down the window blinds and half shut the shutters, while an ignorant nurse will probably shut the remainder of the shutters — especially if it is a bright day — and draw the bed-curtains. We have the positive testimony of a well-known London physician, given in his report to the Netley committee that whenever he enters a sick-room, he takes care that the bed shall be so placed that the patient shall be turned away from the light ... After this, we cannot blame army medical officers for not knowing much about the matter. An acquaintance of ours one day passing a barrack, saw the windows on the sunny side boarded up in a fashion peculiar to prisons and penitentiaries. He said to a friend who accompanied him, "I was not aware that you had a penitentiary in this neighborhood." "Oh!" said he, "it is not a penitentiary — it is a military hospital. There is a great horror of light on the part of certain army medical men. I suppose," he added, "the medical officers are afraid the light will alter the shape of the men." Not a few civil surgeons, also, treat light as if it were an enemy.[7]

Although it would be another two decades before the germ theory of disease was finally proved, Nightingale's *Notes on Hospitals* provided a theoretical and practical framework for hospital design and administrative reform that served to reduce disease-related mortality. Her pavilion plan was first used at the new general hospital at Woolwich, which opened in 1865, and eventually became the standard ward plan for civilian and military hospitals in Britain and many parts of the world.

Infection: Miasma or contagion?

Nightingale's guidelines for hospital design and sanitation reflected her understanding of the prevailing theories of disease transmission. The two chief theories during her formative years were the miasma theory and the contagion theory, neither of which had been scientifically proved.

Advocates of the predominant miasma theory believed that illness was caused by poisonous vapors that were generated spontaneously from putrefying animal or vegetable matter. To back up their theory, they rightfully pointed to the advances in health that had been achieved by sanitary improvements, such as removing dung heaps, providing leakproof drain pipes for cesspools and sewerage, and generally improving cleanliness in homes and hospitals. Although the miasma theory had no scientific basis, common sense encouraged the use of measures that would minimize contamination of food and water, such as maintaining clean kitchens and ensuring cleanliness and adequate ventilation and light in the construction of buildings.

The rival contagion theory held that direct personal contact was the cause of infection. However, no one had any idea exactly what substance passed between persons. Various observers, starting with the Roman poet Lucretius (in the 1st century B.C.), postulated that disease was spread from person to person by direct contact or indirect contact through the medium of invisible "seeds." In the 1830s, an article in the *Lancet* medical journal theorized that in the spread of cholera, "We can only suppose the existence of a poison which progresses independently ... of all conditions of the air and of

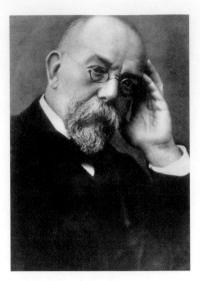

Scientist Robert Koch, whose landmark 1879 paper on the etiology of traumatic infectious diseases confirmed the germ theory of disease

the barrier of the sea; in short one that makes mankind the chief agent for its dissemination."[8] Another writer suggested that clouds of minute insects, too small for the eye to detect, "commissioned by the Divine Omnipotence to this end, are probably wafted in straight lines through the atmosphere."[9]

Prevailing opinion about one theory versus the other was guided not only by medical and scientific inclination, but also by political and economic factors. For instance, the government's response to the cholera epidemic of 1832 was based on acceptance of the miasma theory — not from scientific considerations, but political and economic ones. According to the contagion theory, the logical remedy for the epidemic would have been to quarantine seaports and arriving ships as well as cities where cholera was discovered. However, merchants, bankers, industrialists, civic leaders, and other economic and political leaders balked at the huge costs and crippling of trade and economic prosperity that a quarantine would entail. Cleaning up the town in line with the miasma theory was much more palatable and feasible.

Largely because of such economic and political considerations, and the subsequent development of the sanitary movement, the miasma explanation eventually became the prevailing theory of disease. As late as 1864, the *British Medical Journal* observed that the miasma school "probably embraces the great majority of medical practitioners and the whole of the 'sanitary' public, which teaches that sundry disease poisons are constantly being generated *de novo* by the material conditions which surround us."[10]

Nightingale was among this majority. Like many other "miasmatists" in the sanitary reform movement, she actively opposed the "contagionists" for fear that any gain in their political power or prestige might lessen the public health improvements already achieved by the sanitary reformers and could threaten future advances. In her opinion:

> *In the ordinary sense of the word, there is no proof, such as would be admitted in any scientific inquiry, that there is any such thing as "contagion"... The word "infection" which is often confounded with "contagion" expresses a fact, and does not involve a hypothesis. But just as there is no such thing as "contagion" there is no such thing as inevitable "infection." Infection acts through the air. Poison the air breathed by individuals and there is infection ... if we have a fever hospital with over-crowded, badly ventilated wards, we are quite certain to have the air become so infected as to poison the blood not only of the sick, so as to increase their mortality, but also of the medical attendants and nurses, so that they also shall become subjects of fever...[11]*

It would be another 20 years before microbes were firmly established as the agents of disease. French chemist Louis Pasteur made a major contribution in 1857 when he presented his observations on lactobacilli and the fermentation of milk to the Lille Scientific Society. In December 1858, he read a second paper to the Academy of Sciences in Paris, announcing that he had seen through his microscope small grey globules in fermented substances, which no one had ever noticed before.

These discoveries didn't become known in England until 1865, when Glasgow surgeon Joseph Lister, who was fluent in French, read Pasteur's work. Lister immediately recognized that the microscopic substances that Pasteur described must somehow be related to infection. However, it wasn't until 1867 that Lister, still without fully understanding the etiology of infection, presented his paper on antiseptic procedures. The tide finally began to turn in the late 1870s with Robert Koch's precise scientific exploration of specific and diverse bacteria and their relation to infection. Koch's landmark paper, "The Etiology of Traumatic Infectious Diseases," in 1879 finally confirmed what became known as the "germ theory" of disease.

Praise for Notes on Hospitals

When Dr. James Paget, the eminent dean of St. Bartholomew's Hospital, read Nightingale's *Notes on Hospitals,* he wrote to her: "It appears to me to be the most valuable contribution to sanitary science in application to medical institutions that I have ever read."[12]

Soon after the book's publication, Nightingale began to receive a steady stream of correspondence seeking her advice about hospital construction from committees, hospitals (in England, Belgium, France, and India), and infirmaries. In 1859, the King of Portugal, through Prince Albert, asked her advice on a hospital to be built in memory of his late wife. A second edition of *Notes on Hospitals* was published in 1859 and a third in 1863. In the third edition, she wrote:

> *It may seem a strange principle to enunciate as the very first requirement in a Hospital that it should do the sick no harm. It is quite necessary nevertheless to lay down such a principle, because the actual mortality in hospitals, especially in those of large crowded cities, is very much higher than any calculation founded on the mortality of the same class of patient treated <u>out</u> of hospitals would lead us to expect.[13]*

In the third edition, Nightingale added new chapters on improved hospital plans, convalescent hospitals, children's hospitals, and hospitals for soldiers' wives. She also made another case for keeping uniform hospital statistics to help determine the relative mortality rates and frequency of certain diseases at different hospitals.[14] She clearly understood the possibilities of data manipulation to make mortality rates appear lower than they really were:

> *We have known incurable cases discharged from one hospital, to which the deaths ought to have been accounted and received into another hospital, to die there in a day or two after admission, thereby lowering the mortality rate of the first at the expense of the second.[15]*

She was also aware of the practical challenges involved in the accurate collection and interpretation of data and saw the limitations of naive calculation of surgical mortality rates:

> *... so many operations of such and such a nature, without reference to age, sex, or cause of operation, followed by so many deaths, without reference to age, sex, or complications. Given these elements, divide the one by the other, and you get the mortality ... A statistical procedure such as this can at best lead to very loose approximations. It can convey but a very imperfect idea of the real state of the case. And one thing is quite certain, that it can lead to no practical result whatever, either as regards the true causes of the mortality, or how these might be mitigated.[16]*

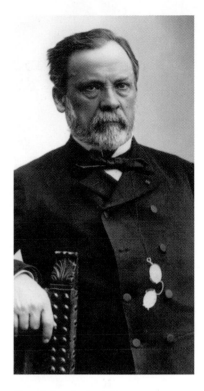

French chemist Louis Pasteur, whose work on fermentation led to greater understanding of the germ theory of disease

Notes on Nursing

Nightingale's next book, though only 79 pages long, was to become the best known of all her works. With Chadwick's encouragement, she began to write *Notes on Nursing* to help people care for themselves, their family, and their friends. She shared early drafts with Sutherland who, with his writing ability and range of experience, offered some practical insights. The advice in the following excerpt is an excellent illustration of the array of complementary talents that Nightingale and her colleagues provided one another:

> *I would soften down the doctrines in the first page because they would be disputed by some men of name, & the general tenor of the criticism would, I fear, set the M.D.s against you and stave off improvements. It is very important not to offend the doctors.*
>
> *If I were you I should go on with it. Get out all your ideas on the subject of nursing & all your experience. Never mind the arrangement. The great thing is to get the ideas into tangible shape ... I should feel disposed also to go more into details & to distinguish between the different classes of nursing, for instance, Hospital Nursing, Domestic Nursing by hired nurses, and Domestic Nursing by mothers, sisters, etc., and I put in a petition for a few words on that kind of nursing that most nearly touches my feelings — namely, nursing the poor in their own homes, and how charitable women could go about quietly, unostentatiously, & without letting their left hand know what is done by their right hand. You might draw such a picture of the work as would draw all hearts to it.*
>
> *If you come to teach nursing to the class of people from whom nurses are taken, you will have to be simpler ... illustrating your precepts when required by a few easy sentences requiring little thought but appealing to the one element that every good nurse must have, namely common sense. This strikes me as the general plan of such a manual ... God bless you and give you strength for such a work. I am yours ever.[17]*

Notes on Nursing, which focused on illness prevention, was designed for use in the home rather than the hospital because that was where most nursing occurred. It covered a broad range of topics, from the general to the particular, including ventilation and warmth, basic sick room management (rules for visitors, decreasing patients' anxiety), noise, light, diet, variety of activities (such as needlepoint, light reading, seeing the outdoors), bed and bedding, cleanliness of rooms and walls, personal cleanliness, and observation of the sick. The book also contained a great deal of Nightingale's theosophical and philosophical ideas expressed in very practical terms.

Nightingale saw healing as a reparative process regulated by the laws of nature, as are all physical phenomena, and as a manifestation of God. She believed that nature alone cures and that the nurse's job is to put the patient in the best condition for nature to act upon him. According to her, disease need not be accompanied by suffering:

> *The thing which strikes the experienced observer most forcibly is this, that the symptoms or the sufferings generally considered to be inevitable and incident to the disease are very often not symptoms of the disease at all, but of something quite different — of the want of fresh air, or of light, or of warmth, or of quiet, or of cleanliness, or of punctuality and care in the administration of diet, of each or of all of these.[18]*

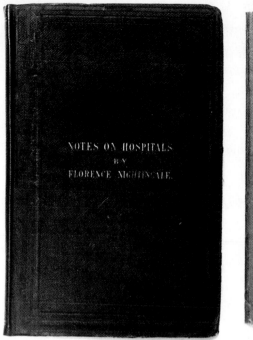

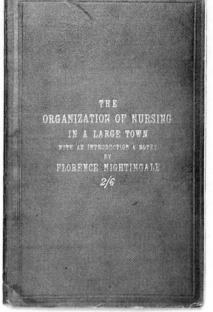

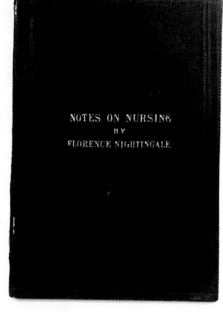

First editions of Florence Nightingale's Notes on Hospitals *(1859) and* Notes on Nursing *(1860), as well as* The Organization of Nursing in a Large Town *(1865), a book about the Liverpool nurses' training program for which she wrote the introduction and was a consultant*

By discovering and practicing the laws of healing, she believed nurses — and women in general — could participate consciously in the restorative process.

The Nightingale legacy

Nightingale's classic *Notes on Nursing* has a modern message. Many of the concepts that she suggested — for example, the healing value of color, light, music, pets, relaxation, nutrition, and exercise — are today being integrated with traditional medicine and referred to as "caring-healing modalities," "alternative therapies," or "complementary therapies." Her great accomplishment was to establish a theoretical framework for nursing practice where none had existed.

Published in January 1860, *Notes on Nursing* was an immediate success and became a touchstone for the emerging profession of nursing. The first printing of 15,000 copies sold out within a month, and the book has been in print ever since. Nightingale realized a considerable profit from *Notes on Nursing* despite the fact that there were no international copyright laws at the time and London publications could be copied with impunity. However, uninterested in personal financial gain, she was merely delighted that the book was being widely disseminated — even as far as the United States — and at no cost to her. Foreign translations soon appeared, further contributing to this groundbreaking book's enduring legacy.

Praise for Notes on Nursing

Nightingale received many congratulatory letters for *Notes on Nursing*. Dr. James Paget was as impressed with this book as he had been with her first book on hospitals: "I am ashamed to find how much I have learnt from the *Notes,* more, I think, than from any other book of the same size that I have ever read." Sir James Clark, nearing the end of his long and distinguished career in reform, said of the *Notes,* "I am delighted with them. They will do more to call attention to household Hygiene than anything that has ever been written."[19]

Her friend Harriet Martineau thought the book was a "work of genius if ever I saw one ... so real and intense, that it will, I doubt not, create an Order of Nurses before it has finished its work." She sent along the comments she had received from a friend in America whose daughter thought that Nightingale's *Notes on Nursing* should be read in churches:

> I thank you heartily for the "Notes on Nursing." It is an admirable book. It is already republished here. I suppose we always like in a book to have it tell us what we already know, & what at the same time is not generally known. We feel stood-by to others, & confirmed in our own minds. I feel in this book still another satisfaction: — it ploughs deep — begins or ends with the idea of health & its conditions, & does not shrink itself up in order to avoid awakening general thought ... What I especially admire is the absence of all professional taint [jargon], while yet every page contains the high ability to bear with, & lead on, & make the best of professors of healing.[20]

In another letter in June, Martineau wrote Nightingale that a friend had told her that the book was on every table wherever they went and that everyone was talking about it. However, not all of the reactions were uniformly positive. The comments of one skeptical young woman indicated the mindset that Nightingale was attempting to break through:

> ... She [Martineau's friend] was ashamed, wherever she went, to hear the women talk. Such conceit, ignorance, such insensibility she could not have conceived ... One young lady seems to have particularly impressed Fan. "That about the skin, & washing, & hot water, & stuff coming off! I don't believe a word of it. Try? ha, ha, I shan't try, I'm sure. I don't believe it is true: & if it is true, I am quite satisfied with my skin, & don't want it any better than it is." — The book has a large work to do among such people; & in time it will do it ...[21]

Nightingale prepared an abridged version of the book, called *Notes on Nursing for the Laboring Class.* It contained a new chapter called "Minding Baby" and was published in 1861.

Congratulatory letters on this condensed edition poured in from all quarters — from doctors, politicians, school mistresses, and the general public throughout the spring and summer of 1861. Edwin Chadwick's daughter Marion requested 300 copies for her schoolmates in 1861.[22] Harriet Martineau was ready with a laudatory review in the *Quarterly Review*:

> There is not a sentence of fine [pretentious] writing, and hardly a superfluous word. The amount of meaning conveyed in the shortest and sharpest way gives the impression of wit [great intelligence]; and the complex influence of this stimulating style, and the pathos of the topic treated, is the genuine operation of genius.[23]

Suggestions for Thought revisited

Between 1858 and 1859, Nightingale was intellectually and spiritually stimulated by Arthur Hugh Clough, who had been helping her with her correspondence since 1857. The son-in-law of Aunt Mai and Uncle Sam, Clough had the capacity to inspire her genius and stimulate her mind with spiritual speculations, as few others did. The two enjoyed discussing the nature of reality, God, and other philosophical and spiritual ideas.

During this period, Clough encouraged Nightingale to revise her *Suggestions for Thought,* the philosophical and religious work she had developed in 1851 and 1852. This three-volume, 829-page work contained Nightingale's ideas on the concepts of God, Universal Law, God's Law and Human Will, sin and evil, family life, spiritual life, and life after death. The first volume, *Law as the Basis of a New Theology,* dealt with her philosophical beliefs. The second volume, *Practical Deductions,* was a criticism of religious dogma and the social life of her day. It also contained her feminist essay "Cassandra." The third volume was a summation of concepts from the first two volumes.

To stimulate her thinking, she reread John Stuart Mill's *History of Logic,* particularly his chapter on "Free Will and Necessity," and *Histoire de mes Idées* by Mill's contemporary, Edgar Quinet, a French historian and political philosopher.

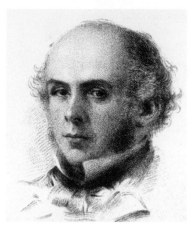

Arthur Hugh Clough (1819-1861), poet, scholar, and husband of Nightingale's cousin Blanche Smith, who served as first secretary of the Nightingale Fund and was Nightingale's assistant and confidant from 1857 until his death in 1861

A gifted soul

Clough's background reveals much about why Nightingale valued his friendship and his suggestions about this work. Clough was a noted poet, one of the outstanding scholars of his day, and a man of great sensitivity who was just a year older than she.[24] At Oxford University in the late 1830s and 1840s, he became interested in the theological controversies of the time and could no longer accept the dogmatic teachings of the Church of England. Clough believed that divine revelation had been given to mankind throughout human history and wasn't exclusive to Christianity.[25] He is credited with coining the term "Broad Church" for those who shared this belief.

Like Nightingale, Clough was distressed with the crisis of faith in midcentury European life. From October 1852 to July 1853, Clough lived in Cambridge, Massachusetts, at the invitation of his friend, the American transcendentalist Ralph Waldo Emerson. He was cordially welcomed by the scholarly community and began lecturing and writing, his articles appearing in the *North American Review* and *Putnam's Magazine.* He also revised John Dryden's famous translation of *Plutarch's Lives.*[26]

Upon his return to England, Clough took up a position as examiner with the Education Office, and the following year married Blanche Smith, eldest daughter of Nightingale's Aunt Mai and Uncle Sam. In the spring of 1856, he was appointed secretary to a commission examining the scientific military schools on the continent. For 3 months, he visited the best schools for artillery and engineering in France, Prussia, and Austria. He was also appointed to examine candidates on English literature.

Soon after Nightingale returned from the Crimea in 1856, Clough became deeply involved in assisting her. Nightingale knew that her *Suggestions for Thought* needed much editing but she didn't have the desire or energy for the task because of her chronic ill-

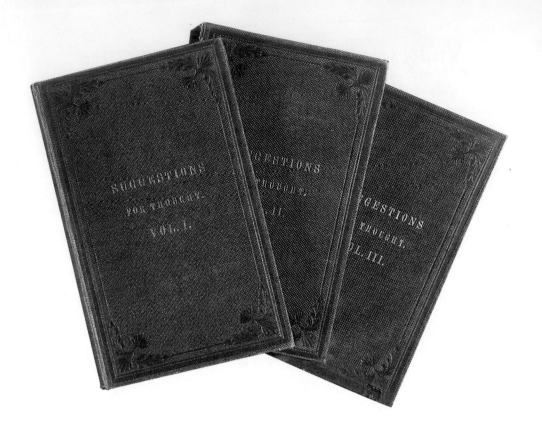

ness and her ongoing work. Aware of the book's deficiencies, she had never wanted it published in her lifetime, at least not with her name on it. Because most of this work had been written when she was in her late 20s and early 30s at different times and places, it lacked the clarity, precision, and logical flow of ideas that marked her later writings. However, at Clough's insistence, early in 1860 she had six copies of the manuscript privately printed and gave them to six people for their critiques: her father, her Uncle Sam, John Stuart Mill, the Reverend Benjamin Jowett (a well-known classical scholar and theologian at Oxford), Sir John McNeill (her old colleague from the Commissariat Commission), and Richard Monckton Milnes (her former suitor and dear friend). Although she received suggestions for various revisions and reorganization from all of these readers, she most valued the comments from Mill and Jowett.

Mill and Jowett's counsel

Nightingale's contact with Mill, whom she greatly admired, had come through Edwin Chadwick, who actually presented the *Suggestions* to him. In her accompanying cover letter dated September 5, 1860, Nightingale told Mill how much his work, *A System of Logic,* had influenced her and explained what had motivated her to write *Suggestions*:

> *... Many years ago, I had a large and very curious acquaintance among the artisans of the North of England and of London. I learned then that they were without any religion whatever — though diligently seeking after one, principally in Comte and his school. Any return to what is called Christianity appeared impossible. It is for them this book was written.*
>
> *I never intended to print it as it was. But my health broken down, I shall never now write out the original plan. I have, therefore, printed the MSS as they were, mainly in order to invite your criticism, if you can be induced to give it ...*[27]

Mill responded to her letter on September 10:

... I should most willingly do my best to be of use to you in the matter which you speak of, if you think that I am a suitable person to be consulted about a work of this kind. In one respect indeed I am very well fitted to test the efficiency of your treatise, since I probably stand as much in need of conversion as those to whom it is addressed. If in spite of this (or perhaps all the more on that account) you would like me to read and give my opinion on it, I will do so with much pleasure ...

It is very agreeable to me that you should have found my Logic *of so much use to you, and particularly the chapter on Free Will and Necessity, to which I have always attached much value as being the uniting issue of a train of thought which had been very important to myself many years before, and even (if I may use the expression) critical to my own development.[28]*

After he critiqued her first volume, she sent him the second, and he responded to her in October 1860 that he would have been sorry to miss the sequel. He made many suggestions for revisions and encouraged her to publish it over her name.

After Jowett read the manuscript, he told Clough, "It seems to me as if I had received the impress of a new mind." Jowett, who possessed one of the finest minds of his era, urged Nightingale to devote time and effort to improving *Suggestions*:

No one can get the form in which it is necessary to put forth new ideas without great labour and thought and tact. It takes years after ideas are clear in your mind to mould them into a shape intelligible to others ... I should not much care if only a comparatively small part of your work is finished. Its greatest value will be that it comes from you who worked in the Crimea. Shall I say one odd and perhaps rather impertinent thing? You have a great advantage in writing on these subjects as a Woman. Do not throw it away, but use the advantage to the utmost. In writing against the World ... every feeling, every sympathy should be made an ally, so that with the clearest statement of the meaning there is the least friction and drawback possible ...[29]

Jowett's primary criticism of the manuscript was that certain parts were too combative and revolutionary in form. Throughout the manuscript he wrote "very good" or "very fine and noble," and then followed with a characteristic comment, such as: "I have ventured to put down the criticisms which occur to me quite badly; they must not be supposed to be inconsistent with the greatest respect for the mind and genius of the writer."[30] Jowett's detailed critique of *Suggestions* and his annotated copy became one of Nightingale's most cherished possessions.

Nightingale and Jowett finally met in 1862, when she asked him to come to London to give her the sacraments during a severe bout of illness when she couldn't leave her room. Jowett later became a frequent visitor and correspondent, and the two remained close friends until Jowett's death in 1893.

For his part, McNeill offered the following:

I doubt whether it is now in such a form as to be extensively studied by the classes for whose use and benefit it is chiefly designed, but I do not doubt that it is a mine which will one day be worked by many hands and that much precious metal will be drawn from it.[31]

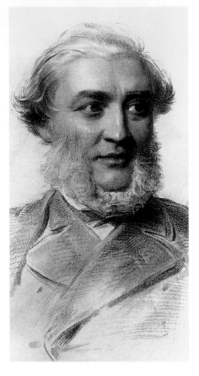

Dr. Henry Bence Jones (1814-1873), physician and chemist at St. George's Hospital, who treated Sidney Herbert for kidney disease

Unfortunately, Nightingale never completed her revision of *Suggestions for Thought*, partly as a result of Arthur Clough's untimely death in 1861. In 1865, she asked Jowett if he would edit it, but he thought the entire work needed to be redone; as it stood it was merely the preparation for a book.

Toward the end of 1860, Nightingale received word of the deaths of two dear friends of earlier years, Christian von Bunsen, the former Prussian ambassador to England who first suggested that she study nursing at Kaiserswerth, and Madre Santa Colomba of the Trinità de Monti Convent in Rome, the woman she referred to as her "spiritual mother." To make matters worse, Uncle Sam Smith and his family wanted Aunt Mai to return home because she had been away a great deal since July 1855, when she accompanied her niece to the Crimea. Nightingale looked on Aunt Mai's departure in March 1860 as an abandonment in the midst of her enormous work. It would be another 20 years before she reconciled with her. At this time Nightingale's cousin Hilary Bonham Carter came to London to take Aunt Mai's place.

"Poor Florence! Our joint work unfinished"

In early December 1860, Sidney Herbert's health began to rapidly fail; he was diagnosed with advanced kidney disease and was placed under the care of Dr. Henry Bence Jones, a well-known specialist in kidney disease and diabetes at St. George's Hospital, London.[32]

Shocked and dismayed, Nightingale refused to accept Bence Jones's grave diagnosis. However, Herbert, aware that he was incurably ill and lacked the strength to continue his many duties, called on her on December 6 to discuss how they could continue to work together as long as possible. Herbert put before her his three alternatives: to retire from public life altogether; to retire from office and keep his seat in the House of Commons; or to keep his Secretaryship of War, leave the House of Commons, and go to the House of Lords. His first choice was to give up his office and retain a seat in the House of Commons, where he had actively served for 28 years as a commanding, eloquent speaker who enjoyed great popularity. For the sake of their unfinished work, Nightingale and others persuaded him to keep his office and resign his seat in the House of Commons. He was then created Lord Herbert of Lea and moved to a seat in the House of Lords.

Nightingale urged Herbert to seek fresh air, rest, proper nutrition — and a second medical opinion. To this end, she suggested many specialists, listing the merits and demerits of each. In a letter to Elizabeth Herbert on December 13, she made an interesting comment completely in line with her philosophy and the miasma theory, that medicine itself doesn't cure, but puts the body in the best position for nature to accomplish its healing:

> I cannot tell you how very glad I was to hear that Mr. Herbert had been "out hunting" and had "slept like a top" after it ... There is another danger which people in general are very little aware of and that is: — the Doctors often produce the very disease they prescribe for — and

often <u>nail the disease upon the patient by assuring him he has it;</u> on the continent, Doctors are much more aware of this than in England.

... This is why it is dangerous to alter a patient's whole mode of life — to impress upon him that he is doomed to die by "that particular disease" and the strong brain is not at all more exempt from this danger than the weak one, on the contrary, it often lays hold of it with greater tenacity. I wish you would tell Mr. Herbert this — sleep, fresh air, regular food, these are the good medicines.

And he <u>must</u> put himself into the way of life to procure these, and no medicine will do any good, if he does not. I always look upon such a patient as doomed not because he has this disease or that, but because he <u>cannot get natural sleep</u> — natural sleep during which all the repair of the body takes place ... if a patient is too weak to take the exercise, fresh air and food necessary to procure sleep, then you may consider anything like recovery impossible.[33]

Resist as she might, by early January 1861, Nightingale saw death written on Sidney Herbert's face. Nevertheless, she was determined not to let his illness or her own prevent her from achieving her mission; there was simply too much left to do. She continued to push Herbert relentlessly. She herself was only able to work for about half an hour at a time. On July 9, 1861, Nightingale saw Sidney Herbert for the last time. He died of kidney failure on August 2, 1861, at the age of 51.

On August 12, Elizabeth Herbert wrote to Nightingale: "Dearest — This is the anniversary of our wedding day 15 years ago. I send you some of his last words — those to you were 'Poor Florence! Poor Florence! Our joint work unfinished.' God bless you E.H."[34]

A cruel blow

Although poor health prevented Nightingale from attending Sidney Herbert's funeral, his death was the severest blow that she had ever suffered. Herbert had been not only a dear friend since they first met in Rome in 1847, but also her closest colleague in the battle for army reform for the past 5 years. Their work together was more important to her than her own life.

Nightingale began to pay tribute to Herbert after his death by referring to him as her "Master." Feeling her life severed, she wrote to her father on August 21:

Indeed your sympathy is very dear to me. So few people know the least what I have lost in my dear master. Indeed I know no one but myself who had it to lose. For no two people pursue together the same object, as I did with him. And when they lose their companion by death, they have in fact lost no companionship. Now he takes my life with him. My work, the object of my life, the means to do it, all in one, depart with him.

Grief fills the room up of my absent master ... it "eats and sleeps and wakes with me." Yet I can truly say that I see it is better that God should not work a miracle to save Sidney Herbert, altho' his death involves the misfortune, moral and physical, of five hundred thousand men, and altho' it would have been but to set aside a few trifling physical laws to save him ...

Now not one man remains (that I can call a man) of all those whom I began work with, five years ago. And I alone, of all men "Most dejected and wretched," survive them all. I am sure I meant to have died ... [35]

Working through her grief and pain, Nightingale confessed to her close friends how hard she had been on Herbert. She wrote to Harriet Martineau on September 24, 1861:

> And I, too, was hard upon him. I told him that Cavour's death was a blow to European liberty, but that a greater blow was that Sidney Herbert should be beaten on his own ground by a bureaucracy. I told him that no man in my day had thrown away so noble a game with all the winning cards in his hands. And his angelic temper with me, at the same time that he felt what I said was true, I shall never forget. I wish people to know that ... all his latter suffering years were filled not by a selfish desire for his own salvation — far less for his own ambition (he hated office, his was the purest ambition I have ever known), but by the struggle of exertion for our benefit.[36]

After Herbert's death, a few negative obituaries began to appear, associating him with the Crimean debacle and various War Office problems while ignoring his achievements. To counter this, Nightingale — at the request of Chancellor of the Exchequer William Gladstone — began writing a true account of Herbert's achievements as a reformer whose goal was the preservation of the physical and moral health of the British soldiers: "This is the work of his which ought to bear fruit in all future time, and which his death has committed to the guardianship of his country." At the end of the document, she wrote: "He died before his work was done."[37] Later, she privately printed her memorandum, *Memorial to the Late Lord Herbert,* for the Herbert family and friends.

Continuing to work out her grief in her letters, Nightingale wrote to her friend Mary Clarke Mohl: "A woman once told me that my character would be more sympathized with by men than by women. In one sense I don't choose to have that said ... Sidney Herbert and I were together exactly like two men ..."[38] To Martineau she wrote: "I supplied the detail, the knowledge of the actual working of an army, in which official men are so deficient; he supplied the political weight."[39]

She also wrote and printed a pamphlet in 1862 entitled *Army Sanitary Administration and its Reform under the late Lord Herbert.* This allowed her to honor her friend's achievements again and still have a voice in agitating the government.

Death of Arthur Clough

Scarcely had Nightingale absorbed the shock of Herbert's death when Arthur Clough's health began to fail, too. Sent to Italy in the summer of 1861 to rest and recover, Clough died in Florence on November 12, at the age of 43, of a severe fever and paralysis.[40] He was buried on a hilltop cemetery outside the city walls. After Clough's death, Nightingale's cousin, Henry Bonham Carter, was appointed Secretary of the Nightingale Fund.

Nightingale grieved for Clough, a man she referred to as "the purest of souls," almost as much as she did for Herbert. To Sir John McNeill she wrote in November 1861:

> He was a man of rare mind and temper. The more so because he would gladly do "plain work." To me, seeing the inanities & the blundering harasses which were the uses to which we put him, he seemed like a race horse harnessed to a coal truck ... He helped me immensely, though not officially, by his sound judgment, and constant sympathy ...[41]

McNeill replied in a letter of deep sympathy:

... His [Clough's] death leaves you dreadfully alone in the midst of your work but that work is your life and you can do it alone. There is no feeling more sustaining than that of being alone — at least I have ever found it so ... To work out views in which no one helped me has all my life been to me a source of vitality and strength. So I doubt not it will be to you, for you have a strength and a power for good to which I never could pretend. It is a small matter to die ... a few days sooner than usual. It is a great matter to work while it is day and so to husband one's powers as to make the most of the days that are given us. This you will do. Herbert and Clough and many more may fall around you but you are destined to do a great work and you cannot die till it is substantially if not apparently done. You are leaving your impress on the age in which you live and the print of your foot will be traced by generations yet unborn ...[42]

Four months after the death of her "dear Master" and a month after the passing of Clough, Nightingale remained emotionally overwhelmed. She stopped delivery of all newspapers because she couldn't bear to read anything negative that might be written about Herbert. Also, there was so much work to be done in Herbert's name.

When Nightingale received a book written by her friend Mary Clarke Mohl on the life of the famed French literary hostess Madame Récamier, she questioned Mohl's proposition that women were more sympathetic than men. For Nightingale, "sympathy" was a quality of shared feeling and commitment to do the work — a quality she had shared with Herbert and her other fellow reformers, all men:

I have read half your book thro' and am immensely charmed by it. But some things I disagree with and more I do not understand. This does not apply to the characters ... But to your conclusions, e.g. you say "women are more sympathetic than men." Now if I were to write a book out of my experience, I should begin, women have no sympathy.

Yours is the tradition. Mine is the conviction of experience. I have never found one woman who had altered her life one iota for me or my opinions. Now look at my experience of men. A statesman [Herbert], past middle age, absorbed in politics for a quarter of a century, out of "sympathy" with me, remodels his whole life and policy — learns a science, the driest, the most technical, the most difficult, that of administration as far as it concerns the lives of men, not, as I learned it, in the field, from the stirring experience, but by writing dry Regulations in a London room by my sofa with me. This is what I call real sympathy.

Another, Alexander (whom I made Director-General), does very nearly the same thing. He is dead too. Clough, a poet if ever there was one — takes to nursing administration in the same way, for me.

I only mention three, whose whole lives were remodelled by sympathy for me. But I could mention very many others, Farr, McNeill, Tulloch, Storks, Martin, who in a lesser degree have altered their work by my opinions. And, the most wonderful of all, a man [Sutherland] born without a soul, like Undine [water spirit in German folklore] — all these elderly men.

Now just look at the degree in which women have sympathy — as far as my experience is concerned. And my experience is almost as large as Europe ... No woman has excited "passions" among women as I have. Yet I leave no school behind. Not one of my Crimean following learnt anything from me — or gave herself for one moment after she came home to carry out

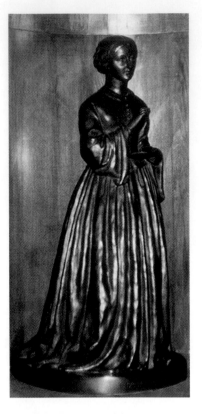

Statuette of Florence Nightingale completed by her cousin Hilary Bonham Carter in 1862

the lesson of that war or of those hospitals. No woman that I know has ever appris à apprendre [learned to learn]. And I attribute this to want of sympathy ... Adieu dear friend. How glad am I to see this miserable year come to a close ...[43]

In the midst of her grief over the death of these two dear friends, Nightingale also felt some remorse about the demands she was making on her favorite cousin, Hilary Bonham Carter. Although Hilary was kept busy with correspondence and errands, Nightingale was concerned that her considerable artistic talent was being wasted. She agreed to sit for a statuette by Hilary that was completed in the spring of 1862. She also granted two sittings for a marble bust by the Scottish sculptor John Steell that had been commissioned by "her dear children," the officers and men of the British army. This marble bust was later placed in the Royal United Service Institution in accordance with Nightingale's will.

In July 1861, Sir James Clark resigned from the Nightingale Fund because of poor health, and Sir Harry Verney, Nightingale's brother-in-law, became the new chairman. Verney served the Nightingale Fund until his death in 1894. In August 1861, Nightingale moved out of the Burlington Hotel because she couldn't bear to remain there after Herbert's death. Several months earlier, Queen Victoria had offered her a residence at Kensington Palace, but Nightingale declined because it was too far from the center of London and would deprive her of her frequent meetings with various officials. She moved temporarily to a borrowed house in Hampstead and then to the Verney house at 32 South Street in London.

Military turns to Nightingale again

When the American Civil War broke out in April 1861, President Abraham Lincoln, Dorothea Linde Dix (Superintendent of Female Nurses for the Union Army), and many army officers found themselves confronted with the same chaos that Nightingale had dealt with in Scutari and the Crimea. Doctors and others soon wrote to Nightingale seeking advice on how to care for the sick and wounded troops.

Harriet Martineau, who had maintained contacts in the North through her New York publisher, asked Nightingale for detailed information that could be sent to the Union army about army organization, army hospital forms, and hospital management of the sick and wounded. Martineau wrote to Nightingale on September 20, 1861:

> *... The reason of my writing now is that I have just heard something that I think will gratify you. Our book ("England & her soldiers") is at present quoted largely & incessantly in American Medical Journals, as a guide in the newness of military management in the Northern States. Before I knew this, I had sent one of two articles (the second goes today) on "Health in the Camp," & "Health in the Hospital," to the "Atlantic Monthly." I don't like magazines, or writing for them: but that very good one has such an enormous circulation that I know & then said "yes" when the proprietors ask me to write. In spite of the war, they have again asked me now, & I thought it a good opportunity to interest their public in saving their citizen-soldiers & health. It is more to the purpose that the medical journals are learning from us; & I am sure you will be glad to hear it ...*[44]

Nightingale wrote back 4 days later, recommending some other publications that Martineau might send to Union officers and giving some advice of a more confidential nature:

> I am really grateful to you for what you tell me about the Northern States. When you speak of their "new ways of military management," it occurs to me, would you like to send them a collection of what might be useful "as a guide" in the Sanitary Service? If you do, I should recommend (& would gladly send you for transcription)
>
> 1. the Royal Comm. "Sanitary Report" of 1858 — written by Sidney Herbert in 1857 — which you know
>
> 2. the Army "Medical Regulations," issued by him, October 1859 — which I think you know — these have now been at work for two years. They were tested in the China War. And the result was that, instead of having fifty out of every 100 die from disease, (as we had in the first winter of the Crimean War) we had only six percent including those killed in action ... These "Regulations" are now considered the best code of any of the armies of Europe — including as they do a whole sanitary service. And I have been applied to more than once by foreign powers for them.
>
> 3. The Army Purveyor's "Regulations," issued by Sidney Herbert in January 1861. These are what this name imports.
>
> 4. The Report (very short) on the Army Hospital Corps & Service of General Hospitals — issued by a Commission called together in 1860 & acted upon by Sidney Herbert in 1861 — not presented to Parliament.
>
> 5. The "Barrack & Hospital Improvement Commission" Report of 1861 of which I sent you a copy as soon as we could (presented in Paris) ...[45]

Nightingale also mentioned a report that had never been sent to Parliament about the benefits of establishing "day rooms" or clubs — supplied with coffee, newspapers, dominoes, and chess — at barracks to keep soldiers from frequenting taverns and prostitutes.

Nightingale's Crimean War accomplishments served as a model for the struggling medical services of both sides in the Civil War. Her old friend Dr. Elizabeth Blackwell, the first woman doctor in the United States, organized the Women's Central Association for Relief in New York, which sent women nurses to serve in military hospitals. Some 600 Sisters from 12 religious orders served as nurses during the war, and many other women and men volunteered as well.[46] In addition, a United States Sanitary Commission was established in June 1861 by order of President Lincoln. The commission, which collected $5 million in cash and $15 million worth of supplies, became a forerunner of the American Red Cross.

Trent affair and Canadian expedition

In December 1861, Nightingale was urgently consulted by the new Secretary of State for War, Lord de Grey (later Lord Ripon, who became her ally in India sanitary reform), when it appeared that England and the United States were on the brink of war. On November 8, 1861, a Union navy frigate had stopped the neutral British ship *Trent* on the high seas and removed two Confederate commissioners, Mason and Slidell, who were seeking the support of England and France for the Confederate cause. Lord Palmerston's government sent the Union an ultimatum demanding an apology and the release of Mason and Slidell. To avert armed conflict, William Seward, Lincoln's Secretary of State, apologized, and the Confederate commissioners were soon released.

While these negotiations were underway, Palmerston ordered that British troops be sent to Canada to reinforce the garrisons there in case war broke out with the United States. To avoid a repeat of the Crimean War debacle with thousands of men dying from winter cold and disease, the government once again turned to Nightingale.

Presented with this new opportunity to serve her soldiers, Nightingale seemed to come alive again and plunged into the work with her usual attention to the minutest detail. She calculated the average dogsled speed in transporting the wounded across the snowbound Canadian terrain. She compared the relative weights and warming capacity of buffalo robes and blankets and recommended the types and amounts of necessary clothing, food, supplies, and water. Doubtless with the Balaclava disaster in mind, she was adamant about establishing a central supply depot and dispensary. She also devised job descriptions for orderlies and medical officers, who were responsible for day-to-day operations.

At the end of 1861, Nightingale sank back into illness and was carefully watched by Dr. Sutherland. In spite of her poor health, she now began some of her most useful and long-lasting efforts on behalf of Poor Law reform, army and civilian sanitation in India, and ongoing nursing reform and development.

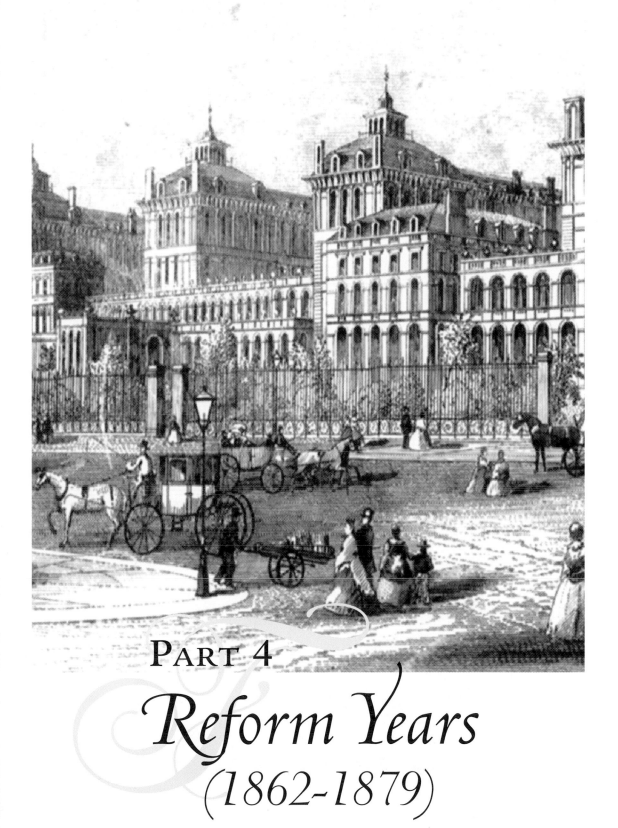

PART 4

Reform Years
(1862–1879)

Chapter 13

Private Life

Sometimes I wonder that I should be so impatient for death. Had I only to stand & wait, I think it would be nothing — tho' the pain is so great that I wonder how anybody can dread an operation. If Paget could amputate my left fore quarter, I am sure I would have sent for him in half an hour.

— *Florence Nightingale to Fanny Nightingale, March 7, 1862[1]*

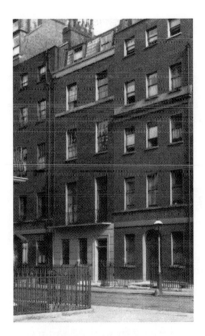

Nightingale's residence on South Street in London, where she lived from 1865 until her death

The nonstop years of prodigious work that Nightingale had begun in the Crimea, compounded by the fever she had contracted there, began to take their toll. During 1861, at age 41, she suffered three severe attacks of symptoms similar to those of her initial fever in 1855. Her physical vitality began to diminish and her illness became chronic. In addition, without her late friend Sidney Herbert to prod the career bureaucrats in the War Office, her life suddenly lost its sense of urgency. Although she was kept informed about her nurse training school, she was not involved in it on a daily basis. Her work on India and Poor Law reform occupied most of her time.

As her work began to take a new direction, family ties became more important to Nightingale. With her parents aging, she was forced to spend much time dealing with their business and domestic affairs in the 1870s, a situation she resented. However, the old bitterness toward her mother and sister gave way to acceptance and affection, especially as Fanny became increasingly ill and feeble and Parthe was now happily married. Nightingale also became very close to the family of her brother-in-law, Sir Harry Verney, and to the children of her cousins, whom she referred to as her nieces and nephews.

Weak and alone

In December 1861, Nightingale developed severe spinal pain (today called spondylitis), accompanied by intermittent depression, that continued over the next 7 years. Dr. Charles Edouard Brown-Séquard, the leading specialist in spinal disease, told her that constant worry had brought on "congestion of the spine which could lead straight to paralysis."[2] He advised rest, not fully aware of her drive and penchant for work.

Time hadn't healed Nightingale's grief over the deaths of Sidney Herbert and Arthur Clough, as family and friends hoped it would. Though she kept busy, devoting a large part of her work to reform in India, she despaired at the emptiness of her life. Illness made her well aware of her advancing age but, even more than that, she keenly felt the loss of direction, support systems, and professional discourse to which she had grown accustomed. In March 1862, weak and alone, she described her loneliness in a rambling letter to her mother:

> I think what I felt most (during my last three months of extreme weakness) is not having one single person to give me one inspiring word or even one correct fact. I am glad to end a day which never can come back; gladder to end a night — gladder to end a month. I have felt this much more in setting up (for the first time in my life) a fashionable old maid's house in a fashionable quarter (tho' grateful to Papa's liberality for enabling me to do so) because it is as it were deciding upon a new & independent course in my broken old age — which I never have been called upon to do even in my vigorous youth. Always before my path was so clear to me, what I ought to do, tho often not how to do it. But now it was quite doubtful to me whether ... I had better not have left the Army altogether...
>
> Poor Mrs. Herbert told me that her chief comfort was in a little Chinese dog of his, which he was not ... very fond of ... but which used to come & kiss her eyelids & lick the tears from her cheeks. I remember thinking that this was childish. But now I don't. My cat does just the same. Dumb beasts observe you so much more than talking beings; & know so much better, what you are thinking of ...[3]

On the anniversary of her arrival in Scutari, she expressed her feelings of loss in a poignant private note:

> It is 10 years today since Inkerman ... 10 years since I arrived at Scutari. It seems to me like 3 lives tho' I have spent 7 of those 10 years in bed. It seems to me like 3 different existences in different worlds. In that time I have lost all and won all 3 different times. The last 3 years have been quite different to me (since Sidney Herbert and Clough left me) as if I had gone to another world.[4]

A permanent home

To be near the hub of political activity and the War Office, Nightingale lived in various rented houses and hotels in or near London in the decade after her return to England. Moves were difficult, requiring that vanloads of papers and government Blue Books be boxed and unboxed. She received help in house hunting and tending to daily household business from Mrs. Sutherland, the wife of her colleague and friend from the Sanitary and Royal Commissions, Dr. John Sutherland, with whom she continued to work almost daily during this period. Mrs. Sutherland also hired Nightingale's servants, including a personal maid, a cook, a maidservant, and a messenger, making sure that each person could meet Nightingale's detailed requirements and schedules.

Despite such help, until the end of her life Nightingale continued her methodical attention to household details, such as purchases of bedding, linen, and food. She reviewed her guests' daily schedules, whom they met and how they were entertained, and the time and place they would dine and take their tea. She reviewed their menus and the

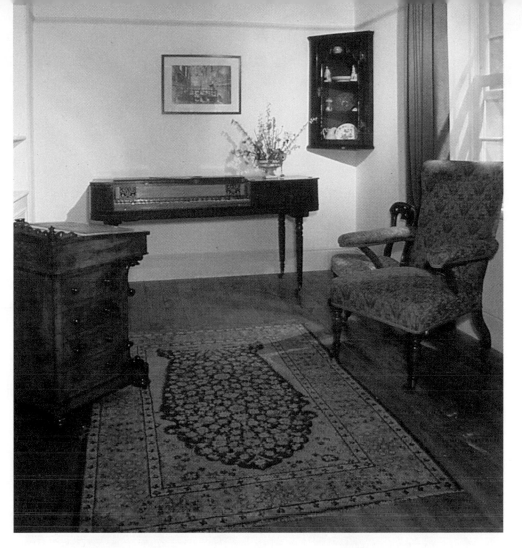

meal preparations and wrote reminders to her cook — for example, regarding a minced veal dish, "Meat hard, and remember that mincing makes hard meat harder." Sometimes she laced her notes with hyperbole to get her point across, for example, "why was the glue-pot used for the stewed cutlets?"[5]

Since her time in the Crimea, Uncle Sam Smith had assisted Nightingale with bookkeeping, bill payments, and other business matters. In one letter to him, Nightingale gives some idea of the financial arrangement they had:

> ... I am afraid I must trouble you for another cheque of £60 tho' I am not quite out. And I propose that in future you should be so good as to send me a cheque on the 1st of each month of £50, or if you are going abroad or away for more than a month accordingly — I send you, if you please, my account as usual, tho' not at regular times to which I am now often unequal. I need not spend the whole £ per month, tho' I am afraid you will think that is but too likely. I fear this will have been a very expensive year – the necessity of going to Hampstead &c — you will see that I have paid 3 bills by cheque. This has been a sadly expensive house also. I propose to take a house (Mr. Remington's) in the row of fine ones of Oak Hill Park from July 23 to October 23, at 8 guineas a week.[6]

In November 1865, Nightingale moved into a house that her father rented for her at 35 South Street (later renumbered 10), which was to remain her residence until her

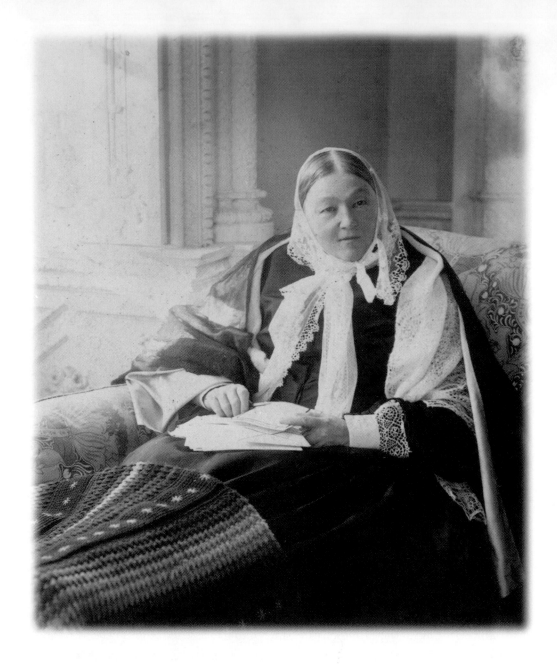

death. From the front windows of the house, she could look west on South Street and see the lovely green spaces of Hyde Park; the back of the house, where her second-story drawing room and bedroom were located, overlooked the gardens of the Dorchester House Hotel. Fresh air, gorgeous trees, lush garden flowers, sunlight and sky, and the birds brought Nightingale tranquility and pleasure, as did her cats. In the spring she placed primroses, anemones, snowdrops, and other seasonal flowers on her balcony.

Nightingale's sparsely furnished drawing room was lined with bookcases filled with government blue books and other reports. On one wall hung an engraving of the ceiling of the Sistine Chapel. A letter to her mother described other pictures that framed her view:

> *Parthe told me you wanted to know whether the Dresden Raphael had come in its new frame. Yes, it did ... The frame is beautiful. It is just what that kind of print wants to lighten it — an*

open frame. I always think good prints are spoilt by framing them in solid wood — & made to look heavy ... Hung up your Dresden Raphael & Murrillo Virgin, Mrs. Bracebridge's Annunciation (from the Papal Chapel), an unframed Guercino Ecce Homo, & Sistine Isaiah — and two Chromolithographs from Roberts & a Norwegian. And Sutherland said I was a "vain thing," to have decorated my room. There are some people who always say the wrong thing.[7]

In the bedroom, light flooded the white walls through uncovered windows. The bed faced a fireplace, and behind the headboard stood a long bookcase topped by lamps. A large chaise longue was placed for Nightingale between two windows. There she sat, when she felt well enough, usually wearing a dark dress, a lace headscarf, and a shawl. On the walls hung several pictures, including a long chromolithograph of the ground around Sebastopol, a watercolor of an Egyptian sunset, and later a photograph of Sir John Lawrence, her favorite viceroy of India. On the mantle stood a framed chromolithograph with the words "It is I. Be not afraid," a reminder of her first Call from God on February 7, 1837.

Here in her bedroom and drawing room, Nightingale held her interviews and did her work. Cut flowers sent weekly from her friend Lady Ashburton and other admirers graced a bedside table.

Nightingale's residence was only a few doors from her sister and brother-in-law, the Verneys, an arrangement that all three found agreeable. Nightingale believed that she could be useful to her sister, Parthe, whose husband, a member of Parliament, was one of her important links to the world of politics, government officials, and the Nightingale School of Nursing. When the Verneys were in London, Sir Harry would visit almost every morning to discuss business and to read a spiritual passage.

The Verneys often entertained Nightingale's many guests at dinner and tea and also took them on carriage rides in the park and to the opera, the theatre, Parliament, and other places at her request. They even provided overnight accommodation. When Nightingale's guests stayed at the Verneys, however, she would send her maid to clean and scrub the guestroom and furnish fresh sheets, bedding, and food. To the fastidious Nightingale, Parthe's housekeeping wasn't up to standards. Despite this "shortcoming," Parthe's marriage to Sir Harry had secured her place in the world and made the relationship between the aging sisters more supportive and amicable.

Helpers, friends, & visitors

After the death of Sidney Herbert and Arthur Clough in 1861, Nightingale's primary assistant in work-related matters became Dr. John Sutherland, one of the last remaining members of her "Little War Office." Sutherland was one of Nightingale's earliest allies in the struggle for army medical and sanitary reform, and he continued to work closely with her on official business until his retirement in 1888. Dr. William Farr no longer came regularly, but she consulted with him by mail. Cousin Hilary Bonham Carter moved to London in 1860 to help Nightingale with domestic affairs, visitors, and correspondence, replacing Aunt Mai, who had returned to her family.

Dr. Sutherland's counsel

Sutherland met with Nightingale almost daily, serving as a liaison to various officials and other visitors. He also served as her personal physician and was best able to evaluate the physical and psychological effects of her illness.

The two colleagues agreed on most matters. With her physical stamina declining, Nightingale depended on him to check her work, particularly government documents and correspondence. When he moved farther away from London in 1865, their work had to be carried on by mail, leading to occasional misunderstandings and delays. With her need for precise answers and aversion to wasting time, Nightingale frequently became impatient and irritable, as evidenced in the following letter:

> I could do the work if it were real work done at the least expenditure to myself. But to do a minimum of work at the greatest expenditure to myself (by driving, pumping, etc.) is now physically impossible to me.[8]

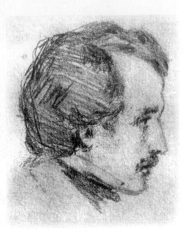

Sketch of John Sutherland by Hilary Bonham Carter, c. 1859

Sutherland handled Nightingale's irritability with patience and good humor. He was unintimidated by the curt notes she would send, such as "Can you answer a plain question?" "I cannot flatter you on your lucidity," and "I do not shake hands until the Abstract is done." He often teased her in return, beginning his letters with "Respected Enemy" or "Dear howling epileptic Friend." When she appeared especially fretful, he consoled the woman he believed was divinely inspired: "I am at your orders in this as in all things" or "All I can say is, I am ready to help."[9]

Their close relationship is evident in this humorous exchange written after Nightingale received the 1871 census form to complete:

> Am I the head of this household?... Occupation column: as I think every body ought to have a defined occupation, I should like to put what mine is, but I don't know how to define it. The last column asked whether the householder was deaf and dumb, blind, imbecile, or lunatic? I shall return Imbecile and Blind, and if everybody did the same, it would be true.[10]

Sutherland needled her in return: "To the head of the household, that is obviously you; as for occupation, it is None."[11]

Hilary: The "purest gold"

Nightingale's cousin Hilary, the best friend of her youth, had never married, instead devoting herself to tending to her parents and siblings. Now she had come to London to devote herself to her famous cousin. Although Nightingale appreciated Hilary's help, she felt that Hilary was wasting her life and her artistic talent. In 1862, Nightingale sent Hilary back home, hoping that she would devote more time to her art. Believing that Hilary would outlive her, she also provided money in her will for that purpose, as she informed her cousin later that year:

> Dearest Hilary, I have left you £1000 in the earnest hope that, though not in possession, it may enable you, at some present sacrifice, to provide yourself with an Atelier or other means of pursuing your Art.[12]

Hilary was overwhelmed and quickly replied:

Your thoughts & your deed are very, very kind. It does not bear much speaking of, but I feel it very gratefully that you wish to furnish my sinew to poor art as well as ardour. And yet I am much convinced you should find some better Institution than this so to endow ...[13]

Another letter of encouragement a year later expressed Nightingale's own driven personality and her understanding of the need for teamwork:

My usefulness in the Crimea ... rested simply on this, that I cooperated with the powers administrative. I did not let up for myself ... All usefulness in work comes out of co-operation of different elements & collusion too. You must have the steel & the flint, or you will have no fire.[14]

Nightingale was delighted when Hilary finally went to Paris to study art and live with the Mohls in May 1863. Along with a letter expressing her happiness, she also took the opportunity to enclose a parcel and asked Hilary to deliver it. This initiative typified Nightingale's focus and her ability to get her own work done, no matter what:

Dearie, You could not have given me a greater pleasure than by your going to Paris! I only hope you will stay longer than a fortnight. Do you know Dr. Shrimpton? If not, would you take this parcel & letter, & send it to him — if yes, give it to him — You can roll up the parcel, if more convenient — tho' it is better to carry it flat. It has taken me odds & ends of time for two years to prepare these forms, simple as they look. For (at least in England) this is the first complete list of operations & of complications (curious as this sounds) that has been made. I had to appeal to every large hospital in London to send me its own list of complications: all imperfect. And the forms had to be sent back to people, revised three times (after they had been looked over each time by our most eminent surgeon), to add in the names of important operations which had been left out. So laborious is it, when you come to do a thing of this sort to include everything.[15]

Although Nightingale's health remained poor, she was nearly always able to marshal the energy to write documents. In those days, even prime ministers and ministers of departments wrote out their own documents and correspondence in longhand, which clerks copied for dissemination as needed. In August 1863, Nightingale expressed her exhaustion to Hilary after a long interval of writing:

I feel so entirely broken down now — having had the <u>whole</u> weight of the correspondence of the Indian Commission upon me 5 weeks tomorrow — & not one single soul has given me the least help ... And people write to me, "Oh I thought the India Commission was done! & you were taking a complete rest!!"[16]

On September 5, 1865, Hilary died at age 44 of cancer. Nightingale wrote to Mary Clarke ("Clarkey") Mohl: "The golden bowl is broken, and it was the purest gold I have ever known."[17] She added that Hilary had never pursued her art because her family had slowly killed her with its demands, fully aware that *she* was as guilty as the rest.

A month later, she received word that Lord Palmerston had died, ending her 9 years of direct access to the Prime Minister. "He was a powerful protector to me ... I have lost, in him, a powerful friend," she wrote to Dr. Farr.[18]

Keeping up with old friends

Nightingale exchanged letters regularly with Elizabeth Herbert, Sidney's widow. She often reminisced about the work she and Herbert had done together and kept Elizabeth informed about her progress on her ongoing War Office reports:

> I have taken this house in order to be near the W. O. & shall be here till autumn, if I am oblig-ed to live so long. He [Sidney Herbert] used to laugh at me & say he would give me lodgings over the W. O. Things are perpetually hanging fire there, mainly owing to that Sir G. Lewis. Sometimes they seem to make some progress. But more often I have not the joy to see his re-forms carried on. I have had many touching letters (from professional men chiefly) speaking of the little paper with the Diagram [on mortality of the army in the Crimean War] on him say-ing "What a work to have done in a short life time," & "what a memorial that Diagram is to that noble man."
>
> The Queen asked for a copy & gave one of her own accord to P[rince] Louis of Hesse. And in return she sent me her book (on Prince Albert [who died in 1861]), with such a touching in-scription. She always reminds me of the woman in the Greek chorus, with her hands clasped above her head, wailing out her irrepressible despair. I think [she] is far from well.[19]

Nightingale always wrote to Elizabeth on the anniversary of Herbert's death to console her — and perhaps herself:

> I can't let this terrible anniversary pass, without a word to you — terrible I call it because the wreck occasioned by his loss is from year to year more complete — not terrible to him, God knows. I cannot write anymore, for I am too ill. I must keep all my strength for his work. I am almost glad to be so suffering as to feel the day less. God bless you! ... I feel everyday more and more, as I feel his loss everyday more and more, how priceless, how noble his memory — how great his service to God — how great the future of an eternity of service to God, before him. God did bless him; and God will bless all who follow in his steps.[20]

Elizabeth Herbert converted to Catholicism in 1865 and began to write books on religious figures and travel books to the Holy Land that were published by church-related publishers. Nightingale had little contact with her after her conversion, except for occasional letters filled with personal news. In January 1869, when Elizabeth became ill, Nightingale's letter revealed a personal change in outlook. She now perceived herself as leading a less hectic but still active life, though still working from her bed:

> Dearest — Indeed, I do know how very ill you have been. There have been those who wished for nothing, neither to die nor to live, except as they fulfilled God's will — who had so strong a feel-ing of their own lives being one with the will of God as to exclude every other feeling, every care, every hope or fear of living or dying How far I am from this — True, it is easier in a con templative life than in an active strife in God's service, such as you & I have to live — But may we not hope that each year of strife may bring us nearer to this absolute one-ness with God's will, making our active life a "spiritual exercise?"[21]

Nightingale's correspondence with Clarkey became more frequent during 1864 and 1865, the two friends exchanging stories about illness, work, and mutual interests.

In the following letter, Nightingale asked her friend to visit on a "terrible anniversary:"

> *You will be doing me a favour if you come to me. August 2 is a terrible anniversary to me. And I shall not have my usual solace, for Mrs. Bracebridge has always come to spend that day with me, and I am sure she would have come this year, but I could not tell whether I should be able to get Sir John Lawrence's things off by that time. It does me good to be with you, as with Mrs. Clive [a noted author and fellow invalid], because it reduces individual struggles to general formulae. It does me harm, intensely alone as I am, to be with people who do the reverse. But it is incorrect to say, as Mrs. Clive does, that "I will not let people help me," or, as others do, that "no one can help me." Any body could have helped me who knew how to read and write and what o'clock it is.[22]*

Clarkey was nearly always a welcome visitor, although even she was sometimes refused admittance. In one letter, Nightingale explained her point of view about her work and her limited time and physical reserves:

> *Clarkey Mohl Darling — How I should like to see you now. But it is quite, quite, quite impossible. I am sure no one ever gave up so much to live, who longed so much to die, as I do and give up daily. It is the only credit I claim. I will live if I can. I shall be so glad if I can't. I am overwhelmed with business. And I have an Indian functionary now in London, whose work is cut out for him every day at my house. I scarcely even have half an hour's ease.[23]*

Living with chronic illness

Nightingale's health remained generally poor throughout the 1860s and 1870s. During the winter of 1864, feeling near death once again, she proposed moving permanently to St. Thomas's Hospital, where she would live in a small ward for the rest of her years. She wrote of her idea to Selina Bracebridge:

> *You know that I always believed it to be God's will for me that I should live & die in Hospitals. When this call He has made upon me for other works stops, & I am no longer able to work, I should wish to be taken to St. Thomas' Hospital, & to be placed in a bed in a 'general' ward (which is what I should have desired, had I come to my end as a Hospital Matron). And I beg you to be so very good as to see that this my wish is accomplished.[24]*

She also instructed Henry Bonham Carter to have all her letters destroyed after her death. However, she later changed her mind about this.[25]

Limiting contact with visitors

To preserve her health and minimize interruptions to her work, Nightingale at this time found it necessary to curtail the constant stream of visitors and the onslaught of mail that had besieged her since her return to England after the Crimean War. Except for family and friends, she decided to meet only people directly related to her work and these by appointment only. In addition, Uncle Sam Smith wrote to the *Times*, explaining that his niece would be unable to answer unsolicited requests for information or favors.

When it came to visitors, Nightingale made no exceptions, even for royalty, as this letter to the Mohls about a proposed visit from the Queen of Holland makes clear:

Would you tell M. Mohl this, if you are writing, about the Queen of Holland's proposed visit to see me. She is a Queen of Queens. But it is quite, quite, quite impossible ... I am so weak, no one knows how weak I am. Yesterday because I saw Dr. Sutherland for a few minutes in the afternoon, after the morning's work, and my good Mrs. Sutherland for a few minutes after him, I was with a spasm of the heart till 7 o'clock this morning and nearly unfit for work all to-day.[26]

In 1867, Nightingale limited her direct contact with visitors even further; she began communicating with them in writing. Nearly all visitors — even the most distinguished — would be greeted by her maid and led to a ground floor sitting room, given a pencil and paper, and asked to clearly and concisely state their desired business with Nightingale. The maid would then carry the visitor's note upstairs to her and return Nightingale's answer to the visitor. If Sutherland were present, he might convey her answers or even write them for her. Only a very few were invited upstairs for a personal interview.

Sleepless nights, painful days

In the mid-1860s, Nightingale's insomnia intensified. She spent many nights writing letters to her friends and reading and taking notes on books unrelated to work. During this time, she carried on a long correspondence with Clarkey's husband, Julius Mohl, about religion and theology, philosophy, politics, and literature. Mohl was a leading Orientalist best known for his translation of Firdausi's Persian epic "Shah Nameh" ("Book of Kings"). Nightingale considered Mohl's studies a significant contribution to theodicy, one of her major preoccupations — the belief that the world as it is remains the best possible world and that the existence of evil is a necessary condition for the existence of the greatest moral good.[27] She asked Mohl to share with her more about Firdausi and the Sufis, their belief in a God, and whether the God was good or bad.

She also asked his opinion on gnosticism, a religious and philosophical movement of the Hellenistic and early Christian world that combined elements of Judaism, Christianity, and other religious beliefs. She often asked his interpretation of certain concepts or words from the Buddhist religion and the meaning of various words in Sanskrit, the language of India's ancient holy texts.[28]

By 1866, Nightingale was in almost constant pain; she couldn't bear her weight and had to be carried from room to room. At times she couldn't tolerate having her position changed for 48 hours at a time. During the winter and spring, she underwent subcutaneous injections of opium — a recognized medical treatment for severe symptoms — which relieved her pain for 24 hours. She monitored the drug's effects, noting that it muddled her thinking. In January 1869, she wrote to Elizabeth Herbert:

Very sick for 17 nights with each attack on my chest that I have been able neither to lie down nor to sit up nor to speak. It would not have significance so much but that, as you know, we are never so busy as at this time of year [closing sessions of Parliament] — and his [Sidney Herbert's] work is always sacred to me — always to be carried on, in spite of everything.[29]

Family affairs

Despite her chronically poor health, Nightingale always set aside time for her father, who visited her often in the early 1860s, particularly on Sundays. He was a source of great joy for her, and they continued to share intellectual interests they had developed since her education as a young girl in the library at Embley. "I shall always be well enough to see you as long as this mortal coil is on me at all," she wrote to him.[30] And again, a few days later: "Dear Papa, I will keep all Sunday vacant for you. I should like to have you twice, please, say at 11½ and 3½."[31]

Although her mother and sister came on occasion, Nightingale didn't encourage their visits because she realized they couldn't comprehend her intense nature or the unrelenting pressure of her reform work. Plus, neither her family nor her friends ever fully grasped the severe effects of her chronic illness and her limited physical reserve.

However, at the urging of her friend Benjamin Jowett, Nightingale spent July through September 1867 with her parents at Lea Hurst. The visit turned out to be rewarding for both Mrs. Nightingale, now age 80, and her daughter. The two women were able to talk about past misunderstandings and, to some extent, heal old wounds. Mrs. Nightingale even admitted her past errors, conceding, "You would have done nothing in life, if you had not resisted me."[32] Nightingale wrote to Clarkey that Fanny was more cheerful and gentle than she ever remembered her.

In the 1870s, a number of people who had been major players in Nightingale's life died. The death of Charles Bracebridge in July 1872 brought back tender memories of this loyal friend who, with his wife Selina, had been more like parents to Nightingale than her own. The next year brought the death of John Stuart Mill, the man she and others regarded as the foremost British philosopher of his time. However, these two deaths were just the beginning.

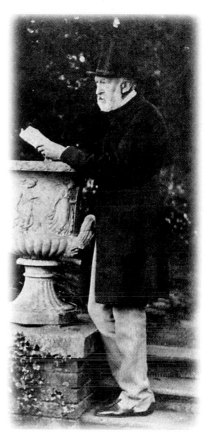

Nightingale's father, William Edward Nightingale, c. 1870, with whom she remained close until his death in 1874

Death of father

Nightingale didn't see much of her father in the early 1870s, but she sent him short letters and kept informed about his health and activities. She was in London when she received word from Parthe that W.E.N., age 80, had suddenly died at Embley on the morning of January 5, 1874. Coming down for breakfast, he had forgotten his watch and started back upstairs when he slipped and fell, hitting his head on the steps. He died instantly. Responding to a letter of condolence from Elizabeth Herbert a few days later, Nightingale wrote:

> ... Yes: my dear Father went home [died] quite suddenly on Monday morning at 8 o'clock: he had got up at his usual early hour: when they ran to him, there was no breath, nothing. I do not feel his death awful for <u>him</u>: it is <u>his</u> New Year: it is what he would have chosen — he was quite ready to part with his life: he always wished to go out of the world quietly: it was part of his single-minded character. I think his was the purest mind & most single heart I have ever known:
>
> But it is very dreary not to have seen him once more: that none of us were by him at the last: not a last word or farewell. But for <u>him</u> it is best so. The Almighty Goodness has done with him what was best. No one knows what a break up it is to us: for me especially: I had only just re-

ceived the idea that I might survive my mother: I never once thought that I should survive him: I thought he had 10 years of life in him: I perhaps not one.

The funeral is on Saturday: a walking funeral — what he would have wished: only the family & the tenants: his cottagers carry him — One of the very last things he did, tho' ailing, was to see after building fresh rooms to a cottage. And the night before he died he carved [meat] for a large family party, including children, as usual. No: his death is not awful for him: he was the truest father to all his people & cottagers: not pauperizing them: but wise & careful: helping them to help themselves: even seeing that the wives kept their husbands' houses tidy himself.

There was hardly a pauper on his places: May those who come after him do as well for those he so loved & cared for: He said a few words, evidently meant as a farewell to us, to one of his nieces that last day — repeated 2 lines about meeting again — which my dear Mother treasures up — Her grief is sweet & gentle: she begged to go in & "kiss him": but yielded when she was told that it was only his "old garment" there: he was not "there" ...[33]

Because of her extreme weakness, Nightingale didn't attend her father's funeral but soon went to Embley to look after her mother and settle her father's estate and business affairs. Because there were no Nightingale sons, the Embley and Lea Hurst estates passed to the next male heir of the Nightingale lineage — William Shore Smith ("my boy Shore"), the only son of W.E.N.'s sister, Aunt Mai. The disposition of family possessions and servants dragged on and made Nightingale miserable. Deciding where her mother should live was another concern. "I am utterly exhausted. Not a day passes without the most acute anxiety and care. Oh the cruel waste of time, of all real work," she wrote.[34]

Shore was exceedingly kind to both his cousin and aunt. He increased Nightingale's annual income to £2,000 (approximately £95,000 and US$157,000 in current values[35]). In July, Fanny went to live with him and his family, then at Lea Hurst. Nightingale spent much of the summer and autumn with her mother. By this time Fanny was 86 years old, senile and nearly blind, and a great source of concern to Nightingale. The constant barrage of domestic worries kept Nightingale from her work and made her feel trapped. This was the first time since her return from the Crimea that family matters, rather than work, were determining where and how she should live. "... Stranger vicissitudes than mine in life few men have had: vicissitudes from slavery to power: and from power to slavery again," she wrote to Clarkey.[36]

A 2-month visit to Claydon with her mother in the autumn brought a brief respite. She wrote to thank Sir Harry and Parthe, who were away, "I should be very sorry to leave your beautiful place, its silence, and peace, its trees and these lovely and comforting rooms. I have not been down to the library: but I have been into Emily's [Sir Harry's daughter] old room and daily hold communion with her."[37]

More friends gone

Just a few weeks after her father's death, Nightingale suffered another great loss when her old friend Selina Bracebridge died. "She was more than mother to me," she wrote to Elizabeth Herbert from Embley on February 3, 1874. "What should I have been without her?"[38] In a letter to Clarkey, Nightingale reflected on the places that she had been with the Bracebridges and what the couple — "the Creators of my life" — had meant to her:

... she had qualities which no Greek God ever had — real humility (excepting my dear Father, I never knew any one so really humble), and with it the most active heart and mind and buoyant soul that could well be conceived ... He and she have been the Creators of my life. And when I think of him at Scutari, the only man in all England who would have lived with willingness such a pigging [lowly] life, without the interest and responsibility which it had to me, I think that we shall never look upon his like again. And when I think of ... all the places that I have been with them, of the immense influence they had in shaping my own life — more than earthly father and mother to me — I cannot doubt that they leave behind them, having shaped many lives as they did mine, their mark on the century — this century which has so little ideal at least in England. They were so immeasurably above any English "country gentry" I have ever known.[39]

To the end of her life, Nightingale held sacred the memory of her beloved friends. Though they had both long since died, she still wrote of them in her will: "To my beloved and revered friends, Mr. Charles Bracebridge and his wife, my more than mother, without whom Scutari and my life could not have been, and to whom nothing that I could ever say or do would in the least express my thankfulness, I should have left some token of my remembrance that they, as I expected, survived me."[40]

February brought the death of Adolphe Quetelet, Nightingale's statistical mentor. She expressed her appreciation of him in a letter to her fellow statistician, Dr. Farr:

I cannot say how the death of our old friend touches me, the founder of the most important science in the whole world, for upon it depends the practical application of every other and of each art, the one science essential to all political and social administration, all education and organization based on experience, for it only gives exact results of our experiences.[41]

In July 1874, Nightingale received word that her old opponent Lord Panmure, the former British Secretary of State for War from 1855 to 1858, had died. She wrote to Clarkey that Panmure had been both an enemy and a friend and that his death represented "the last ghost disappearing of my Sidney Herbert life."[42]

In the fall, a close friend and admirer, Paulina Irby, spent some time with Nightingale and her mother at Claydon. Irby was a Christian missionary and teacher who provided aid to the persecuted Christians of Bosnia and Herzegovina, then a part of the Turkish Ottoman Empire. She had come to England to collect money for her work in Bosnia but had ended up spending months at Embley, helping to care for Fanny. Nightingale was tempted to keep Irby on as a companion to Fanny but decided that her work in Bosnia was more important. The two women corresponded at length between 1876 and 1879, and Nightingale contributed to Irby's Bosnian relief fund.

In 1876 and 1877, Nightingale lost two more close friends — Harriet Martineau, who for 20 years had been a key figure in helping her shape public policy, and Clarkey's husband, Julius Mohl, whose correspondence and friendship she had enjoyed for nearly 40 years.

One bright note in this difficult period was her correspondence with her favorite nieces and nephews. In 1876, she sent a special New Year's gift to Shore's granddaughter, May Coape Smith: "I hope you will not like it the less because it has been through the Crimean War with me, nor because my father gave it ... I do not use a watch now, because I am not moveable."[43]

During the remainder of the 1870s, Nightingale spent a lot of time finding people to care for her mother. Fanny had become increasingly senile since W.E.N.'s death, and it seemed that wherever she went to live, she would soon become unhappy. All of these troubles took their toll on Nightingale, whose letters during this period reveal her exhaustion and exasperation. "Do you know what have been the hardest years of my life?" she wrote to Clarkey in September 1879, "Not the Crimean War. Not the 5 years with Sidney Herbert at the War Office when I sometimes worked 22 hours a day. But the last 5 years and three quarters since my father's death."[44]

While embroiled in these domestic matters, Nightingale was in the throes of her work on India sanitary reform, which she had begun in the early 1860s and considered a sacred mission: "How to create a public health department for India; how to bring a higher civilization into India. What a work, what a noble task for Government ... that would be creating India anew."[45]

Chapter 14

Sanitation for a Subcontinent

> *T*he British race has carried with it into those regions of the sun its habits, its customs, and its vices,
> without considering that under a low temperature man may do with impunity what under a higher
> one is death. Our vast Indian Empire consists of many zones, of many regions, of many climates ...
> The observance of Sanitary laws should be as much part of the future régime of India as the holding
> of Military position or as Civil government itself. It would be a noble beginning of the new order of
> things to use hygiene as the handmaiden of civilization.
>
> — Florence Nightingale, flyleaf to Notes on the Army, 1857[1]

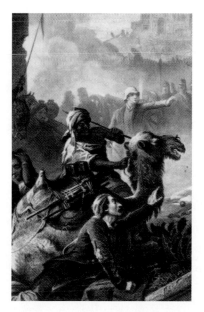

*Detail of "The Relief of
Lucknow" on page 268*

When Florence Nightingale turned her attention to India, it marked the beginning of a
monumental work that would occupy the rest of her active life. She would begin by leading the movement for sanitation reform, first in the military stations and then in all of
India. She would personally educate five viceroys and, toward the end, would work with
the leaders of the early Indian nationalist movement, one of whom was the political
mentor of Gandhi. In the course of these events, the phrase "public health" that we
know today would begin to gain usage.

Nightingale's work in sanitation would be instrumental in two major areas: the
technical, political, and administrative aspects of sanitation itself; and the influence of
increased public awareness on political powers in Britain. Her interests would grow to
include irrigation, rural land finance and tax reform, famine relief, and reduction of the
salt tax, among other topics.

When news of the Indian mutiny against British rule, which broke out in May
1857, reached Nightingale, her first impulse was to answer a new call to arms and return
to the field. However, it was only an impulse; poor health precluded such an action.
Sidney Herbert firmly reminded her that she already had undertaken a great deal of
work in home army reform, in which she had enlisted his service, and that she must help
him finish what they had jointly begun.

*"The Relief of Lucknow,"
depicting the triumphant
meeting of Sir Henry Havelock,
Sir James Outram, and Sir
Colin Campbell in November
1857 during the Great Mutiny,
painted from sketches and
portraits done on the spot*

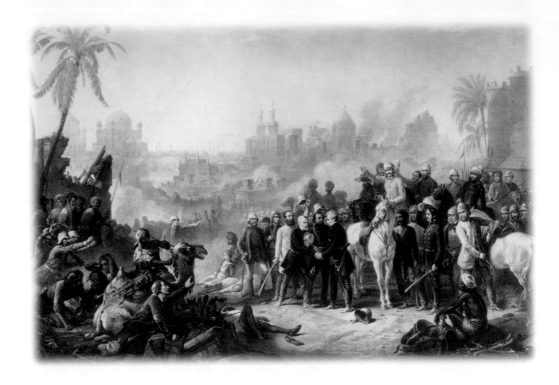

Nightingale instinctively realized that the sanitation campaign, now underway on the home front, must be extended to India. Appalling reports on the sanitary condition of the Indian army had surfaced during the Royal Commission army inquiry, and she already had received firsthand reports of sanitation problems in the campaign to subdue the mutineers and rebels.

She wrote in late 1857 that "a certain earnest, energetic Officer appointed a sanitation inspector to attend to the cleansing of a captured city, and to the burial of some thousand dead bodies of men, horses, asses, bullocks, camels, and elephants, which were poisoning the air." Yet the Bombay government wouldn't sanction the action "because there was no precedent for it." She noted that "it ought to be the duty of the Indian Government to require no precedents for such procedure."[2]

Although Nightingale would never go to India, relatives, friends, and colleagues who were there provided her with firsthand information. Her cousin Lothian Nicholson, now a major of the Royal Engineers, had been sent to join Sir Colin Campbell's expedition to relieve the siege of Lucknow. Nightingale also corresponded with the former head of her governing committee at Harley Street, Lady Charlotte Canning, whose husband had gone to Calcutta as Governor-General of India in 1856. Another invaluable resource was Sir John McNeill, her friend from the Crimean days, whose first career post was as a surgeon with the East India Company in Bombay. However, it was Nightingale's ability to develop a statistical picture of sanitation in India that gave her a perspective unmatched by anyone.

The British in India

England's presence in India dated from the last day of the year 1600, when Queen Elizabeth I granted a monopoly on trade to the East India Company. By the end of the

17th century, the English had surpassed the Dutch and the Portuguese, and had established three centers of power — at Bombay, Calcutta (Bengal province), and Madras — which came to be known as "the presidencies." In the mid-1700s, shifting alliances in Europe precipitated an Anglo-French struggle in India, but by 1761 Britain had triumphed and stood as the dominant European power on the subcontinent.

As British trade and influence gradually spread out from the three presidencies, conflicts arose among the British and the hundreds of native rulers of the interior and the unconquered coasts. Around 1800, the desire on the part of the East India Company for the economies of peaceful trade, coupled with a concern for any Napoleonic venture, fostered an expansionist policy with the goal of political control of the subcontinent.

By the early 1800s, British hegemony over India was complete. The country was governed in two ways by the East India Company acting for the government: direct rule by a British governor (as in the case of the three provinces of Bombay, Bengal, and Madras, over which the British government had supervisory power) and indirect rule through "subsidiary alliance" treaties with hereditary native princes. The British guaranteed military security for the native rulers in return for heavy payments and loyalty to the Crown; a British Resident, or Agent, was stationed in each princely state.

India was used to being governed in this manner, inured to the idea of political overlordship. The religious, cultural, ethnic, and linguistic diversity of the subcontinent

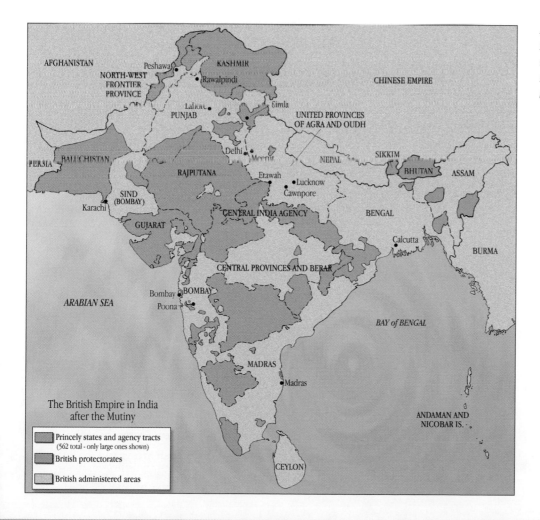

Areas directly governed by the British after the 1857 mutiny when some of Nightingale's sanitation reforms were implemented

made its inhabitants vulnerable to external aggressors for centuries. In effect, the British government was a paternalistic despot that retained the traditional regional structures of Indian administration — an effective civil service and army.

The mutiny and its legacy

The 1857 mutiny, also known as the Great Mutiny or the Sepoy Rebellion, stemmed from rising discontent over the increasing westernization of Indian culture and daily life, especially by the railroad, telegraph, and postal service as well as the influx of Christian missionaries. Other factors that contributed to the conflict were the outright annexation by the British of princely states when a native ruler died — a violation of traditional arrangements — and the introduction of low-caste soldiers into the native army.

The flashpoint occurred when sepoy ("soldier" in Hindu) troops at Meerut, northeast of Delhi, were jailed for refusing to use a new type of musket cartridge, reputedly greased with cow and pig fat, which violated both Muslim and Hindu religious practice. Native troops released their jailed compatriots and killed the British officers, then rode the 45 miles to Delhi and massacred Europeans in the streets. The uprising and similar atrocities quickly spread over northern India in May and June of 1857.

When the mutineers surrounded the British residency at Cawnpore, Nana Sahib, a local ruler and former darling of London drawing rooms, guaranteed the British officials safe passage and then reneged and slaughtered 250 British men. When his soldiers refused to kill the 400 women and children, the Nana brought in assassins who butchered them with knives and threw their remains down a well.

Enraged by these massacres, the British suppressed the rebellion with a vengeance unmatched in English history. Tens of thousands of natives died; mutineers at Cawnpore were forced to lick up the blood on the floor of the butchery room before being executed; Indians who turned their backs on the British troops as they marched through the countryside were shot on the spot; and rebellious sepoys were shot, hung, or blown apart by cannons. By November 1857, the British had regained control of key positions, and cleanup operations continued into 1859.

The Great Mutiny of 1857 marked a turning point in the British rule of India, not only in political arrangements, but also in the deep-seated feelings of betrayal and anger that lasted on both sides for many years. The British attitude of paternalism that had prevailed before the mutiny changed to a control mentality with racial overtones. The Indians never forgot the degradations they suffered, and the British never again felt completely secure.

Government of India Act

Against this backdrop in August 1858, Parliament passed the Government of India Act, which transferred political control from the East India Company, which was generally blamed for the mutiny, to the Crown. The bill provided for a new Secretary of State for India; converted armies of the East India Company to the British army; and mandated a higher ratio of British troops to Indian troops, roughly 1:2 instead of the previous 1:5.

The Secretary of State for India was a member of the cabinet and presided over the India Office in London. A 15-member Council of India, which came to be known as the India Council, advised the Secretary on financial affairs and provided other assistance.

The Governor-General of India, referred to as the viceroy when acting as a direct representative of the Crown, was headquartered in Calcutta, where he ran the largest imperial bureaucracy in the world. Reporting to him were the province governors, lieutenant governors and — the backbone of the British government in India — the 1,500 district officials of the famed Indian Civil Service. Although the Governor-General reported to the Secretary of State for India in London, the British officials running India enjoyed substantial autonomy because they controlled their own purse strings — all government revenues were raised in India, three-fourths in heavy land taxes.

To calm feelings and promote peace after the mutiny, Lord Canning, the Governor-General, announced several new policies: There would be nonintervention in native religious beliefs and perpetual support of native princes, as long as the rulers swore their allegiance to the Crown. As a result, about one-fourth of the Indian population and 40% of the subcontinent remained under the autocratic control of 562 princes, an arrangement that endured for the remaining 9 decades of British rule.

The India Sanitary Commission takes shape

Within months of Lord Stanley's appointment as the first Secretary of State for India in 1858, Nightingale had begun trying to convince him of the need for an India Sanitary Commission. Stanley agreed and the delicate process of selecting the most effective members began.

Nightingale had met Stanley in early 1857; her dear friend and former suitor Richard Monckton Milnes had arranged a dinner to introduce her to "the best man you could get in the House in whatever you wish to be done."[3] Stanley, an admirer of John Stuart Mill and already a champion of such causes as women's rights to own property and obtain divorce, had told Nightingale then that he lived in hope of receiving "future instructions" from her. From that moment on, he kept her informed on Parliamentary issues and asked questions at her suggestion on the House floor.

Even before their first meeting, Stanley had spoken at the public meeting in 1855 announcing the creation of the Nightingale Fund. In recounting Nightingale's accomplishments in the Crimea, which reflected his own values, he clearly understood the obstacles to reform that they would also face in India:

> The best test of a nation's moral state is the kind of claim which it selects for honour ... It is not easy everywhere, especially in England, to set about doing what no one has done before ... in this case custom was to be violated, precedent broken through, the surprise, sometimes the censure of the world to be braved. And do not under-rate that obstacle. We hardly know the strength of those social ties that bind us until the moment when we attempt to break them.[4]

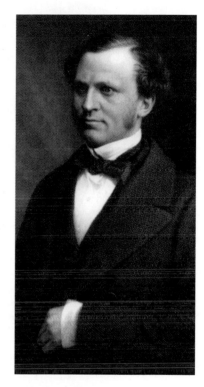

Lord Stanley, Britain's first Secretary of State for India and a faithful supporter of Nightingale's policies

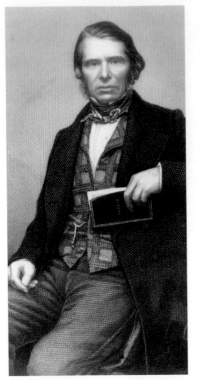

Sir Charles Trevelyan, Governor of Madras in 1859, who supported Nightingale's effort to obtain data on sanitary conditions at all of the Indian military stations

Although Stanley was the head of the India Office in London, he arranged for the Royal Sanitary Commission to operate under and report to the War Office. The War Office was now open to suggestions for improving health in the Indian army in the interests of military efficiency and reduced costs.

Over the next several months, all those involved agreed on the makeup of the new Sanitary Commission: three sanitarians, a statistician, and two members of the India Council, the advisory group recently formed under the Government of India Act. The first four spots went to members of Nightingale's inner circle who had been involved in home army reform: Dr. John Sutherland, Dr. Ranald Martin and Dr. Thomas Alexander as the sanitarians and Dr. William Farr as the statistician. Sidney Herbert was chosen as chairman, but stepped aside in June 1859 when he became Secretary for War; Stanley then assumed the chairmanship. The other three members — two from the India Council and, at the queen's request, a person with India experience — were all acceptable to the reformers.

Canvassing the Indian military

The Royal Warrant establishing the India Sanitary Commission was issued on May 31, 1859, but Nightingale had already gone to work. In early May, finding that no meaningful records or statistics existed regarding sanitation issues in India, she designed a circular of inquiry, a questionnaire to send to every military station on the subcontinent to gather information.

She submitted her early drafts to Sir John McNeill and requested his thoughts on the general direction the inquiry should take. She wrote to Sir Charles Trevelyan, now Governor of Madras, and enlisted his support; as Assistant Secretary to the Treasury during the Crimean War, he had provided her with every assistance possible. She also sought information from all other well-placed medical and military men she knew or to whom she could obtain an introduction.

One of Nightingale's great talents in administrative politics was her ability to set the stage for discussion and debate. She surveyed the available data and statistics, conceptualized what would be needed to advance her position, and then designed the instrument and managed the physical gathering of facts that would help her win her arguments. She needed data on health and sanitary conditions in India to fully understand the problem and formulate policy recommendations and — as in her British army reform — to influence public and political opinion.

In addition to sending out the questionnaire, she asked the 200 largest military stations for copies of all regulations relating to sanitation and administrative issues. This last was a prescient request; when the reformers requested a copy of the Indian Medical Service regulations from the East India House, the London headquarters for the now moribund East India Company, they were informed that only one office copy existed, and they must send to India for the needed material. As usual, Nightingale was already one step ahead.

Despite the effort required to complete her lengthy questionnaires, two-thirds were returned with hard facts. Each of the papers returned to her was signed by the command-

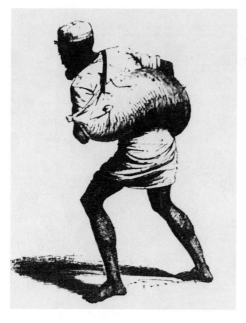

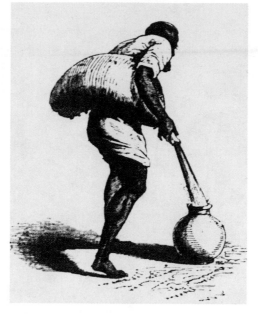

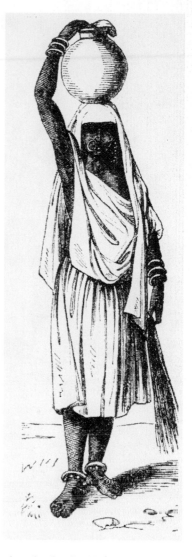

ing officer, the engineer, and the medical officer for each military station. The returned questionnaires, which filled an entire room in Nightingale's house and required two vans when she moved, provided the only database available for the India Sanitary Commission to accomplish its work; no official government statistical survey of India was conducted for another 13 years.

Sanitary Commission report

Nightingale worked hand in hand with Farr and Sutherland to analyze the questionnaires and develop the commission report. Because she had conceived of the undertaking and developed the bulk of the information, the commission formally invited her to submit her comments. These were included as a 24-page section entitled "Observations by Miss Nightingale."

To make her section of the report more vivid to readers, Nightingale, who had obtained rough sketches from her India contacts, asked her cousin Hilary Bonham Carter to help with a few illustrations:

> My dear, I ... ask you to do the following for my Indian Evidence ... 1. An Indian bheestie (or water carrier) with his skin of water over his shoulder; 2. An Indian scavenger (or sweeper) carrying off the refuse on his head or in whatever way he does carry it. (These two I presume could be found in any Indian illustrated book.) 3. One of the vast Indian barrack rooms of more than 100 men, an interior view, with all the men talking on their cots during the hot hours — a day view.[5]

The Treasury Department was horrified at the thought of spending extra money to enhance a government Blue Book, but allowed Nightingale to print the illustrations at her own expense.

The completed India Sanitary Commission report, issued in May 1863, totalled 2,028 pages in two volumes, the second of which contained only the completed ques-

Three sketches that Nightingale commissioned from her cousin Hilary Bonham Carter to illustrate her section of the India Sanitary Commission report. Nightingale jokingly referred to the two Indian water carriers (above left and center) as the Indian system of water supply and drainage — the man on the left was the "beginning of water pipe" and the other man, the "end of water pipe." The other drawing is of a female sweeper (scavenger or garbage collector) carrying refuse on her head.

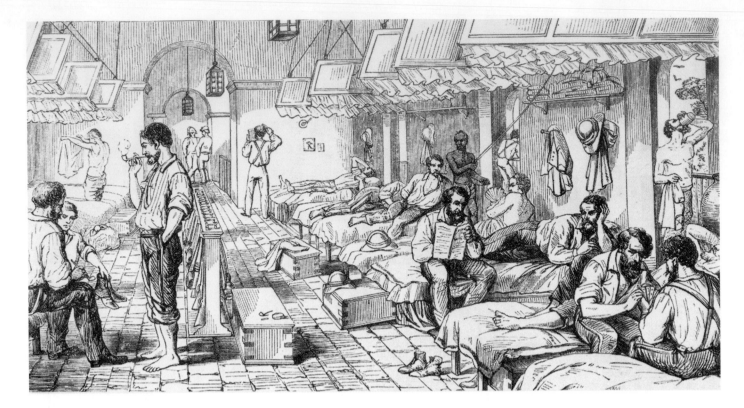

Sketch by Hilary Bonham Carter of an army barrack showing means of occupation and amusement during the heat of the day when the soldiers were confined to quarters

tionnaires. Just as Nightingale's statistics had formed the irrefutable proof of unsanitary hospital conditions at Scutari and in the Crimea, so they established the indisputable case for India.

The information was shocking. Since 1817 the annual death rate of British soldiers in India had reached 69 per 1,000, more than three times higher than the death rate of British troops at home before the 1857-to-1861 army reforms. Nightingale's analysis revealed that 9 per 1,000 had died of natural causes, while 60 per 1,000 had died from causes related to poor sanitation. Ultimately, one company per regiment had been sacrificed every 20 months to maintain British control of India. Nightingale calculated that the annual cost of preventable sickness in the British army in India came to £388,000 per year (approximately £16,000,000 or US$30,000,000 in current values[6]).

The causes of sickness had little to do with tropical conditions. The situation was the same as in the Crimea: Typical camp diseases were prevalent, mostly because of poor site selection for the military stations and poor sanitary practices. Nightingale wrote that "where tests have been used, the composition of the water reads like a very intricate prescription, containing nearly all the chlorides, sulphates, nitrates, and carbonates in the pharmacopoeia, besides silica and quantities of animal and vegetable matter, which the reporters apparently consider nutritive." As to drainage, she wrote that "there is *no* drainage, in any sense in which we understand the word. The reports speak of cesspits as if they were dressing-rooms."[7]

Barracks were constructed with "floors of earth, varnished over with cow-dung: a practice borrowed from the natives. Like Mahomet and the mountain, if men won't go to the dunghill, the dunghill, it appears, comes to them." The barracks were hopelessly overcrowded. One report stated that the men (300 per room) "are generally accommodated in the barrack without inconvenient overcrowding." "What is *convenient* over-crowding?" Nightingale asked rhetorically.[8]

However, the problem was greater than the army stations alone; India was a country of more than 200 million people, scattered mostly among 500,000 villages, all living in primitive conditions. With the army camps next door to the towns and villages, Nightingale realized that ensuring the health of the army, now numbering some 65,000 men, required sanitation for *all* the people of India. Sir Charles Trevelyan, who had initiated valuable reforms as Governor of Madras and aided administrative reform and development of public works as finance minister for India, confirmed Nightingale's analysis:

> In this case you are doing much more than providing for the health of the Troops; for, to be effectual, the improvement must extend to the civil population, and thus another great element of Civilization will be introduced.[9]

The final recommendations of the India Sanitary Commission were broad in scope. Each of the three largest provinces governed directly by the British was to establish a sanitary commission for military affairs. Two Indian representatives were added to the existing Barracks and Hospital Subcommission, which had been created in the earlier army reforms. Sutherland was a permanent member of this commission, so at least all army sanitation affairs in India would pass through his hands.

Nightingale had advocated establishing a Sanitary Department in the India Office in London to provide technical support and oversight for the whole of India, hoping to accomplish some improvements for the civilian populations, both in the directly governed provinces and in the indirectly governed princely states. However, bureaucratic rivalry between the War Office and the new India Office at home, and between the civilian and military elements of the government in India, precluded this at the time.

It was a beginning. Nightingale was asked to develop suggestions for sanitation improvements and rules and regulations, which could be sent to India and used as a basis for a sanitation code.

The "little red book"

Nightingale was delighted with the final report issued by the Sanitary Commission, but clever and effective bureaucratic obstruction by lower-level administrators threatened to override its effect. A clearer example can hardly be found of the maneuvering employed by the antireformers to thwart positive change, and the meticulously detailed tactics that Nightingale successfully employed to overcome such footdragging.

An attempt to gut the report came from an unexpected quarter — the secretarial staff. Without consulting the commission members, the clerk — a minor official appointed by career bureaucrats — printed a shortened and heavily edited version of the report. Gone were the entire second volume consisting of the Military Station questionnaires, Nightingale's "Observations," and a 91-page Abstract of the Station Reports appearing under Sutherland's name, which he and Nightingale had coauthored. To replace this excised material, the clerk wrote a "Précis of the Evidence" that was so incompetent that it contained confusing references to excised material. It was this watered-down, incomplete version that was to be distributed to Parliament and made available to the public.

Only 1,000 copies of the complete two-volume report had been printed; the type had already been broken up. These volumes were available only to members of Parliament, who had to apply for a copy at the Burial Board office, where the clerk for the Sanitary Commission held a full-time post.

Nightingale took immediate steps to make sure the unabridged report would not be buried. She wrote to all members of Parliament with whom she was acquainted, told them the facts, and urged them to apply for the original copy at the Burial Board. For the first time in history, there was a run on a government Blue Book. One reply she received was from Lord Shaftesbury, a veteran at overcoming bureaucratic obfuscation:

> *I will immediately apply for the copy of evidence you mention, but ought we not to insist when Parliament meets that it be fully circulated like any other document? Sir C[harles] Wood [who succeeded Lord Stanley as Secretary of State for India] may have made a "mistake," but a far greater mistake would be to bury this important matter in the "tomb of all the Capulets" ... You have achieved very grand things; and you must thank God that He has called you to such a work, and has so blessed it. I have much to talk to you about.[10]*

Farr and Sutherland, equally indignant, arranged for a private printing of Nightingale's "Observations." Bound in red cloth, it became known as "the little red book" and enjoyed brisk sales, prompting a round of favorable reviews. Edward Stanford, the publisher, placed a prefatory note in the little book:

> *On a subject of the highest interest to the country, it appears desirable that Miss Nightingale's views should be placed in the hands of the public, both in England and in India. Those who have Miss Nightingale's other volumes will thus be able to add to them a book which is second to none in charm of style, and will promote the reform of the sanitary condition of the British Army, as well as conduce to the well-being of the natives of India.[11]*

Many years later, when asked what started the movement for sanitation reform in India, Sir Bartle Frere, who was Governor of Bombay when the India Sanitary Commission report was published, replied that it was neither of the government Blue Books, but rather a certain little red book "which made some of us very savage at the time but did us all immense good."[12]

Plans for an army lavatory in a tropical region, which Nightingale noted did not have a drain for the cesspool

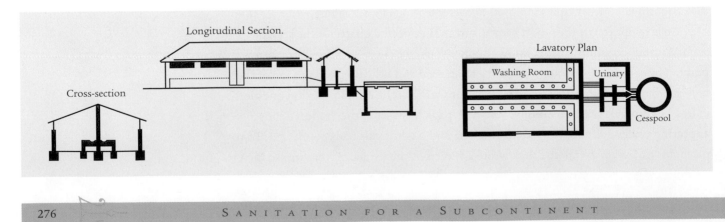

At the time, however, Nightingale was concerned that there was no mechanism to officially ensure that the India Sanitary Commission's report would reach the Indian Civil Service officials and military officers throughout the subcontinent who were in a position to directly implement change. She wrote to her friend Lord de Grey, Secretary of State for War, pointing out that the clerk's abridged version had excluded all the work she had accomplished at official government request. She offered to amend this abridged version, including all of the necessary data and comments that had been deleted. Cleverly playing her departmental rivalry card, she added that "surely Sir Charles Wood will be very grateful to you for remedying his mistake."[13]

As she had done before, Nightingale offered to underwrite the cost of printing to save the Treasury Department any unnecessary expense; de Grey agreed to the project completely. Her original work on the India Sanitary Commission report had taken nearly a year of her time in 1861 and 1862. In the fall of 1863, she spent another 3 months rewriting 140 pages of the "Abstract of the Evidence" to repair the damage to the original report.

As a final safeguard to ensure official attention, she prevailed on de Grey to write the preface to her amended version; the Secretary of State for War noted that Nightingale's version of the report was circulated "with a view of affording information on the subject to Commanding, Engineering, and Medical Officers."[14] Nightingale, through personal contacts, then generated publicity for this final edition with a series of articles that appeared in the *Times* on the need for sanitation reform in India.

Friends in high places

The fact that Lord de Grey was now in a position to assist Nightingale and the reformers was due in part to Nightingale's earlier efforts to help secure his appointment as Secretary of State for War. She was always alert to any opportunity to help place allies in key political or administrative positions.

Sir George Lewis, the former Secretary of State for War, had died suddenly on April 13, 1863. The next day Nightingale's brother-in-law, Sir Harry Verney, informed her that de Grey was one of three men being discussed as Lewis's probable successor. With the army reforms at home already begun, and the report of the India Sanitary Commission due the following month, Nightingale leapt at the opportunity to help secure a proven sanitation reformer as the new head of the War Office.

Born at 10 Downing Street during his father's brief tenure as prime minister, de Grey first became actively engaged in politics as a liberal member of the House of Commons in 1852 at the age of 25. Three years later, he voted in favor of the Roebuck inquiry into army conditions in the Crimean War. He supported open competition, by means of an examination, for civil service posts. After his father's and uncle's deaths in 1859, he moved into the House of Lords with two titles, Earl of Ripon and Earl de Grey, and advanced rapidly in public life. As under-secretary to Sidney Herbert from 1859 to 1861, he sought Nightingale's counsel on reorganization of the War Office, the Army Medical School, soldiers' reading rooms, and the Trent expedition to Canada in 1861.

Telegram from Florence Nightingale to friend Harriet Martineau, urging her to use her Daily News *column to "Agitate, agitate for Lord de Grey" to succeed Sir George Lewis as Secretary of State for War*

To gain positive press coverage and influence public opinion, Nightingale sent a telegram on April 16 to her journalist colleague Harriet Martineau, urging her to "Agitate, agitate" for Lord de Grey.[15] Martineau's column appeared in the next edition of the *Daily News* announcing that the appointment of Lord de Grey was expected.

Nightingale then wrote a letter of support, listing de Grey's strengths for the position, and asked Verney to take it to Lord Palmerston, with instructions that he read it immediately to the prime minister. Palmerston carried the letter to Windsor Castle, where he read it to the queen. On April 22, Queen Victoria approved the appointment of de Grey as Secretary of State for War.

A new ally as Viceroy

In the summer months of 1863, following the release of the India Sanitary Commission report in its various forms, there was a huge outcry against the proposed changes from the entrenched bureaucrats at the War Office and the India Office in London as well as from government officials in India. Although sanitary progress in both army and civilian affairs had become more acceptable at home, there was considerable resistance to change in India, especially among Indian Civil Service officials.

However, in November 1863, Sir John Lawrence, former Chief Commissioner of the Punjab, was appointed Viceroy of India after the death of Lord Elgin. Lawrence, one of the greatest of India's civil servants and a staunch reformer, was the first civilian in 90 years to be appointed Viceroy. His military talents were equal to his administrative abilities. When the 1857 mutiny broke out, he quickly disarmed the sepoys, raised 34,000 loyal Punjab troops, and sped relief columns to Delhi, reversing the tide of the rebellion.

Nightingale admired this energetic, stern, determined, and dedicated man, who had learned firsthand about the life of the Indian people and ways to improve their lot. Deeply religious and rigorously honest, he possessed "a certain heroic simplicity."[16] Although sometimes hot-tempered and rough-mannered, he cultivated intimate relationships with the native people wherever he was stationed. His mastery of Bengali, Urdu, and Persian languages enabled him to communicate directly with the native leaders in their villages, which fostered personal loyalty from them and gave him a firsthand understanding of local problems.

Like Nightingale, Lawrence's capacity for work was enormous, even to the point of damaging his health. In 1859, suffering from neuralgia and near-blindness, he had retired from the Punjab, saying that except for 1 month, he hadn't had "a day's rest for nearly 16 years."[17] He returned to England in 1859 a popular hero, and was made a Knight Grand Cross of the Bath, awarded the Freedom of the City of London, and created a baronet and member of the Privy Council, the Crown's historic advisory group. The moribund East India Company voted him an annual pension of £2,000, and Oxford and Cambridge awarded him honorary degrees. He was appointed to a seat on the new India Council but found board work constricting and thought the council essentially powerless. When he was offered the viceroyalty in November 1863, he immediately accepted.

On the day after Lawrence's appointment, Lord Stanley wrote to urge Nightingale to meet the new viceroy. "Why should not he see you? The plans are in the main yours; no one can explain them better: You have been in frequent correspondence with him ... Let me repeat — you must manage to see Sir John Lawrence ... Your position in respect of this whole subject is so peculiar that advice from you will come with greater weight than from anyone else."[18] Stanley was assiduous in promoting the meeting; he even dropped by South Street unannounced and sent up word asking if Lawrence was coming.

Nightingale had met Lawrence 2 years earlier, when he had called while she was working on the Military Station Reports. At Stanley's prompting, she now invited him for an interview in the 10 days remaining before he sailed for his new post. On December 4th, 1863, the new viceroy, whose career already spanned a quarter century in India, called on the invalid lady who had never been to India personally, but whose facts and figures on sanitation provided her a unique overview.

Lawrence, who was noted especially for his financial administrative expertise, now received the best of sanitation advice. The interview lasted for several hours; he asked Nightingale to provide him with full statements and plans as well as suggestions for membership in the three presidencies' sanitary commissions. Before Lawrence sailed, Nightingale met again with Stanley, and correspondence flowed among the three reformers. Lawrence also requested that the Barracks and Hospital Subcommission, with its two new members from India, begin formulating specific sanitation goals and objectives for India. Far from considering the Sanitary Commission's report exaggerated, as did some who opposed reform, Lawrence considered it under the mark.

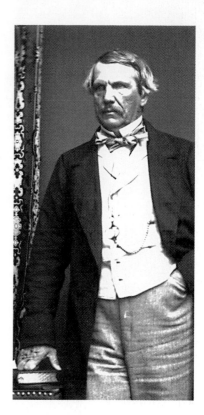

Sir John Lawrence, Viceroy of India from 1863 to 1869, who, when his physician told him not to return to India, said, "If I can't live in India, I must go and die there."

Lawrence was the first of five viceroys who, between 1863 and 1888, would meet and confer with Nightingale on sanitation issues before heading to India. Many other less influential officials with sanitation interests also called. In the end, Nightingale's influence from her "Little India Office" at South Street was greater than her power from the "Little War Office" when Sidney Herbert was Secretary at War. Lawrence was by far Nightingale's favorite viceroy. In her later years, his picture occupied a permanent place in her bedroom, and she attended his funeral in 1879.

A beginning in India

Shortly after Sir John Lawrence arrived in India, he wrote to Nightingale in early February reporting his first steps toward implementing the recommendations of the India Sanitary Commission:

> I write a line to say that we have commenced work by establishing our Sanitary Committees for Calcutta [Bengal], Madras, and Bombay. They are composed of five members. A Civilian is at their head, and a Medical Officer as Secretary. I hope that you will expedite the transmission to India of the codes and rules and plans which have been approved of for home and the colonies. We shall then have an idea in a practical shape of the main features of the sanitary system, and can readily adapt it to the peculiar circumstances of the country.[19]

Once more there was departmental wrangling to overcome at home. In the same month that Lawrence had visited Nightingale, Lord de Grey asked her to proceed on a draft code of sanitation suggestions for India — "the codes and rules and plans" in Lawrence's query. Nightingale, working with Dr. Sutherland and Dr. Farr, as well as Sutherland's colleague from the Crimea, the civil engineer Robert Rawlinson, completed the report, entitled *Suggestions in Regard to Sanitary Works Required for the Improvement of Indian Stations,* in January 1864 and submitted the report to Lord de Grey at the War Office.

Not until early summer, after a delay of several months, was the report finally issued by the Barracks and Hospital Subcommission. The problem, it turned out, was that the India Office felt that it was being dictated to by the War Office. Lord Stanley interceded with a semantic and political compromise: On the title page of the Blue Book issued by the subcommission appeared a statement that the *Suggestions* had been prepared "in accordance with Letters from the Secretary of State for India in Council."

Although the sanitary commissions for the three provincial governments of Bombay, Bengal, and Madras were supposed to address military issues, Nightingale styled their responsibilities in the broadest manner possible; they were charged to "consider and afford advice and assistance in all matters relative to the health of the Army, and to supervise the gradual introduction of sanitation improvements in Barracks, Hospital, and Stations, as well as in Towns in proximity to Military Stations."[20]

Although Lawrence had inherited a difficult situation, he pushed forward where he could. In February 1864, he wrote that "I am doing what I can to put things in order out here; but it is a very uphill work, and many influences have to be managed and overcome."[21] He had to contend with tight budgets, burdened as the government was with paying off the military expenses incurred to quell the 1857 mutiny and deal with British civil servants who now harbored animosity toward the people they ruled.

When the government officials made their annual summer retreat from Calcutta to Simla, over 900 miles away in the cooler and dryer foothills of the Himalayas north of Delhi, Lawrence reported to Nightingale on the condition of all the military stations he passed through and requested assistance on special points.

Both the need and the worth of Nightingale's vision were evident in a letter she received from Sir Hugh Rose, Commander-in-Chief of the army in India, saying that he had introduced regimental workshops and soldiers' gardens at the military stations. In one instance, the gardens served a threefold purpose. At a station where cholera had raged for 2 years, newly arrived soldiers were told by the departing battalion that "they would never come out alive. However, the entering battalion ... made gardens with such good effect that they had the pleasure, not only of eating their own [uncontaminated] vegetables, but of being paid for them too by the Commissariat ... and not a man had cholera."[22]

Other improvements at the military stations included the establishment of savings banks, libraries, and recreation rooms that provided games and refreshments. Heavy drinking was curbed by a new law imposing a heavy fine or imprisonment for the illicit sale of alcohol near military camps, and the regulation two drams were reduced to one.

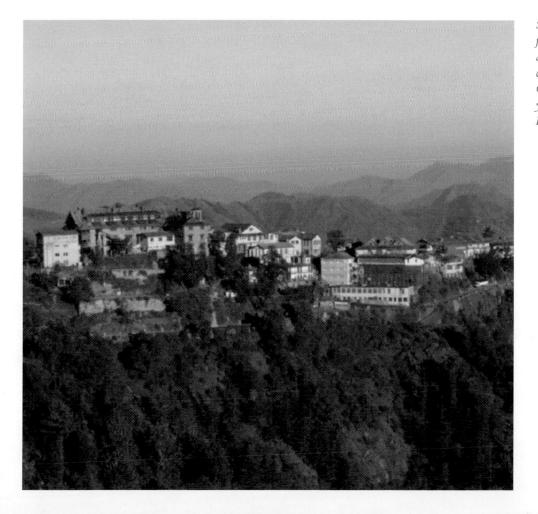

Simla in the Himalayan foothills, where British officials and their families went to escape the summer heat of Calcutta and which became a year-round home for many British

Nightingale in the details

Nightingale also addressed many other concerns, which reflected the myriad issues medical officers dealt with — conflict between military, civil, and native populations; unsanitary conditions of bungalows near the river; problems with supplies at the Commissariat; and census errors in soldiers' death rates at 43 stations from 1859 to 1862. She took particular interest in a health problem called the Delhi boil, or Delhi ulcer, a widespread affliction among soldiers as well as civilians. Her brother-in-law, Sir Harry Verney, conveyed a report that one regimental officer had 80 boils on his body.[23] Nightingale queried one of her regular correspondents, Dr. J. Pattison Walker, who was Surgeon-Major in the Bengal Indian Army and Secretary of the Bengal Sanitary Commission. A long response from one of Walker's colleagues provided her with descriptive details on the Delhi ulcer and its local treatment, the ingredients of which were kept secret for generations in Indian families as a means of gaining personal acclaim and livelihood. Data on all these concerns became the foundation for Nightingale's continued work in India and the articles she published from 1864 to 1883.

Nightingale found occasion to work directly with members of the three newly formed provincial sanitary commissions. When Mr. Ellis, the Chairman of the Madras Sanitary Commission, visited England, Nightingale arranged for him to meet with Lord Stanley. She discussed with him proposed changes in the membership of the sanitary commissions, about which she was corresponding with Lawrence. While Ellis was in London, she welcomed him to her house, and dispatched Sutherland to accompany him on his inspections of hospitals and barracks.

The Secretary of the Bengal Sanitary Commission wrote to her seeking information on reliable tests for water purity. Nightingale contacted Dr. Angus Smith, who had developed a similar test for air, and Smith authored a pamphlet on procedures to test for water purity. Nightingale printed the pamphlets at her own expense and received approval from the War Office Sanitary Committee (the renamed Barracks and Hospital Subcommission) to distribute copies in India.

The construction or improvement of infrastructure for sanitation projects, such as new buildings and drains and sewers, always had to compete with military priorities, especially roads and fortifications. Nightingale was elated when Lawrence, who had asked for £10,000,000 to improve the army barracks throughout India, received final approval for £7,000,000 (approximately £300,000,000 or US$500,000,000 in current values).[24] In February 1865, a deeply satisfied Nightingale wrote to Harriet Martineau:

> How well it looks — six noughts after a 7 — £7,000,000. Like the man henpecked by his heiress wife, who is used to retire to comfort himself with her Banking book, I am married to the Indian Office confound it. But I retire to comfort myself with the look of my dear millions.[25]

Nightingale articulated goals in sanitation reform for India that far exceeded the system's capability for change. Her priority for the health of the individual soldiers, other Europeans, and the natives in their 500,000 villages was for her the "product of a real civilization." At one point Nightingale wrote to Lawrence:

Your Bengal Sanitary Commission is doing its work, like men, like martyrs, in fact. And what a work it is! All we have in Europe is mere child's play. Health is the product of a real civilization ... In India your work represents not only diminished Mortality ... but increase of energy, increase of power, of the populations. I always feel as if God had said, mankind is to create mankind. In this sense, you are the greatest creator of mankind in modern history.[26]

Such a vision was often at odds with the priorities of business and government officials, who were usually driven by concern for profitable activities that benefited only select interests.

Stanley, temporarily out of office but still a formidable member of Parliament and chairman of the India Sanitary Commission, clearly understood the strategic importance of Nightingale's work. He admired her patience and restraint in the face of delays by the antireformers — "the savage tribe" — and cautioned her, as did many others, against the perils of overwork. From his political perspective, he wrote in 1864 that he was convinced of two things:

First, the vast influence on the public mind of the Sanitary Commissions of the last few years – I mean in the way of speeding ideas which otherwise would have been confined to a few persons; and next, that all this has been due to you, and to you almost alone. [27]

Side step to Australia

While Nightingale was toiling over the circular of inquiry for India in 1859 and 1860, Sir George Grey, former private secretary to Queen Victoria and Governor of New Zealand, sought her advice on a similar social concern: the declining numbers of aboriginal peoples, particularly in New Zealand, Australia, and Canada. As British colonization spread, indigenous peoples were suffering as native environments were destroyed and customs altered. Grey suspected that imposing formal education and a European school system might be a factor in the disappearance of the aborigines, but he could find no supporting data.

Nightingale developed a new circular of inquiry and sent it to the Colonial Secretary in London, who then dispatched copies to colonial schools and hospitals in those areas where aborigines were encountered. As replies came in, the Secretary forwarded them to Nightingale for analysis. Statistics on sanitation and conditions were returned from 143 schools in Australia, Ceylon, Africa, and Canada; from colonial hospitals that treated natives in South and West Africa; and from two hospitals in Canada. In 1863, Nightingale submitted a paper comparing diseases that were common in the schools with those that were prevalent among adults. The paper was printed in *Transactions of the National Association for the Promotion of Social Sciences.*

Nightingale's conclusions on native colonial hospitals and the causes of the disappearance of native races mirrored her conclusions about death rates in the Crimea — bad water supply and drainage, imperfect agriculture, lack of cleanliness, and other bad habits such as alcohol. She suggested proper provision of land for tribes, admonished the British for selling intoxicating drinks to those who had never known them, and emphasized that education among the natives should be conducted in a very different manner than in England. According to her, every colony where native races were declining could furnish a report, but it wasn't mandatory: The injustice was a common one, and so should be the remedy.

Nightingale's second paper, "Note on the Aboriginal Races of Australia," was read at the annual meeting of the National Association for the Promotion of Social Science at York in 1864 and published in 1865. In it, she concluded that sanitation education in native colonial schools was important, but that cultural beliefs and habits must also be considered because many native customs were healthy and practical. Referring to a paper by Bishop Salvado of Port Victoria, she wrote:

> ... as soon as native habits and customs begin to undergo change under European influences, the work of destruction has at the same time begun. "Few sick aborigines ... are restored to health," whereas, under similar circumstances, "few Europeans would die." The native appears to have little or no chance of recovery from the moment he sets foot within a house or hospital and comes under medical treatment. He longs to return to the bush; he escapes; "and yet that dying native, a few weeks afterwards, when every one that knew him believed him to be dead and buried, is as strong and healthy as ever, having traveled perhaps fifty or more miles on foot ...[28]

Although Nightingale ultimately was unsuccessful in stopping the decline of the aboriginal races, she did bring scientific data to the attention of the government. This led to further study and some measure of protection.

Progress by "fits & starts"

By early 1867, Sir John Lawrence reported to Nightingale that "the death-rate among the English troops for 1866 was only 20.11 per thousand, while it was 24.24 per thousand in 1865."[29] Although this was a solid beginning to improve the lives of the 65,000 British troops, these figures didn't include wives and children of these soldiers, the 140,000 natives in the Indian army, or the 200 million peasants and townspeople of India — all of whom Nightingale thought should enjoy the blessings of "civilization."

Although there had been many improvements, Nightingale wrote that "whatever has been done in the way of improving the Public Health, has been done by fits & starts — & without any system."[30] There still existed no administrative organization and mechanism to ensure continuing progress after Lawrence finished his term of office. Even with his personal leadership, internal opposition had reduced the sanitary commissions in the three presidencies from the original five members to two each, a president and secretary, on the grounds of reducing expenses.

Three organizational goals

In 1867, the need for tamper-proof administrative machinery, coupled with the emergence of two new allies in key positions, opened the door for Nightingale to push for her original administrative design to ensure continuing action for sanitation in India. Her goals were:

1. a Sanitary Department in India that would be responsible for all projects and report directly to the Governor-General

2. a Sanitary Department at the India Office in London to oversee, evaluate, and control the work

3. an annual publication describing the measures adopted for sanitary improvement in India, which would serve two purposes: first, the public and politicians would be informed, which would provide a valuable incentive for officials in India to work diligently; second, the report itself would provide an opportunity for criticism and suggestions.

Sir Bartle Frere at her side

In 1867, the return to London of Sir Bartle Frere, the recently retired Governor of Bombay, opened the door to the India Office for Nightingale. An ardent reformer and brilliant administrator, Frere had been appointed to the India Council upon finishing his term as governor.

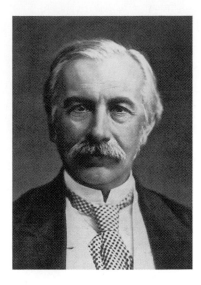

Sir Bartle Frere, Governor of Bombay (1862-1867), member of the India Council, and frequent correspondent on Indian sanitation reforms, who told Nightingale, "Men used to say that they always knew when the Viceroy had received a letter from Florence Nightingale: it was like the ringing of a bell to call for sanitary progress."

Frere had begun his Indian career in 1834 and had risen rapidly through the ranks. He was known for his genuine human concern for the welfare of the people, whose lives he greatly improved wherever he was posted. Like Lawrence and other Indian civil servants of his generation, he acted from the same Benthamite utilitarian principles that had contributed to the great changes in England. In 1850, he became Chief Commissioner for the province of Sind. There, he introduced education for soldiers' children and native orphans, aided the development of local government, built roads and canals, made sanitation improvements, established surveys and judicial codes, organized trade fairs, and promoted land and tenant reform.

Frere called on Nightingale in June 1867, and she found in him a like-minded ally who also possessed vast experience and profound insight into the details of administrative governance in India.

> We had a great talk. He impressed me wonderfully — more than any Indian I have ever seen except Sir John Lawrence; and I seemed to learn more in an hour from him upon Indian administration and the way it is going than I did from Ellis in six months ... or from Indian Councils (Secretaries of State and Royal Commissions and all) in six years.[31]

Frere thoroughly agreed with her ideas for administrative reform and pledged to help her win over Sir Stafford Northcote, the new Secretary of State for India. He vowed to "make [Nightingale's house at] 35 South Street the India Office while this affair is pending."[32] He not only became one of her main correspondents over the next 5 years, but he and his family became close friends of W.E.N. and Fanny, visiting often at Embley.

As for Nightingale, she had found a man to head the office for the second of her three administrative goals. She wrote to her cousin's husband, Captain Douglas Galton, her quiet confederate on the War Office Sanitary Committee, with whom she conferred on these plans. Her note included a new term: "If only we could get a Public Health Department in the India Office to ourselves with Sir B. Frere at the head of it, our fortunes would be made."[33]

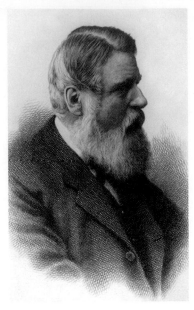

Sir Stafford Northcote, Secretary of State for India, who helped Nightingale realize one of her goals — to establish a Sanitary Committee in the India Office in London

Sir Stafford Northcote takes up the cause

Frere's enlistment opened the door to the new Secretary of State for India, Sir Stafford Northcote, whom Nightingale had never met. Fortunately, Northcote, who had been a Balliol scholar with Arthur Clough, was conscientious and worked hard at Indian affairs.

Within a few weeks after their first meeting, Nightingale had drafted a letter, approved by Frere, in which she asked Northcote to "put the Indian Health Service once and for all on a satisfactory footing."[34] Frere, as one of the members of the Indian Council created to advise the Secretary of State, delivered the letter to Northcote in person.

After exchanges of correspondence, Northcote called on Nightingale in late August 1867. He was convinced of the need for a Sanitary Committee at the India Office, as Nightingale had suggested, with Frere as chairman. Acutely aware of departmental jealousies, he asked Nightingale's opinion on how relations between the War Office Sanitary Committee and the new India Office group should be structured. She advised, and he agreed, that the India Office committee should be the controlling body and the War Office group should be consultative. Nightingale had now accomplished the second of her three organizational goals.

The first goal remained out of reach, but there was improvement. Lawrence had suggested that principal health officers be appointed in each local government, with their salaries to be paid by the central Indian government in Calcutta. Although it wasn't a separate Public Health Department, as Nightingale originally conceived, it was a substantial advance.

Northcote asked Nightingale to make suggestions at large, which allowed her to secure her third organizational goal. As a result of her suggestions, in April 1868 Northcote ordered an annual Report on Sanitary Progress. These reports were collected each year and printed in a government Blue Book, along with other papers, which formed the first of an annual series of Indian Sanitary Reports.

Assisted by Frere and Galton, Nightingale had achieved two of her three organizational goals. More importantly, Nightingale became the unofficial editor for the annual reports on sanitary progress, a position that enabled her to stay abreast of India affairs. Frere, as head of the India Office Sanitary Committee, instructed that all the material received for each report be submitted to Nightingale for her review. She wrote or outlined the introductory comments, edited the abstracts of local reports and, with Sutherland, discussed the details of each report.

Nightingale was elated to be working with departmental colleagues and allies. In May 1869, the clerk for the committee, Mr. Plowden, who became another of Nightingale's friends, wrote to her: "I forward a sketch of the Introductory Memorandum ... the greater part of it is copied verbatim from a memorandum of your own that Sir Bartle Frere handed over to me for this purpose."[35] Frere wrote to her in July, "I can never thank you sufficiently for all the kind help ... I feel sure it will leave its mark on India."[36]

Lawrence's retirement

Although Nightingale held Lawrence in the highest personal esteem, he didn't see, or understand, the necessity of establishing an independent Public Health Department in the Indian government, which was the first of her goals. Toward the end of his term, he wrote to her:

> It may seem to you, with your great earnestness and singleness of mind, that we are doing very little, and yet in truth I already see great improvement, more particularly in our military [stations], and doubtless we shall from year to year do better. But the extension of sanitation throughout the country among the people must be a matter of time, especially if we wish to carry them with us.[37]

Nightingale continued to urge Lawrence to make the changes she envisioned before he left India in January 1869, but he had neither the leeway nor an administrative style suited to an increasingly complex era. His viceroyalty wasn't marked with sweeping reform, as Nightingale had wished. To be fair, though, he had inherited a staggering deficit due to military expenses incurred during the mutiny; when he tried to cut back on expenditures, he was severely criticized in England as well as in India, particularly by the governors who were trying to improve their provinces.

Lawrence and Nightingale remained great friends and mutual admirers, and he told her, "You initiated the reform which initiated Public Opinion which made things possible, and now there is not a station in India where there is not something doing."[38]

Health missionaries for India

From 1868 through 1874, Nightingale edited and contributed to each annual government Blue Book, which summarized the army station reports and outlined sanitary progress in India. Sir Bartle Frere, as head of the Sanitary Department at the India Office in London, met with her frequently. After Nightingale analyzed the compiled data, it was given to Mr. Plowden or another clerk at his office, who then issued the official report from the India Office.

During these years, much new data was gathered from the cholera inquiries, which sparked increasing interest after Dr. John Snow published his 1855 paper linking the cholera outbreak in London to the Broad Street pump. Nightingale had long ago outlined effective sanitary measures to prevent cholera, yet they still weren't being carried out at the local level in India. Frustrated, she began to meet with governors and health officers from India as well as native Indians through her contact with Frere.

Lord Napier of Madras

One of these governors was Lord Francis Napier, Governor of Madras, who became another of Nightingale's allies in India. She had met him first on her arrival at Scutari in 1854 when he was secretary to the British Ambassador to Turkey, Lord Stratford. He valued her ideas and implemented them in India, making significant improvements in urban drainage and sewer systems. When Nightingale recommended that he send some

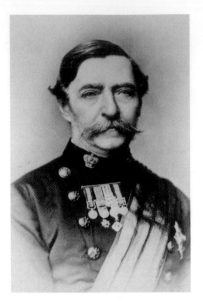

Lord Robert Napier of Magdala (1810-1890), Field Marshall and Commander-in-Chief of the British army in India

engineering officers to London to study sanitation works, he responded quickly, sending two professionals in the field.

Napier began to introduce Nightingale's ideas of sanitation on a small scale in a Madras hospital for women, focusing on specific diseases; his wife became interested in a lying-in (maternity) hospital and several orphanages. He also introduced a taxation bill to finance improvements in local roads, primary education, and sanitation.

Lord Napier of Magdala

In December 1869, ever alerting Nightingale to influential people who might aid her cause, her London ally Frere asked her to meet with another Napier, Lord Robert Cornelius Napier of Magdala:

> *... Lord Napier of Magdala is in town ... & writes to say that it would make him very happy if he could have the privilege of paying his respect to you before he leaves London ... He is likely to serve again, in India and elsewhere. I am sure he would be the better able to aid, in all you have so much at heart if he has the advantage of being personally known to you — & he has infinite stores, if he would only unpack them, of what would interest you, & you know how devoted he is to the good cause.[39]*

In January 1870, before they could arrange to meet, Napier was indeed appointed to serve in India, as Commander-in-Chief of the Indian army. Soon after, Nightingale began discussions with him on the priority of reforms in India. Napier agreed with her about the possibility of improving the moral and physical condition of the soldiers by means of recreation and suitable employment. In March, having spent his last morning in England in discussions with Nightingale, he sailed for India with her directives fresh in his mind. Encouraged, she wrote to Julius Mohl about their meeting:

> *[We] were like a brace of lovers on our Indian objects or rather passions & even our rages ... And I sent away the C. in C. [Commander-in-Chief] to India without anything to eat! He said he had too much to talk about to waste his time in eating.[40]*

New opportunities with Bengalis

After Napier's departure, more avenues to Indian reform opened for Nightingale. She was elected an honorary member of the Bengal Social Science Association, whose members were primarily native Indians interested in furthering the practical application of sanitation science in the villages. This membership allowed her the opportunity to correspond and meet with dedicated men in India who could effect change at the local and village level. In a cordial letter of appreciation, she wrote:

> *For eleven years what little I could do for India, for the conditions on which the Eternal has made to depend the lives and health and social happiness of men, as well Native as European, has been the constant object of my thoughts by day and my thoughts by night.[41]*

Her new Bengali connection proved a fortuitous one. Her work on a tract to India's village elders, laying out a vast plan for sanitation reform, was translated into Bengali and, through Sir Bartle Frere's efforts, into several other Indian languages. It became her most widely circulated address to the people of India. Her faithful assistant, Dr. John Sutherland, as was their practice, had submitted a rough draft for her to put into her own words. In his view, the finished paper was probably the most important contribution she had made on the question of sanitation. Frere was thrilled with this paper as well and wrote:

> ... your paper for the Calcutta Social Science Association ... has acted on me, & will, I am sure act on many more, as a cordial or tonic — much needed in these days when, morally as well as physically, one may say that all the sky is brass, & all the earth is iron. May I keep a copy to have it translated into Mahavatti [Marathi] & Guzerratti [Gujarati]? The Calcutta people will have it translated as well into Bengali, through which you may speak to 40 million. The Mahavatti speaking people are probably barely 20 million and the Guzerratti perhaps 10 or 12 but they are the most advanced in intelligence & most likely to profit of any nations in India — and many more will follow. I have tried to criticize — but can really pick no holes, nor suggest any additions; & it might I am sure be read in any of the Indian vernacular languages, and every word of it, intelligible to any decent headman of any ordinary village.[42]

In the spring of 1873, Nightingale was invited to submit a paper to the Meeting of the National Association for the Promotion of Social Science. This association, founded in 1857, included male and female members and was one of the most important groups influencing public policy in England. Nightingale's paper, "Life or Death in India," was a 10-year summary of her work on Indian reform and sanitation. The following year, it was published as a pamphlet titled *How Some People Have Lived and Not Died in India*. When the American Statistical Association made her an honorary member in 1874, she sent an acceptance letter along with copies of her papers "Annual Sanitary Report of the Indian Office" and "Life or Death in India."

At home Nightingale's work continued apace, but Benjamin Jowett was alarmed at her overworked state and wasted no time reminding her of their mutual contracts:

> We have three compacts: first, you are to give an hour a day to writing or some unprofessional occupation (& not to overwork — I excuse the letter to the Presidencies, but would rather it did not happen again) in return for which I will observe hours and days (I have only broken the hours once) ... Second, we have a minor compact not to be observed so strictly; not to speak evil of others — not to "bring a railing accusation"; this, however, may be occasionally broken when human nature can endure no longer ... Third, we will have a great compact that every year is to be calmer, happier, & more efficient & productive of results ...[43]

Voice for the people

For many years, Nightingale had been frustrated with the British government's treatment of the people of India. By August 1878, specifically, she was outraged at the government's failure to enforce policies that would address the continuing problems of drought and famine. She couldn't tolerate the abuse of the peasants by landlords, many of whom were also moneylenders and shopkeepers. By now, some British businessmen

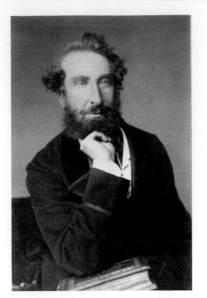

Lord Lytton, Viceroy to India, who placed political control of the subcontinent above issues of reform

had become absentee landowners, living in grand style far away from their holdings and leaving the supervision to local agents.

To address these injustices, Nightingale wrote an article, "The People of India," that lambasted Britain for its shoddy rule of the country. She began, "We do not care about the people of India" and went on to condemn Britain for the oppressive salt tax, the virtual slavery of the people to landowners, the death of 6 million people by starvation, and much more. Published in a new magazine, the *Nineteenth Century,* her article shocked the British people and raised considerable support for her cause.

Some people at the India Office thought Nightingale had exaggerated the problems. The current viceroy, Lord Edward Robert Lytton, acknowledged that the issues were political and social and that appearances had to be kept up; Britain's hold on the Indian colony, he said, depended less on reform than on political consolidation.

Nightingale cared little for political policies that were despotic and cruel. She was appalled at the atrocities suffered by the peasants at the hands of landowners. She wrote three articles that were published in the popular periodical *Good Words* in July, August, and September of 1879. The first article and part of the second described the current Indian famine and the relief efforts that fell short of bringing about change. The second article discussed the evils caused by the moneylenders in connection with the agrarian riots. The third described the work of the Sanitary Commission, particularly the work accomplished in Bombay.

In these articles, Nightingale masterfully integrated principles of disease prevention, public administration, and health promotion. She also discussed environmental degradation, pointing out the evils of deforestation and the resulting devastation during the monsoon season. She realized that irrigation, though necessary, had its limits. Cutting forests without replanting new growth was, to her, alarmingly shortsighted for the future of the peasants and the country. Her second and third article praised Sir John Lawrence. Although she often felt that Lawrence could have done more in his viceroyalty, she acknowledged that he had done the best he could under the circumstances.

In June 1879, on the afternoon that Lawrence died, a note from him was delivered to her along with some Indian famine papers. That they cared for each other and the mission despite their differences was clear. With her brother-in-law Sir Harry Verney, she attended Lawrence's funeral at Westminster Abbey, one of her very few public appearances.

Chapter 15

Nursing Reform &
Progress for Women

*T*he whole reform in nursing both at home and abroad has consisted in this; to take all power over the nursing out of the hands of the men, and put it into the hands of one female trained head and make her responsible for everything (regarding internal management and discipline) being carried out ...

— Florence Nightingale to Mary Jones, May 1, 1867[1]

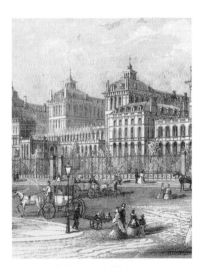

The new St. Thomas's Hospital, which became the home of the Nightingale School of Nursing in 1871

The nursing revolution that Nightingale had pioneered by her example at Scutari, and for which she had established a theoretical framework with the publication of *Notes on Nursing,* now began to spread slowly into the two categories of civilian hospitals that existed in England — the "voluntary," or private, hospitals and the "workhouses," which were designed as public shelters for the jobless poor, but which also had come to serve a crude hospital function. Wealthy people were still treated at home.

Before the Nightingale reforms, hospital administration was shared by lay administrators and the medical staff. The matron was primarily a housekeeper, who reported to the administrators and played only a small role in nursing management. The doctors dictated to the nurses, who usually came from the ranks of domestic servants and tended to remain in the same wards continuously.

Nightingale's introduction of a trained superintendent, or matron, and trained nurses created a tripartite administrative structure, though not without a struggle. The matron centralized the administration of nursing affairs and assumed some of the responsibilities previously given to the lay administrators and doctors. It was a battle of the sexes — the woman superintendent against the male administrators, the male doctors, and the male governors (guardians or board of directors).

In the voluntary hospitals, such as St. Thomas's, this reform spread fairly quickly for several reasons. The activist women who sought power moved in the same social circles as the governing committees and could personally influence change. In addition, trained nurses provided a higher standard of care than the old-style nurses and at less cost. Furthermore, these hospitals were increasingly staffed by a new generation of doctors who had come to recognize the value of trained bedside care.

By 1861, the voluntary hospitals had some 11,000 patients throughout England, were supported by charitable contributions, and were governed by the donors, leading citizens, and doctors.[2] Patients in the countryside gained admittance on recommendation from this group, but in London patients tended to be selected to meet the needs of research and teaching. For the sick poor, the only alternative to wasting away in a slum or on the street was to enter a workhouse. Here they lived in virtual barracks and could hope for some medical treatment. However, it was only a hope, for the workhouses had not been administratively or physically designed for the sick.

During the 1870s and 1880s, Nightingale devoted much of her time to improving the situation in the workhouses, promoting the training of workhouse nurses and district nurses, and campaigning for the establishment of an army nursing service. She also took a more active role in the affairs of the Nightingale School of Nursing and in the lives of the nurse probationers.

Workhouse nursing

The workhouse was one of Britain's early experiments in public welfare to deal with the jobless poor, known today as the structurally unemployed. In the first part of the century, each parish (similar to a county) had aided the poor out of locally collected taxes, a system that was greatly abused.

The amended Poor Law of 1834 required all persons seeking public aid to enter a workhouse, where they would be provided bed and meals in return for performing various menial tasks. The official policy was to make the workhouses austere and harsh to separate the lazy from those with no other alternative. Families were broken up by sex and age, and residents lived in prisonlike conditions. The 15,000 parishes were formed into 643 "Poor Law unions," each responsible for its own "union workhouse."

The workhouses rapidly filled not only with the jobless poor, but with the elderly, sick adults and children, the blind, the mentally ill, the disabled, and those with chronic and incurable diseases, such as epilepsy, tuberculosis, venereal diseases, and skin conditions. The voluntary hospitals were interested in treating only curable cases and used the workhouses as dumping grounds for undesirable patients.

By 1861, the workhouses throughout England contained some 150,000 poor people, of whom 50,000 were medical patients.[3] In London alone, 40 workhouses contained 21,150 patients.[4] The level of medical care was abysmal; workhouse doctors received low wages and there were only a few trained or paid nurses.

Although her time was consumed by her army and India reform work, Nightingale had long been aware of the terrible workhouse conditions:

> I have always felt workhouse patients were the most neglected of the human race — far more so than in Hospitals ... I remember years and years ago when I used to visit at Marylebone Workhouse feeling how hopeless those depths of misery were to comfort — and that visiting did nothing, but break the visitor's heart.[5]

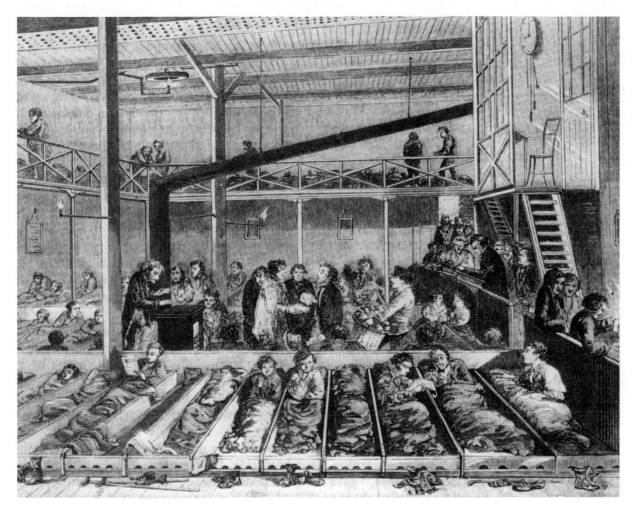

Leadership in Liverpool

William Rathbone, a wealthy merchant and philanthropist from Liverpool, was appalled by the conditions of the Liverpool Workhouse Infirmary, which housed 1,200 paupers. In January 1864, he wrote to Nightingale asking for her help in providing trained nurses for the workhouse. He guaranteed financing for the project if Nightingale would act as a consultant and help him find a qualified lady superintendent, which both agreed was crucial to the success of the project.

Rathbone had already been successful in establishing the Liverpool Training School and Home for Nurses, using Nightingale's advice, in 1862. This school provided nurses for the Royal Infirmary, to which it was physically connected, and for the district nursing program. Despite Rathbone's proven track record, influence, and financial support, negotiations with the workhouse bureaucracy were long and tedious. The board agreed to the project after 3 months, but another year passed before it actually began. During this period, Rathbone published his book *The Organization of Nursing in a Large Town,* to which Nightingale wrote an eight-page introduction.

Twelve trained Nightingale nurses and their superintendent, Agnes Elizabeth Jones, began work at the Liverpool Workhouse Infirmary on May 16, 1865. In the history of modern nursing in England, this date is second in importance only to the opening of the Nightingale School at St. Thomas's Hospital on June 24, 1860. Nightingale and Rathbone's introduction of trained nurses into the workhouse infirmary laid the foundation for government provision of health care services for the poor.

The occasion was so important to Rathbone that he wrote to Nightingale a few days earlier on her birthday, May 12, expressing his wish to send her flowers regularly for her room (which he did until his death in 1902):

> *... I beg to be ... your gardener to the extent of doing what I have longed wished—providing a flower-stand for your room and keeping it supplied with plants. I hope you will not be offended with my presumption or refuse me the great pleasure of thinking that in your daily work you may have with you a reminder of my affectionate gratitude for all you have done for our town and for me. If the plants will only flourish, as the good seed you have planted here is doing, they will be bright enough; and as for my personal obligations, you can never know how great they are to you for guiding me to and in this work.[6]*

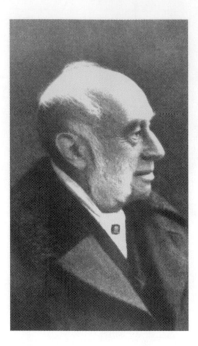

William Rathbone (1819-1902), the philanthropist and reformer who, with Nightingale's help, introduced trained nurses into workhouses

Agnes Jones: Workhouse nursing pioneer

Recognized as the pioneer of workhouse nursing, Agnes Jones was the niece of Sir John Lawrence, the Viceroy of India and a favorite ally of Nightingale. Jones had been inspired to go into nursing by Nightingale's work in the Crimea and had trained at Kaiserswerth and St. Thomas's Hospital. Nightingale described her as attractive, rich, and witty, but intensely religious and devoted to her work. In 1863, Mrs. Sarah Wardroper, the matron of St. Thomas's, praised Jones as by far her best nurse probationer.

Jones was at first reluctant to go to Liverpool but, after her interview with Nightingale, came to believe that it was God's will. Upon first entering the wards, with all their filth, drunkenness, and disease, she compared them to Dante's *Inferno*. After 2 years of hard work, Jones and her staff had turned the inferno into one of the most orderly infirmaries in the country, and the trained nurses were seen as a complete success, despite some bureaucratic disputes that Nightingale and Henry Bonham Carter, the Nightingale Fund Secretary, had to smooth over.

Unfortunately, Jones died in February 1868 after a severe 2-week bout of typhus. Several other nurses sent to replace her were deemed incapable of filling the position. Rathbone asked Nightingale to send another team of nurses from St. Thomas's, but there weren't enough trained nurses to send. However, Nightingale nurses eventually did return to the Liverpool Workhouse Infirmary and furnished most of the staff.

In June 1868, Nightingale anonymously wrote "Una and the Lion" as a eulogy to Jones:

> *... She [Jones] was always filled with the thought that she must be about her "Father's business." She could do, and she did do, more of her Father's business in six hours than ordinary women do in six months, or than most of ever the best women do in six days. But, besides this and including this, she had trained herself to the utmost — she was always training herself; for this is no holiday work. Nursing is an art; and, if it is to be made an art, requires as exclusive a devotion, as hard a preparation, as any painter's or sculptor's work; for what is the having to do with dead canvas or cold marble, compared with having to do with the living body — the temple of God's Spirit? It is one of the Fine Arts; I had almost said, the finest of the Fine Arts.[7]*

Nightingale gets involved

When the *Times* reported the death of a young boy from filth due to gross neglect in a London workhouse in December 1864 under the headline "Horrible Treatment of a Pauper," followed by a similar case a few months later, a huge public outcry quickly followed. Nightingale wrote to Charles Villiers, president of the National Poor Law Board, describing the Liverpool Workhouse Infirmary project then being developed, and suggested that similar reforms in London could save the government further bad publicity.

Villiers met with Nightingale in early January 1865 to discuss her ideas for comprehensive reform of workhouse administration, which she believed was the necessary precursor to improvements in medical and nursing services. He assigned H.B. Farnall, Poor Law Inspector for the Metropolitan District, to work directly with Nightingale in gathering data and preparing their case. Although Villiers and Farnall were reformers at heart, they were a minority in the bureaucracy they sought to change.

The organizational and administrative structure of the workhouses, as set forth in the amended Poor Law of 1834, guaranteed mediocrity, if not downright incompetence, in medical matters. The national board of three commissioners had only advisory powers. The governing board of each urban workhouse, called the guardians, was usually composed of tradesmen, shopkeepers, or retired businessmen, some of whom had once been paupers themselves. The driving force in workhouse management was to keep expenses at a minimum so that local tax rates would remain low.

Nightingale's entry into the workhouse debate helped tip the scales in favor of the reformers, who had gained momentum in recent years because of their increased participation in public affairs. The Workhouse Visiting Society, begun by Louisa Twining, an acquaintance of Nightingale, had grown to 140 members by 1860; these ladies read to, instructed, and gave comfort to workhouse residents. The National Association for the Promotion of Social Science, founded in 1857, publicized workhouse scandals and became one of the most important groups influencing public policy.

In addition to Farnall's internal investigation for the National Poor Law Board, the *Lancet* medical journal sponsored an inquiry in 1865 by a committee of doctors, which evolved into the Association for the Improvement of London Infirmaries. Their findings were printed in successive issues. Finally, three-fourths of the frustrated medical officers who actually practiced in the workhouses established a reform group to deal with any "departmental trickery."[8]

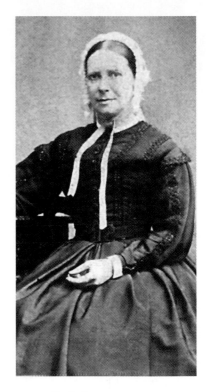

Agnes Elizabeth Jones, a graduate of the Nightingale School who became first lady superintendent of the Liverpool Workhouse Infirmary

A chilling story

The various investigations found that, with few exceptions, the 40 London workhouses were overcrowded, poorly ventilated, and lacking even the basic amenities, such as enough beds and towels. At one workhouse paupers were sleeping on the floor, and in another 40 young girls shared 13 beds. Mattresses were a rare commodity. People with contagious fevers were placed amid the general population, and at two workhouses, some of the sick were "found washing in their chamber pots." Thirty inmates at one workhouse used a single towel, and eight syphilitic women at another shared one towel a week. Every investigator criticized the preparation and provision of food for the sick.[9]

The data on medical conditions told a chilling story. There was one medical officer for each workhouse, a ratio of one doctor for every 530 patients. There were only 142 paid nurses for 21,150 sick people. Thirty-five of the paid nurses were employed at two of the better institutions, which held 3,150 patients. The other 107 paid nurses, scattered among 38 workhouses, ministered to 18,000 sick people, a ratio of one paid nurse for every 168 patients.[10]

Most of these paid "nurses" had received no hospital training; they were nurses in name only, having come from the ranks of maids, laundresses, and other laborers. Their low wages were supplemented by board and allotments of beer. Their main duty was supervising the large number of "pauper nurses," workhouse residents assigned to do the brunt of the nursing. While a few of these pauper nurses performed adequately, drunkenness was common because the pauper nurses also received an allowance of beer — with gin for night duty. Many were overworked, old, and feeble and stole food and stimulants from patients. Very few could read; doctor's instructions were ignored and medicine was given with "systematic irregularity."[11] The *Lancet* committee summed up the situation this way:

> *Patch up the present system as we may, it will still continue to be a scandal and a reproach ...*
> *The State hospitals are in the workhouse wards. They are closed against observation, they pay*
> *no heed to public opinion; they pay no toll to science. They are under the government of men*
> *profoundly ignorant of hospital rules ... To perpetuate 39 bad hospitals when half a dozen good*
> *will suffice would be an act of gross and dangerous misgovernment.[12]*

The ABC's of reform

All the reform groups agreed on a few basic issues, such as isolating fever patients, but Nightingale, with her gift for large-scale systems analysis, saw that the problem originated with the administrative structure and intent of the Poor Law:

> *So long as a sick man, woman, or child is considered administratively to be a pauper to be*
> *repressed, and not a fellow-creature to be nursed into health, so long will these most shameful*
> *disclosures have to be made. The care and government of the sick poor is a thing totally*
> *different from the government of paupers. Why do we have Hospitals in order to cure, and*
> *Workhouse Infirmaries in order not to cure?[13]*

Working with Farnall and colleague Dr. John Sutherland, Nightingale developed an overall plan for legislative reform; she summarized the main points of the plan, which she called the "ABCs," in a letter to former Poor Law administrator Edwin Chadwick in July 1866:

> *A. To insist on the great principle of separating the sick, Insane, infirm & aged, incurable,*
> *imbecile, & above all the children from the usual pauper population of the Metropolis ...*
> *B. To advocate a single central administration.*
> *C. To place all these classes (especially those suffering from any disease, bodily or mental)*
> *under a distinct & responsible administration, amenable directly to Parliament — these are*
> *the A.B.C. of the reform required.[14]*

The "ABCs" were distributed not only to Poor Law commissioners, but also to newspapermen and other government officials and allies, such as John Stuart Mill, who sat on a Parliamentary committee on local government. Nightingale's visionary administrative blueprint presaged the structure of modern public health services:

• The sick, insane, incurable, and children must be separated from the general population and placed in institutions specially designed for each group, where professional medical and nursing services would be available. A modern system of data collection and classification must be implemented.

• There must be a central administration to manage and train personnel, allocate bed space and other resources, and contain costs, rather than 40 different local governing boards that didn't communicate with each other.

• Underlying the whole plan was the issue of public finance. For the population in need of medical services, a general tax rate should be levied and equalized for the entire London metropolitan area. Consolidation of services and a general tax rate went hand in hand to ensure professional administration.

Metropolitan Poor Act of 1867

Villiers decided to adopt Nightingale's plan and began to prepare legislation, but in June 1866 the Whig government — and Villiers — went out of office. His successor, Gathorn Hardy, moved slowly and cautiously on the reform issues before him. However, a consensus had developed on the need for fundamental change, and in February 1867 Hardy introduced in Parliament the Metropolitan Poor Bill.

Lacking a clear majority, Hardy worked out a compromise that incorporated Nightingale's core administrative principles. Under the Metropolitan Poor Act of 1867, all workhouse districts were combined into one Metropolitan Asylum District for cases of fever, smallpox, or insanity — paid for by a Common Fund supported by equalized rates from all districts. For the noninfectious sick, the Common Fund would pay for all medical and nursing salaries as well as medicine, medical equipment, and any other treatments. Children were removed from the workhouses and placed in separate institutions.

The Metropolitan Poor Act was a milestone in English social history, and Florence Nightingale had crafted the administrative framework. For the first time, the state acknowledged its explicit responsibility to provide hospitals for the poor, a responsibility that culminated in the National Health Service Act some 80 years later.

One of the first Poor Law unions to respond to the passing of the Metropolitan Poor Act was St. Pancras Union, whose guardians asked the Nightingale Fund to provide a superintendent for a new 500-bed hospital to be built for noninfectious patients in Highgate. The woman chosen, Elizabeth Torrance, was a born leader. In 1870 with the help of the Nightingale Fund, she set up a program to train pauper nurses. Torrance and the St. Pancras medical officer, Dr. Dowse, did the training because her head nurses were incapable of giving instruction. The program was successful because Torrance took a real interest in her nurse probationers.

Unfortunately, in 1872 the Nightingale Fund sent Torrance back to St. Thomas's to be an assistant to Mrs. Wardroper, who was overwhelmed with work. Several other trained nurses were sent to Highgate Infirmary to serve as superintendent, but they didn't have Torrance's leadership ability. By 1877, the Nightingale Fund had withdrawn its support from workhouse nurse training because it had neither enough trained nurses to send nor enough money to support the training plan.

The situation had improved by 1881, when the Nightingale Fund Committee agreed to send a superintendent and a group of nurses and to provide some funds for a workhouse nurse training program for St. Marylebone as well as other hospitals. For the next 10 years, the fund had an enormous influence on workhouse nursing by supplying trained nurses to these facilities.

District nursing

District nursing, also called home nursing, evolved to meet the needs of sick people who needed trained nursing care in their homes. During the mid-1860s, critics were assailing the Nightingale Fund for devoting most of its efforts to hospital nursing, which only benefited St. Thomas's Hospital. Nightingale herself had for some time been questioning the benefit of hospital care for sick people. In June 1867, she wrote to Henry Bonham Carter that "the ultimate destination of all nursing is the nursing of the sick in their own homes. I look to the abolition of all hospitals and workhouse infirmaries. But it is no use to talk about the year 2000."[15]

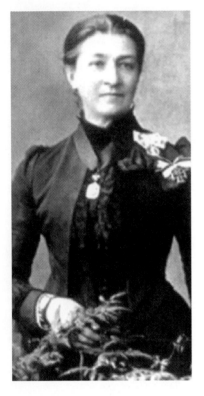

Florence Lees, whom Nightingale considered the inventor of district nursing

Home nursing up to this time consisted mainly of ladies' voluntary committees, which collected money to buy medical supplies for poor people and hired untrained "nurses" to provide basic unskilled care for people in their homes. Nightingale, in contrast, wanted home nurses to have real training. To achieve her objectives, however, she needed data. As usual, there was no uniform system of data collection on home nursing cases, so she designed her own forms and sent them to many cities and towns.

However, as with her earlier reform plans, Nightingale faced an uphill battle. The lady volunteers were opposed to nurses filling out her home nursing care forms, and they preferred hiring untrained women because they were less likely to challenge the ladies' ideas about patient care. Over the next 5 years, many district nursing programs sprang up around the country, each with its own system of administration. Most of these programs had untrained but paid nurses and untrained lady superintendents from the local ladies' voluntary committees.

District nurse training established

In the late 1870s, Nightingale began to promote district nursing in London and corresponded frequently with the Metropolitan and National Association for Providing Trained Nurses for the Sick and Poor, which had been established in 1875. Fortunately, her friends William Rathbone, Henry Bonham Carter, and Dr. Henry Acland, a professor of medicine at Oxford, were on the association's committee, so she could feel confident that her ideas would be considered.

With her usual flair for statistics, she prepared a questionnaire to ascertain all the types of nursing being used in the London area — including hospitals, workhouses, and district nursing — the nurses' training, and the nursing practices of the different sister-hoods, religious organizations, and other associations. The results were printed in 1876 in a 119-page booklet called *The Report of the National Association for Providing Trained Nurses for the Sick and Poor*. The survey revealed that there were 26 district nursing institutions, but only 11 with trained nurses. It provided little information on the work or value of the existing training programs but emphasized the need for district nursing.[16]

After this report, a central home for training district nurses, sponsored by the Metropolitan and National Association, was set up in Bloomsbury Square and subsidiary homes soon followed in Holloway and Paddington. To Nightingale, a central training home was essential because district nurses weren't affiliated with a hospital and had little supervision. From 1877 to 1881, the Nightingale Fund paid for the training of dozens of district nurse probationers, many of whom were Nightingale nurses.[17]

Florence Lees, who had trained at the Nightingale School and served as a nurse in the Franco-Prussian War, became the first superintendent of the Metropolitan and National Association. Lees's superintendency was plagued by personality clashes with various committee members, and her views on what kind of training district nurses should receive soon differed from Nightingale's. In spite of these problems, Lees is considered the founder of district nursing.

After Lees's marriage in 1878 to Rev. Dacre Craven, a well-known activist for Poor Law reform, the ties between the Nightingale Fund and the Metropolitan and National Association weakened. Lees resigned as superintendent of the association but continued to work for Poor Law reform and district nursing. Her husband became a member of the Nightingale Fund Council in 1888.

Nightingale's strong interest in district nursing is evident in a brief address written for the Association in 1878:

> ... *District Nursing, so solitary, so without cheer and stimulus of a big corps of fellow workers in the bustle of a public hospital, but also without many of its cares and strains requires what it has with you, constant supervision and inspiration of a genius of nursing and a common home. May it spread with such a standard all over London and over the whole of the land.*[18]

The Nightingale School of Nursing

When the Nightingale School of Nursing was still located in its temporary quarters at Surrey Gardens, Nightingale had little contact with the school's management because of other compelling work, particularly Poor Law and India reform. However, from 1870 to 1890, she became more involved with the training program and its students.

The training program originally had been financed largely by the Nightingale Fund. However, as the cost of training increased, St. Thomas's Hospital was forced to gradually assume a greater part of the financial burden. By the late 1800s, the Nightingale Fund was serving more like a foundation, providing funds for different types of nurse training programs.

After the death of Arthur Clough in November 1861, Henry Bonham Carter, Hilary's 34-year-old brother, became the secretary of the Nightingale Fund, a position

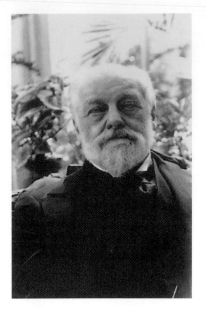

Nightingale's cousin Henry Bonham Carter, who served as Secretary of the Nightingale Fund for 38 years and helped her run the nurse training school at St. Thomas's

BELOW: *Surrey Gardens, the temporary home of St. Thomas's Hospital and the Nightingale School of Nursing from 1861 to 1871*

he held until 1899. He stayed on the council until just before his death at age 93 in 1921, when his son Walter became secretary until 1947.

The two cousins worked closely together in overseeing the operations of the fund and corresponded almost daily. Nightingale would send him a letter in the morning, and her messenger would wait for his response. Nightingale relied on him to address the fund's financial concerns and confided in him about all matters related to the school — superintendents, nurse probationers, doctors, and other key people. Bonham Carter, a barrister, eventually gave up his law practice and took a salaried position with an insurance company so that he could devote more time to the Nightingale Fund. Much of Nightingale's success with various nursing reforms was due to his diligent work and good mind for business.

Nightingale had emphasized from the start that her nurses were to be trained in all aspects of nursing and, once trained, would be sent to other hospitals to work and to teach; they weren't being trained merely to staff St. Thomas's. Nightingale's insistence on the spread of instruction to other hospitals is what characterized the Nightingale training school and led to the dispersal of Nightingale nurses throughout the world.

To Nightingale, the purpose of her school was to create for nurses a respected profession combining both "art and science" as well as an opportunity to serve God by serving mankind. She believed that everyone, regardless of vocation, had a role to play in God's plan and that performing one's job well was a way of attaining divine perfection:

> *...God sent them [human beings] into the world expressly for the purpose of doing the business of the world ... the object of the statesman, the lawyer, the doctor, the merchant, the shopkeeper, the day labourer are as sacred as those of the priest ... when the scavenger cleans the street or the stockbroker sells shares, or the publican serves his customers, he is discharging a divinely imposed duty and playing his part — and an essential part too — in a divine scheme, as much as a priest administering the sacrament to a dying man.[19]*

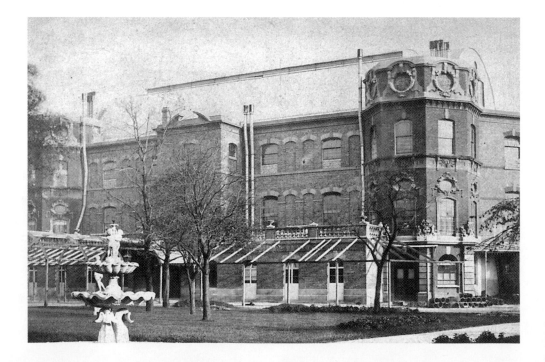

NURSING REFORM & PROGRESS FOR WOMEN

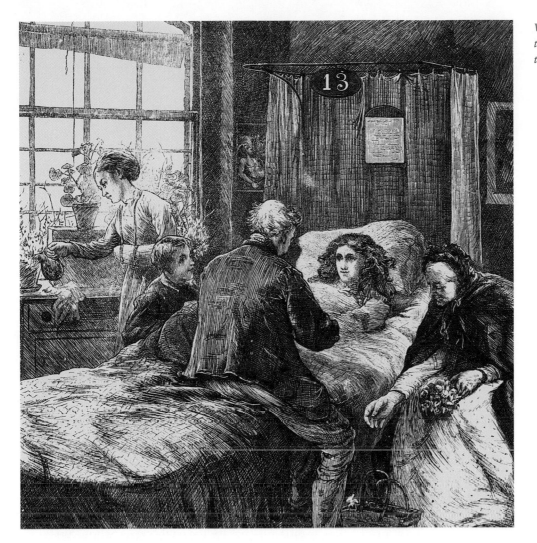

New home

In 1868, Queen Victoria laid the foundation stone for the new St. Thomas's Hospital with the assistance of Richard Whitfield, the hospital's Resident Medical Officer, who had also been hired as lecturer for the nurse probationers. Although Nightingale didn't attend the groundbreaking ceremony because of her chronic illness, her popularity soared as the Nightingale School of Nursing moved to its new location in Lambeth, directly across the River Thames from the Houses of Parliament. The move meant that more young women could now enter the nurse training program. The new St. Thomas's Hospital was formally opened on June 21, 1871, with the queen again in attendance, and patients were admitted in September.

Although poor health kept her from attending opening day ceremonies, Nightingale monitored the probationers' progress and curriculum from her South Street home. As part of their training requirements, the probationers were expected to keep diaries about patient care and their daily activities in the wards. These diaries, along with Nightingale's famous record sheet — "Monthly State of Personal Character and Acquirements of Nurse During Her Period of Service" — on each probationer, were brought to her by the head matron, Mrs. Sarah Wardroper, or by her assistant.

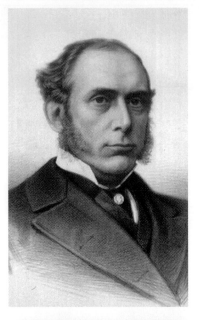

Nightingale was dismayed by the educational levels she perceived in the diaries. The students' entries on patient care indicated inadequate patient assessments and very little scientific knowledge or training in practical skills. For example, an entry might read simply "bed sore dressed" without providing an assessment of the bed sore or the patient's general state, the treatment, how often the dressing was changed, or whether there were any signs of wound healing.

Nightingale wrote frequent letters to both Whitfield and Wardroper about her concerns and also to Bonham Carter, urging him to enforce stricter rules. To learn more about what was going on at the school, she began to invite the nurse probationers to her home for tea. Over the years, Whitfield had disagreed with Nightingale on many points of her curriculum, and by the late 1860s, he was failing to provide basic nursing information. The probationers complained to Nightingale about his poor teaching. One of them, Rebecca Strong, wrote an account of her training after graduating in 1867, noting that she hadn't received a single lecture in anatomy or physiology and wouldn't recommend the program to anyone.

In 1872, Whitfield began to criticize Nightingale's whole nurse training program, charging that her expectations and ideals were too high. He also quarreled with Dr. John Croft, a member of the senior surgical staff and a lecturer whom Nightingale respected. Nightingale demanded Whitfield's resignation in October 1872. Croft assumed the lecturer's job and made changes in the curriculum that pleased Nightingale. He assigned required reading for probationers, printed his lectures, and invited other members of the medical staff to lecture the students.

A difficult beginning

The first 10 years, 1860 to 1870, were difficult ones for the Nightingale School, primarily because there weren't enough suitable applicants to meet the demand for trained nurses. Another challenge was how to implement Nightingale's new standard of patient care when so many hospitals and others institutions refused to accept it.

By 1867, there were five distinct classes of probationers:
• nurse probationers ("Ordinaries"), who received £10 per year
• "Free Specials" — usually clergymen's daughters or educated women left in difficult situations — who received no salary
• "Free Specials" who received a small salary
• "Specials" who paid £30 yearly for their room and board
• "Specials" who paid £52 yearly and didn't sign a contract.[20]

The "Specials" were educated women with leadership abilities who were expected to become a superintendent at the end of their training year. They received the same training as the ordinary probationers but with varying pay scales, depending on their financial needs. If an ordinary nurse probationer was found to be exceptional, every effort was made to help her succeed to the next level.

The first four groups were required to sign a 4-year contract stating that they would spend 1 year in training and then 3 years at whatever position was found for them after graduation. Because the fifth group paid for their own education and room

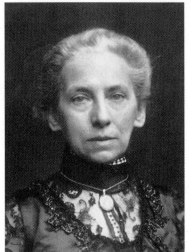

ABOVE: *Dr. John Croft (1833-1905), Resident Surgeon at St. Thomas's, who replaced Mr. Whitfield as instructor for the nursing students in 1873*

BELOW: *Rebecca Strong, who wrote a critical but helpful account of the Nightingale school upon graduating in 1867*

and board, they weren't required to sign a contract. After 1872, the 4-year contract was reduced to 3 years because so few of the graduates completed the 4-year requirement. One of the reasons for this was the program's insistence that applicants had to be single or widowed. Nightingale believed that nurses' responsibilities were so great that they wouldn't have any time to care for a family. As a result, many promising candidates were forced to drop out of the program when they opted for marriage.

By the end of 1870, of the 196 probationers who had successfully completed the first year of training and been entered on the register as a "certificated" nurse, fewer than 60 were still nursing; of the others, 66 quit for personal reasons (such as marriage or poor health), 4 died, and 64 were dismissed for reasons ranging from insobriety and drug addiction to syphilis and tuberculosis.

As a result of the rapid changes in medicine, most London teaching hospitals had training schools for nurses by 1870. These schools, which had less rigid contracts for their nurses, competed with the Nightingale School for qualified applicants. However, the better-educated, upper-class women were attracted to St. Thomas's because of the prestige associated with Nightingale's name.

To ease some of the pressure on Mrs. Wardroper, who was in poor health and overwhelmed by her management responsibilities, in 1872 Nightingale created a new position — assistant to the matron — which later came to be called "home sister." Elizabeth Torrance, the successful superintendent at St. Pancras's Highgate Infirmary, was

The new St. Thomas's Hospital, which opened in 1871, was built using Nightingale's pavilion floor plan. The Houses of Parliament and Big Ben can be seen across the Thames.

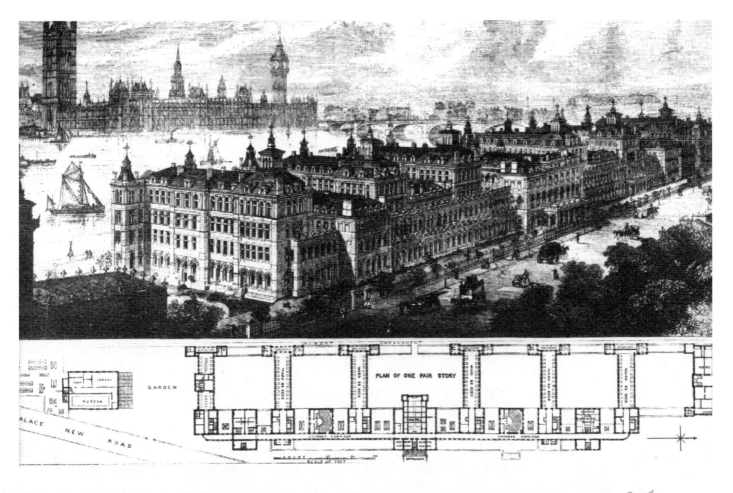

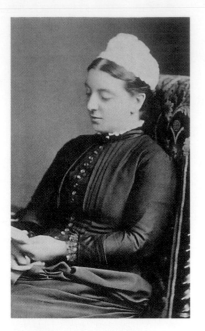

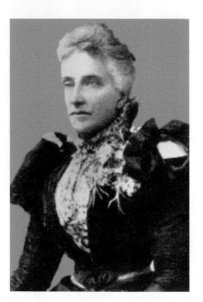

Two of Nightingale's favorite nursing students, Angelique Pringle (top), who later became Superintendent of Nurses at the Edinburgh Royal Infirmary, and Rachel Williams, who later became Superintendent of Nurses at St. Mary's Hospital in London

recruited back to St. Thomas's to serve in this subordinate position. Torrance remained in the post until December 1873, when she married and fell from Nightingale's graces. Maria Machin, another Nightingale favorite, succeeded Torrance and stayed until 1875, when she went to Canada.

The first woman to really make an impact as home sister was Mary Crossland, a former governess, who held this position until her retirement in 1895. Crossland was in charge of the probationers' residence, their religious and moral training, checking of their diaries and lecture notes, instruction on the wards, and special tutoring for less educated probationers.

Favorite students

Despite the numerous problems in the early days of the Nightingale School, there were many rewarding aspects for Nightingale. She took special pride in her best and brightest nurses. Her favorites received invitations to dine and sleep at her house and were lavished with letters, praise, and gifts.

They also received the best assignments. Elizabeth Barclay, a well-educated Quaker, was sent to the Edinburgh Royal Infirmary with nine nurses in October 1872. Angelique Pringle, whom Nightingale called "Little Sister" or "the Pearl," became Barclay's assistant. Unfortunately, Barclay was forced to resign in November 1873 because of alcohol and opium addiction.

Pringle took over as superintendent of the Edinburgh Royal Infirmary and ran a successful training program for 14 years. She had to resign when she converted to Catholicism in 1884, but she remained very close to Nightingale and was the last visitor outside of the family to visit Nightingale before her death in 1910.

Another Nightingale favorite was Rachel Williams, an outspoken and temperamental Quaker whom Nightingale sometimes called "Goddess" for her beauty. Williams, who had been at Edinburgh with Pringle, became superintendent at St. Mary's Hospital, a London voluntary hospital, in 1876. She had many problems at St. Mary's with the doctors, who were accustomed to an untrained matron who obediently followed their orders. Williams finally resigned in 1885, but Nightingale later sent her to serve as superintendent of nurses during the Egyptian campaign. After her return from Egypt, she married and became superintendent of a nursing home in Cannes until her death in 1908.

Nightingale's addresses to her nurses

Alarmed at the lack of moral training of her nurses and probationers at St. Thomas's, Nightingale began writing annual addresses to them in 1872 and continued the practice until 1900. These letters were usually read aloud to the women by her brother-in-law, Sir Harry Verney, the chairman of the Nightingale Fund. Each nurse also received a printed copy, marked "for private use only," of the handwritten address in which Nightingale shared her philosophy, ideals, and guidelines.

The letters, addressed to her "dear children" or "dear comrades," were written from the point of view of both a nurse and a person with a chronic debilitating illness. They contain universal themes found in all the major world religions: There is One God, speak the truth, God is love, it is more blessed to give than receive, love thy neighbor, heaven is within, conquer with love, blessed are the peacemakers, examine thyself, do no harm, the Golden Rule, as ye sow so shall ye reap, man does not live by bread alone, it is blessed to forgive, be slow to anger, and a man is known by his deeds and not his religion. Woven throughout was her loving message of self-healing with quiet time, prayers, self-discipline, and becoming aware moment by moment of how to deepen one's inner knowledge of the interconnectedness with self, others, nature, and God.

Her 1874 address spoke of the importance of good assessment and note taking and reminded her nurses that they were role models for Christian ideals:

> *How can we be "stewards of grace" to one another? By giving the "grace" of our good example to all around us ... Do we look enough into the importance of ... keeping careful Notes of Lectures, of keeping notes of all type cases ... so as to improve our powers of observation: all essential, if we are in future to have charge? Do we keep in view the importance of helping ourselves to understand these cases by reading at the time books where we can find them described, and by listening to the remarks made by Physicians and Surgeons in going round with their Students? (Take a sly note afterwards, when nobody sees, in order to have a correct remembrance.)*
>
> *So shall we do everything in our power to become proficient, not only in knowing the symptoms and what is to be done, but in knowing the "Reason Why" of such symptoms, and why such and such a thing is done: and so on, till we can some day TRAIN OTHERS to know the "reason why."*
>
> *Many say: "We have no time; the Ward work gives us no time." But it is so easy to degenerate into a mere drudgery about the Wards, when we have goodwill to do it and are fonder of practical work than of giving ourselves the trouble of learning the "reason why" ... Take ten minutes a day in the Ward to jot down things, and write them out afterwards ... It is far better*

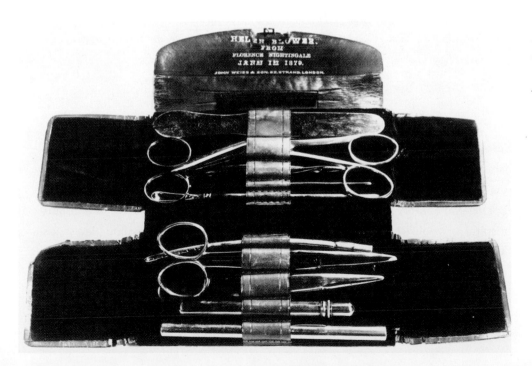

Instrument kit that Nightingale gave to Helen Blower, a graduate of the Nightingale School for Nurses, when she left for Montreal General Hospital in 1879

to take these ten minutes to write your cases or to jot down your recollections in the Ward than to give the same ten minutes to bustling about.

... It is of ourselves and not of others that we must give an account. Let us look to our own consciences as we do to our own hands, to see if they are dirty. We take care of our dress, but do we take care of our words? It is a very good rule to say and do nothing but what we can offer to God ... It is example which converts your patients: your ward-maids; your fellow-Nurses or charges; it is example which converts the world ...

... A woman, especially a Nurse, must be a missionary, not as a minister or chaplain is, but by the influence of her own character, silent but not unfelt ... A Nurse is like a traveller, from the quantity of people who pass before her in the ever-changing wards ... The traveller may call himself a missionary or not, as he likes. He is one, for good or for evil. So is the Nurse ...[21]

In her 1875 address, she criticized "the sentimental view of nursing":

Above all, let us pray that God will send real workers into this immense "field" of Nursing, made more immense this year by the opening out of London District Nursing at the bedside of the sick poor at home. A woman who takes the sentimental view of Nursing (which she calls "ministering," as if she were an angel), is, of course, worse than useless; a woman possessed with the idea that she is making a sacrifice will never do; and a woman who thinks any kind of Nursing work "beneath a Nurse" will simply be in the way. But if the right woman is moved by God to come to us, what a welcome we will give her, and how happy she will soon be in a work, the many blessings of which none can know as we know them ...[22]

Her 1878 address urged her nurses to "stick together" like the ancient companies of Roman soldiers under one commander:

... And what were those soldiers not able to do? They would hold a post till the last man of them had died at it — each man forgetting himself, each man standing by the others, no man saying, "oh this is hard." These were the men who conquered the world. And not alone among the Romans were such men to be found ... We have our own men, of whom it was written: "Forward the Light Brigade: O the brave charge they made!" And I say: Forward the Light Brigade of St. Thomas: God will back you, if you look to Him, against any "charge" of any day. He loves a brave woman, a magnanimous heart ...[23]

Military nursing

Since returning from the Crimea in 1856, Nightingale had campaigned for the establishment of an army nursing service as well as for new military hospitals. Although she was unsuccessful in stopping the outmoded corridor design from being used in the first general military hospital (the Royal Victoria Hospital at Netley), the new military hospital at Woolwich, which opened in 1865, was built using the pavilion plan that she favored. At Nightingale's urging, it was renamed the Herbert Hospital.

Nightingale and Sidney Herbert had envisioned a comprehensive army health service, and many of the improvements they had suggested in the 1861 Royal Commission subcommission report were enacted. Some of these were the improved record keeping and statistics in the army's Medical Department, army medical training of doctors, implementation of job descriptions and regulations for orderlies, and creation of recreational facilities for recuperating soldiers.

On many occasions since her return from the Crimea, Nightingale had written the War Office about the importance of using educated, disciplined, and properly trained women nurses in military hospitals in peacetime. The War Office finally was persuaded, and the Nightingale Fund became actively involved in finding the first superintendent of nurses for the Royal Victoria Hospital and later at the Herbert Hospital.

Two early army nursing superintendents

Nightingale persuaded Lady Jane Shaw Stewart, who had gone to the Crimea with the Mary Stanley party, to accept the superintendent's job at the Royal Victoria Hospital. Shaw Stewart had served valiantly as superintendent of nurses at the Castle Hospital in Balaclava; after the war, Nightingale arranged for her to receive additional surgical training at St. Thomas's. Also, when Nightingale had felt near death in 1857, she had recommended Shaw Stewart to Herbert as the only nurse capable of developing a training program with the Nightingale Fund.

In 1863, Shaw Stewart and five nurses began work at the Royal Victoria Hospital, where they had trouble almost from the beginning. Shaw Stewart's reputation among some military officers, doctors, and patients for being demanding and quick-tempered had followed her from the Crimea. Some were antagonized by her insistence on having complete control of her nurses and the running of the ward, according to the Nightingale model of superintendent. Shaw Stewart compounded her problems because she was task-oriented and lacked people skills. She was also accused of "Anglicanism" (proselytizing) and not following military protocol. The situation came to a head in 1869 after Shaw Stewart forbade a night orderly from entering a certain ward and a patient died. She was accused of manslaughter and forced to resign in November 1869. However, she and Nightingale remained friends.

Jane Deeble, a 40-year-old widow of an army surgeon, succeeded Shaw Stewart as superintendent after training at St. Thomas's. On their way to the Royal Victoria Hospital in 1869, Deeble and six ward nurses went to visit Nightingale, who offered them words of encouragement and advice on work regulations. One nurse wrote of the visit:

> That I have seen Miss Nightingale will be one of the white mile-stones on my road, to which I shall often look back with feelings of gratitude and pleasure. I trust that I shall never forget some of the things you said to me.[24]

The medical staff at the hospital were cordial to Deeble because she didn't insist on independent rules for the nurses. However, she still had a high rate of nurse turnover and many other challenges in establishing a female nursing presence in the military.

In 1879, Deeble took a group of trained nurses to the Zulu War in South Africa, the first time that trained army nurses had served overseas. By 1883, the War Office had sent trained female nurses to serve in other military hospitals at Cambridge, Devonport, and Malta. Deeble, who retired in 1889, is regarded as having laid the foundation for the Queen Alexandra Royal Army Nursing Service.

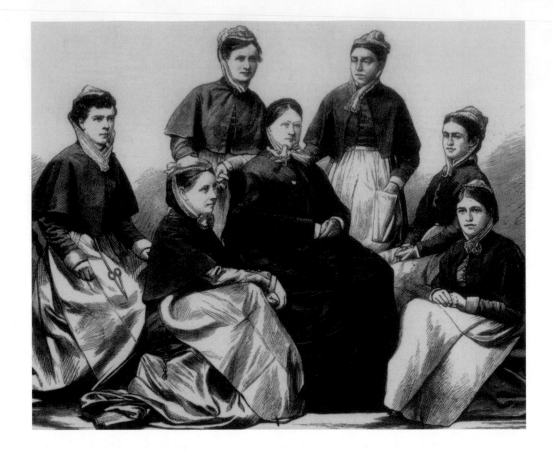

Nightingale was also contacted to help rescue the Army Medical School, which had moved to Netley in 1863 and was being threatened with peacetime budget cuts in 1876. Nightingale persuaded the Nightingale Fund Council to intervene; letters and meetings were held and the Army Medical School was spared. By 1877, the War Office became responsible for army nurse training and the Nightingale Fund was no longer involved.

Nightingale was never successful in implementing the type of military nursing service she proposed in her 1858 *Subsidiary Notes as to the Introduction of Female Nursing into Military Hospitals in Peacetime,* but her efforts weren't wasted. Her ideas for necessary reform eventually became a reality in World War I; the matron-in-chief was responsible directly to the War Office and all nurses were first trained in civilian hospitals before entering military nursing.

Midwifery nursing

At the beginning of the 19th century, childbirth was seen as a natural, female-focused, home-based event. Lay midwives delivered most of the babies in rural England as well as in the cities. Older midwives taught apprentices female anatomy, herbal pharmacology (such as ergot to stop bleeding after childbirth), and general care of the mother and baby during and after the birthing process.

In the early 1800s, London had eight lying-in (maternity) hospitals, which were used primarily to teach medical students; these hospitals were used only by charity cases because wealthy Victorian women delivered their babies at home. Obstetrics developed apart from mainstream medicine in the 1800s; it was considered a separate profession that required a separate apprenticeship. Lectures in midwifery weren't part of the medical curriculum until the 1850s.

By the mid-1850s, the development of new instruments (such as forceps), increased demand for painless childbirth using chloroform, and an increase in the number of lying-in hospitals had led to the "medicalization" of childbirth. Childbirth came to be seen not as a natural process but as a pathologic condition that required medical intervention with forceps, chloroform, and pain medications. In the large cities, physician accoucheurs (doctors specializing in childbirth) began to replace midwives after the licensing act gave them control of drugs, primarily chloroform.

Puerperal fever: A national health problem

The increased use of chloroform during childbirth, which required hospital admission, led to a huge increase in the number of cases of puerperal fever (childbirth fever) and, consequently, in the mortality rate associated with childbirth. Because the germ theory still was not understood, medical students often came to deliver babies directly from the dissection wards, without washing their hands or changing their aprons. Although the use of chlorine washing was known to decrease the incidence of puerperal fever as early as 1822, doctors refused to believe that they could be carriers of infection.

The medical evidence that puerperal fever was spread by doctors' hands was first presented in 1843 by Oliver Wendell Holmes in his essay "The Contagiousness of Puerperal Fever," now considered a medical classic. Holmes asserted that physicians who had conducted postmortem dissections or treated women with puerperal fever should not take care of women about to give birth. The next person to link high maternal mortality rates with doctors' careless sanitary practices was Ignaz Semmelweis, assistant director of the Lying-in Clinic of Vienna. In 1847-1848, Semmelweis noticed that maternal death rates were highest on wards where medical students practiced, and he attributed this to the students' going from the dissection table to the delivery ward without washing their hands. In his classic treatise *The Cause, Concept, and Prophylaxis of Childbirth Fever,* not published until 1861, he showed that the maternal death rate dropped from 10% to 1% when doctors washed their hands before delivering children.

In the 1860s and 1870s, Holmes and Semmelweis's theories were still widely criticized by the medical establishment and the high mortality rate associated with childbirth continued to be a major health problem in England. Even when Louis Pasteur finally identified the streptococcus organism that caused puerperal fever in 1879, routine hand washing still wasn't widely accepted. In 1883, Joseph Lister acknowledged Semmelweis's work as a forerunner of his own theory of antisepsis.

Midwife training program

Florence Nightingale never considered childbirth a pathologic condition requiring medical care. She believed that properly trained midwives could deal with even difficult deliveries but that they first required formal instruction. Unfortunately, midwifery in England was subsumed under medicine, not nursing, until the early 1900s.

In 1861, Nightingale decided to set up a new branch of her nurse's training school that would instruct women from parishes to become trained midwives. Her intent was to offer proper childbirth services to poor people in rural areas, where trained midwives were sorely needed, and to create a prototype national midwifery training program that would ultimately become a responsibility of the government. The Nightingale Fund Committee arranged with the authorities at St. John's House, an Anglican sisterhood, to set up the program at King's College Hospital.

The midwifery training program opened in October 1862 with Nightingale's friend Mary Jones, an experienced midwife, as superintendent. Jones, the spiritual head of St. John's House (an Anglican sisterhood) and the superintendent of nurses at King's College Hospital, had sent six nurses to serve under Nightingale during the Crimean War, and Nightingale considered her the best teacher of moral character that she knew.

The probationers would have no obligations to the Nightingale Fund Council after their training, but they were asked to sign a contract with their parish stating that they would return to serve the rural poor for 4 years. The parish would pay them £20 a year and provide adequate housing if their services were satisfactory. If the midwife married or failed to fulfill her 4-year term, she would have to pay a penalty of £40 less £5 for every completed year of the contract.

The midwifery probationers were to follow the rules of St. John's House. The Nightingale Fund agreed to pay the hospital £500 a year for total training expenses and to furnish and maintain 10 lying-in beds on this ward. Healthy women ages 26 to 35 of good character would undergo a 6-month training program, Nightingale explained in a letter to Harriet Martineau in September 1861. The Fund would pay each probationer £12 to help with the boarding cost, and each probationer would pay 8 to 9 shillings to complete the cost of boarding.[25] The physician-accoucheurs agreed to teach the probationers for free in the lying-in ward.

In 1863, Nightingale published the third edition of *Notes on Hospitals* with a short appendix called "Notes on Different Systems of Nursing," which she later published separately as a short pamphlet. In this publication, she reviewed the different types of sisterhoods that had been set up specifically for nursing. Most were linked to the Anglican Church, such as St. John's House. She particularly praised St. John's, where nurses were under their own spiritual head and under a separate secular governing body. However, after the religious problems that later developed at King's College Hospital, she changed her mind about sisterhoods.

More religious controversies

In 1866, Mary Jones decided that, in addition to being superintendent, she should also be the spiritual head of nurses at King's College Hospital, instead of the chaplain. She wanted to establish an altar and have the sacraments displayed; if she couldn't have her way, she threatened to take her Sisters elsewhere. Around this time, Nightingale learned that Jones was secretly a Roman Catholic. Many Anglicans were converting to Catholicism, and both groups were very suspicious of each other. Nightingale was extremely distressed by these events and thought that Jones was acting irrationally.

The next year Jones and her Sisters resigned from St. John's House to set up their own private program. With no qualified replacements to take Jones's place, Nightingale withdrew the Nightingale Fund's support from the program. In February 1868, the Midwifery Training Program was officially closed; the official reason given was the high death rate from puerperal fever — 20 out of 781 deliveries (or 25.6 deaths per 1,000) — but the death rate in other hospitals was higher. Although Nightingale and Jones remained friends and continued to consult each other about the training of nurses, this incident convinced Nightingale to never again become involved with hospitals affiliated with religious orders.

Introductory Notes on Lying-in Institutions

Because of the high death rate from puerperal fever in the midwifery training program and throughout England and Europe, Nightingale published *Introductory Notes on Lying-in Institutions* in October 1871. This book contained the results of her statistical analysis on the causes of death in home deliveries and lying-in hospitals, and provided suggestions for improving the construction and management of these facilities. She dedicated the book to Socrates's mother, who had been a midwife.

Nightingale's 110-page book is a remarkable work in applied statistics that filled an important gap in medical knowledge in the 1870s. Midwifery statistics at this time were still in their infancy. Lying-in institutions kept some records, but standard mortality data on childbirth-related deaths were virtually nonexistent in Britain. Nightingale pulled together the best data of the time on childbirth, synthesized it, and then drew her conclusions from it.

The *Introductory Notes* contain a detailed classification of causes of mortality in home deliveries and lying-in facilities as well as "secondary influences" that affected mortality: the mother's age, number of pregnancies, duration of labor, the state of delivery (for example, short or difficult), her general state of health before the delivery, social class, the general conditions of the place of delivery, and the amount of time in the midwifery wards before and after delivery.

Nightingale had expected to find that women who delivered in workhouses had a higher death rate — because of poverty and poor health — than those who delivered in lying-in institutions, but her data showed the opposite; the death rate for women who were delivered by physician-accoucheurs or medical students in lying-in wards was higher. She concluded that the cause was the accoucheurs' and students' failure to take basic sanitary precautions. Based on these findings, Nightingale advocated banning medical students from delivery rooms and closing all lying-in wards connected to hospitals to prevent the spread of infection.

Nightingale was also astonished to discover that home deliveries by accoucheurs resulted in 1 death per 128 deliveries (almost 8 deaths per 1,000), compared to 2.17 deaths per 1,000 for home deliveries by midwives. She wrote:

> ... *One feels disposed to ask whether it can be true that, in the hands of educated accoucheurs, the inevitable fate of women undergoing, not a disease but an entirely natural condition, at home, is that one out of every 128 die?*[26]

Most of the book focuses on personal and ward hygienic procedures. Even though the germ theory of disease was still unproven, Nightingale had always been aware of the importance of institutional and personal cleanliness. Based on simple common sense and good sanitary principles, she created a standard for hand washing in *Notes on Nursing*:

> *Every nurse ought to be careful to wash her hands very frequently during the day ... Compare the dirtiness of the water in which you have washed when it is cold without soap, cold with soap, and hot with soap. You will find that the first hardly removed any dirt at all, the second a little more, the third a great deal more ... that by simply washing or sponging with water you do not really clean your skin. Take a rough towel, dip one corner in very hot water, — if a little spirit be added to it will be more effectual, — and then rub as if you were rubbing the towel into your skin with your fingers. The black flakes which will come off will convince you that you were not clean before, however much soap and water you have used ...*[27]

Nightingale's plans for improving the construction and management of lying-in wards included the use of small, separate delivery rooms to lower the high mortality rate and the installation of more sinks than other hospital wards. She also provided detailed instructions for the mother's and baby's baths as well as for the cleaning of bed linen, beds, ward furniture, floors, and walls.

Introductory Notes was a major contribution to the understanding of childbirth and its risks. She summed up her beliefs in the following words:

> *In short, the entire result of this enquiry may be summed up, in a very few words, as follows: — A woman in ordinary health, and subject to the ordinary social conditions of her station, will not, if delivered at home, be exposed to any special disadvantages likely to diminish materially her chance of recovery. But this same woman, if received into an ordinary lying-in ward, together with others in the puerperal state, will from that very fact become subject to risks not necessarily incident to this state. These risks in lying-in institutions may no doubt be materially diminished by providing proper hospital accommodations, and by care, common sense, and good management. And hence the real practical question is, whether it is possible to ensure at all times the observance of these conditions.*[28]

Dispute over licensure of midwives

To meet the growing demand for trained midwives, the Obstetrical Society, formed in 1862, proposed the establishment of a licensing system to regulate midwifery. The society proposed to offer examinations four times a year that would cover female pelvic anatomy, mechanisms and management of the birthing process, recognition of abnormalities, how to handle emergencies, and how to work with doctors. To be eligible for the examination, the midwife would have to document attendance at 25 supervised deliveries and present evidence of good moral character. After successful completion of this process, she would receive a diploma stating that she was a skilled and competent midwife capable of performing a normal delivery.

Nightingale was opposed to this plan because it didn't require a formal midwifery training program based on uniform standards that included moral training. She felt

The following table gives the actual facts and dates:—

Midwifery Statistics, King's College Hospital.

Year	Total Deliveries	Fatal Cases				Deaths to Labours
		Date of Birth	Nature of Labour	Cause of Death	Date of Death	
1862	97	Nov. 6	Natural	Puerperal peritonitis	Nov. 25	
		,, 30	Twins	Phthisis and puerperal fever	Dec. 27	1 in 22·3
		Dec. 10	Natural	Puerperal peritonitis	Dec. 20	
1863	105	Jan. 10	Natural. Child still-born	Puerperal fever	Jan. 16	1 in 32·5
		April 29	Natural	Puerperal fever	May 20	
1864	141	Feb. 16	Natural	Puerperal fever	Feb. 25	
		April 14	Induced	Pyæmia	April 29	1 in 47
		Dec. 1	Born in cab	Hæmorrhage	Dec. 7	
1865	163	Jan. 30	Natural	Embolism	Feb. 12	
		Feb. 8	Natural	Puerperal fever	Feb. 18	
		June 24	Forceps	Puerperal metritis and pelvis cellulitis	July 30	1 in 32·6
		Oct. 20	Forceps	Laceration of perinæum, puerperal fever	Nov. 3	
		Oct. 29	Natural	Puerperal fever	Nov. 9	
1866	150	Jan. 10	Natural	Gastro-enteritis	Jan. 20	
		Mar. 24	Natural	Retained placenta, puerperal fever	April 10	
		Oct. 8	Placenta prævia. Turning	Emphysema and bronchitis	Oct. 10	1 in 30
		Nov. 10	Forceps	Peritonitis	Nov. 15	
		Dec. 4	Natural	Puerperal fever	Dec. 31	
1867	125	Jan. 10	(Had erysipelas when admitted*)	Puerperal fever	Jan. 30	
		Feb. 7	Natural	Considerable hæmorrhage, puerperal fever	Feb. 22	
		,, 8	Natural	Puerperal fever	Feb. 22	
		April 12	Turning	Puerperal fever	April 22	
		May 18	Natural	Pyæmia	May 27	1 in 13·8
		June 4	Natural	Puerperal fever	June 19	
		July 26	Natural	Puerperal fever	Aug. 11	
		Nov. 5	Twins: 1st dead, 2nd by turning	Puerperal fever	Nov. 10	
		,, 8	Forceps	Laceration of vagina, puerperal fever	Nov. 14	
Total	781	—	—	—	deaths: 27	1 in 28·9

* 'So was confined in No. 4 ward.'

TABLE XVI.—Proposed Registry of Midwifery Cases.

Column headings (form fields): Name | Age | Residence | Married or Single | No. of Pregnancy | Date when last Child was Born | Date of Admission | Period of Gestation | Date of Commencement of Labour | Duration of Labour, in hours | Nature of Delivery | Presentations | Complications of Delivery | Operation, if any | Accidents or Diseases, if any, after Delivery (Nature of Accident or Disease | Date of Attack | Duration | Result and Date) | Births: Single, Twins, or Triplets | Infant Born Living or Dead | Sex of Child | If Infant Dead after Birth, Cause of Death, and Date | Date of Removal from Lying-in Department | No. of Days in Lying-in Department | Date of Discharge from Institution | Remarks

NOTE.—Should any death take place in a woman discharged from the institution within a month from the time of her delivery, a record of this death, its date, and cause, to be entered in the column of Remarks. In the same column should be entered remarks on abnormal conformation, or on abnormal conditions of health which might influence the result of the delivery.

that documenting attendance at 25 deliveries was insufficient to prove that a woman was properly trained and that passing an examination would demonstrate only minimal competence and show nothing about moral character.

Her friend Dr. Henry Acland, a member of the General Medical Council, contacted Nightingale about granting certificates to various disciplines connected with medicine and midwifery, later called paraprofessionals. However, Nightingale saw midwifery as a part of nursing — not medicine. She was firm in her opinion that the nursing profession shouldn't get mixed up with the medical profession. Her reply to Acland was right to the point:

> ... Experience teaches me that nursing and medicine must never be mixed up. It spoils both ... if I were not afraid of being misunderstood I would say that the lesser knowledge of medicine that the hospital matron has the better (1) because it does not improve her sanitary practice, (2) because it would make her miserable and intolerable to doctors.[29]

LEFT: *Some of the midwifery statistics from King's College Hospital that Nightingale compiled and used in her Introductory Notes on Lying-in Institutions*

RIGHT: *Proposed Registry of Midwifery Cases (upside-down, as it appeared originally), which Nightingale hoped would encourage midwives to record significant observations*

Despite Nightingale's objections, the Obstetrical Society began a registry of midwives in 1873. Nightingale's 1861 Midwifery Training Program eventually became a prototype for a government training program. Although there were many dissenting voices, particularly those of male obstetricians, the Midwives Act of 1902 secured a place for trained and licensed female midwives who delivered infants in homes and lying-in hospitals and provided well-baby care.

Nightingale nurses abroad

As word of the Nightingale School spread, numerous requests were made for more information on the training program as well as on the availability of nurses to be sent to hospitals throughout the Empire. There weren't enough trained nurses or superintendents to send to all of the countries that made inquiries, but Australia and Canada did receive nursing contingents.

Australia

When Sir Henry Parkes, the colonial secretary of New South Wales, Australia, wrote to the Nightingale Fund in 1866 requesting that nurses be sent to Sydney, Nightingale felt obligated to respond since so many Australians had contributed to the Nightingale Fund. Lucy Osburn, a distant cousin of Nightingale's who had nursed in Holland, Kaiserswerth, Jerusalem, and Vienna, applied for the position of superintendent of nurses.

In December 1867, after briefly training at several workhouse infirmaries at her own expense, Osburn sailed to Sydney with five nurses chosen by Mrs. Wardroper; Nightingale provided them with textbooks and supplies for the long journey. According to the terms of her 3-year contract, Osburn was to be paid £150 as superintendent and each of the nurses was to receive £50, which included room and board. If the 3-year contract was successfully completed, a return fare to London would also be paid.

Upon arriving at Sydney Hospital, Osburn immediately encountered problems with the doctors and lay administrators. The terms of the superintendency had been clearly defined by the Nightingale Fund. The superintendent was to be directly responsible to the medical officer for all patients' medical treatments but directly responsible to the hospital board of governors for such matters as diets, cleanliness, and ventilation. She was to have total responsibility for any women engaged as nurses, and male nurses were to be discontinued.

The doctors and lay administrators objected to the new superintendent's power because former matrons had been totally subordinate to them, making no decisions on their own. In addition, as in the Midwifery Training Program, a controversy with religious overtones arose when Osburn tried to have her title changed to "Lady Superior" and the head nurses to "Sisters," changes that the staff immediately perceived as a Roman Catholic plot.

Shortly after Osburn's arrival, Queen Victoria's son Alfred, Duke of Edinburgh, was wounded in an assassination attempt while visiting New South Wales. The queen

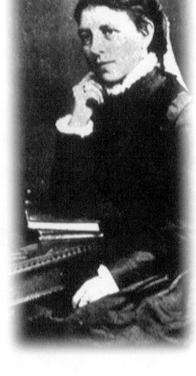

Lucy Osburn, Superintendent of Nurses at Sydney Hospital, who is considered the founder of the Sydney Nurse Training School

later wrote a letter of thanks to the nurses for their excellent care of her son. When Osburn's uncle in London had the queen's letter privately printed for circulation, Nightingale and the Nightingale Fund Committee were shocked. Osburn offered to resign her post, but the letter was suppressed and she withdrew her resignation. However, Nightingale never trusted Osburn after this incident.

Osburn stayed on as superintendent at Sydney Hospital for another 25 years and is considered the founder of the Sydney Nurse Training School. Of the five nurses who accompanied her, one finished her contract and returned to Edinburgh, where she had a successful nursing career; another married; and the other three were dismissed. Osburn never requested more nurses from the Nightingale Fund.

Canada

The Nightingale Fund sent a second team of nurses abroad in 1874, this time to Canada. The administrators of the Montreal General Hospital wanted to begin a training program for nurses similar to the one at St. Thomas's. Unknown to Nightingale, they had already made arrangements for a 32-year old native of Quebec, Maria Machin, to become their new superintendent. The administrators appealed to the fund for four trained nurses to accompany Machin.

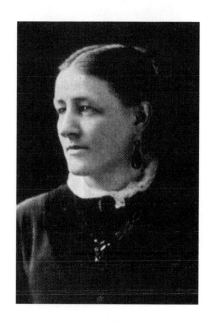

Maria Machin, a Nightingale-trained nurse, who became superintendent at Montreal General Hospital

Machin, a Nightingale-trained nurse, had a rough start during her first winter in Montreal. Of the four Nightingale nurses who were sent to Canada, only one was a good nurse; one died of typhoid, one married, and the fourth had too little education and couldn't cope. Of the two replacements sent from England, one developed typhoid and the second couldn't conform to the discipline.

In 1877, Machin asked Mrs. Wardroper at St. Thomas's to send two better-qualified nurses to replace the last two, offering to cover their travel expenses. Machin wrote that she was moving forward with her plans for the training program, but this never happened. In the meantime, she became secretly engaged to a doctor at the hospital.

Although she was criticized by the board of governors for incurring unnecessary costs and for failing to start the formal training program as stated in her contract, Machin's tenure was successful on the whole. The medical staff was pleased with the increased quality of the nursing service under her leadership. However, after Machin's fiancé died of diphtheria in September 1877, she returned to England and became superintendent at St. Bartholomew's Hospital. In 1885, Machin and Rachel Williams were sent to serve in the Egyptian campaign. Machin later married and moved to South Africa where she nursed during the Boer War and helped established a hospital at Bloemfontein.

The shortage of trained probationers limited the Nightingale Fund's ability to send nurses abroad. In its first 20 years, the fund sent only two Nightingale nurses — Osburn and Machin — abroad to serve as superintendents. By the 1900s, the Fund made no more attempts to send nurses abroad because there were other organizations — such as the Indian Nursing Service and the Colonial Nursing Service — who could meet nursing needs abroad.

Advances in women's rights

Florence Nightingale was a feminist long before the word was coined. All her youthful struggles had stemmed from the need to free herself from the imprisonment of upper-class domestic life and find a meaningful vocation. Her singular example in the Crimea and the founding of the Nightingale School for Nurses forever shattered the old myths of helpless women and helped foster the new paradigm in which women began to organize and agitate for their rights.

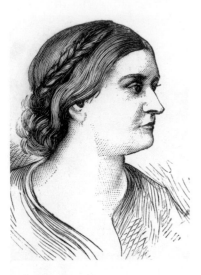

Nightingale's cousin Barbara Smith Bodichon, who was an early activist in the women's rights movement

When women's suffrage became the subject of public debate in the mid-1860s, it was only one of many rights and privileges that women hadn't yet obtained, such as the right to own property, to obtain a divorce for the same reasons as a husband, to obtain a college education, to attend medical school and become a licensed doctor, and to obtain better jobs and wages. The right of women to vote was much more than another political issue; it represented radical social change. In 1865, only 1 person in 22 had the right to vote, all of them men. Even of the men, only those who owned property of a certain minimum value qualified for the ballot. This amounted to 1 in 10 men.

The women's suffrage movement was not one of Nightingale's top priorities. She was more interested in improving economic conditions and believed that providing greater opportunities for education and meaningful employment was a better path to improving the lot of women. Coincidentally, though, two of the most active advocates in the early fight for women's rights had connections to Nightingale. One was her own first cousin, Barbara Leigh Smith (later Bodichon), the daughter of Fanny's shunned brother Benjamin Smith. The other was the philosopher John Stuart Mill, who had critiqued Nightingale's *Suggestions for Thought* in 1860.

Right to own property

From a legal standpoint, a married woman in England in the mid-1800s was the property of her husband. Her children, possessions, earnings, liberty, and even her conscience legally belonged to her husband. Sir William Blackstone, the English legal authority, summed it up in his famous dictum: "My wife and I are one, and I am he."[30] Her only escape from marriage was death.[31]

In 1855, just as Nightingale was becoming a household name throughout Britain, Barbara Smith wrote and published a pamphlet called "A Brief Summary in Plain Language of the Most Important Laws Concerning Women," which argued that the most important issue for women was not the right to vote but the right to make wills and own property.[32] To change the laws, public meetings were held and committees were organized. By 1856, 26,000 signatures of men and women had been gathered.

The Married Women's Property Bill was introduced in Parliament in May 1857 but was co-opted by government-sponsored legislation that provided only minuscule advances. The opposition to any such rights for women was summed up by the *Saturday Review*, which editorialized that such proposals "set at defiance the common sense of mankind, and would revolutionize society. There is besides a smack of selfish independence about it which rather jars with poetical notions of wedlock."[33]

The committee work for the unsuccessful Married Women's Property Bill had brought together a new generation of activists who, led by Barbara Bodichon, in 1857 took offices in Langham Place and started the *Englishwoman's Journal*. The "Langham Place Circle," as it became known, was the midwife of the women's movement. For the first time, women — rich or poor, married or unmarried, titled or commoner, rural or urban — had a place to come for help and networking. Soon there was a Women's Employment Bureau, a Lady's Institute, the Educated Women's Emigration Society, a Society of Female Artists, and the Victoria Press. Whether it was the push for higher education, classes for bookkeepers, or monitoring the divorce courts, everything was reported in the *Englishwoman's Journal*, and the new ideas spread swiftly through English society. The full Married Women's Property Bill was finally passed in 1882.

The vote

When John Stuart Mill was invited to stand for Parliament from Westminster in 1865, he placed the vote for women among his top priorities and helped raise the debate to a new level. Mill's earlier works on political and legal reform, such as *On Liberty* (1859) and *Considerations on Representative Government* (1861), brought weight and credibility to the issues of women's suffrage, parliamentary reform, and proportional representation.

In *The Subjection of Women*, begun in 1861 but not published until 8 years later, he considered the full range of political and human consequences caused by the submission of women. He wrote that "we have had the morality of submission, and that of chivalry; but the time is now come for the morality of justice."[34] One of his arguments borrowed directly from Nightingale's essay "Cassandra":

> ... If he [a man] has a pursuit, he offends nobody by devoting his time to it; occupation is received as a valid excuse for his not answering to every casual demand which may be made on him ... [A woman] must always be at the beck and call of somebody, generally of everybody. If she has a study or a pursuit, she must snatch any short interval which accidentally occurs to be employed in it. A celebrated woman in a work which I hope will some day be published [Nightingale's Suggestions for Thought] remarks truly that everything a woman does is done at odd times. Is it wonderful, then, if she does not attain the highest eminence in things which require consecutive attention, and the concentration on them of the chief interest of life.[35]

When the petition from the first Women's Suffrage Committee, organized by Bodichon, was carried to Westminster Hall in June 1866, it marked the beginning of over a half-century of struggle until English women would fully gain the vote (in 1918). Although Nightingale's signature was at the top of the list of some 1,500 names, along with those of Harriet Martineau and Mary Somerville, she didn't become an activist in this campaign for several reasons. The most important reasons were that she was a 45-year old invalid; her areas of expertise were nursing, sanitation, and hospital and medical reform; and her great talent was administrative politics, not electoral politics, which required a different set of skills and motivation.

The issue of the women's vote raised fierce resistance among many men who were open to change in other areas, such as education and professional careers. Nightingale

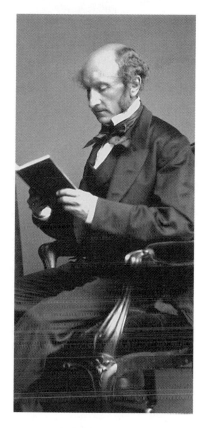

Distinguished philosopher John Stuart Mill, a strong supporter of the women's rights movement in the 1860s

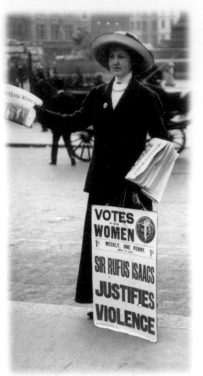

English activist selling the newspaper Votes for Women *at the height of the militant suffragette campaign in 1912, 6 years before women obtained the vote*

understood the deep resistance to fundamental social change and correctly foresaw that it would be years before women obtained the vote. When Mill asked her to serve on the board of the National Society for Woman's Suffrage in 1867, her reply reflected her practical attitudes toward women's rights:

> *That women should have the suffrage, I think no one can be more deeply convinced than I ... But it will probably be years before you obtain the suffrage for women. And, in the mean time, are there not evils which press much more hardly on women than not having a vote? And may not this [the vote], when obtained, put women in opposition to those who withhold from them these rights, so as to retard still farther the legislation necessary to put them in possession of their rights? I do not know. I ask the question very humbly and I am afraid you will laugh at me.*
>
> *Could not the existing disabilities as to property and influence of women be swept away by the legislature as it stands at present? — and equal rights and equal responsibilities be given as they ought to be, to both men and women? I do not like to take up your time with giving instances, redressible by legislation, in which women, especially married poor women with children, are most hardly pressed upon now. I have been a matron on a large scale the greater part of my life, and no matron with the smallest care for her nurses can be unaware of what I mean e.g. till a married woman can possess property there can be no love and no justice.*
>
> *Is it not possible that, if woman-suffrage is agitated as a means of removing these evils, the effect may be to prolong their existence? Is it not the case that at present there is no opposition between the two elements of the nation — but that, if both had equal political powers, there is a probability that the social reforms needed might become matter for political partizanship — and so the weaker go to the wall? I do not know. I only ask and very humbly ...*
>
> *I have been too busy for the last fourteen years ... to wish for a vote — to want personal political influence. Indeed I have had, during the 11 years I have been in Gov't offices, more administrative influence than if I had been a Borough returning two M.P.s ... I have not time to serve on the society you mention, otherwise, there is scarcely anything which, if you were to tell me that it is right to do politically, I would not do. But I could not give my name without my work. This is only personal (I am an incurable invalid.) I entirely agree that women's "political power" should be "direct and open." But I have thought that I could work better for others, even for other women, off the stage than on it.[36]*

Despite her preference for anonymity, Nightingale joined the National Society for Woman's Suffrage in 1868 and allowed her name to be placed on the General Committee in 1871. She subscribed annually to the Society Fund. In 1878, the Society's publication printed the following statement by her:

> *... It seems a first principle, an axiom; that every householder or taxpayer should have a voice in electing those who spend the money we pay, including as this does, interests the most vital to a human being — for instance, education. At the same time I do not expect much from it, for I do not see that, for instance in America, where suffrage is, I suppose, the most extended, there is more (but rather less) of what may truly be called freedom or progress than anywhere else. But there can be no freedom or progress without representation. And we must give women true education to deserve being represented. Men as well as women are not so well endowed with that preparation at present. And if the persons represented are not worth much, of course the representatives will not be worth much.[37]*

Medical education

Barbara Bodichon was instrumental in opening the door to medical education for women when she invited Dr. Elizabeth Blackwell, the first woman medical doctor in the United States, to deliver a series of lectures in England in 1859. Blackwell, a friend of both Bodichon and Nightingale, became the first woman to have her name placed on the British Medical Register in 1859, although holders of foreign degrees were excluded the following year.

One of those attending the first lecture in London in March 1859 was Elizabeth Garrett, who worked with Bodichon in the women's movement. After being turned down for admission to various medical schools, she trained as a nurse at Middlesex Hospital in 1860 and then discovered a loophole in the Society of Apothecaries charter. She gained her apothecaries' license in 1865 and opened a small dispensary for women and children. (An apothecary in the mid-19th century was a general practitioner.) In 1869, she became the first English woman to obtain a medical degree in England and have her name placed on the British Medical Register. Others tried to follow in Garrett's footsteps, but in 1867 the authorities closed the loophole that had allowed her to obtain an apothecaries' license.

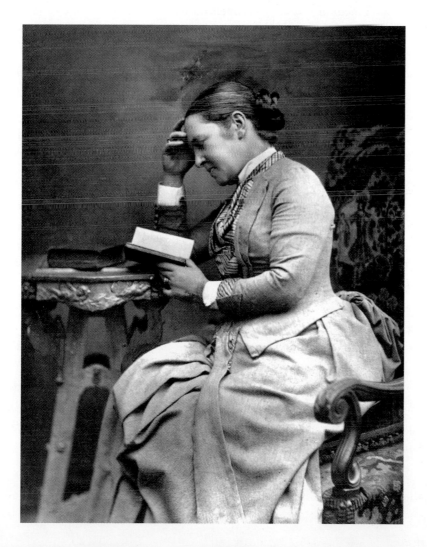

Elizabeth Garrett (later Anderson), the first English woman to obtain a medical degree in England and to be listed in the British Medical Register in 1869

One of the other pioneers in women's medical education in Britain was Sophia Jex-Blake. While in Boston studying education, she met Dr. Lucy Sewell, one of Elizabeth Blackwell's protégées, and decided to become a doctor. She returned to England in 1868, determined to carry out her plan. She finally gained admittance, along with five other women, to the University of Edinburgh for a special course in medical instruction in 1869. Over the next 3 years, however, resistance to the women increased and, in 1872, the University refused to graduate them, offering instead "certificates of proficiency" which wouldn't qualify them for the Medical Register or for practice.[38]

Undaunted, Jex-Blake returned to London and found a few sympathetic professors at the teaching hospitals who were willing to give lectures to women medical students. In 1874, she opened the London School of Medicine for Women. Elizabeth Garrett Anderson, by then married, joined the staff for the first round of fall classes, and Elizabeth Blackwell soon became professor of gynecology. In 1877, the school reached an agreement with a cooperating hospital and was able to offer clinical training.

In 1876, Parliament passed the enabling act allowing universities to examine and accredit women. Although the University of Edinburgh still refused to cooperate, Jex-Blake secured certification from the Irish College of Physicians in 1877 and had her name put on the British Medical Register. The barriers had at last been broken down, and other medical schools soon opened their doors to women. By 1881 there were 21 registered women doctors in England, and by 1895, there were 264.[39]

Nightingale didn't initially approve of women becoming doctors for several reasons: She thought there was a greater need for women to go into nursing; she thought that women were more concerned with acquiring a doctor's license than a good medical education; and she considered the "Medical ladies" she had met as arrogant as the male doctors. She summed up her opinions, including her differences with Garrett, in a letter to Sir Harry Verney in April 1867:

> 1. She [Garrett] starts on the ground that the summum bonum for women is to be able to obtain the same Licence or Diploma as men for medical practice. Now I start from exactly the opposite ground. Medical education is about as bad as it possibly can be. It makes men prigs [arrogant]. It prevents any wise, any philosophical, any practical view of health & disease. Only a few geniuses rise above it. It makes a man a prig, it will make a woman a prig-ger ...
>
> It is quite true that every Oculist, Dentist, Accoucheur, practises much better for having had a general Medical education. But Miss Garrett does not say this. She does not say: how can we give women the best general Medical education? She says — how can we satisfy the "Examining Boards"? Now — every old fogey, like me, knows that ... what makes a man pass is memory ... that "Examining Boards" are just so many charlatans ...
>
> The great error of these Medical ladies appear to me to be: that they not only put the cart before the horse, but that they expect the cart to drag the horse. How is a woman to get a man's Diploma? — that is all they ask. It is just the same as if I, instead of qualifying myself to assist Sidney Herbert in the War Office, had bent all my energies to: how is a woman to become a Secretary of State?[40]

Nightingale felt that women who wished to become doctors should concentrate on midwifery or diseases specific to women or children and not try to compete with men.

In the same letter, she lauded the Parisian model of midwifery training, which was superior to the English system even though it didn't offer a specific license:

> How do people in Paris do these things? for 50 years there has been a succession of Lady Professors at the Maternité, who rank … much higher than Simpson [eminent obstetrician] or Locock [first physician-accoucheur to the queen] here. Their works are quoted as authorities all over Europe … There is no struggle with the men-Doctors. How have they done all this? Not certainly by trying for men's Diplomas — not by a paper war, not by struggling to get into men's colleges. Simply by working a female School on female Patients to perfection & letting all controversy alone.
>
> But then … an "eleve sage-femme" [student midwife] cannot be certified under 2 years, instead of in one month, as in England … The [second year] eleves sage-femmes are made to help in training the [first year] eleves sages-femmes. No Medical School of men ever known is anything to be compared to its perfection in point of instruction, both practical & scientific. And all this they have done — how? Not by aping a man's Medical School. Just the reverse. By simply doing the very best to form good Midwives & not thinking about men at all.
>
> … If I were forming a Female Medical School in England, I should just cut the Gordian knot at once, & avoid all collision with men, by beginning as closely as possible on the Parisian model, & then afterwards, if you extend it to all diseases of women & children, so much the better — or even to a more general education still.
>
> … As long as Medical ladies go on in England in this way, I have no hope. One sensible woman, like Miss Garrett, may now & then win her way to practice. But even she is as senseless as the others about Female Medical Schools. Let women begin by that branch of the Profession (Midwifery) which is undoubtedly theirs. Let them do it as well as possible — let them conquer their place in it — instead of, as now, as it seems to me, lady Doctors affecting to despise it. All the rest will follow. But none of the rest will follow, if their only aim is to be to extort from men a man's place.[11]

By the mid-1870s, when the first women's medical college had been established, and the politics of admittance, examinations, licensure, and certification were beginning to be the same for women as for men, Nightingale took a modern view:

> But whether this idea [that women should enter medicine] be right or wrong, shall we not do more harm than good in shutting out women? Let them try: Once we have "free trade" supply and demand will, will they not, adjust themselves: it will be seen by the simple test of utility, of profit and loss, whether women doctors can get practice and deserve practice.
>
> Fortunately for them they cannot make us legislate that the Public shall employ women Doctors: any more than we can legislate that the Public shall employ men-Doctors from what we think are the best schools. Give us free trade: & let the Public decide.[42]

So drastically did Nightingale eventually change her stance on women doctors that in her later years she was cared for by a woman doctor. By the end of the decade, several more milestones in women's education had been achieved. In 1878, the University of London admitted women for the first time and Oxford allowed women to attend lectures.

Nightingale was a role model for the women's movement. She didn't compromise her stance and worked behind the scenes in the way that made the most sense to her.

Her major contributions to this movement were in political theory, social criticism, administrative reform of the Poor Law, applied statistics, and particularly in midwifery, all of which are part of her enduring legacy. Women were major players with her on all of these issues.

The army and prostitution

In the early 1860s, another issue was to unite many women in Britain — opposition to government regulation of prostitution. Ever since the Crimean War, Nightingale had given much thought to the problem of venereal disease in the army. In July 1862, officials were debating a number of proposals dealing with "regulation of vices" (venereal disease).

Nightingale's colleague Edwin Chadwick, the sanitary reformer, was among those advocating that Britain adopt the French method of containing venereal disease in the army, which was known as the Continental system. This system required known or suspected prostitutes to undergo a painful compulsory internal physical examination to determine if they had a venereal disease; those who did were placed in a locked hospital ward for treatment. The proposed British legislation was known as the Contagious Disease Act.

Nightingale, Harriet Martineau, and Dr. Elizabeth Blackwell were among those who vehemently opposed the Contagious Disease Act and worked hard to block its passage. Many women believed that the physical examinations were a form of rape — both cruel and unnecessary. For her part, Nightingale believed that the French system was tantamount to state-organized prostitution for the armed forces, which was not only immoral but ineffective in controlling venereal disease. She believed that if the soldiers were offered more healthy outlets during their free time, there would be less prostitution, and thus less venereal disease.

As she had done earlier, Nightingale once again turned to statistics to make her case. She sent her statistics to Sir George Lewis, the Secretary for War, and supplied them to Martineau to use in her *Times* and *Daily News* articles in the hopes of turning public opinion against the Contagious Disease Act. She also printed and circulated a private paper called "Note on the Supposed Protection Afforded against Venereal Disease by Recognizing Prostitution." Dr. John Sutherland was listed as the sole author, but all those who received the paper knew who its real author was.

Despite these efforts, the Contagious Disease Act was passed by the House of Commons in 1864. Nightingale was asked to help with the selection of medical officers who would conduct the physical examinations, but she flatly refused. Having failed to stop the legislation, she now pushed even harder for more diversionary outlets for the soldiers, such as recreation and reading rooms, clubs, and other facilities to stem boredom and isolation. She drew up a list of the appropriate furniture, books, and other supplies and even bought some on her own and shipped them to various regiments. At the request of Lord de Grey, now Secretary for War, she wrote a paper on the subject of employing soldiers in meaningful trades, such as shoe repair, baking bread, and basic carpentry.

Meanwhile, opponents of the act lobbied for its repeal. In December 1869, the *Daily News* printed a petition for repeal signed by 2,000 women, led by Martineau and Nightingale. The act was finally abolished in 1886.

Formation of the Red Cross

The problem of inadequate medical and nursing care for wounded soldiers was not confined to the British in the Crimean War — it existed in most of the world. Inspired by Florence Nightingale's heroic nursing efforts in that war, one man decided to launch a broader humanitarian mission.

Swiss banker and philanthropist Jean Henri Dunant had witnessed the bloody Battle of Solferino, one of the decisive battles in the Italian War of Independence, in 1859. Appalled by the inadequacy of medical care behind the front lines — only two doctors to treat 6,000 wounded and no nursing services whatever — Dunant began a 5-year effort to garner support from the governments of Europe for a new international humanitarian organization that would provide volunteer medical and nursing aid to all wounded soldiers, regardless of nationality. He called this proposed organization the Red Cross.

In August 1864, representatives from 12 governments convened in Geneva to develop the principles of the new organization. A month earlier, Lord de Grey at the British War Office called on Nightingale to help draft position papers that would be presented at the Geneva Convention by the British delegates, Dr. Thomas Longmore and Dr. Rutherford, both noted professors of military surgery at the Army Medical School.

The Treaty of Geneva, signed on August 22 by all 12 representatives, established the neutrality of all soldiers wounded in battle and guaranteed them medical treatment. The organization's international symbol, a simple red cross on a white background (in Muslim countries, a red crescent on a white background) became the emblem of neutrality in time of war, guaranteeing protection for wounded soldiers, hospitals, ambulances, doctors, nurses, and volunteers, both professional and nonprofessional. The guidelines also had provisions allowing volunteers to offer humanitarian aid to either side of a conflict.

Although Nightingale supported the neutrality principle of the Geneva Convention, she objected to the focus on volunteers to care for the sick and wounded. Since the Crimean War, she had looked upon each government as responsible for its own sick, wounded, and injured; she feared that the emphasis on voluntary measures might relax the government's responsibilities. In addition, she doubted that the signing of a document could ultimately guarantee humane treatment and expressed her concerns in a letter to Longmore:

> *... It is like vows: people who keep a vow would do the same without the vow, and if people will not do it without the vow, they will not do it with. England and France will not be more humane to the enemy's wounded for having signed the convention, and the convention will not keep semi-barbarous nations ... from being inhumane ...*[43]

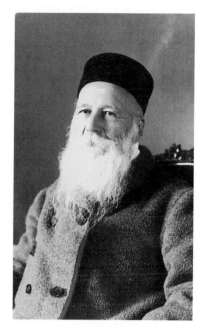

Jean Henri Dunant, Swiss founder of the Red Cross, who credited Nightingale's work in the Crimean War as his inspiration

But Nightingale's political opinions did not stand in the way of her aiding the wounded. During the Franco-Prussian War in 1870-71, she sent nurses to serve on both sides and advised both the French and the Germans about hospital construction, administration, medical aid, technical support, nurses, supplies, and various other details. After the war, both countries recognized her humanitarian contributions; she received the Prussian Cross of Merit from the Emperor and the Bronze Cross from the French Société de Secours aux Blesses.

England did not sign the Treaty of Geneva until 1870. On August 7, 1872, Dunant — in London to deliver a paper — acknowledged his debt to Nightingale:

> Though I am known as the founder of the Red Cross and the originator of the Convention of Geneva, it is to an Englishwoman that all the honour of that Convention is due. What inspired me to go to Italy during the war of 1859 was the work of Miss Florence Nightingale in the Crimea.[44]

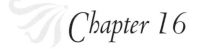

Chapter 16

Spiritual Surrender & Mysticism

*W*here Shall I find God? In myself. That is the true Mystical Doctrine. But then I myself must be in a state for Him to come and dwell in me. This is the whole aim of the Mystical Life, and all Mystical Rules in all times and countries have been laid down for putting the soul into such a state.

— *Florence Nightingale*, Notes from Devotional Authors of the Middle Ages, *1872*[1]

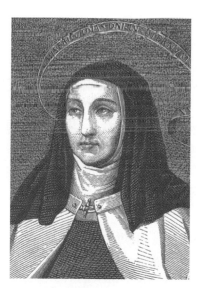

St. Teresa of Avila (1515-1582), Spanish mystic and founder of the Reform Carmelite order, whose life and writings inspired Nightingale

Ever since her Call from God on February 7, 1837, Nightingale had felt that her purpose in life was to serve God. She frequently referred to herself as his handmaid, his missionary, and his coworker. Her mysticism wasn't associated with trances, renunciation of the world, or visions of an afterlife, rather, it was an active and passionate mysticism that focused on creating a better life for mankind here on earth through social action. It was this passion for social action that gave her life meaning.

For Nightingale, the "true doctrine of the Mystics" was "not devotion, but work and suffering for the love of God."[2] She believed that God created man with the ability to achieve perfection and that the way to achieve it was by working to lessen human suffering, a process she called "mankind creating mankind." She also believed that each person had the ability within himself to experience God's presence; individuals didn't require religious rites or the clergy "to draw near to God."

After the deaths of Sidney Herbert and Arthur Clough in 1861, Nightingale had entered the next phase of the mystic's spiritual development, Surrender, also called the "Dark Night of the Soul" or the "Obscure Night." In this move toward a higher level of purification, the mystic learns to detach from the personal satisfaction derived from things of the spirit and to surrender individuality and will completely in preparation for the unitive state. Motivated and energized by Divine Will, the mystic labors arduously toward the perfection of his or her vision.

Surrender often brings with it a period of fatigue and lassitude after a period of sustained mystical activity, and Nightingale's experience was no exception. Driven by her quest to serve God's will, her superhuman labors since the Crimea — compounded by her chronic poor health — had left her exhausted. Because of this, she often felt herself an "utter ship-wreck" and overpowered by a sense of failure. However, her belief in a benevolent God, full of love, goodness, forgiveness, and patience, carried her through this dark period.

By the mid-1860s, the political climate in England was changing and significant reform was taking place. With the deaths of Sidney Herbert and Lord Palmerston, Nightingale's direct links to the highest government offices were broken, except for those involved in India reform. Now, her friendship with Mother Mary Clare Moore of Bermondsey and Professor Benjamin Jowett of Oxford provided emotional and spiritual sustenance as she moved into her own "Dark Night of the Soul."

Reverend Mother & the Dark Night

Nightingale's correspondence with Reverend Mother Mary Clare Moore, her loyal friend from the Crimean period, ranged over discussions of God, their work, and the lives of medieval mystics and saints. Their letters reveal a close friendship between two women who were united by their love of God and their commitment to serve God and mankind. Replying to one of Mother Moore's letters, Nightingale expressed the strong bond they shared as a result of their common nursing background and their experience at Scutari from 1854 to 1856:

> One of the bright jewels in your crown will be your conduct in the Crimean War (to use St. Gertrude's phraseology) ... I always felt you ought to have been the superior and I the inferior and it was not my fault that it was not so — that I always felt how magnanimous your spiritual obedience in accepting such a position — and how utter my incapacity in making it tenable for you — and how I should have failed without your help — that I always wondered at your unfailing patience, sweetness, forbearance, and courage under many trials peculiar to yourselves, beside what was common to all. If I did not express this more, which I always felt, it was because I wondered so much that you could _put up_ with me — that I felt it was no use to say to your face, either then or since, how I admired your ways. As for you having ever shown "temper" to me, I don't like to write the word, I can't conceive what you are thinking of.[3]

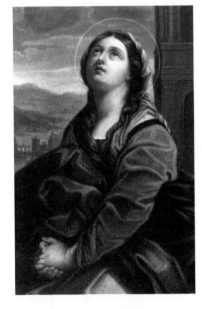

A 16th-century drawing of St. Catherine of Siena, a nurse and mystic of the 14th century with whom Nightingale identified

Many of Nightingale's spiritual guides, who were the subjects of many of her letters to Mother Moore and of books the two women shared, also had been successful leaders in politics and administration. St. Teresa of Avila, who also suffered health problems most of her life, founded the Reform Carmelite order in Spain in 1562 and was a prolific writer of religious treatises. St. Catherine of Genoa, noted for her financial management skills, rose to the post of administrator of the well-known Pammetone Hospital in Genoa and took emergency measures to combat the plague in 1493. The charismatic St. Catherine of Siena, who began nursing at the age of 16, wrote one of the great mystical works in Italian literature, _The Divine Dialogue_, and journeyed to Avignon in 1377 to persuade Pope Gregory XI to return the Holy Church to Rome. In their experiences, Nightingale found a common thread:

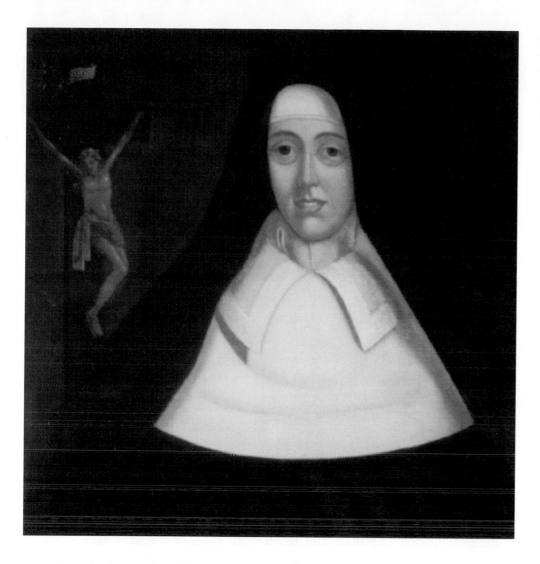

"St. Teresa's strength and that of the whole school of Mystic Ascetics was not in their doctrine of a God ... but in their absolute purity of intention ... their absolute linking of themselves in the idea of service ...[4]

As St. Catherine of Genoa says, when she thinks that "God became man in order to make man into God", I like those words so much ... that belief in perfection ... I often say that prayer of St. Catherine of Siena "I offer and recommend to you my very beloved children, for they are my soul ... to you eternal father, I unworthy, offer again my own life for them ... that when and ever it shall please your goodness, you take me from my body and return me to the body with even greater pain ... provided that I see the reformation of the Holy church." St. Catherine did not see the reformation she desired and I shall not see the reformation of the Army.[5]

When Nightingale received word in December 1863 that Mother Moore was ill, she commiserated with her friend and reflected on her own illness and lack of strength:

To hear of your feverish attacks always makes me uneasy. And I must write to know how you are ... I have all your dear letters. And you cannot think how much they have encouraged me. They are almost the only earthly encouragement I have. I have been so very ill — and even the little change of moving knocks me down for a month. But God is so good as to let me still struggle on with my business.

I return the life of S. Catherine of Genoa. I like it so much. It is a very singular and suggestive life. I am so glad she accepted being Directress of the Hospital ... I am quite ashamed to keep St. Teresa so long. But there is a good deal of reading in her — and I am only able to read at night — and then not always a large, close printed book ...

My strength has failed more than usual of late. And I don't think I have much more work in me — not, at least, if it is to continue [to be] of this harassing sort. God called me to Hospital work, (as I fondly thought, for life) — but since then to Army work — but with a promise that I should go back to Hospital — as I thought as a Nurse, but as I now think, as a Patient.[6]

Later that month, on Christmas Eve, remembering other Christmas Eves spent in the Crimea, Nightingale wrote of the soldiers she would never forget:

May we all believe in Our Lord's "goodwill towards man" ... I do strive to believe that God's "goodwill towards" the 500,000 men, who are like sheep without a shepherd, is the same now as when He gave them that good friend, Sidney Herbert — now they have no friend but a poor creature like me — that He will lead and guide them ...

... whatever I have known our Lord to desire of me, I have never refused Him (knowingly) anything. And I can feel the same now. Pray for us then, dearest Revd. Mother, that we may know of God's <u>goodwill</u> towards us.[7]

During the early winter of 1865, Nightingale had a return of what she called "rheumatism in the spine," which made her "more helpless than usual." Although the pain hampered her ability to write, she kept at her work so as not to fall behind. According to her, the rheumatism:

... seemed to fix itself in my right elbow, of all places, which is the only sound place I have in my body. But it disappeared from there almost as suddenly as it came, and I was most thankful to God. For as all my business is writing, I might almost as well have lost my head ... I could hardly wash my face, or crook my finger and thumb to hold my pen. However I never did interrupt my writing for a single day — if I did my arrears would be quite hopeless ...[8]

In matters of her "lending library," Nightingale was indeed in arrears. When returning another book, she lamented and then embraced the possibility of her own journey into the "Obscure Night":

I am quite ashamed of keeping S. John of the Cross so long. But I kept St. Teresa much longer. I feel like a child who excuses itself for being naughty by telling how much naughtier it is sometimes. I hope to send back the 2nd Vol. soon. I am often afraid that I have not so much as entered into the first Obscure Night. Yet that Obscure Night does seem so applicable to me. I have never found S. John of the Cross mystical or fanciful. On the contrary, he seems to have the most wonderful practical knowledge of the ways of God in the heart of man.[9]

In keeping with the practice of many mystics, Nightingale sometimes recorded the moments when God had called her to service. Five days before her 47th birthday, she recorded the memorable dates in her journey of faith:

This is the word of the Lord unto Thee, London May 7, 1867. It is 30 years since I called thee unto my service [at] Embley [on] February 7, 1837. It is 15 years today since I called thee to the perfection of my service (to be a savior) [at] Tapton, May 7, 1852. How hast thou answered? What opportunities have I not given thee since then? I entered thee at Harley St. Aug. 12, 1853. I entered thee at Scutari Nov. 4, 1854. I entered thee with Sidney Herbert.[10]

In September 1868, Nightingale wrote to Mother Moore after a series of August anniversaries. She was fully aware of her own shortcomings in doing God's work, and her letters were often self-exhortations to do better:

> ... *Alas! dear Revd. Mother, you ask after me — I feel as if I was only quite in the infancy of serving God — I am so careful and troubled and have such a want of calmness about His work and His poor — as if they were my work and my poor instead of His. I have not learnt yet the first lesson of His service. I* think *I seek first the kingdom of God and His righteousness. But I am sure I don't succeed in being filled with His righteousness — And so I suppose that I regard too little Himself and too much myself — I should like to try to listen* only *to His voice as to what He wishes me to do, among all His poor.*
>
> *It is 12 years last August 7 (do you remember?) since we came to you at Bermondsey, returning from the Crimea. It is 11 years last August since I have been a prisoner more or less in my room. It is 7 years last August since Sidney Herbert died. You know what a terrible break-up that was to what we were doing in the War Office. Still God has pleased to raise up the India work and the Poor Law work since that. And I ought to be very thankful.*
>
> *But it does me good, I assure you it does (tho' I can't bear myself,) if I think that your dear Reverence is offering me to God, that whatever He wills may be carried out in me. I have so little of the only true patience.*[11]

In December 1874, Nightingale learned from one of the Sisters at the convent of Bermondsey that Reverend Mother Mary Clare Moore, her loyal friend from the Crimean days, had died. In her copy of *Narrative of the Demolition of the Monastery of Port Royal des Champs*, she wrote the following private note:

> *Dec. 18/74. To see God — to see Him without eyes and hear Him without ears, as we see and hear with eyes and ears, to know Him, what He is doing, and be able to help Him and to know His thoughts, His plans, in its infinite purity and Holiness — this is all my desire now — this is my hope for another world — this is what Rev'd Mother is doing now ...*[12]

Benjamin Jowett's friendship

Noted theologian and professor of Greek at Oxford, Benjamin Jowett had been introduced to Nightingale's work in 1860, when their mutual friend, Arthur Clough, suggested Jowett as one of the persons to critique her *Suggestions for Thought*. They began their correspondence shortly after the deaths of Herbert and Clough, but it was another 2 years before they met in person.

The Oxford don and the "lady with the lamp" had much in common. Jowett was a noted scholar and educator, a leader in university and educational reform, and a prominent liberal theologian. Although his professorship was in Greek, his main field of study and interest was theology. His belief in freedom of thought and discussion pitted him against the religious establishment. At Oxford, he was among the minority who

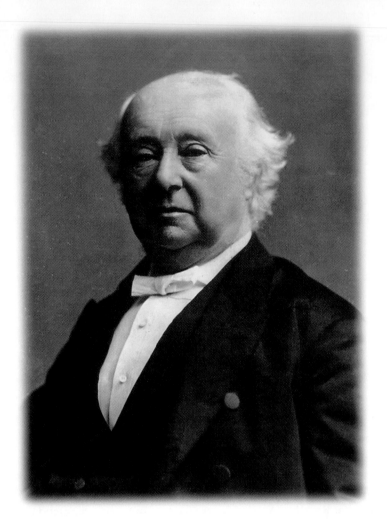

Benjamin Jowett (1817-1893), theologian, professor of Greek, and later Master of Balliol College at Oxford, who shared an interest in spiritual and philosophical issues with Nightingale for 33 years

fought to rid the university of its outdated religious restrictions. Convinced that "not a twentieth part of the ability in the country ever comes to the university,"[13] he worked unceasingly to modernize the curriculum, establish scholarships for needy students, promote university extension to secondary schools and local communities, and provide university support for successful candidates for the Indian Civil Service examinations.

Born in 1817 in Peckham, the third of nine children, Jowett was raised in a modest family with Evangelical views. An outstanding Latin scholar, he was awarded a scholarship to Oxford's Balliol College in 1836, elected a Fellow of the college while still an undergraduate — a rare honor — and appointed a Tutor in 1842. He took deacon's orders in 1842 and was ordained in the Anglican church in 1845. His reputation as both a scholar and a theologian spread beyond Oxford, and in the early 1850s, Sir Charles Trevelyan (later Governor of Madras) began consulting with him on the Indian Civil Service examinations. In 1855, now known for his progressive views, Jowett was appointed Regius Professor of Greek by Lord Palmerston, though he would have preferred the chair in Divinity. In 1870, he became Master of Balliol College.

Jowett and Nightingale's 33-year relationship began with a mutual respect for each other's work and progressed to an enduring, lifelong friendship with religious discussions at its core. Jowett's feelings for Nightingale may have run deeper than friendship at one time. According to Cornelia Sorabji, one of his Indian students at Oxford in the

1890s, Jowett once confided to her that he had asked Nightingale to marry him in the early years of their friendship.[14]

Both Jowett and Nightingale were introverts whose brilliance was tempered by common sense. Jowett was painfully shy and rarely spoke in groups; it was in his sermons and lectures and in his letters to Nightingale and other friends that the full range of his intellect and compassion was revealed.

In their early correspondence regarding *Suggestions* and other topics, Jowett was the tutor guiding the student, just as he had mentored hundreds of undergraduates at Oxford. He hoped that Nightingale would recast her "stuff," as she referred to these writings, in a form that people could understand. He believed that the work should put forth the "central light of all religion" — that is, Divine Justice and Truth. From the beginning, he was a constant source of support and encouragement, which comes through in a letter she wrote to him in July 1862, while immersed in her India reform:

> *You are so good as to enquire after the "stuff." There has been nothing done to it (or about it) since you heard of it last. But my War Office life is drawing to a close, and then, if I have any life left, I shall turn to the "stuff," and if I do anything with it, it will be owing to your encouragement. (It is a year today since Sidney Herbert's resignation of office a fortnight before his death), and in one short year Sir G. Lewis has dragged down the War Office to the position of contempt, out of wh[ich] S.H. was 5 long years in dragging it up ...*
>
> *I could not go on for the sake of mankind doing the immeasurably little I can for them, if I did not believe myself part of a plan by which God is doing the immeasurably much for them. If I did not believe God's plan intended the ultimate perfection of every human being ... I could not work. For otherwise, it would seem as if I had been trying to work for God and he to thwart my work (I have often told him so). He brought about the most extraordinary combination, one wh[ich] could hardly ever happen again, by which a woman obtains all the practical knowledge of Army organisation, and a Secretary of State is willing not only to listen to her, but to devote every instant of 5 years to it — and he breaks this up ...[15]*

Jowett and Nightingale's first meeting occurred in 1862, when he was 45 and she was 42. During an episode of excruciating spinal pain, which made her feel that she was near death, she asked Jowett to come to London and administer "the Sacrament," the term many of her dear Crimean soldiers had used for communion. He did so on October 26, with the Nightingales, Selina Bracebridge, and several other friends present. Over the years, Jowett made many visits to South Street, Embley, and Lea Hurst, during which he frequently administered communion to Nightingale. Nightingale's family and friends came to refer to him as "that good man" and "that true saint."

When Nightingale confided to Jowett the opinion of others that she might have worked Herbert and Clough to death, Jowett wrote to reassure her after a visit with Clough's widow, Blanche:

> *No one says anything unkind about you to me. Indeed, I am sure no one ever could say anything which could shake my faith or admiration. Mrs. Clough did not appear to me to entertain the painful impression to which you refer ... I consider you a sort of Royal personage, not to be gossiped about with any one.[16]*

At odds with the Church

Jowett's liberal position on theological matters created a good deal of controversy in church circles. In a collection of essays on St. Paul's epistles that he published with Arthur P. Stanley in 1855, Jowett scandalized Evangelicals and High Church Anglicans by questioning the doctrine of Atonement. His appointment as professor of Greek that summer prompted religious conservatives to seek retribution. They found an obscure ecclesiastical statute on which to accuse him of heresy, but their power was waning, and Jowett was merely forced to sign again the Thirty-Nine Articles, the articles of faith that in 1563 had defined the Church of England after its split from Rome. If he had written 10 years earlier, he might have been driven from Oxford for his liberal views.

Jowett was harshly attacked again in the early 1860s, when his essay "Interpretation of Scripture" appeared in *Essays and Reviews* with the work of several other liberal theologians. The essayists contended that the same critical analysis applied to other academic disciplines must also be applied to theology, including scientific and historical investigations. Jowett had written that "the healthy tone of religion among the poor depends upon freedom of thought and inquiry among the educated."[17]

A letter to Nightingale in December 1862 shows Jowett trying to remain optimistic in the face of the new charges:

> *My prosecutors have not troubled me as yet and I rather hope they will not do so. They have to set in motion a rusty old Court in which such a cause was never tried, and which has to proceed by the forms of Common Law. Then again the Statute seems expressly to say that they can only try me for what I have said as a Professor in lecturing, and not for any book and writing ... There is a statute of limitation of 2 years in the Ch[urch] Discipline Act which I am told will be held to apply ... The Delegates to whom the appeal has to be made are very liberal in their sentiments. These are the chances of escape before the cause begins. So you see that I am a fortunate criminal ... There is some amusement, is there not, in fighting a battle? At least I suppose there is no harm in trying to find amusement in doing so.[18]*

Jowett and two of his fellow essayists were found guilty of heresy by the ecclesiastical court in February 1863, but a civil court dismissed the charges, thus dealing the Church of England a serious blow. The fact that six of the seven essayists were ordained churchmen suggests that more liberal religious thinkers were finding a place in the established church. When religious antagonists again brought heresy charges against Jowett, the charges were once again dropped; the tide of liberalism and freedom had become obvious.

In April 1864, Garibaldi, the Italian patriot and revolutionary, requested a meeting with Nightingale to seek her advice about various administrative matters facing his new government. Nightingale was a longtime supporter of Garibaldi's and had contributed funds to the Ladies' Philanthropic Association he had formed to help the needy. When Nightingale informed Jowett of the proposed meeting, he wrote back with advice that indicated the depth to which he understood the world around him. The unification of Italy required new political talents and skills from those who had excelled as military leaders, and Garibaldi's fitness for his new role was a topic of the day:

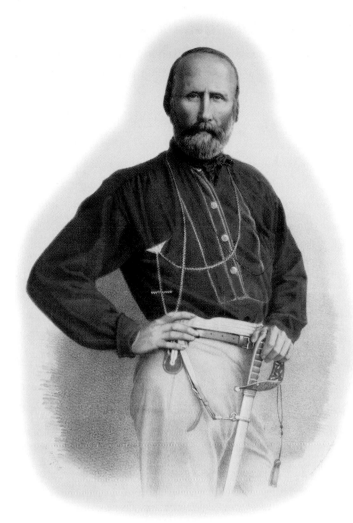

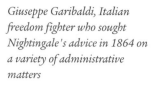

Giuseppe Garibaldi, Italian freedom fighter who sought Nightingale's advice in 1864 on a variety of administrative matters

I think we may trust God to give us his own calmness and clearness on any great occasion, such as this is. I hope you will inspire G[aribaldi] for the future and not pain him too much about the past. Ten years more of such a life as his might accomplish anything for Italy in the way of military organization and sanitary and moral improvement — if he could only see that his duty is not to break the yet immature strength of Italy against Austrian fortresses.

I think we must allow great men to be very different — Cavour for one use and Garibaldi for another — both of them almost enemies in life and yet both of them to be regarded from a higher point of view as carrying out a common work. I am not disappointed in Garibaldi for I do not expect from a man of genius who is impressible, a strong will. There are many ways and many instruments by which the world is carried on.

I should have been sorry if you had not seen him. I am sure you can do him good — if you can only make him see that more and something of a different kind is required of him in the remaining years of life. I sometimes think that in one point, the expedition to Naples, the foolishness of G. was wiser than the wisdom of Cavour.[19]

After her meeting with Garibaldi, Nightingale commissioned a bronze bust of the Italian patriot. She presented it to the Grosvenor Hotel, which owned the building where she was living at the time and where it can still be seen today.

"Behold the handmaid of the Lord"

Nightingale's letters to Jowett over the years often included her ruminations on mysticism. Her comments in the following letter reveal her progress in the process of purification at the stage of Surrender:

> Behold the handmaid of the Lord: be it unto me according as Thou will. 1. What a wonderful favour to be chosen before as many thousands to be the handmaid of the Lord. 2. What return does God expect from me — with what purity of heart & intention should I make an offering of myself to Him — And when that offering is made, what a life ought I to lead? 3. I give myself up entirely to Him that He may do with me whatever it pleases Him — and I earnestly desire that He will never think of sparing me and let no occasion pass of mortifying my pride & trying my temper. 4. God forbid that I should glory save in the Cross of our Lord Jesus Christ ... We really love God if we desire to do his Will. I make it my earnest prayers that I may live so as to have fulfilled the will of God in every thing.[20]

In August 1871, Jowett told Nightingale that he was going to write about the religions of the world. She was very pleased and began a series of letters on God:

> I am overjoyed that you are going to write an Essay on the "religions of the world," and "then make applications of them to ourselves." You ask me what I have to "say about it." And as I am naturally a patient and obedient beast (I do not look into your face for fear of seeing that you don't agree on this point), this is what I have to say.
> 1. Let what comes out of them all be: the search after a Perfect God — i.e. how far the search after Him comes out of each.
> 2. Let what comes out of them all be: the search after Truth — that there is a truth, we are to find it — not that we are "speculating" or "criticizing" or exercising our "private judgment" or being "liberals" or illiberals or "Pantheistic" or "Deistic" — but that, if there is a God at all, He is an existence outside of us, (perhaps the only real existence there is) — & we have to find Him out — an absolute Truth, not depending upon "Church" or "private judgement" either — upon what "I think," or upon what "you think" ...
> The search after the Perfect God. If He is perfect, He has a plan for bringing us all to perfection ... If there is a plan for bringing us all to perfection, surely the most momentous study of Theology is to discover what this is & of Religion to second it ...[21]

In another long letter to Jowett a week later, Nightingale again explores "the character of God":

> What is the character of God? Not to look to good intentions without requiring practical wisdom to allow blunders their full consequences in evil, as well as sins; to require that is, the same search, study, earnest and wise endeavour, patient investigation of laws in discovering and reforming in the moral world as in the material. (All that jargon about "forgiveness," salvation — & the reverse — is as much jargon in the moral & spiritual world as it would be in the Material, where people now have too much experience to use it.) Intellect may be enough for the pursuit of Science, the "God revealed in nature" — but for the pursuit of Moral Science, as, e.g. the knowledge of the character of God — all, all our faculties, intellectual, moral, emotional, (or affectional) & spiritual are wanting — are essential ...[22]

The letter goes on to reiterate her belief that individuals working together can improve life for mankind:

> *Mankind must discover the character of God. Mankind must find out God — I cannot by my-self find out God — Mankind must create Mankind — You said to me last year, "I don't know what you mean by mankind, &c." This is all I mean: viz. that human (Mankind's) experience must come to be the "grounds on which we believe the anticipations" of our "Reason & Conscience," and mighty little we have as yet of that experience! with all our Criticism.*[23]

Nightingale's frequent use of terms such as "character of God" prompted Jowett to complain in October 1872 that "during the ten years & more that I have known you, you have repeated to me the expression "character of God" about 1,000 times, but I cannot say that I have any clear [idea] of what you mean, if you mean anything more than divine perfection."[24] Apparently, her use of this term had frustrated Jowett in the past because a year earlier Nightingale had written to him: "I don't at all plead guilty to your accusation that I 'speak of the character of God, without coming to the point.'"[25]

Nightingale's quest to understand the deeper levels of Divine Reality continued to the end of her life and was woven into her letters to her nursing students; her work-house nursing and India reform; her drafts for *Notes from Devotional Authors of the Middle Ages,* which she worked on in the 1870s but never completed; and her in-depth study of the Bible and related works.

Literary criticism

Nightingale had encouraged Jowett while he was working on his five-volume translation of the works of Plato, and he sought her help when he was about to begin the second edition. Because Nightingale was familiar with Plato and knew Greek, Jowett asked her to critique his introductions and summaries and to offer ideas for his second edition. She tackled this project in her characteristic way, devoting an enormous amount of thought, time, and energy to it.

The two exchanged many lively letters about man's place in nature. In one exchange, they clashed on the question of whether the physical good is sometimes at variance with morality. To support this thesis, Jowett pointed to Plato's claim that the chief principle in marriage should be the parents' health and strength, regardless of whether they were married, and that the laws of physical improvement required that society get rid of sick and deformed infants. Nightingale's caustic but humorous answer followed:

> *I am quite scandalized at your materialism. (I shall shut up you and Plato for a hundred years in punishment in another world till you have both obtained clear views.) Is it for an old maid like me to be preaching to you, a Master in Israel, that even "on physical principles" there are essential points in marriage (to turn the best order of children), which, being absent, the perfection of "health and strength" in both parents is of no avail even for the physical part of the children? ... (My son, really Plato talks nonsense about this) ... As Plato says, the mind informs the body, owns the body, the body is the servant of the mind. How can the owner and the master be the limit? We must pray for your conversion.[26]*

When Jowett received two parcels of Nightingale's notes on *The Republic* in 1874, he wrote her a short note of thanks: "It is not everyone who has the advantage of being criticized by the Goddess Athene."[27] Although Nightingale's name wasn't mentioned in the acknowledgments to the second edition, published in 1875, her suggestions are evident in any comparison of the two editions and in her letters to Jowett.

Battling feelings of despair

In June 1872, feeling worn down by years of chronic illness, despair, and frustration about the slow pace of reform, Nightingale again considered moving to St. Thomas's Hospital as a live-in patient. Jowett responded with a witty plea not to do so: "(1) Because it is eccentric and we cannot strengthen our lives by eccentricity. (2) Because you will not be a patient but a kind of Directress to the Institution, viewed with great alarm by the doctors."[28] On a more serious note, he told her that living as a patient would kill her — that she needed to live in a place where she could do her best work and try to remain independent.

A few months later, Nightingale expressed a sense of futility about her many years of hard work:

... You tell me to look back on the good that has been done. I cannot. It is not in me. I am just as much stripped of my past life, "stand naked there" on the brink of the grave, as if it had really been done in another life ... I cannot remember, still less "think of" my life in the Crimea or my 5 years' incessant work with S.H. [Sidney Herbert], or my 9 years' Indian work — more than if it had been really the life of others — indeed much less — for I am sure that I think much more of what Mr. Jowett has done than of what I have done ...

If I am forgotten it is not more than I have forgotten myself. If I am like a dead man out of mind, it is not more than a dead man is out of his own mind. And F.N. is not less stripped out of anyone else's mind than she is out of her own ... To hope is for me like brandy. One feels all the weaker afterwards. I cannot & do not wish "to hope" for what I know will not come. "Pray for time to finish your work." You are at the pinnacle of your power, thank God. [You] only want time to finish. [I] with an utterly shattered body have to begin all over again.[29]

Many people have characterized the many self-pitying comments in Nightingale's diaries and letters as Victorian melodrama and exaggeration. However, her intense mental and spiritual suffering were a classic element in the Surrender phase of the mystic's spiritual development. Nightingale was impatient and frustrated with herself because she felt she wasn't doing enough for God, and her study of the lives of the mystics made her even more aware of her own imperfections. Jowett was a true friend to whom she could pour out her pain; he understood, but encouraged her to continue to do the things she could do well.

Self-Knowledge & Bible annotations

Nightingale's Surrender phase was not a giving up; it was a deeper exploration of experiencing God, which allowed her to feel more connected to all things. Her intense study of the Bible was a vehicle for self-knowledge, a process that continued for most of her life and that is revealed in the many annotations she wrote in her King James Bible.

Nightingale had studied the Bible since childhood, and the many notes she wrote over the years in her Bible reveal much about her journey on her "Dark Night of the Soul." Her annotations appear in Greek, Latin, Italian, German, and French. In many places, she identifies with major prophets, apostles, and other people on their journeys of faith. She often challenges the masculine imagery of God. (In *Suggestions for Thought*, she had written "The next Christ will perhaps be a female Christ."[30])

The most heavily annotated sections are the Psalms and Isaiah in the Old Testament as well as the gospels of Matthew, John, and Acts, and the book of Romans in the New Testament. Few passages are dated, but changes in her handwriting allow the reader to differentiate earlier annotations (from the 1840s and 1850s) from those made later in life. The earliest recorded date is 1844 and the last is 1875.

In the following examples, Nightingale's dated passages and her comments reflect her spiritual struggles at different stages of life:

A page from Nightingale's annotated Bible, showing comments — written in both English and French — that reflected her own spiritual journey over the years

• Isaiah 57:10 — Beside the passage "Thou art wearied in the greatness of the way ... thou hast found the life of thine hand; therefore thou wast not grieved," Nightingale wrote the date "14 September 1845" and "He is to give her employment." (During this period, she was struggling to understand how she could carry out her chosen work of nursing and be of service to God and mankind. It would be another 8 years before she began her work as superintendent at Harley Street.)

• Zechariah 12:5 — Beside the passage that reads "the inhabitants of Jerusalem shall be my strength in the Lord of hosts their God," she wrote "The nurses shall be her strength."

• Psalm 18:4-6 — "The sorrows of death compassed me about ... The sorrows of hell compassed me about. The snares of death prevented me. In my distress I called upon the Lord and cried unto my God." Beside this passage, she wrote and underlined in red "This world is hell — 1862." (This was written soon after the deaths of Sidney Herbert and Arthur Clough, a period of intense physical and emotional pain.)

• Genesis 45:5 — From the story of Joseph being sold into slavery, "Now therefore be not grieved nor angry with yourselves that ye sold me hither: for God did send me before you to preserve life," she wrote in large bold print "Be not grieved nor angry with yourselves — for God did send me — to preserve life." At Genesis 45:8, she rewrote and added feminist imagery: "So now it was not you that sent me hither but God: And he hath made me a mother to many. March 30, 1873."

• Acts 9:16 — Next to the passage where Jesus prophesies the suffering that Paul will experience, she rewrote the passage, adding the feminine reference: "See how great he (or she) must suffer for my sake. Sept. 23, 1867, Jan. 7, 1872, Jan. 2, 1873, June 7, 1873." (All these dates indicate when Nightingale reread this passage: in 1867, she was working incessantly for India; in 1872 and 1873, she was critiquing the introductions and summaries in Jowett's *Plato*, beginning her *Notes from Devotional Authors of the Middle Ages*, more active in the nurses' training program at St. Thomas's, and continuing her work for India.)[31]

A flurry of writing

Aware of Nightingale's frustration over Indian reform efforts, and hoping to keep her occupied, Jowett suggested in 1871 that she write treatises on theology, Poor Law reform, women's education, and other topics, drawing from her *Suggestions for Thought*:

> *I think that you are quite right in not propounding schemes of Army Reform at the present time. But there remain a great many interesting subjects on which you have thought & had experience …*
>
> *I. Theology — a) you must work out your notion of Divine perfection, especially showing that this may be consistent with the appearances of evil in the world — b) of the vanity of free thinking & criticism, & their purely negative use.*
>
> *II. Social life — the ideal of the family: Education of women —Sisterhoods & their true principles. The employment of women; (you might rewrite in a more consecutive manner some part of those volumes which you used to call the "Stuff").*
>
> *III. The poor law — beginning with a Study of Political Economy & showing how there is still a place for humanity.*
>
> *IV. Sanitary or theological tracts for the poor, "How people may live & not die." These are the subjects which appear to me most suited to you. But if you will supply the outlines & materials of any others I will work them up for you, not in my own style but as far as I can in yours, which is much better & more striking … The great point is to be moderate & consecutive. I think that you should try the form of short papers or Essays, because these depend least upon the form, & admit even of an imperfect expression of the idea.[32]*

Intrigued, Nightingale submitted three articles to *Fraser's Magazine*, a progressive literary journal. In the first paper, "A Note of Interrogation," published in May 1873, she defined her concept of God as a God of Law whose character could be learned from social and moral science. She defended her concepts against some Christian church ideas on the one side, and against Auguste Comte's philosophy of positivism on the other. According to Comte, positive knowledge must be based on natural phenomena and their properties, as verified by the empirical sciences; theology and metaphysics were only imperfect modes of knowledge. Although Nightingale agreed with what could be learned from science, she was critical of the positivists, particularly their atheism. She disagreed with the notion that positivism was a substitution for the idea of a personal God. To her, scientific inquiry could offer new ways of thinking about how to use God's laws to help mankind.

Her second paper, "A Sub-Note of Interrogation: What Will Our Religion be in 1999?" published in July, centered on her belief that, although history unfolded according to certain laws, man could make a difference in the future of mankind:

> *Monday, May 26, 1873.*
>
> *The eclipse of the sun has begun. 7.36 A.M.*
> *The eclipse of the sun is at its full. 8.28 A.M.*
> *The eclipse of the sun has ended. 9.24 A.M.*
>
> *After this a dearth of great eclipses of the sun visible in this country succeeds for years. On August 11, 1999, at 12 minutes 20 seconds to 10 A.M., "local time," the next total solar eclipse in England is to occur, we are told.*
>
> *Supposing us to study the laws under which the Political and Moral World is governed, as we study those under which the solar system, the Material World, is governed, could we arrive at something of the same certainty in predicting the future condition of human society? How it will be with Europe? How it will be with England? How it will be with any one of our homes or institutions on August 11, 1999, at ten o'clock in the morning? (for I would not be particular to a minute).*
>
> *One thing is certain, that none who now live will then be living here. (Perhaps by that time we may have sufficiently mastered the laws of moral evidence to say with equal certainty that every one who now lives will then be living — Where?) Another thing is certain, that everything ... is so governed, by laws which can be seen in their effects, that not the most trifling action or feeling is left to chance, and that any who could see into the mind of the "All-Ordering Power," as manifested by His laws or thoughts, could of course predict history.*
>
> *All will be Order, not chance. But whether it be the Order of Disorder, so to speak, or the Order of Good Order, depends upon us. And this is practically what we have to consider.*
>
> *What will this world be on August 11, 1999? What we have made it.*[33]

The editor rejected her third article, "On What Government Night Will Mr. Lowe Bring Out Our New Moral Budget? Another Sub-Note of Interrogation," calling it "unfocused." In this plea for social reform, which was strongly linked to her religious philosophy, she used statistics to expound her concepts of social and moral science. The first article drew praise and criticism. Her rejection of eternal damnation had some critics declaring that they would pray for her conversion. Author Thomas Carlyle faulted her second paper, comparing its author to "a lost lamb bleating on the mountain."[34] Nightingale complained, in a provocative postscript to her third, unpublished article, that many of her critics had read reviews of the article rather than the article itself.

Children's Bible

Nightingale had suggested to Benjamin Jowett that he compile a children's Bible in the hope that children would no longer be told lies in the parables; she also believed that more appropriate Bible stories could be chosen. Jowett accepted the challenge and helped his friend William Rogers write and edit a Bible for children. The two men then sent the manuscript to various friends, including Nightingale and the poet Algernon Charles Swinburne, for their suggestions on what should be included.

This project was a natural for Nightingale because she was quite familiar with the Bible and had been critiquing it since her youth, pointing out incorrect translations of the original and what was real and what wasn't. She was critical of the preliminary selections for the proposed children's Bible; to her mind, it came up short in the following ways:

> *(a) Matters of <u>universal</u> importance, moral and spiritual (<u>e.g.</u> the finest parts of Isaiah, Jeremiah, Ezekiel and the New Testament); (b) Matters of <u>historical</u> importance (<u>e.g.</u> which embrace the history of great nations, Egypt, Assyria, Babylon. The petty wars of the petty tribes seem to take up quite a disproportionate space); (c) Matters of <u>local</u> importance, which have acquired a <u>universal moral</u> significance (e.g. Jonah is entirely left out: yet Jonah has a moral and spiritual meaning, while Samson, Balaam and Bathsheba have none); (d) Matters of <u>merely local</u> importance, with no significance but an <u>immoral</u> one (<u>e.g.</u> the stories about Abraham, Isaac and Jacob, almost all Joshua and Judges, and very much of Samuel and Kings). The story of Achilles and his horses is far more fit for children than that of Balaam and his ass, which is only fit to be told to asses. The stories of Samson and of Jephthah are only fit to be told to bull-dogs; and the story of Bathsheba to be told to Bathshebas. Yet we give all these stories to children as "Holy Writ." There are some things in Homer we might better call "Holy" Writ — many, many in Sophocles and Aeschylus. The stories about Andromache and Antigone are worth all the women in the Old Testament put together, nay, almost all the women in the Bible.[35]*

Jowett adopted most of her selections with little change. The children's Bible was published in 1873 as *The School and Children's Bible Prepared Under the Superintendence of the Rev. William Rogers*. Jowett wrote to Nightingale: "I blessed you every time I took the papers up, especially in the Prophets ... [I] have adopted your selection almost entirely, with a slight abridgment."[36]

During this period, Jowett also used many of her suggestions for the sermons he preached at Oxford and other places. Some of the themes she suggested were "God the Lord," "God the Father," "God the Judge," "God the Friend," and "the Way of the Cross." The topics often had to be altered because of the political climate at Oxford.

In 1873, Jowett began complaining to Nightingale of his isolated life at Oxford and his failing memory. Nightingale couldn't bear to see her friend's health failing. She suggested a "holiday" contract, just as Jowett had once written a regimen of work and rest for her:

> *I, B. Jowett, agree to take an entire holiday doing nothing for 3 weeks at the present time — for not less than 3 weeks at Easter — & for not less that six (6) weeks on the Long Vacation.*
>
> *I agree to take two days in every week during Term Time (Sunday & one other day) of entire holiday, doing nothing except when I have a sermon to write.*
>
> *I agree to give not more than two lectures a week during the present year & to register all this in an Almanac.[37]*

Notes on the mystics & devotional authors

Nightingale had begun to read the works of the mystics, such as Meister Eckhart, St. John of the Cross, St. Teresa of Avila, and St. Francis of Assisi, in her late twenties, and she shared her thoughts about these works with Mother Mary Clare Moore and Benjamin Jowett during the 1860s and 1870s. She was particularly inspired by the life of the great medieval mystic Thomas à Kempis (1380-1471), whose book *The Imitation of Christ* she reread during the 1870s. His classic words detailing the saints' inner joy and freedom — "[they are] free, and nothing can hold them" — resonated with Nightingale.[38]

She particularly empathized with the point of view of some saints that they were "not for Church but for God" and that they "lived for God alone." Although Nightingale believed that Christianity was the last and most perfect manifestation of God, she had realized since her twenties that to know God, one must also learn about and try to understand the practices and beliefs of the other world religions: "You must go to Mohametanism, Buddhism, to the East, to the Sufis & Fakirs, to Pantheism, for the right growth of mysticism," she wrote in March 1853.[39] One of her favorite works was an ancient Persian prayer:

> *Four things, O God, I have to offer Thee*
> *Which Thou hast not in all Thy treasury;*
> *My nothingness, my sad necessity,*
> *My fatal sin & earnest penitence*
> *Receive these gifts & take the Giver hence.*[40]

From 1872 to 1875, Nightingale read and reflected on a book about the suffering of French Catholic nuns, *Narrative of the Demolition on the Monastery of Port Royal des Champs*. She heavily annotated her own copy, writing notes or dating passages about the nuns' spiritual struggles and reflecting on her own spiritual journey.

During this same period, Nightingale worked on the first drafts of a book called *Notes from Devotional Authors of the Middle Ages, Collected, Chosen, and Freely Translated by Florence Nightingale*. Although she never finished this book, she certainly intended it for publication because she added her name to the title. Her drafts show her intense reflection about and understanding of the practice of mysticism and the lives of male and female medieval saints and mystics whom she intended to include in the book: Blessed Angela of Foligno, Ste. Jeanne Francoise de Chantal, St. Francis of Assisi, St. Francis Xavier, St. John of the Cross, St. Peter of Alcantara, Father Rigoleuc, St. Teresa of Avila, and Father Surin.

The preface provides an excellent summary of her thoughts on mysticism:

> *It may seem a strange thing to begin a book with:— this Book is not for any one who has time to read it — but the meaning of it is: this reading is good only as a preparation for work.*
>
> *That Religion is not devotion, but work and suffering for the love of God; this is the true doctrine of Mystics, as is more particularly set forth in a definition of the 16th century: "True reli-*

gion is to have no other will but God's." Compare this with the definition of Religion in Johnson's Dictionary: "Virtue founded upon reverence of God and expectation of future rewards and punishments"; in other words on respect and self-interest, not love. Imagine the religion which inspired the life of Christ "founded" on the motives given by Dr. Johnson!

For what is Mysticism? Is it not the attempt to draw near to God, not by rites or ceremonies, but by inward disposition? Is it not merely a hard word for "The Kingdom of Heaven is within"? Heaven is neither a place nor a time. There might be a Heaven not only here but now. It is true that sometimes we must sacrifice not only health of body, but health of mind (or, peace) in the interest of God; that is, we must sacrifice Heaven. But "thou shalt be like God for thou shalt see Him as He is": this may be here and now, as well as there and then. And it may be for a time, then lost, then recovered, both here and there, both now and then.

Christ Himself was the first true Mystic. "My meat is to do the will of Him that sent me and to finish His work." What is this but putting in fervent and the most striking words the foundation of all real Mystical Religion?, which is that for all our actions, all our words, all our thoughts, the food upon which they are to live and have their being is to be the indwelling Presence of God, the union with God; that is, with the Spirit of Goodness and Wisdom.

A page from Nightingale's Notes from Devotional Authors of the Middle Ages, *in which she reflected on the lives of saints and mystics*

That the soul herself should be heaven, that our Father which is in heaven should dwell in her, that there is something within us infinitely more estimable than often comes out, that God enlarges this "palace of our soul" by degrees so as to enable her to receive Himself, that thus he gives her liberty but that the soul must give herself up absolutely to Him for Him to do this, the incalculable benefit of this occasional but frequent intercourse with the Perfect: this is the conclusion and sum of the whole matter, put into beautiful language by the Mystics. And of this process they describe the steps, and assign periods of months and years during which the steps, they say, are commonly made by those who make them at all.

The way to live with God is to live with Ideals, not merely to think about ideals, but to do and suffer for them. Those who have to work on men and women must above all things have their Spiritual Ideal, their purpose, ever present. The "mystical" state is the essence of common sense.[41]

To the end of her life, Nightingale explored spiritual issues and sought the presence of God in her work and everything she did. She recognized a force greater than herself and a power that heals. During these years of chronic pain and insomnia, she spent many hours alone, wrestling with her failures, contemplating, and praying, as many mystics had done before her. Contemplation led her to be honest about her struggles and her lack of perfection, and to come face to face with the parts of herself that needed healing. This striving for perfection was at the core of her spirituality and the driving force that guided her lifelong pursuit of public health, nursing reform, and India reform.

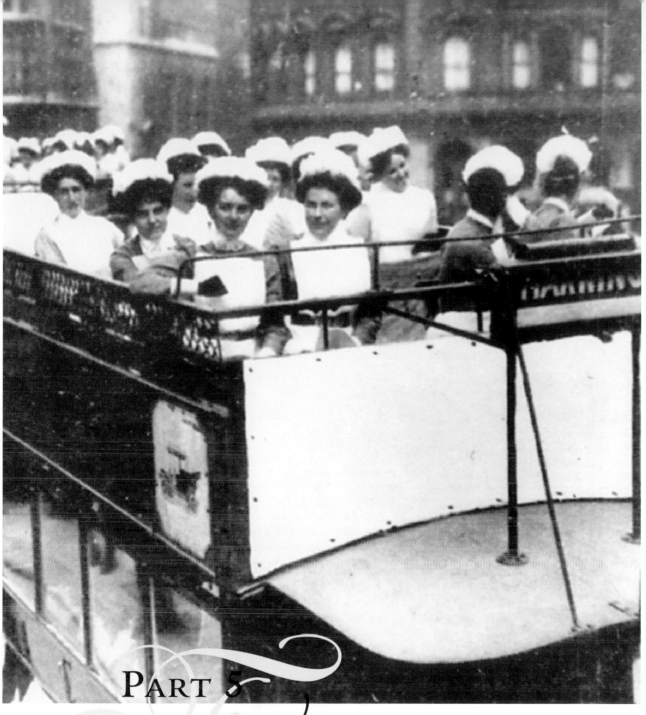

PART 5

Later Years

(1880-1910)

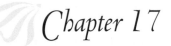
Years of Loss

Death comes to set thee free, O meet him cheerily as thy true friend; and all thy cares shall cease, and in eternal peace thy troubles end.

— Florence Nightingale to Sir Harry Verney, 1889[1]

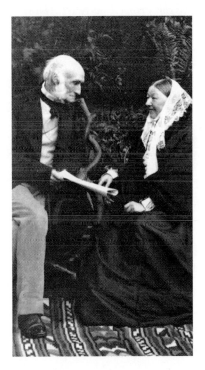

Sir Harry Verney and Florence Nightingale at the Verneys' estate, Claydon, c. 1880

The 1880s were a decade of loss for Nightingale as more of the people who had been important in her life died, beginning with her mother in 1880. The next to go were Mary Clarke Mohl, one of her oldest friends, and Dr. William Farr, her statistical advisor since her return from the Crimea, both of whom died in 1882. Sir John McNeill, a father-figure who had been one of her staunchest allies in the battle for army reform, died in 1883. A year later, Sir Bartle Frere, who had worked with her closely on Indian affairs, died after a long illness.

Her former suitor, Richard Monckton Milnes (Lord Houghton), who had remained a lifelong friend, advisor, and loyal supporter, died in 1885. By 1890, her sister Parthe, her Uncle Sam and Aunt Mai Smith, Selina Bracebridge, Lord Panmure, Rev. Mother Mary Clare Moore, Harriet Martineau, and Julius Mohl would all be gone.

Nightingale had considered herself old since the mid-1870s. Chronic illness and overwork had kept her from healthy physical activity, and she began to assume a more matronly appearance. Yet her gentle, round face, often framed by an elegant Buckinghamshire lace scarf tied at the chin, now revealed a kindly radiance.

With her former connections to the halls of power gone, Nightingale became less intensely focused on her social action or on the outcome of her labors than before. As she mellowed, she found more time for her personal interests. On her visits to Claydon, the estate of her sister and brother-in-law, she often felt well enough to take walks in the garden. Back at South Street, she loved feeding the birds from her balcony and studied the different varieties and their eating habits. She also found great enjoyment in the antics of her cats, a family of Persians. She named one "Barts" after St. Bartholomew's Hospital, and the other "Tom" after St. Thomas's Hospital. She wrote about their intelligence and affectionate natures. She sometimes treated them as if they were her guests and allowed them to dine from plates on a tablecloth.

Death of mother

Fanny's health had been failing ever since W.E.N.'s death in 1874 and, on February 2, 1880, just before her 93rd birthday, she died, with William Shore Smith, who had inherited the Nightingale estate, by her side. Shore wrote to his cousin that in Fanny's final hours, she had listened to and repeated her favorite hymns and prayers and smiled, as if to say, "I'm dying. It's all right." At 9 p.m., she folded her hands, closed her eyes, and lay down. In 3 hours, she was gone to a "Greater Love than ours."[2]

Nightingale received many notes acknowledging her mother's death; the nurses from St. Thomas's sent a beautiful wreath in her memory. Worried that her mother's funeral would become a spectacle, she quickly notified her brother-in-law, Sir Harry Verney, that she wanted only a few family members and loyal servants to follow Fanny's casket to the grave:

> There are many strong reasons to my feeling why those who should follow my dear mother to the grave should only be Shore and his wife and yourself. I would not ask any of my "Cousins" — not one — If Wm. Coltman & Sir Harry B. C. like to offer let them — But pray do not let us do anything to prevent Louisa going with Shore. It is converting a lovely act of love into a farce to ask the "Cousins": is it not? The people she would like would be: — yourself, Louisa, Shore — Coachman & Charles—and Morris, if she would like it; no one else.[3]

Nightingale herself was too ill to attend the service. On February 6, she wrote a sweet note to Parthe: "The accompanying flowers, dear Pop, taken out of my mother's coffin by dear Louisa's care are for you. I have a long letter to write to you about darling Mother, which I will today, if only possible."[4]

On February 13, Queen Victoria sent a message of sympathy, and Nightingale wasted no time in responding. She addressed the letter to the "Empress of India" and wrote about conditions there, making a plea on behalf of the Indian people. The Queen didn't respond but sent Nightingale a copy of the *Life of the Prince Consort,* a biography of her late husband, who had died in 1861.[5]

In the aftermath of their mother's death, the two sisters spent a lot of time debating the proper wording for the death announcement and the gravestone inscription. Nightingale made an effort to take into account the wishes of both Parthe and Sir Harry. In earlier years, she might not have considered Parthe's comments, but she now treated her sister with more respect and kindness, qualities the sisters shared in their last years together.

The emotions and activities surrounding her mother's death left Nightingale exhausted. Her doctors told her that she was near a nervous collapse and ordered sea air and a year's rest from her responsibilities. That, of course, was impossible, but she did go to a seaside resort for 3 weeks and wrote to Parthe from there:

> I am "not worse," my dear P. And I like looking at the "white horses" [white-capped waves] coming in, which I have not seen for 24 years. But the place is too London-y & I don't like acting the "lady." I hope Sir H. did not feel cold at the Station. My love to him for coming with me ...[6]

In late March 1880, Nightingale asked her cousin Henry Bonham Carter to settle Fanny's estate and was surprised to find that her mother had bequeathed to her two daughters about £1,000 and a small amount of stocks.[7] When Nightingale and Parthe offered to pay their devoted cousin for his legal help, he sent the following reply:

I have been remiss to respond to your kind proposal that I should accept £100 as an acknowl-edgment of your and Parthe's appreciation of what I may have done in the way of help in your mother's affairs. To accept this would not my dear Flo be agreeable to me — detracting as it would from the pleasure which is afforded by being able to be of some service in a matter which could not perhaps have been so conveniently and easily done by another. If you had had a brother such business affairs would have fallen upon him ... and I hope that you will both, in this respect, allow me to stand in the position of one ...[8]

Closer ties to the Verneys

After Fanny's death, Nightingale became much closer to her sister and brother-in-law as well as to the Verney children. She began to visit the Verneys at Claydon more often, and Parthe and Sir Harry asked her to consider it her country home. There she had her own bedroom and parlor, called the "F wing" in her honor, with her own bell in the servants' quarters so she could call when she needed assistance.

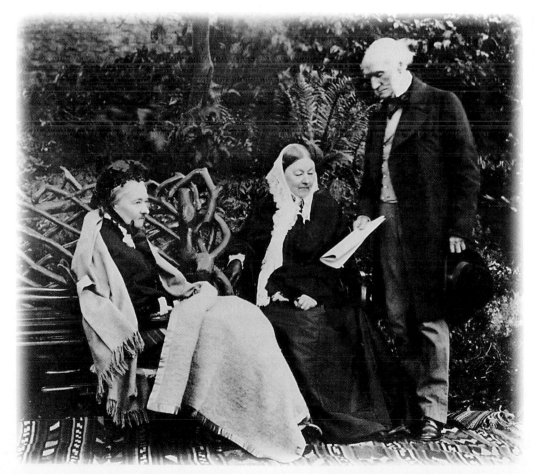

(Left to right) Parthenope Verney, Florence Nightingale, and Sir Harry Verney at Claydon, c. 1880

A belated birthday letter to "dearest Pop" in April 1880 reveals the sisters' renewed love and respect for each other:

> ... The wide-winged Lea birds overhead chuckle in their flight, & say: None but us, none but us can sit on the cliffs. Perhaps they are going up the Channel as far as Dover: & I will entrust one with a letter, under his wings, of love to thee, my dearest Pop, which, as he says he cannot carry a serenade, shall take a more prosaic note, with best earthly birthday blessings and heavenly. I feel that I have nothing now to do but to work the work of Him that sent me while it is called to-day. I so prepare for the Immediate Presence of God. Pray for me that I may do it less badly ... I would if I could send you & pick as of yours an Embley nosegay of lilacs from the American garden always out on thy birthday.[9]

After her marriage, Parthe continued painting and sketching; she also wrote essays and tales on various topics, including British and American life,[10] women in medicine, nature, country life, the Franco-Prussian War, the education of women in France, and peasant life in the historic French mountain district of Auvergne.[11] She also compiled the Verney family letters in a book titled *Memoirs of the Verney Family during the Civil War*, which she edited and illustrated.[12] In spite of Parthe's severe rheumatoid arthritis, she was able to entertain friends and family at Claydon with assistance. Among the occasional visitors were Nightingale's nurse probationers from St. Thomas's.

A perfect hostess

Nightingale was extremely concerned about the Verneys' comfort and well-being. When the couple were in London, she would send a maid almost every day, weather permitting, to their house, just down the street, to see if Parthe had the shades up and the windows open in all the rooms. Whenever Nightingale traveled to Claydon, she would do the same. She would also stroll down the hall at appointed times to visit Parthe in her living quarters, depending on her state of health as well as Parthe's.

Nightingale was also an excellent hostess at her home in London; she never took meals with her guests but had her maids and servants tend to their every need. She often asked the Verneys if her guests could stay with them or arranged for accommodations at the Grosvenor Hotel. In January 1881, she enlisted Sir Harry's help in planning a "little spread and party for her maids," complete with ale and music. Ever the able administrator, she made detailed plans for every activity and sent them to the Verneys:

> 1. Would you kindly send me the address where you get your Hams? at once. The program of our Wednesday's entertainment is as follows:
>
>> Company come at 7 p.m. (a little tea and cake)
>> Dancing 7:30 till 9
>> Supper 9
>> Disperse at 10
>> Break up at 11
>
> 2. I would be extremely obliged to Morey [one of Verney's servants] with your permission if he would take the head of the table at supper & if he would order from Grosvenor Hotel a sufficient number of bottles of Bitter Beer or Ale for about 17 or 18: & dispense it himself. (Three

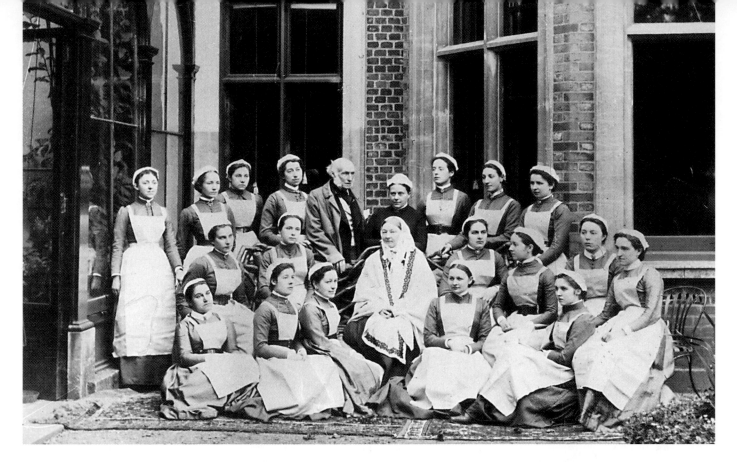

Sir Harry Verney, Florence Nightingale (seated with scarf), and the Nightingale nurse probationers at Claydon in 1886, with Mary Crossland, home sister for the probationers, standing behind Nightingale

out of my 4 maids are not allowed Beer by Doctor's orders. I don't want to forbid it on this festive occasion: but I only want moderation.)

3. I should be extremely obliged to Morey if, with your permission, he will engage a fiddle to come at 7, & play dance music. I don't like to ask Morey to play dance music, but we shall hope to have his music too & Bond's both before & after supper. We hope to have from your house Morey, Julie, Leonard, Phoebe the housemaid, & Bond. And if you would look in upon the festivities, (as I can't) it would more than double their value.[13]

Reconciliation with Aunt Mai

Uncle Sam Smith's health had been failing throughout 1880 and, in early November, he was very ill at Embley; his son Shore was also ill and was being nursed by his wife, Louisa, at Lea Hurst. Uncle Sam died at the end of November at age 86 and, at Aunt Mai's request, received a quiet funeral service. Her uncle's death prompted Nightingale to make peace with Aunt Mai after a 20-year rift.

Nightingale and her aunt had become estranged in 1860 after Aunt Mai left the Burlington Hotel, where she had been taking care of her niece since 1857, and returned to her family at Combe Hurst. Nightingale saw Aunt Mai's departure, which came at one of the most crucial points of her work, as a desertion and a betrayal. For the next 20 years, she refused to communicate directly with her aunt, although she frequently inquired about her in letters to Uncle Sam and other family members. Now Nightingale addressed her letters once again to "dearest Aunt Mai" and signed them "your loving Flo." They quickly resumed their earlier relationship with an affectionate correspondence consisting of philosophical and theosophical discussions.

Amidst the chaos of family illnesses, Uncle Sam's death, and her own infirmity, Nightingale found time to establish a coffee room at the railroad stop of Whatstandwell, near Lea Hurst, because she felt the village workers needed informative reading materials on sanitation and health.[14]

Medical consultation

Although she sometimes felt well enough to take a walk outdoors, Nightingale's health was still poor, for the most part. Her most common symptoms were palpitations, insomnia, headaches, and depression. At the end of 1887, she sought the advice of Dr. Thomas Lauder Brunton, an eminent doctor and lecturer at St. Bartholomew's Hospital in London, for severe joint pain caused by her chronic, debilitating illness.[15] Brunton had first gained recognition in 1867 for his classic paper in the *Lancet*, "On the Use of Nitrite of Amyl in Angina Pectoris."[16]

Nightingale probably became aware of Brunton through her friend Dr. James Paget, who also practiced at St. Bartholomew's and was well aware of her chronic illness. In 1886, Brunton served on the commission reporting on Pasteur's new vaccination treatment for hydrophobia (rabies), and he was the leading authority on chloroform, which was of great interest to Nightingale. As she kept abreast of all the commissions that were being planned for service to India, she must have known about Brunton's appointment in 1889 to the Hyderabad Chloroform Commission. Brunton had prescribed massage for Nightingale's joint pain and, on December 18, she reported to him:

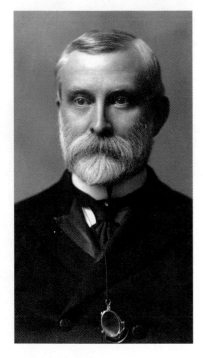

Dr. Thomas L. Brunton, who treated Nightingale for severe joint pain

> ... I have just had my first seance [session] from your Swedish masseuse, Miss Brinck, I arranged with her, thank you, to come down to me every evening at Pine Acres, Sunnydale, [home of Fred Verney, Sir Harry's son] whither I go on Tuesday for two or three weeks. And I hope you will allow me to send for you when I come back. I need your most kind help.
>
> Do you know that I feel doubtful of being able to take the Bromide? I took yesterday the dose in the morning, I was so cold, and my brains so m[ixed] after it that I could hardly do anything. I took one dose of the Comp. Spirit chloroform in the afternoon because I had a heavy appointment. I could scarcely get thro' it. It has never had that effect upon me before...[17]

Many of Brunton's medical lectures at this time focused on diet, exercise, massage, cupping, and bleeding as treatments for various disorders.[18] Nightingale's reference to "Bromide" was potassium bromide, which Brunton commonly prescribed as a sedative. At that time, potassium bromide was also prescribed for epilepsy, tetanus, nymphomania, delirium tremens, and seizures. The compound spirit of chloroform was given orally primarily for painful abdominal disorders and as a sedative.[19]

In addition to the medical therapy and massage, Nightingale also made use of other therapies — what today are commonly called alternative therapies — to help relieve pain, such as singing songs to herself, placing beautiful flowers in her room, opening the windows for fresh air and sunlight, listening to the birds and feeding them, playing with her cats, having occasional visits from close friends and her special nurses to stimulate her mind, and writing long letters to her friends, particularly Benjamin Jowett.

Nightingale's letters reveal that she received enough relief from her massage treatments while at Fred Verney's home to take walks in and outside the house, to sit at the kitchen table and compose a letter, and to marvel at nature.

Deaths of Aunt Mai & Parthe

Nightingale and Parthe's almost daily letters to each other in the late 1880s were filled with affection and focused on routine daily matters, such as the health of various family members. "Only out of bed once these 2 months long enough to have my room 'done,'" Nightingale wrote in April 1888.[20] That same month, Sir Harry fainted at Nightingale's house and she wrote about the incident to Parthe:

> Sir H. was very poorly indeed here this morning and fainted on the floor. I was first in line to catch him — and let him down quite easily and he was not in the least hurt ... please have him rest and keep him perfectly quiet ... for otherwise this might be the beginning of an illness ...[21]

On Parthe's birthday in the same month, she wrote:

> This is the day that gave you to the world. I have not lilacs and baby mums to lay upon your altar as we always had at Embley — Excuse a prosaic £25. I pray God that, in the midst of an intense trial of pain and suffering, heroically home, you have still, dearest Pop, much happiness.[22]

Nightingale's years of severe, chronic joint pain helped her to better understand Parthe's severe rheumatoid arthritis pain, as shown in a December 1888 letter:

> Grieved you are so bad ... I do think of you and Sir Harry with my whole heart to our Father, who is Almighty Love. I don't like the Commandments, it is all, "you shall not, you shall not" till Christ explained them. Negatives never gave love. love to each other and to God. And I don't like the (perpetual) perfection of having no other will but His. That is only another negative — a strong will, to second His: that is the real end and perfection, and I think you do. Dear Pop — I am always thinking of you ...[23]

Aunt Mai, whose health had been failing for some time, died in January 1889. To the Smith family, Nightingale referred to Aunt Mai as "Dearest Friend ... loving, loving soul; humble mind of high and holy thought."[24] And in a private note, she wrote the following tribute:

> Farewell, farewell, our dearest friend
> And it does fare well with thee
> O lovely, lovely soul
> O humble mind of high and holy thoughts
> gone home unto thy Maker
> Unto the high and lofty One that inhabiteth Eternity
> that dwelleth in the high and holy place within them also that are
> of a humble and contrite Spirit
> to thy blessed memory this Cross and Crown
> Mary Smith [25]

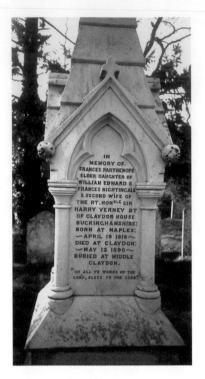

Parthenope's inscription on the Nightingale family grave marker at St. Margaret's Church, East Wellow, Hampshire, written by Florence

This was followed by another private note later that month:

Aunt Mai — born Feb 4 1798 — died at Embley Jan 17 1889. How impressive to me is the belief that every one of us, since our Father constitutes us as the actors in His vast organization, including all that lives and feels, are to be helped not only to be the actors, but to desire with all our hearts to serve God's ends in that organization. Of all the best, most humane people how few, it seems to me, feel continuously this connection with the Father — more perhaps in past times. Yet God will lead us to its being so for us all — Farewell, dear friend for today — A change may go on as it has done so gradually, or quickly bring the last change in this world. "Is there any final farewell?" asks Walt Whitman. "None" we will answer with grateful hearts.[26]

By early 1889, Parthe was also extremely ill and Nightingale was overwhelmed with removing the last of the family's personal belongings from the Embley estate. She wrote to Sir Harry:

Your letters are very precious to me — How often I think of those first two verses of Romans XII, where first he "beseeches" us, not from fear but "by the mercies of God," to give ourselves a living sacrifice, holy, acceptable unto God; our reasonable service. And then he goes on to ask himself to be acceptable to God — whether He is acceptable to us — prove, he says, what is that — good & acceptable & perfect will of God — And then he reminds himself & us that even this we cannot do without having our minds renewed, & being transformed. So we must ask that Almighty Love will come & dwell in us — & watch for the answer. I will not write any more today — My mind is very full of you & Parthe. But Embley makes it over full. Parthe will tell you ... I am afraid Parthe is very suffering.[27]

Parthe's last year was filled with great physical pain, but she was mentally alert and strong until the end. The two sisters last saw each other on Sunday, May 4, 1890, when Parthe was carried into Nightingale's room at South Street. A week later, on May 12, 1890 — Nightingale's 70th birthday — Parthe died at Claydon. The Nightingale family marker at St. Margaret's Church in Hampshire indicates that she was buried at Claydon.

Although she reduced her workload in the 1880s and 1890s, Nightingale still took an active interest in nursing matters — particularly the controvery over nurses' registration — and the politics of the growing Indian nationalist movement. Old age was no impediment to her correspondence and other efforts on behalf of issues that were important to her.

Chapter 18

The Birth of Indian Nationalism

*W*e are watching the birth of a new nationality in the oldest civilisation in the world ... How critical will be its [the Indian National Congress's] first meeting at Poona. I bid it God-speed with all my heart.

— *Florence Nightingale to Sir William Wedderburn, September 27, 1885*[1]

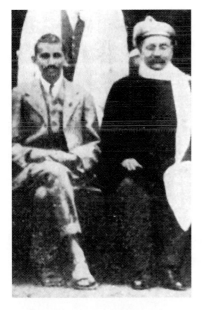

Mohandas K. Gandhi (left) and Gopal Krishna Gokhale, two of India's early Nationalist leaders, in South Africa in 1912 (detail of photograph on page 371)

Although Nightingale suffered many personal trials and the deaths of loved ones and friends in the 1870s and 1880s, she never forgot about the pain and suffering of the Indian people. From her bedroom window overlooking the Dorchester gardens, she may have been struck by the contrast between the privileged gentry promenading under her window and the impoverished people of India, particularly in the villages, who were enduring physical and political hardships exacerbated by the British government. She did not ask why there was poverty but how it could be overcome.

Since 1862, while continuing to work for improvements for British soldiers and their wives and children at British military stations in India, Nightingale had also tried to use existing political frameworks to improve civil sanitation at the local level. The traditional village ruling council, known as the Panchayat, consisted of five or more elected adult men representing the major castes in each village. Nightingale envisioned that the head men in each village could be empowered to educate villagers on sanitary issues and improve sanitation. She continued to campaign for elimination of landowners' abuse of the *ryots,* the tenant farmers who lived in poverty and starved by the millions during famines.

Practical education

Before there were enough educated young Indians working in India, Nightingale corresponded with anyone who had practical ideas and was interested in furthering the education of the Indian people. For years, she had prodded the British government to give top priority to India and its problems. She recommended an official corps of agricultural advisors and the establishment of agricultural colleges and model farms that would be directed by well-paid Indians.

As was her modus operandi, she became a master networker, bringing together people who might synergistically make change happen at the local level in India. For instance, she introduced W. R. Robertson, Principal of the Agriculture College and Superintendent of the Government Farm at Sydapor, to the provincial governor. Her understanding of the complexities of the Indian people, their nationalities and religions, and the British government's refusal to recognize the problems in India are evident in a letter to her brother-in-law, Sir Harry Verney, in November 1880:

> ... *Mr. Robertson was not only "in command" of that Farm, Agriculture College, and Institution, and had practical & moral knowledge of his Students, Brahmins, Pandoors & others — of their abilities, caste, prejudices, and the way they manage them & turn them to good — also of the people & agriculture of Madras — but he has Government agriculture tours in Comibalore, Bombay Presidency & elsewhere. He knows the state of the land & people of Southern India.*
>
> *There is perhaps one who could give His Excellency the Governor more intimate information as to the causes of deterioration of the land as to the ways by which the attention of the native "Gentlefolks," or the higher class of Cultivators or of the class which now all "runs" to Government clerkships, could be called to the improvement of their lands ... None into making them good farmers, good landlords or landlord agents, none into making them "better" the main industry of India Agriculture. And the 9 tenths who fail in becoming Government clerks become Home Ruler and write seditious nonsense in native newspapers in India.[2]*

By 1882, Nightingale was glad to see some progress made; candidates selected for the Indian Civil Service were offered a year's training at Oxford. Unfortunately, most of these students still received the typical classics-oriented education rather than a practical education that would have a direct impact on improving the life of Indian villagers.

At Nightingale's insistence, Benjamin Jowett, then Master at Balliol College, who had been involved in Indian Civil Service affairs since the 1850s, established classes following her specific curriculum. She impressed upon Arnold Toynbee, the Balliol College tutor whom Jowett had assigned to students interested in Indian affairs and those undertaking Indian Civil Service appointments, that if the students were to make a difference as true missionaries to India's millions, they needed to learn agriculture, chemistry, botany, and geology to promote soil conservation and water supply. Her list also included forestry to better understand fuel and rainfall as well as animal physiology to learn about cattle diseases, breeds, and fodder.

Hardening attitudes

Nightingale and her colleagues encountered growing resistance to their efforts to improve the lot of the common people. The rigidity of British attitudes toward the people of India in the aftermath of the 1857 mutiny was inexorable and pervasive. Nightingale deplored the new British attitude of racial superiority, which increasingly alienated India's millions of darker-skinned people.

Gone were the informal days of the first half of the century when British officials serving in the Indian Civil Service, usually unmarried and almost a 6-month sail from home, had more daily interaction with Indians. The old patronage system had produced a superior civil servant — the Lawrences, Freres, and Trevelyans — who improved the lives of India's masses. These men were steeped in the Benthamite ideals of reform taught at Haileybury College, the East India Company's own training school.

However, the new generation of Indian Civil Service officials reflected a new political attitude. They had gained their positions by the competitive civil service examinations and were educated at different colleges after Haileybury closed in 1859; they tended to be politically conservative and shared neither the earlier group's values nor their breadth of vision and experience gained in the frontier wars. As steamships reduced the travel time home to a matter of weeks, more English women and children arrived in India to join their husbands and fathers. As a result, British officials spent more time with their families and in their clubs, and grew more detached from the natives.

With the rise of a classic colonial economy, India became an exporter of raw goods and an importer of English manufactured items. Before 1800, India had been the largest exporter of finished cotton fabrics in the world; now only cotton bales were shipped, and natives were clothed in Lancashire-produced goods. Local village weaving and other handicrafts vanished as railroads delivered cheap manufactured goods from England. The economic benefits of cotton exports and tea plantations — and the fact that investment bonds in India brought a higher return in London than any other similar instruments — led Indian government officials to promote improvements that would benefit business interests: roads, expanded railroads, irrigation, commercial agriculture instead of food crops, and policies that favored British manufacturers.

As more entrepreneurs, planters, and managers appeared in India, they combined with the common soldiers to form a group of lower class Britons who had little sympathy for native customs and often abused and insulted the Indians, a problem recognized with increasing alarm by responsible higher officials. The native Indians, whether local aristocrats or village rice growers, found themselves treated with increasing contempt while subjected to worsening economic conditions. Nightingale was among the small number of English reformers who supported the emerging political developments that would eventually lead to self-rule in India.

The seeds of self-rule

Following the postmutiny transfer of power to the British government in 1858, many educated young Indians sought employment in the Indian Civil Service and in the professions of journalism, law, and education. Increasing numbers graduated from the universities in Bombay, Calcutta, and Madras, which the East India Company had established in 1857 for the purpose of providing an English education.

Like Nightingale and their British mentors, these politically ambitious, Western-educated Indians were reared on the reform ideas of Jeremy Bentham and utilitarianism. They were also steeped in the political philosophy of proportional representation and parliamentary reform developed by John Stuart Mill, who headed the examiner's office of the East India Company until his retirement in 1858. Following their apprenticeships and formal education, these latent nationalists were convinced that they could eventually make a difference in the British Indian government.

However, in the aftermath of the mutiny, British bureaucrats devised ingenious ways to bar Indians from permanent "covenanted" positions in the Civil Service, so called because the appointee signed a covenant to perform faithfully and honestly. These positions were the key to promotion and pay raises. Another obstacle was that the open qualifying examinations for the Civil Service, begun in 1853, were given only in London. For Hindus, such a journey would be not only a physical and financial burden, but also a violation of caste rules, which forbade travel to the land of Untouchables. As a result, only 12 Indians joined the Service between 1861 and 1885; from 1886 to 1910, there were only 68 Indians compared to 1,235 Europeans. Only in 1920 was the examination finally held in India as well as London. The only Civil Service jobs truly open to Indians and other non-British nationals were "uncovenanted" positions (later termed the Provincial Civil Service), temporary slots whose holders were poorly paid and could be fired without cause.

The Indian Civil Service was the exclusive ruler of the subcontinent. At its head was the Viceroy, followed by the governors and commissioners; fanned out across India were the roughly 1,500 covenanted district officers, who were all-powerful as civil authorities, revenue assessors and collectors, magistrates, and judges. In the background was the reorganized Indian army, capable of quickly quelling any civil unrest or violence. The revenues for the Indian government derived from India, and the civil service was responsible to no constituency save its own bureaucracy. Excluded from their own governance except in menial positions, native Indians of all religions now had a common oppressor, the British government, and a common cause, Indian self-government.

Key early players

During the 1870s and 1880s, Nightingale followed the work of the early Indian nationalist leaders and the sympathetic Anglo-Indians (British residents in India), who promoted the formation of provincial political associations. She hoped that they would share her view of what the country needed and begin to define a practical path for India.

Banerjea, Ranade, Gokhale, and Tilak

One of the first graduates to pass the Indian Civil Service examination was a brilliant man named Surendranath Banerjea (1848-1925), who was unfairly dismissed for what was later acknowledged to be insufficient cause. He became a Calcutta college teacher and editor of *The Bengalee* and founded the Indian Association in Calcutta. Nightingale approved of the Indian Association because she believed it was essential to the improvement of the plight of the peasants. Also, it provided a political alternative to Bengal's professional elites and the large landholders who resisted rent and tenure reform.[3]

In 1883, Banerjea convened the first Indian National Conference in Bengal. He would later receive national acclaim as the leader of the *swadeshi* ("of our own country") movement, which promoted the use of Indian-made goods and the boycott of British-manufactured products.

THE BIRTH OF INDIAN NATIONALISM

On the other side of India, Mahadev G. Ranade (1849-1901) founded the Poona Sarvajanik Sabha (Poona Public Society) in 1870. The Sabha was a true grassroots organization; each member had to gather the assent of 60 people to speak for them in public affairs. After graduating with honors from Bombay University, Ranade was employed in the educational department of Bombay, taught at Elphinstone College, wrote historical and other essays, edited the magazine *Indu Prakash,* and helped start the Hindu reformist Prarthana Samaj (Prayer Society) in Bombay. He later became a barrister and was appointed to the Bombay High Court.

Ranade's brilliant disciple was Gopal Krishna Gokhale (1866-1915), whom Nightingale would meet in 1897 and with whom she shared many interests. Gokhale, who had earned a degree in mathematics and received the best in English education, was noted for his excellent written and spoken English. Although he passed the law examination in 1885, Gokhale decided to join the New English School in Poona as an assistant master. He and the other staff members, styling themselves as "Indian Jesuits," had a missionary zeal to bring English education to the Indian people. Gokhale started as a lecturer in English literature but later taught mathematics and then history and political economy.

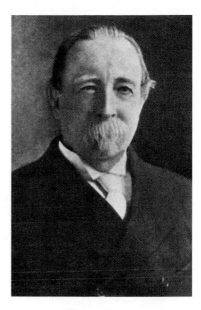

A.O. Hume (1829-1912), the "father" of the Indian National Congress, whose efforts on behalf of the Indian cause Nightingale supported

Both Nightingale and Gokhale had authored best-selling books at a young age. Her most successful book had been *Notes on Nursing,* his a mathematics text for high school students that was reprinted by Macmillan Company in 1896. Like Nightingale, he was an avid and accomplished statistician who pored over statistical tables and government documents. His fine memory and study of economics, statistics, and history gave him great insight into India's contemporary problems, and his speeches and articles revealed great precision, analysis, and suggestions for reform.

Another early reformer was Bal Gangadhar Tilak (1856-1920), who represented the more radical stance against British rule. Tilak had no faith in British government and agitated against it and in favor of restoring swaraj ("self-rule") to India. He was the most popular journalist in Poona and became the leading literary thorn in Britain's side with his vernacular newspaper *Kesari* ("Lion"). He exhorted Indian nationalists to take an interest and pride in their cultural, religious, and martial history and brought many non-English–educated Hindus into the nationalist movement. However, Tilak's orthodox Hindu character and his revolutionary approach alienated many Indian Muslims, which exacerbated tensions between the two groups. When he was jailed in 1897 for his writings encouraging orthodox Hinduism and Maratha history as the sources for Indian nationalism, he became known as Lokamanya ("Revered by the People").

Allan Octavian Hume

Early on, the nationalist movement also attracted two forward-thinking Britons: Allan Octavian Hume and Sir William Wedderburn. Nightingale had much in common with Hume (1829-1912), a wealthy man who was the son of an English radical politician. Educated at Haileybury College and London University, Hume joined the Indian Civil Service at the age of 20 and was appointed the Etawah district officer in the North-West province in 1849. He distinguished himself during the 1857 Mutiny and was awarded the Commander of the Bath in 1860.

In 1870, the Viceroy, Lord Mayo, appointed Hume secretary to the Revenue and Agriculture Department of the central government. Because his radical opinions were disagreeable to many officials, Hume was removed from this position in 1879 and sent back to his former post, where he remained active until his retirement in 1882. He later lived in Simla, studying birds and theosophy.

Hume joined the Theosophical Society in London in 1881 and found strong links between the principles of theosophy and Indian philosophy, as did many young Indian nationalists. The Russian-born cofounder of the Theosophical Society, Helena Blavatsky, went to India in 1879, where she became a disciple of the Swami Dayananda Sarasvati (1824-1883). The swami called upon Hindus to return to the original purity of Vedic life and thought — "back to the Vedas" — and to reject such corrupting ancient practices as the caste system, idolatry, and infant marriage. His reformist Hindu society, the Arya Samaj, founded in Bombay in 1875, finally took root at the start of the 1900s and became the leading nationalist organization. Blavatsky soon left to start her own prayer society outside of Madras city. The most famous leader of the Theosophical Society, the Englishwoman Annie Besant (1847-1933), succeeded Blavatsky and, in 1917, became the first and only British woman to serve as president of the Indian National Congress.

By the end of his career, Hume was convinced that India needed its own parliamentary system. On March 1, 1883, he wrote a letter to the graduates of Calcutta University, whom he called the "salt of the land," encouraging them to push for greater economic freedom and management of their own country. He also recognized the need for a representative body of educated Indians to serve as the voice of the Indian masses. In this undertaking, Hume received great support from his colleague, Wedderburn. Under Hume's guidance and with his financial support, this representative body eventually became the Indian National Congress. Hume not only helped form the Congress but was the only official British delegate to the first session in 1885.

Sir William Wedderburn

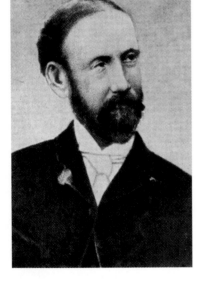

Sir William Wedderburn (1838-1918), the respected and successful Indian civil servant who started the Indian Parliamentary Committee in London in 1893, and with whom Nightingale worked directly from 1885 until her last years

Sir William Wedderburn (1838-1918) began his professional career in the Indian Civil Service in 1860 at age 23. His father, Sir John Wedderburn, was the retired Accountant General in Bombay. Young Wedderburn held many administrative and judicial posts: a secretary to the government of India, Judicial Commissioner of Sind, Judge of the Bombay High Court, and member of the Governor's Council. Like Nightingale, Wedderburn constantly sought out plans to improve the life of the rural poor, such as working for the education of girls. As Indian leaders became aware of his interests in Indian affairs, they began to befriend him. In 1885, he presided over a meeting in Poona, which decided to organize the Deccan Education Sabha. He befriended the Hindu Indian nationalist leader, Ranade, and the Parsi leader Dadabhai Naoroji. Both were freedom fighters and liberal thinkers who commanded the respect of their countrymen and provided continuity in leadership.

Upon his early retirement and return to England in 1887, Wedderburn (a baronet) could have settled for a life of leisure. However, he decided to take up the Indian cause. He had seen the problems and poverty in India, befriended many educated Indians, and

THE BIRTH OF INDIAN NATIONALISM

lost patience with his increasingly conservative colleagues in the Indian Civil Service. He opted to support his friend Hume and the work of the British Parliamentary Committee of the Indian National Congress in London. For his efforts, he was invited to preside over the fifth session of the Indian National Congress in 1889.

Lord Ripon at the helm

When William Gladstone returned as Prime Minister in 1880, he brought back from retirement Nightingale's ally of past years, Lord Ripon (George Frederick Samuel Robinson, also Lord de Grey, a double title inherited after the deaths of his father and uncle), and appointed him Viceroy of India. His appointment once again gave Nightingale hope because Ripon, while at the War Office, had supported her reform ideas and was known for his ability to get things done. Ripon was sympathetic to the educated young Indians and their desire for more involvement in local governments. Like Nightingale, his work was driven by a spiritual core.

Nightingale had recommended that Ripon take Gen. Charles George Gordon to India as his private secretary because she thought that Gordon would be able to deal with the contentious Anglo-Indian community. She was impressed with this mystical "Bible-Soldier" who had fought bravely in the Crimean War and had earned the nickname "Chinese Gordon" for his role in the Taiping Rebellion in the early 1860s. During the 1880s, Gordon kept Nightingale informed about conditions at the various military outposts to which he was stationed.

As soon as he arrived in Bombay, Gordon wrote to Nightingale, confirming the hardening attitudes of some high-level British officials who he thought had little sympathy for the Indian people, hated their jobs, and wished to work only until they qualified for a pension. He noted that the old-style official:

> ... was bound in some way to consider the sympathies of the natives. The governors are [now] sent out for reward for services in England, often they are physically unfit for the country. India is a pasture land for them. They are too high in rank, too imbued with the idea that things will last their time.[4]

Gordon abhorred the new patronizing attitudes he encountered in the administration and resigned within weeks of arriving in Bombay.

Exerting influence from London

During Ripon's viceroyalty, Nightingale wrote him many letters asking him to institute better management and ward training at India's military station hospitals. Patient care at these hospitals was still carried out primarily by untrained military orderlies who oversaw the work of equally untrained coolies who did the actual care — if any was done at all.

In April 1881, Nightingale reminded Ripon about the deplorable conditions outlined in the 1863 *Report of the Royal Commission on the Sanitary State of the Army in India* and urged him to ensure that all the military hospitals in India were supplied with properly trained attendants and cooks:

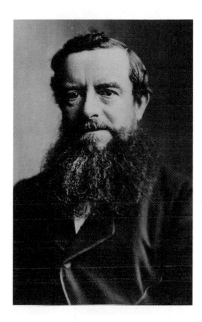

Lord Ripon (1827-1909), Viceroy of India from 1880 to 1884, a Nightingale supporter and lifelong reformer

The orderlies that did the actual nursing had no accountability for anything and had no supervision. The ward coolies or nurses ... had no uniforms or decent places to rest or sleep. The wants of the present system, or no system, of Hospital attendance in India were so enormous: the name even of Nursing was such a farce: the ward coolies who are the Nurses at 4 rupees a month & are not even enlisted — any day they may desert — seem there merely to be "kicked" [coolies were often literally kicked and abused] by the European soldier, who ... didn't know the coolies wear no uniform, & cannot be recognized in the Bazaar if they abscond, which they are always doing.

There is absolutely no supervision of these Nurses: When the Medical Officer is not there the Indian Hospital is deserted. You hear, Coolie! Coolie! Coolie! called but no Coolie is there ... But when in the Wards the Coolie Nurse seems to be there only to be gentle & to be "kicked." This is the real state of things in a Military Hospital in India in time of peace ... These Ward Coolies or Nurses may be children of 10, old men of 80, crippled, blind; in short any one who will come for 4 rupees a month. No other inducement is given: no promotion; no reward; no good conduct pay; no increase of pay for long service; no camp equipage. The Nurses lie for shelter under the walls of the Hospital tents during the bitter cold nights. In a cholera camp in the monsoon they are sometimes roasted & sometimes drowned.

In a word, there is no training of native Hospital servants, no ranking, no uniform, no supervision, no responsibility, no organization, & very little pay: of course, no esprit de corps ... Nursing is the worst ... in any existing Army & threatens often to become no Nursing at all. The cooking is as bad. But all this will now be altered by your beneficent arrangements ... I ask the favor ... for you to send me the further arrangements and particulars of your new Army Hospital Corps. May I remind you of the Recommendations 26, 27, 28 of the R. Commission on the Sanitary State of the Army in India, of which Sidney Herbert first & Lord Stanley (Lord Derby) next were the head & which reported in 1863 ... May God speed your great, your immense work in India, with 200 million of our fellow creatures. May its difficulty be your opportunity. I cannot say what I feel about this ...[5]

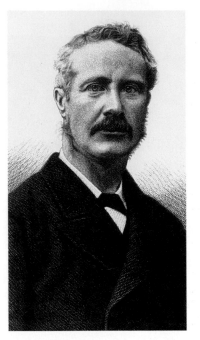

Gen. Charles George Gordon (1833-1885), who began a friendship with Nightingale in 1880 before being posted to India as private secretary to the new Viceroy, Lord Ripon

Nightingale's entreaties failed to bring about the desired changes, but her concern didn't abate; she continued to discuss these ideas with Sir Frederick Roberts, the newly named Commander-in-Chief of the army in Madras. Appointees continued to call on Nightingale to benefit from her expertise. Roberts came to her in 1881, en route to his new post, to get information on the introduction of female nurses in India. Sir Mountstuart Grant Duffy also called on her before he left for his post as Governor of Madras.

The Ilbert Bill

In 1883, Ripon's government introduced the Ilbert Bill, aimed at empowering Indian judges to try Europeans for criminal offenses. The bill quickly ignited a firestorm of protest; British and European planters, and virtually the entire Indian Civil Service, unanimously opposed the proposal.

The sponsor of the bill, Sir Courtney P. Ilbert, a former student of Jowett at Balliol College, had visited Nightingale to discuss his proposed legislation before sailing for India as a judicial member of Ripon's Executive Council. The early signs of demand for self-rule and legislative and judicial reform prompted strident editorials against the bill in the British press, which caused an uproar.

Nightingale was one of Ilbert's key supporters in England, and she also rallied support among her allies in India. Although she refused to join pro–Ilbert Bill committees, she did write many private letters to key prominent Liberal party leaders in support of the bill. She wrote to Gladstone praising Ripon's administration and asking the Prime Minister to put more emphasis on India in his speeches. Gladstone sent her a cordial reply, promising that he would forward her recommendations to the India Council.

Ripon felt the heat of the controversy over the Ilbert Bill and kept Nightingale informed. She urged him not to succumb to the raging storm around him, and he assured her that he would stand firm. Both recognized, as did native Indians, that the opposition to the Ilbert Bill was not only racially motivated but also an attempt to block equal-employment opportunities for Indians and progress toward self-rule. This "white mutiny" was a valuable lesson for the Bengali Hindu intellectuals because they saw the attention gained from effective, well-organized agitation for grievances in street demonstrations and printed protests.

In July 1883, Nightingale's paper, "The Dumb Shall Speak, and the Deaf Shall Hear; or, the Ryot, the Zemindar, and the Government," was read by Sir Harry Verney's son, Fred Verney, at a meeting of the East India Association chaired by Sir Bartle Frere. It was later printed in a journal of the East India Association and also as a pamphlet. In August 1883, the magazine *Nineteenth Century* published her article "Our Indian Stewardship," a defense of Ripon's progressive policy. She had received much help with this paper from her loyal Anglo-Indian colleague, Sir William Wedderburn; in fact, she considered it more his paper than hers. On its publication, she wrote him the following note, longing for the same anonymity as her cats, whose paw marks sometimes could be found on her papers:

> *The more you are so kind as to correct and alter, the better pleased I shall be. Please do not let me be impertinent to the India Office, nor to the departments. It is so very unbecoming of me to be governessing the government. I feel inclined to sign myself "Cat Paw."*[6]

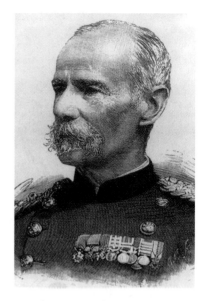

Sir Frederick Sleigh Roberts (1832-1894), reform-minded Commander-in-Chief of the Madras army, and later the Indian army, one of many British officials who stopped to consult with Nightingale before taking up positions in India

Changing of the guard

The Ilbert Bill finally passed in January 1884 with the modification that Europeans tried by certain native judges should have the right to trial by jury, of which half were European. Nightingale felt that Ripon had done the right thing by agreeing to the compromise. However, feeling fierce opposition, Ripon no longer considered himself effective and decided to resign before his term was over. Despite conservative opposition to his liberal views, Ripon was able to push through land reform bills in the Bengal and Oudh provinces, ensuring the peasants' protection from landowners. Nightingale was also pleased with Ripon's establishment of the Agricultural Department in Bengal and his backing of local self-government legislation.

In 1884, Nightingale was greatly saddened by the death of Sir Bartle Frere, one of her most trusted and valued friends who had brought so many good people to her doorstep. With his passing, she saw more of her connections to India fading away but she still continued to work behind the scenes.

In December 1884, Lord Dufferin replaced Ripon as Viceroy. Before his departure for India, Dufferin made an appointment to be briefed by Nightingale. In preparation for their meeting, Nightingale wrote an urgent note to Dr. John Sutherland on a Friday, asking for papers on certain sanitary matters from him by Monday. However, since the 1883 discovery of the cholera bacillus by German scientist Robert Koch, Sutherland had been studying the organism. Not intimidated by Nightingale, he informed her that he would be occupied the entire weekend and thus the Viceroy must wait. Her retort: "If you did a little on Sunday, the Recording Angel would drop not a tear but a smile."[7] Sutherland countered that if Dr. Koch's cholera bacillus turned out well, this knowledge would save more lives than Dufferin. Nightingale and the Viceroy waited.

In the end, Dufferin's trip was delayed by several days, and Nightingale and Sutherland had time to collaborate on a formidable list of priorities for the new viceroy. Dufferin was the fourth viceroy whom Nightingale educated on Indian problems, such as sanitation in and near army military stations as well as irrigation, land tenure, civil service, and agriculture. In his first letter to her en route to India, he expressed his gratitude for the briefing: "... one of the pleasantest 'sweets of Office' I have yet tasted has been the privilege I acquired of coming to pay you that little visit."[8]

Nightingale was particularly pleased with Dufferin's wife. When Lady Dufferin reached India and began to see the country's problems, her own experience confirmed what Nightingale had told her about the need for sanitation and sanitary education in the villages. Compelled by a strong sense of duty to help the people of India, Lady Dufferin founded the National Association for Supplying Medical Aid to the Women of India; she even studied several Indian languages and wrote a few short papers on sanitation that were translated for distribution to the village women.

With Sutherland's assistance, Nightingale began sending books to Lady Dufferin for use in her village education work. The work was extremely difficult because few villagers could either read or write, each village had its own grammar and literature, and there were over 200 dialects. Although Lady Dufferin and Nightingale had good intentions, their efforts with these translations had little immediate effects. Even so, their ideas of grassroots reform were far ahead of their time.

Continuing the sanitary agenda

Nightingale, true to form, appealed to Dufferin to implement the reforms outlined by the Indian Sanitation Commission of 1865. In August 1887, a proposal she had first presented to Sir John Lawrence 22 years earlier finally became a reality. The government of India sanctioned the employment of female nurses in military hospitals at Umballa and Rawalpindi, with a female superintendent of nursing and 18 nurses at each hospital. The Surgeon General, Arthur Payne, consulted with Nightingale before he made the final nurse selections.

Although Nightingale had lost some of her powerful allies on India affairs, she believed that the time was ripe again to lobby for a sanitary department for India as long as she still knew a few people in power. With her usual zeal, she began consulting with her influential friends, starting with Ripon. She had also been corresponding with Sir

Harry Cunningham, a nephew of Sir Harry Verney, on legislative reform matters. As a judge of the High Court of Calcutta, Cunningham had been active in sanitation matters for the city, which had the largest population of any city in India. He prepared a policy memorandum, and Sir Henry Yule, a Nightingale ally who had replaced Sir Bartle Frere on the Indian Sanitary Council in London, wrote another. Nightingale's contributions to these two memoranda are evident. She also continued to meet with Anglo-Indians returning to England after retiring from the Indian Civil Service.

Assessing Dufferin's effect

After 1885, Dufferin kept Nightingale informed about his efforts on behalf of sanitary reforms and other matters. By 1887, his frustration over the lack of cooperation from district and province officials in solving local sanitation problems was evident in his letters to Nightingale. However, he persisted, urged on by her optimism and faith in God. Finally, in July 1888, the Indian government created a sanitary board in each province with a mandate for the local authorities to inform the Indian government about sanitary progress in written reports to the executive agencies.

When Lord and Lady Dufferin left India at the end of his term in 1888, they left behind improvements in irrigation and water purity. Dufferin wrote to Nightingale about the 1888 Annual Report of Sanitary Measures in India, which contained the history of the movement that was launched in her second Royal Commission Report in 1863 and was full of the "Nightingale influence."

Dufferin was succeeded by Lord Lansdowne (Henry Charles Keith Fitzmaurice), who had been one of Benjamin Jowett's favorite students at Oxford. In March 1888, Jowett had the honor of introducing the new viceroy to both Nightingale and Ripon. Jowett sent Nightingale a note that he had received from Lansdowne, asking her to write in simple words the principal issues which he should address and the titles of some books that he should read.[9]

Before Lansdowne left for India, he met with Nightingale twice to discuss Indian affairs, particularly sanitation. Jowett had told her that she had the ability to educate him to be the best viceroy ever — the fifth to receive her instructions and to benefit from her historical perspective regarding improvements in India's army barracks, sanitation, and other matters related to its military stations and their nearby villages.

The National Congress convenes

During his Viceroyalty, Ripon had written to Gladstone, then Prime Minister, that a new era was dawning in India in which "new ideas are springing up; new aspirations are being called out; and a process has begun which will go on with increasing rapidity from year to year."[10] Ripon urged the government to approve advances in local self-government, which would be followed by steps toward representative councils at the provincial and national levels. Because the British government was reluctant to grant these concessions, more Indian nationalists and educated Indians began to claim their voice in Indian affairs, which eventually led to the first Indian National Congress in 1885.

Many members of Parliament opposed the growing fervor for self-government in India. However, Nightingale became one of its earliest and most ardent supporters; her work wasn't for political gain but for social and administrative progress. Nightingale, the futurist, believed that the formation of the Indian National Congress was the beginning of an India independent of Britain. Enthused, she wrote to Sir William Wedderburn, who was to attend the inaugural session of the Indian National Congress:

> This National Liberal Union (one of the names suggested), if it keeps straight, seems altogether the matter of great[est] interest that has happened in India, if it make progress, for a hundred years. We are watching the birth of a new nationality in the oldest civilisation in the world. How critical will be its first meeting in Poona! I bid it God-speed with all my heart.[11]

A.O. Hume, along with prominent professional Hindus, convened the first National Congress in Bombay on December 28, 1885. (The site had been changed because of a cholera epidemic in Poona.) Hume was the only official British delegate, although Wedderburn attended as an observer. Every province of British India was represented, including 73 official representatives and 10 unofficial delegates; 54 delegates were Hindus (nearly all Brahmans), two were Muslims, and the rest were Parsis and Jains — the most recognized religions of India. All spoke English; more than half were lawyers with the rest of the delegates composed of businessmen, landowners, professors, and journalists.

This first Congress was dedicated to peaceful political action; it passed resolutions calling for economic and political change. One such resolution called for the election of unofficial representatives to the provincial and supreme legislative councils. Another aim was to give Indians an equal chance to enter the Indian Civil Service in covenanted positions by requiring that examinations be given in India as well as Britain.

By 1881, it was obvious that the British meant to exclude Indians from permanent, higher-paying Civil Service jobs: the number of covenanted civil servants had shrunk to 873 — nearly all British — and the number of uncovenanted, or provincial, had risen to 4,082, mostly Indian. The Congress also called for reduction of "home charges," which included the entire India Office budget, the pensions of British officials living in India, military expenditures, and administrative expenses. Dadabhai Naoroji (1825-1917), the "grand old man" and eventual three-time president of the Indian National Congress, argued for the popular economic "drain argument," which blamed India's poverty on British exploitation of the colony's raw materials, gold, and silver. His support increased nationalist fervor in the Congress.

Most Britons in India and in England ignored the demands of the first Congress and believed this group was a minority and didn't represent the diversity of the Indian millions. However, support for the Congress increased and within 2 years there were 600 delegates. In 1888, on the eve of his departure from India, although Lord Dufferin dismissed the group as still a minority voice of India, there were 1,243 delegates at the third annual Congress.

The great significance of the first Congress was that it marked the beginning of the idea of Indian national unity and the emergence of a unified national consciousness, whereas before there had existed only local or provincial political, religious, or other interests. There was no hint of disloyalty to the British, although the Indian delegates called for major changes.

A problem that the Congress never solved was its inability to attract Muslims, who were outnumbered six-to-one by Hindus, and who soon realized that they had fallen behind in a critical area — that because of their inadequate education, their needs and views weren't being represented. Attacks by Hindu reformers against important Muslim issues, such as religious conversion and cow killing, further increased their fears of being poorly represented. Many Muslims saw loyalty to the British government as better than working with the Congress leaders. Extreme diversity among India's Muslims presented a further obstacle to their working in a cohesive manner. Not until the turn of the century would the Congress emerge as an all-India political organization. The arrogance and indifference of another viceroy, Lord Curzon (1899-1904), would fuel the fire of Indian nationalism.

Following the first meeting of the Indian National Congress, an Indian newspaper commented hopefully that Wedderburn's presence at the first Congress was a guarantee that the people's voice would be heard. However, not everyone in England had the same high hopes that the paper and Nightingale held for Wedderburn's rapport with Indian political reformers and the Congress. Lord Randolph Churchill, then the Secretary of State for India and father of Winston Churchill, informed Dufferin that Wedderburn couldn't be given a permanent seat on the bench of the Bombay High Court because he was a political incendiary and difficult to work with. Ultimately foiled after serving 27 years in the Indian Civil Service, Wedderburn sought early retirement at age 50 and returned to England in 1887.

Instead of retiring, though, Wedderburn met with Nightingale and joined the fight alongside Hume. In 1888, Nightingale met with Hume and several others who felt the need for establishing a committee to represent the Congress in London. In 1889, the British Committee of the Indian National Congress became a reality with Wedderburn as chairperson and the driving spirit of the group; their journal *India* reported their work. For his efforts, Wedderburn was invited in 1889 to preside over the fifth session of the Indian National Congress.

Supporting the pioneers

Nightingale was kept informed by Indian nationalists and Anglo-Indians alike, who corresponded with her on Indian reform or came to visit her before they took their Indian assignments or when they returned to England on leave. One important visitor was P. K. Sen, a young Indian lawyer and leader in rent law reform, who was determined to devote his life to "giving the people practical education and teaching to improve methods of agriculture."[12] She also received correspondence from Calcutta lawyers, such as Surendranath Banerjea, who convened public meetings to advance rent-law reform and the problems faced by tenant farmers.[13] There was much opposition in Parliament to this fervor for self-government in India. However, Nightingale believed in the future of India as these activists took their first steps toward greater representation and a more meaningful role in their own civic affairs.

In a letter to Sir Harry Verney in April 1888, Nightingale voiced frustration over the frequent changes in government; with each turnover of leadership, the new political party had its own administrative agenda and seldom moved forward on reforms started in the previous administration. She warned that delays in government policy and action would in no way slow the rising Indian nationalist movement:

> [We can] say we will take up such & such measures or not as we please — & when we please. We might just as well say we will turn back the rising tide in the Atlantic.
>
> Everyone of the measures that has caused such out-cries has come from the Govt. of India in the course of business. It could not be turned back. Besides, India is no longer a "geographical expression." She is becoming a nationality (see e.g., the 3 National Congresses). We have done this unwittingly.
>
> He will be the wise Viceroy who will give to the reasonable aspiration of the educated Hindoos a wise satisfaction — in reasonable time before it is too late ... There are 188 million Hindoos to 30 millions Mahometans, 27 millions Buddhists, Sikhs, Parsees all together ...[14]

Following Dr. John Sutherland's retirement from the Army Sanitary Committee in June 1888, Nightingale was concerned that this loss of a paid member and friend on the committee would hinder the progress that had been made in army barrack sanitation improvements. She sought advice from her former colleague Sir Douglas Galton, who was on the committee. However, he had many responsibilities as well as a hectic travel schedule and often couldn't fulfill her requests or answer her questions. Despite Nightingale's efforts, there was no replacement for Sutherland on the Sanitary Committee until 1890 when the Committee was reorganized. Galton remained a member, Dr. J. Marston was appointed as the new paid member to succeed Sutherland, and Surgeon General J.W. Cunningham, the former Sanitary Commissioner with the government of India, was named as the Indian expert on the committee. J. J. Frederick at the War Office, Nightingale's friend from the post-Crimean years, retained his post as Secretary.

Although the Bombay Village Sanitation Act passed in early 1889, Nightingale and other proponents of India reform realized that work remained to enforce the recommendations for proper sanitation. As usual, she continued to draft articles, letters, and her gospel on Health Missionaries for Rural India. In February 1889, her letter to the Joint Secretaries of the Bombay Presidency Association on the Bombay Village Sanitation Bill was printed. On April 5, 1889, a similar letter addressed to the Joint Secretaries of the Poona Sarvajanik Sabha was printed in the *Bombay Gazette Summary*.

Events were taking shape on several fronts important to Nightingale. During the summer of 1891, at age 71, she helped to organize the festivities for the Indian delegation arriving for the fifth International Congress of Hygiene and Demography to be held in London. With Galton as chairman of the organizing committee, she had no difficulty getting him to organize an Indian section. The Native Association in Bombay submitted papers and representatives at her request. New energy infused South Street as she heard about the Congress's activities from participants and read their notes. She arranged for Sir Harry Verney to invite the Indian delegation to Claydon.

Following the meeting, she put together a formal memorandum that pleaded again for every cesspool in India to be cleaned up and anything that could lead to cholera and typhoid to be eliminated. She dispatched the memorandum to Lord Lansdowne, who circulated the paper to the local governments. Other papers on prevention also went out to the local governments and the people.

Nightingale continued to converse with her Anglo-Indian and Indian friends and mounted a campaign to support the provincial sanitary boards' resolution for India to improve village sanitation. In August 1894, she wrote an 8-page pamphlet, "Village Sanitation in India," that was read at the Tropical Section of the eighth International Congress of Hygiene and Demography at Budapest. In December 1896, the journal of the British Committee of the Indian National Congress, *India,* published her article "Health Missionaries for Rural India." Although she recognized her limitations in trying to effect radical changes in distant India from the confines of her bedroom, she never gave up on the important message that local governments must focus on sanitation, clean water, and education. She never lost an opportunity to urge a practical beginning, however small, and often used the metaphor of the mustard seed that germinates and roots itself.

Indian Parliamentary Committee

From 1890 to 1892, Wedderburn was frequently in touch with Nightingale, Ripon, and other Liberal statesmen. After his election to Parliament in 1893, he took the lead in organizing the Indian Parliamentary Committee. Like Nightingale, he affirmed that the interests of the British officials in India were at odds with the Indian taxpayers. In a speech in the House of Commons in 1893 he said, "Every good thing done for the people of India has arisen out of an inquiry in this House for reform."[15]

Nightingale supported Indian nationalists who were seeking election to Parliament. When Parsi leader Dadabhai Naoroji, who lived in England and visited India frequently, was elected as the member of Parliament from Finsbury in 1892, followed by Sir William Wedderburn in 1893, they formed the Indian Parliamentary Committee in London. Nightingale wrote and met with the London group as well as others and shared relevant documents and statistics with them. In preparing their own papers, they used her documents to bolster their arguments.

Nightingale found the early successes of the Indian Parliamentary Committee promising. In 1893, the committee was able to carry through the House of Commons a resolution that supported holding the Indian Civil Service examination in India, which would make the selection process more equitable. In 1894 this committee pressed for a parliamentary inquiry on Indian expenditures and for a redistribution of financial burdens between India and Britain. In 1895, the Royal Commission on Indian Expenditure was announced, and Naoroji and Wedderburn were two of the 13 members appointed to the commission.

The battle was mostly uphill, but impressive progress had been made since the beginning a decade earlier. In an August 1896 letter, Nightingale wrote to the disheartened Wedderburn, encouraging him to carry on his work with the Indian National Congress, and alluding to Isaiah 40:31:

... but they who wait for the Lord shall renew their strength, they shall mount up with wings like eagles, they shall run and not be weary, and they shall walk and not faint.

You have no business to be low-spirited about the future. There is Providence still. It is 40 years this month since I came back from the Crimea. See how poor I have been helped, tho' I have lost all my friends, among Ministers.

You know quite well that you are the only M. P. who knows anything really about India now — You should hold on.

> *"And courage in the evil hour*
> *His heavenly aids impart —*
> *You should fly like the eagle."*

When I am low-spirited, I read about the D[uke] of Wellington in the Battle of Waterloo or in the Peninsular War. And I see how he held on thro' every obstacle & forsaken by our Govt. "Alone he did it!" And what was the end? He saved Europe. So it will be with you — You will save India ... you have divine unconquerable courage.[16]

Nightingale continued to support Wedderburn, who was regarded by some of his former colleagues in the Indian Civil Service and British social circles in India as a traitor or a faddist. However, he had faced these people before in his official capacity in India. Despite the criticism from his colleagues, he was ultimately proud of his ability to further the rights of the people and his record for tackling issues.

Nationalism gains strength

Nightingale was encouraged by the earnestness of the Indian nationalists. In 1896, liberal leader Mahadev Ranade, a judge and a formidable force in the Indian National Congress, was denied an invitation to the commission on Indian expenditures because the Indian government felt that he wasn't acceptable to Europeans in India. Ranade suggested that his disciple, Gopal Krishna Gokhale, then age 30, represent the Deccan Education Sabha on the Royal Commission.

Gokhale took his responsibilities on the Royal Commission very seriously. He spent 10 days at Solapur discussing financial and economic matters with authorities and received his final briefing from Ranade before leaving for London. He was accompanied by fellow committee members representing the three Indian presidencies — D. E. Wacha, a good friend of Gokhale, selected to represent Bombay; Banerjea, representing Calcutta; and G. Subramania Iyer for Madras. Naoroji wrote to Wacha that a supreme effort had to be made at this time to work for the Indian cause because such an opportunity might not come again for another generation. When Gokhale left for England in March 1897, Ranade wrote to Nightingale's friend Wedderburn urging him to take care of his young disciple:

Prof. Gokhale is a young man who has been very successful as Honorary Secretary to the Poona Sarvajanik Sabha ... He has been acting under my advice for the last ten years and I have found that he possesses a very high order of natural talents and scholarship. He is a Professor of English & History ... He is also one of the few good speakers we have on this side of India ... Prof. Gokhale goes fully equipped on the points on which he gives evidence. He is,

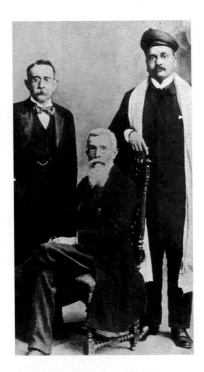

D.E. Wacha (left), Dadabhai Naoroji (seated), and Gopal Krishna Gokhale, representatives to the Royal Commission on Indian Expenditures, which took place in London in 1897

however, a young man and you, Mr. Caine and Prof. Dadabhoy shall have to do your best to see that his examination is conducted in a spirit of fairness ... As he is a good speaker, I would very much like that some arrangements be made to enable him to visit the chief towns where he might speak with great freedom on general questions.[17]

The meeting of Wedderburn and Gokhale began a fruitful relationship between two brilliant men of different generations and cultural backgrounds. In time, Gokhale's leadership and political influence became formidable. Even Mohandas K. Gandhi came to look upon him as his political mentor; in October 1896, Gokhale met with Gandhi, the 27-year-old Gujarati barrister, who had traveled to Poona to seek his support for the Indian immigrants in South Africa where he then lived. The humble and politically in-experienced Gandhi's description of his first encounter with Gokhale was "love at first sight;"[18] he later wrote of that meeting:

> *Gokhale closely examined me, as a schoolmaster would examine a candidate seeking admis-sion to a school. He told me whom to approach and how to approach them. He asked to have a look at my speech. He ... assured me that he was always at my disposal.[19]*

Gandhi returned to South Africa and asked Gokhale to raise questions on behalf of the Indians in South Africa in the Imperial Council in Calcutta and the British House of Commons. This meeting in 1896 between Gandhi and Gokhale started a friendship that forever changed the history of India in ways that Nightingale would have wished.

Nightingale and her like-minded colleagues were now fully aware that the tide was turning in India. Gracious as always with advice and help, she opened her home and convened interviews and meetings with the Indian delegation to the British Royal

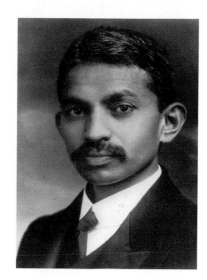

Mohandas K. Gandhi (1869-1948), as a young man at the beginning of his political career, c. 1900

BELOW: *Gandhi (fourth from left), Gokhale (fifth from left), and members of the Reception Committee, Durban, 1912*

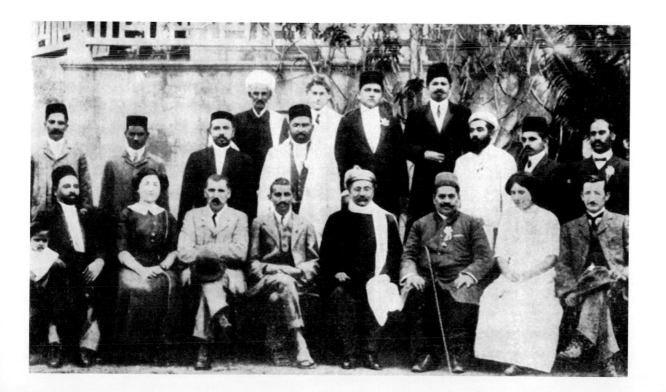

Commission on Indian Expenditures. Although Nightingale hadn't collected the data for this Royal Commission, she helped them organize their presentation.

However, Gokhale almost didn't make it to London and the presentation. Aboard ship crossing the English Channel from Calais, a heavy door swung into his chest, causing serious injury, but Gokhale chose not to reveal his discomfort. He didn't want to disappoint Naoroji, who expected him to meet with other Indian delegates preparing for the Royal Commission. Eventually, Gokhale's pain became so unbearable that he had to tell Wacha about the injury. The injury was diagnosed as a severe contusion of the heart that could have been fatal if he hadn't received medical attention. Realizing that he probably wouldn't be well enough to attend the first session, Gokhale dictated his evidence to the other delegates. However, he was well enough in a short time to appear before the Commission on April 12 and 13.

Gokhale spoke as a scholar and economist, but his passion for nationalism occasionally broke through his self-restraint. He spoke movingly of disasters caused by the 1896-1897 famine, which affected 97 million people, and presented other grievances that three subsequent generations of passionate Indian leaders from Naoroji to Nehru would bring to the world's attention. Gokhale fervently painted a picture of Indians living in an atmosphere of inferiority created by the British and the landowners, in which they were forced to use their talents to serve the despotic British system. A friend, commenting on Gokhale's zeal, said, "You have made a name for yourself in the history of India when words instead of swords are to be wielded."[20] In reply, Gokhale countered that he was "no more than a conduit pipe and Edison's phonograph."[21]

Most importantly, Gokhale clearly refuted the public assertions by the commission members that British economic policy was healthy for India. By speaking out in his first public appearance abroad, he not only gained in self-confidence and a quiet militancy, but also increased his standing in the eyes of his colleagues and especially Wedderburn, who was elated at his performance. Wedderburn, 30 years older than Gokhale, had been searching for younger men to take up the work of the aging Naoroji, Bannerjea, and others. He invited Gokhale to his country home, educated him in the intricacies of British politics, and introduced him to key politicians and administrators. A new link to the future had been forged.

The Nightingale of India

By the 1890s, much to Nightingale's delight, more students from India were entering Oxford. In 1892, Jowett arranged a meeting with a promising young Indian student, Cornelia Sorabji, for whom he had high hopes. He told Nightingale that Sorabji was determined to return to her native India "on a mission something like your own fifty years ago."[22] Sorabji returned to India in 1894 as a lawyer and became known as "the Nightingale of India."

Born into a well-educated Parsi family, Sorabji was raised in English style and in a Christian home with English manners, language, furnishings, and education. Her father had converted at a young age from Zoroastrianism to Christianity to avoid persecution.

Sorabji and her sisters learned about their Persian heritage but wore saris and the family considered themselves Indians. Just as Nightingale's family cared for the poor villagers near their homes, Sorabji's mother frequently visited the nearby villagers, caring for them and teaching them proper sanitary and health practices.

At age 8, Sorabji made the decision to become a lawyer after hearing the distressing story of an Indian woman whose property had been stolen from her because she could not read or write. Sorabji's mother said Cornelia must decide how she could help people like that, and Sorabji determined to study law. She obtained admission to Oxford where she met Jowett, who became one of her mentors. After graduating, she moved to London but often visited Jowett at Oxford. He arranged for her to meet with Nightingale. Sorabji wrote to her family of that meeting:

> I called by appointment on Miss Florence Nightingale. She is such a sweet creature. The dearest old lady in the world with the brightest of faces and the rosiest cheeks and such a twinkle in her eye ... talking to her was like breathing fresh air, it made me feel so strong for what might be in the future for me and she put her hand on my hand and blessed me when I was coming away and said, "I am sure God is sending you to your work my child. Don't be afraid to go in his strength. He will bless you and use you to work his purpose. And she kissed my hands and my forehead.[23]

Shortly after the visit, Sorabji had lunch with Jowett and described her meeting with the "little lady with rosy cheeks in a frilled nightcap whom I saw in bed, surrounded with flowers, her birds singing their hearts out in the aviary by the windows." Sorabji later wrote:

> When I lunched with him [Jowett] after this visit, he said suddenly, indicating the only picture of a woman in his study — it hung on the wall, a girlish figure in a short-waisted dress standing beside a pedestal on which sat the figure of an owl ... "Would you recognize that for the little old lady in a frilled night-cap whom you saw last week?"
>
> I was silent, not knowing what to say, and Jowett continued:
>
> "When she was like that, I asked her to marry me."
>
> Needless to say, I was struck dumb; one had never thought of the Master in human terms, as having had a mother or sisters, for instance, or as dressing like other folk, or having been at any other age or in any circumstance save that at and wherein one knew him.
>
> Jowett spoke again ... in his small abrupt voice: "It was better so."
>
> When the Life of Florence Nightingale was published [in 1913], a cousin of hers showed me an entry in F. N.'s Diary, which was surely a reference to this episode:
>
> "Benjamin Jowett came to see me. Disastrous! Nothing more."[24]

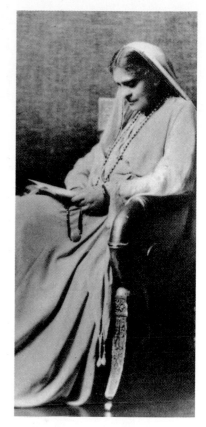

Cornelia Sorabji (1866-1954), a well-educated Parsi from India, who studied at Oxford with Benjamin Jowett and met Nightingale before her return to India in 1894

Passing the torch

The fact that the young Cornelia Sorabji could attend Oxford as well as have lunch with Benjamin Jowett and share his deep feelings for Nightingale, was in itself an indicator of the incipient social and political advances toward freedom that were slowly but inexorably coming to India.

The "dearest old lady in the world," who stood at the center of Jowett's affections, occupied a singular position among the band of British reformers who nursed the Indian National Congress in its infancy. More than one Indian scholar has found it remarkable that Florence Nightingale, when writing about the first Congress in 1885, uttered the phrase "new nationality."[25] Very few at the time possessed that breadth of vision.

The generation of men who had helped establish the British presence before the mutiny, under the aegis of the East India Company — Mill, Lawrence, Trevelyan, Frere, and others — had believed in and governed with a real concern for the people of India. In the conservative backlash after the rebellion, Nightingale provided a seamless stream of statistics and data to her liberal Viceroys to enable them to continue sanitation reform for India.

The British government and economic establishment grudgingly began to yield control of India after the turn of the century. However, during the final harsh years of the 19th century, Nightingale and her British and Indian colleagues kept the embers of Benthamite reform and the ideals of modern democracy burning. Their numbers were small and the obstacles enormous, but their cause was undeniable.

Hume, Wedderburn, Nightingale, and many others had assisted the Indian intelligentsia in the revolution of rising expectations. The fertile ground was well prepared for the day when the moral and political genius of the man in the white loin cloth, Mahatma Gandhi, would energize the Indian National Congress with the voice and vote of the impoverished millions and bring independence to India.

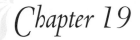

Chapter 19

Nursing Moves Forward

We are only on the threshold of nursing. In the future, which I shall not see, for I am old, may a better way be opened! May the methods by which every infant, every human being, will have the best chance of health — the methods by which every sick person will have the best chance of recovery, be learned and practised!

— Florence Nightingale, "Sick-Nursing and Health-Nursing," 1893[1]

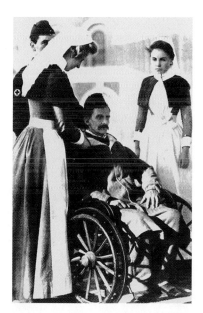

Army nurses with a patient at the Royal Victoria Hospital at Netley in 1897

Although Nightingale complained of failing eyesight in the 1880s, her correspondence, in her characteristic flowing handwriting, was still voluminous. She wrote hundreds of letters to her own graduates, some of whom received up to 50 in 1 year, and received numerous letters from nurses, public health and government officials, and ordinary people from around the world. She continued to take an active interest in her nursing students and graduates, and in a myriad of other health-related and social issues, from compulsory vaccination to the future of boys in reform schools.

Three decades after she made nursing an honorable profession for women, Nightingale could see the fruits of her labors all around her. By the late 1880s, nurses and nurse-superintendents trained at the Nightingale School of Nursing were working at dozens of hospitals and infirmaries throughout Great Britain and had been sent as far away as the United States, Canada, and Australia; other training schools modeled on the Nightingale School had been established; and district nursing had become a reality.

In 1883, Nightingale and another nurse, Jane Deeble, were the first two recipients of the Royal Red Cross Medal commissioned by Queen Victoria. Deeble had served as superintendent of the Army Nursing Service at the Royal Victoria Hospital at Netley from 1869 to 1889; in 1879, she was sent with a party of nurses to the Zulu War in South Africa as part of the National Aid Society endeavor, the first time that trained army nurses had served overseas. Nightingale didn't attend the award ceremony at Windsor Castle because of her work load, but she wrote a letter of thanks to the Queen.

Despite her accomplishments and honors, Nightingale believed there was a lot more to be done in the field of nursing and public health. Among the subjects that most occupied her in the 1880s and 1890s, aside from her Indian nationalist concerns, were her nursing students and graduates, some of whom had been sent to serve in military campaigns abroad; the health missioners program, aimed at educating the rural populace; and opposition to nursing registration.

Rare public appearances

By 1881, Nightingale's letters reveal that she was feeling less pain than in previous years; in fact, she even ventured outside the house on occasion, for example, to attend the funeral of Sir John Lawrence in 1879. On January 27, 1882, Nightingale finally visited her training school and inspected one of the wards at St. Thomas's Hospital. She had been expected to visit 2 years earlier, on the school's 20th anniversary, but had felt too ill to attend. Mrs. Wardroper, the school's superintendent, wrote to her shortly after her visit:

> *Just a week has elapsed since you honored us with your more than welcome presence, and I cannot go to bed to-night until I have thanked you for all the admiration in which you speak of your Home and the pretty Alexandra Ward. No words of mine can ever express the delight it gave us to welcome you, our dearly loved Chief, to the Home and School which has for more than 20 years borne "her honored name."[2]*

At the end of 1882, Nightingale made two other public appearances. Sir Harry Verney persuaded her to go to Victoria Station to witness the return of the Foot Guards from the first Egyptian campaign on November 13. His nephew, Colonel Philip Smith, was a commander of the returning Grenadiers regiment. She later described the soldiers:

Doctors and nurses in a ward at St. Thomas's Hospital in 1909. At left foreground, a child in a croup tent is receiving a breathing treatment.

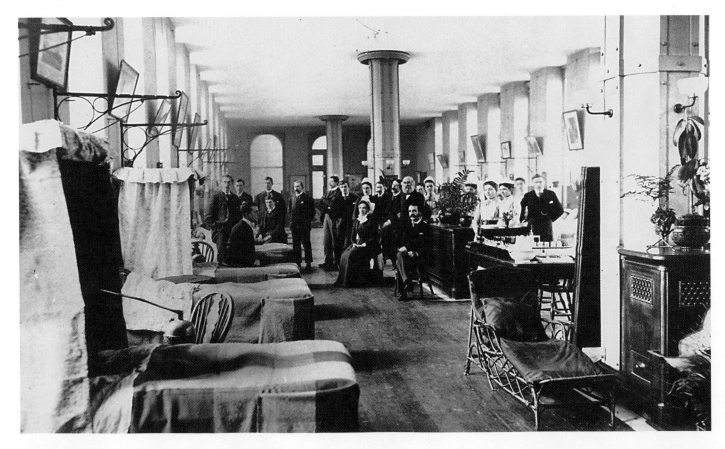

NURSING MOVES FORWARD

... Anybody might have been proud of these men's appearance — like shabby skeletons, or at least half their former size — in worn but well-cleaned campaigning uniforms; not spruce or showy, but alert, silent, steady ... A more deeply felt and less showy scene could not have been imagined.[3]

A few days later, she sat on the royal review stand in the Prime Minister's garden between Prime Minister Gladstone and his wife for the Horse Guards Parade of other troops returning from Egypt, where Nightingale nurses had served. It was reported that "there were tears in dear Miss Nightingale's eyes as she saw the poor ragged fellows march past."[4] Having noticed her presence, the queen sent her a note commenting on how well she looked and inviting her to the opening of the Law Review Court on December 4. Nightingale declined.

Mentoring the Nightingale nurses

Nightingale frequently gave advice to her nurses at various posts, writing lengthy letters about professional concerns as well as their personal health, as seen in a letter to Ella Pirrie, a promising nurse in Belfast:

... How deep is my interest, how intense my feeling for you and your work I need not tell you; every woman must feel the same. You have done a noble deed in beginning. God will grant you success. You have already done great things. But to know that you may have, and that soon, a trained Lady to speak to in the form of a Nightingale Supt. tugs at my heart and that hereafter no vacancy shall occur among the nurses but shall be filled up with a trained nurse. I rather deprecated your having nurses from us, on the ground that Irish don't like English nurses. To help you must be the desire of us all ...

Pray, for all our sakes, observe some regularity in exercise and meals The Infirmary ground is yet unplanned. It seems ridiculous to offer you rhododendrons from England. But if you think well, might we send you some? We have furnished the grounds of two London Workhouse Infirmaries with rhododendrons which did well.

Is there any Flower Mission in Belfast? If one can get in flowers, and plants, a canary or living bird in a cage, a tame cat which will not hurt the canary, it is a civilizer is it not? ... I hope you have these cheerful things in your own rooms.

You wished for a book in Nursing. I am sorry to say that Smith's lectures on Nursing which I sent for are out of print. I send two others which I hope may be useful ...

I will not say farewell, or rather I will say fare you well, fare you very well, and hope that our friendship is only begun ... God bless you: and He will help you ...[5]

One of her most frequent correspondents in the early 1880s was Rachel Williams, the matron at St. Mary's Hospital in London and one of Nightingale's favorite former students. Known to have a quick temper, Williams was having trouble with the doctors, demanding a salary increase, and threatening to resign her post. Nightingale urged her not to resign, but she did so in January 1885. Later Nightingale arranged for Williams to serve in Egypt with the National Aid Society. When Williams got engaged after the Egyptian campaign, Nightingale was depressed to lose one of her favorite nurses to marriage.

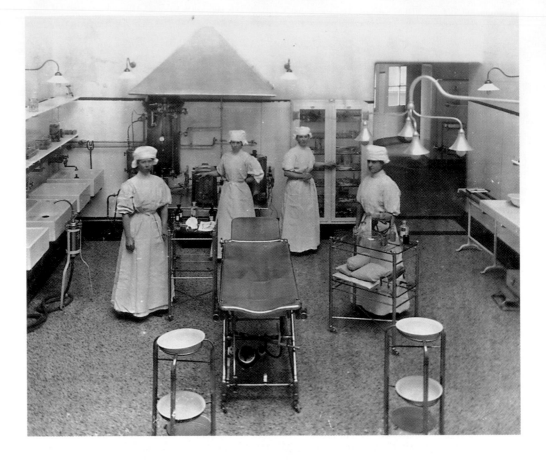

In 1887, Nightingale lost another of her favorite nurses, Angelique Pringle, who had decided to convert to Catholicism. Pringle, who had become superintendent of the Nightingale School earlier that year after Mrs. Wardroper's retirement, was now forced to resign her position. Although Nightingale's letters reveal that Pringle's departure was one of the greatest sorrows of her life, next to the deaths of Sidney Herbert and Arthur Clough, she did not "excommunicate" Pringle, as she had others who had converted in the past.

After Pringle's departure, Louisa Gordon, a former pupil from Leeds, took over as head of the Nightingale School. Although Nightingale had fought so hard to develop the position of a strong and independent matron, during Gordon's superintendency, she came to believe that matrons now had too much power. "I am not sure that the nursing ought to be so entirely in the matron's hands now," she wrote to Henry Bonham Carter in 1894. "We have no dominance over her now. We have recommended people lately who ought not to be in a mile of the hospital."[6] In 1895, Miss Crossland, the home sister, retired on a pension after 21 years of service to the school; nearly 600 nurses had completed their probationary course under her supervision.

Nurses serving in colonial conflicts

From 1879 to 1881, Nightingale was preoccupied with the state of the Army Medical Service, particularly as it related to South Africa and Egypt, where British troops were engaged in various regional conflicts. With her nurses and superintendents at the battlefront, Nightingale now had access to first-hand information about the army's medical operations abroad. Many of the reforms that she and Sidney Herbert had recommended between 1856 and 1861 still had not been implemented. For example, in South Africa, the Purveyor's Department had been abolished, which led to general supply problems; nutritious food wasn't available; and orderlies were often drunk. When a court of inquiry was appointed to investigate these problems in 1882, Nightingale provided the War Office with suggestions for witnesses and elaborate briefs for examination. She was in constant communication with Captain Douglas Galton, now Director of Public Works for the army, urging him to keep the problems of reform in the headlines.

In 1883, Nightingale reacted bitterly to the revised regulations issued by the army Medical Department concerning the superintendent of nurses. The new regulations allowed the superintendent to be appointed by the Secretary of State for War on the recommendations of the Director-General, rather than basing the appointment on the nurse's training. Nightingale believed that her 20-year struggle to promote nurses' training and obtain independent power for the nursing superintendent still had not been achieved and that too much power remained in the hands of medical officers.

Thirty years after the Crimean War, Nightingale was still expressing concern about the readiness of army supplies and troops both at home and abroad, as in this letter to Sir Harry Verney in May 1888:

> *... in reference to what we were talking of this morning, if you were to ask ...*
>
> *(1) whether at Aldershot the personnel & materials, all complete, of a Camp or War Hospital is exercised, not pitch-forked together, as it would act if it had to act in a real campaign, with its complete Staff of Medical Officers, Hospital N. C. Officers & Hospital Orderlies, &*

Helen C. Norman, Lady Superintendent at the Royal Victoria Hospital at Netley, with a group of her nurses in 1897

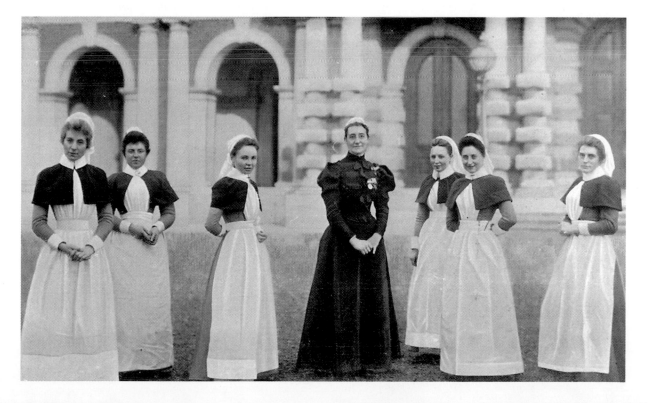

Equipment, etc. etc. complete, so that the Officers know all their men & the men each other and their Officers. So that the men could not only unpack their Equipment but pack it up again (which has not always been the case) it would be a great thing.

(2) then whether every District in England has now such a War Hospital with Staff, material & personnel complete which would be ready to embark in War time — having been regularly exercised — at a few days or even a few hours' notice?

(3) or whether, as hitherto, when they had embarked in war time, no one officer knew any of his men, and no one man the others' — & no man was familiar with his material?

(4) Are the campaigning Hospitals ready to be mobilized at a few days' notice? Or have they then, when on the point of embarkation, to be organized? & brought together in haste.[7]

In 1899, Nightingale urged Henry Bonham Carter, the Nightingale Fund Secretary, to talk to the War Office about sending nurses to serve in the Boer War. She saw this as a good opportunity to gain more recognition for the nurses' training program and to draw more educated women to the nursing profession: "I believe if we could get more government engagements like Sydney ... we could attract a higher class of women than we can get to serve under piddling committees like the workhouse of Liverpool."[8]

At the turn of the century, several female members of the royal family lent their support to the cause of military nursing. In 1897, the Princess Christian (formerly known as Princess Helena), Queen Victoria's third daughter, began the Army Nursing Service Reserve. During the Boer War, 1,400 of these reservists joined the small number of regular army nurses in South Africa. In March 1902, Queen Alexandra, wife of Edward VIII, formed Queen Alexandra's Imperial Military Nursing Service.[9]

Developments in midwifery

In March 1883, Nightingale once again heard from her old friend Dr. Elizabeth Blackwell, the first female doctor in the United States, about the founding of a midwifery school. The midwifery training program that Nightingale had started at King's College Hospital in 1861 had closed in 1868 after its superintendent, Mary Jones, and her nurses left because of religious conflicts and started their own program. Blackwell had been approached by a group of women who had drawn up plans to start a midwifery school on a small scale. Blackwell, now age 62, ended her letter to Nightingale:

You see therefore, dear friend, that we are very far yet from being able to put your admirable plans into force; but they will be a valuable guide for future work, I hope, and I am sure it will encourage future workers to know of the deep and lifelong interest you have taken in this subject.[10]

Eventually, a small school was established. Nightingale's interest in midwifery continued throughout the decade, as evident in this 1889 letter to Ella Pirrie in Belfast:

I hear of your desire "to give all your probationers" "Midwifery training" with fear and joy ... Forgive me for asking questions — it interests me so very much. (You know we had a training school for midwifery nurses for six years and a half).

What is the average number of lying in with you?

What is the average death rate among Mothers? Babies?

What is the average number of puerperal fever cases, or septicaemia, if any?

You have I understood, a good old-fashioned midwife, and her assistant, with both of whom you are satisfied. [Strictly between you and me, the really old-fashioned midwife is sometimes a more useful and thorough person than the three months' practitioner "trained" as they please to call it for 3 months in a Lying-in Hospital here — since she probably sees nothing like the number of cases that you have. You have doubtless a Doctor to call in for the abnormal cases and the sick cases].

What is your proportion of normal? And what of abnormal cases?

Does he come in from the Medical and Surgical wards to the Lying-In Ward, and go out from it to those other wards? After good thorough 3 months' practical training such as you can approve in your wards under a good midwife, do your probationers have any outdoor practice among women lying-in at home?

The examination and certificate of the Obstetrical Society which you mention, is doubtless excellent as giving your candidates a standing but you and I beware of thinking that it is anything more — that it teaches anything. A young woman of good education — used to get up subjects, and put her knowledge into wards — can pass the examination triumphantly, and get a first rate certificate, and know little more what to do in practical midwifery and how to do it than an ignoramus (all this is strictly private) or at least far less than the good experienced old-fashioned midwife who could not pass the Obstetrical Society's Examination to save her life ...[11]

Although the Nightingale Fund didn't establish a permanent midwifery training program during Nightingale's lifetime, it did focus public awareness on the suffering and needs of the poor and on the problems that trained midwives could have prevented. Midwifery training continued to be stymied by the powerful medical profession, which blocked most of the drafted Parliamentary bills. Not until 1902 did the Midwives Act finally ensure proper training and regulation of midwives.

Nightingale's Jubilee Year

In 1887, Jubilee celebrations were underway for the 50th anniversary of Queen Victoria's reign. Nightingale also considered 1887 her own Jubilee Year because it marked the 50th anniversary of her Call from God at Embley. As part of the Jubilee celebration, the public was asked to make donations to the Women's Jubilee Gift Fund. The queen decided to use the bulk of the money collected to fund the Queen Victoria Jubilee Institute for Nurses, which would be devoted to a cause close to Nightingale's heart — district nursing, the care of the sick poor in their own homes.

Nightingale had contemplated the role of district nurses and the best training for them since the 1870s, when the Nightingale Fund helped establish a central training home in London in conjunction with the Metropolitan and National Nursing Association. Because the poor couldn't afford to see doctors, Nightingale saw the role of district nurses not only as patient caregivers, but also as health educators who could teach patients and families about illness prevention and sanitary measures to promote healthier environments.

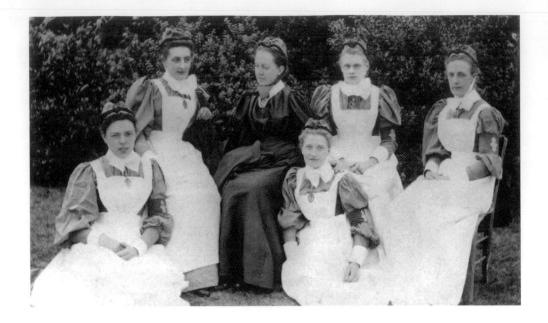

In an 1882 pamphlet titled *Training of Nurses and Nursing the Sick*, Nightingale proposed that every district nurse should complete a year of hospital nursing and then 3 or more months of training in the field, followed by a return to the hospital every 2 years for a 3-month refresher course. Although this proposal wasn't carried out in her lifetime, the pamphlet was very important because it stressed the need for a female superintendent who would supervise the nurses from each District Home and it enforced the notion of nurses functioning as nurses and not as almsgivers.[12]

The Jubilee Gift Fund eventually collected £70,000 (about £3,236,448 or U.S. $5,372,504 in today's values[13]). Queen Victoria took a keen interest in "her nurses," designing a distinctive uniform and a badge worn as a pendant, of which Nightingale disapproved. It bothered her that nursing was becoming a fashionable job, not the "calling" that she had intended. She feared that the Institute would take shortcuts in training and even referred to its nurses as "nothing but a register of quack nurses."[14]

In spite of Nightingale's objections, the Jubilee Institute did much to promote uniform standards of district nursing, which were a distinct improvement over the independent associations controlled by Ladies Welfare Committees. Dame Rosalind Paget, a trained nurse from the London Hospital, a midwife, and the niece of William Rathbone, became the first General Nursing Superintendent and Inspector of the Institute. A Nightingale-trained nurse, Amy Hughes, became the second superintendent (from 1887 to 1894) and is credited with further advancing the role of district nurses.[15]

Health missioners

In 1888, Nightingale became very interested in the County Council Act, which mandated that all county councils spend money on health education. For years, she had envisioned a program of health educators for the English countryside, trained women who would teach country folk about health and sanitation, not unlike those who went out to the rural areas of India to teach villagers these subjects. Now she worked to extend this concept to the villagers of England.

Nightingale spent close to 3 years compiling an exhaustive syllabus on the subjects that should be taught. The first lectures were on basic physiology and hygiene. Subsequent lectures followed this outline:

I. Our Homes
    1. The Bedroom.
    2. The Kitchen and Parlour.
    3. The Back Yard and Garden.
II. Ourselves
    4. The Skin, and how to keep the body clean — Washing.
    5. The Circulation, and how to keep the body warm — Clothes.
    6. The Digestion, and how to nourish the body — Food.
III. Extra Lectures
    7. What to do till the Doctor comes, and after the Doctor has left.
    8. Management of Infants and Children.[16]

Those who passed an examination received a certificate as a "Health Missioner" and were sent out to teach in the spring of 1892. Nightingale described their work as "the skillful hand, directed by the cool head, and inspired by the loving heart."[17] The health missioners were the prototype for today's British Health Visitor program.

At the 1893 Women Workers' Conference at Leeds, a paper written by Nightingale on rural hygiene was presented. The idea she proposed — sanitary inspectors for the villages — was accomplished the following year.

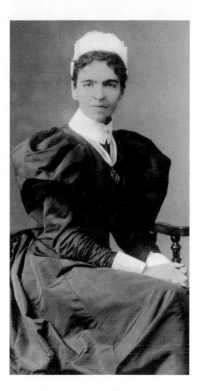

Dame Rosalind Paget, first General Nursing Superintendent of the Queen Victoria Jubilee Institute for Nurses

Battle over nurses' registration

The battle over nurses' registration was Nightingale's last big nursing challenge, one that would occupy her for 7 years. By the mid-1880s, many hospitals and other institutions in the London area and other large towns had their own nurse training programs, yet the training at these facilities varied widely. Some programs had Nightingale-trained superintendents who followed the Nightingale curriculum (18 as of 1887).[18] Those programs without Nightingale-trained superintendents had no allegiance to the Nightingale program.

As more nurses graduated from the different programs, each with its own nursing curriculum, a need arose for clear guidelines to establish who qualified as a trained nurse. The British Hospital Association, which already had a directory listing nurses who had completed 1 year's training in a hospital or an infirmary and who had a good character, appointed a committee of inquiry in 1887 to look into the idea of establishing a General Registry of Nurses based on stricter criteria, including increased education and the passing of an examination.

The controversy over registration split the nursing world into two camps. In the fall of 1887, a majority of the inquiry committee resigned from the committee in opposition to the idea of registration. The minority, spearheaded by the powerful Mrs. Bedford Fenwick, favored the idea of registration and created the British Nurses' Association to carry out the plan. As Ethel Gordon Manson before her marriage, Fenwick had

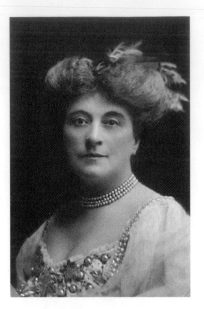

Mrs. Bedford Fenwick (1857-1947), matron of St. Bartholomew's Hospital from 1881 to 1887, who championed the cause of nurses' registration in Britain

been the youngest matron ever of St. Bartholomew's Hospital from December 1881 to October 1887. She was not a Nightingale-trained nurse and had no allegiance to the Nightingale circle.

The purpose of the British Nurses' Association was to raise the standards for trained nurses and to unite all qualified British nurses under one organization. From 1887 to 1889, the association was willing to register nurses who had had only 1 year of training, a group that included the Nightingale nurses. However, after 1889, in order to become registered, a nurse would have to have graduated from a 3-year training program, have passed a qualifying examination, and pay a 5-guinea registration fee (equivalent to about one-fourth of the first year's salary).

Fenwick, one of the new generation of nurses and a born leader, fought to take the nursing profession far beyond the limits that Nightingale found acceptable.[19] Although Nightingale was not against further training, she opposed an examination because she believed that no test could determine a person's character — and character was as essential to a proper nurse as clinical training. Her lifelong doubts about the efficacy of examinations to determine competence were rooted in her earlier observations that such tests for aspiring doctors were simply exercises in memory and rote learning and bore little relationship to real medical knowledge and competent medical care. She had always insisted that nursing was a calling, not just a job, and that this calling could not be tested on an examination. However, she was well aware that the profession was evolving and that standards beyond certification must be created to ensure competence.

Nightingale addressed this subject in her 1888 letter to her nurse probationers:

...We hear much of "Associations" now. It is impossible indeed to live in isolation: we are dependent upon others for the supply of all our wants, and others upon us.

Every Hospital is an "Association" in itself. We of this School are an Association in the deepest sense, regulated — at least we strive towards it — on high & generous principles: through organizations working at once for our own & our fellow Nurses' success. For, to make progress possible, we must make this inter-dependence a source of good; not a means of standing still ...

...We must never forget that the "Individual" makes the Association. What the Association is depends upon each of its members ... Yet, if the individual allows herself to sink to a lower level, it is all but a tinkling "cymbal" for her. It is how the circumstances are worked that signifies. Circumstances are opportunities ...

Every Nurse must grow. No Nurse can stand still, she must go forward, or she will go backward, every year. And how can a Certificate or public register show this? Rather, she ought to have a moral "Clinical" Thermometer in herself ...

Nursing work must be quiet work — An individual work — Anything else is contrary to the whole real-ness of the work. Where am I, the individual, in my utmost soul? What am I, the inner woman, called "I"? — That is the question ...[20]

From 1889 to 1891, the British Nurses' Association made several attempts to obtain a Royal Charter for the organization, which would establish the queen's support for the concept of registration. After Nightingale and her allies presented a petition against the move, the Board of Trade denied the request. In 1891, the association asked the Princess Christian to become its patron, which strengthened the group's hand in the fight for registration, especially among doctors and surgeons. The queen was again petitioned for a Royal Charter — this time by her own daughter.

Nightingale was highly irritated when she heard that the charter idea had gained the support of prestigious doctors:

In all my strange life through which God has guided me so faithfully (O that I had been as faithful to Him as He to me) this is the strangest episode of all — to see a number of doctors of the highest eminence giving their names to what they know nothing at all about. Sir James told me himself that the names were asked for at a Court Ball — following each other like a flock of sheep; to see their Council of Registration made up of Sirs, only one of whom knows anything about nurse-training.[21]

In 1892, a committee of the House of Lords, which had been set up to investigate nurses' responsibilities in metropolitan hospitals, recommended that nurses' training be increased to 3 years and that shifts be limited to 8 hours, but it did not mandate compulsory registration. In May of 1893, the Privy Council granted the British Nurses' Association the right to keep a list of nurses with 3 years' training, although the nurses could not call themselves "chartered" or "registered." In June, the association was granted a Royal Charter.

Although the pro-registration group thought it had the upper hand with a royal princess as its leader, by mid-1893, the anti-registration group had greater numbers because most hospitals still had only a 1-year training program. Believing that her side had won the battle, Nightingale tried to foster good will between the two groups. Fenwick continued pushing for a 3-year training period as a standard for nurses' registration. In 1914, 4 years after Nightingale's death, the Nightingale Fund Council agreed to establish a 3-year training program at St. Thomas's Hospital. Parliament eventually approved a bill calling for nurses' registration in 1919.

Advances in medical knowledge

The explosion of new medical and surgical discoveries, techniques, and procedures in the late 1870s through the 1890s had a direct effect on nursing. The discovery of organisms responsible for diseases such as cholera and tuberculosis paved the way for vaccinations and eventually led to widespread acceptance of the germ theory of disease. Joseph Lister's development and continuing refinement of antiseptic surgery revolutionized surgical procedures and helped to dramatically reduce surgical mortality rates. Some of the new developments, such as the establishment of the Royal Army Medical College (formerly the Army Medical School) in 1902, were a direct result of Nightingale's lobbying over the years.

Among the most important medical developments were:
• 1879 — Robert Koch's landmark paper on "The Etiology of Traumatic Infectious Diseases," which confirmed the germ theory of disease
• 1880 — Louis Pasteur's discovery of the streptococcus, staphylococcus, and pneumococcus organisms; discovery of the typhoid bacillus
• 1881 — Pasteur's creation of a vaccine against anthrax; Koch's introduction of solid

cultures for growing bacteria; creation of the Government Animal Vaccination Establishment, which provided live animals for use in medical experiments
- 1882 — Koch's discovery of the tubercle bacillus, the cause of tuberculosis
- 1883 — discovery of the bacilli responsible for diphtheria, cholera, and infectious conjunctivitis
- 1884 — discovery of the tetanus bacillus
- 1886 — introduction of the concept of sterilized milk for infants and establishment of the Royal Institute of Public Health in London
- 1887 — discovery of *Brucella melitensis*, the organism that causes Crimean fever (now recognized as Malta or Mediterranean fever)
- 1891 — Koch's opening of the Institute for Infectious Diseases in Berlin and Lister's opening of the Institute for Preventive Medicine in London; William Halsted's introduction of rubber gloves for surgery
- 1893 — passage of the Isolation Hospital Act, which required infected patients to be isolated; founding of the Society of Anesthesia in London
- 1894 — discovery of the plague bacillus.

Although Nightingale, like many leading doctors of the day, slowly began to accept the germ theory of disease, she continued to insist on the importance of good sanitation and health education — her message for more than 30 years. As evidenced by the introduction of rubber gloves for surgery and the Isolation Hospital Act of 1893, this message was finally becoming recognized — though not universally accepted — by the medical establishment. Even doctors who wore gloves for surgery seldom wore clean gowns, and surgical masks were yet to come.

The International Medical Congress held in London in 1881, the largest such gathering to date, was important in two respects: It gave physicians and surgeons from many countries the chance to learn about the new science of bacteriology from speakers such as Louis Pasteur and Robert Koch, and it was an opportunity for medical scientists to argue the case for using live animals in medical experiments. Among the prominent physicians attending the Congress were Joseph Lister, P. John Wood, William Jenner, William Osler, and Nightingale's friends James Paget and William Bowman.

Lister and antiseptic surgery

Although Lister had been developing his theories of antiseptic surgery since the mid-1860s, much of the medical establishment in the 1870s and 1880s still viewed his work with skepticism. Lister had begun developing his antiseptic method while a surgeon at Glasgow's Royal Infirmary, where the mortality rate from infection in amputation cases ran as high as 50% in the early 1860s. Building on Pasteur's work on fermentation and putrefaction, Lister became convinced that to reduce surgical mortality rates, it was necessary not only to kill infective agents already present in wounds (antisepsis) but also to prevent such agents from entering wounds (asepsis).

Lister eventually developed a six-part technique involving the use of carbolic acid to clean wounds, which he first performed successfully on a compound fracture of the tibia in 1865. In March 1867, he published the results of further successful trials in the

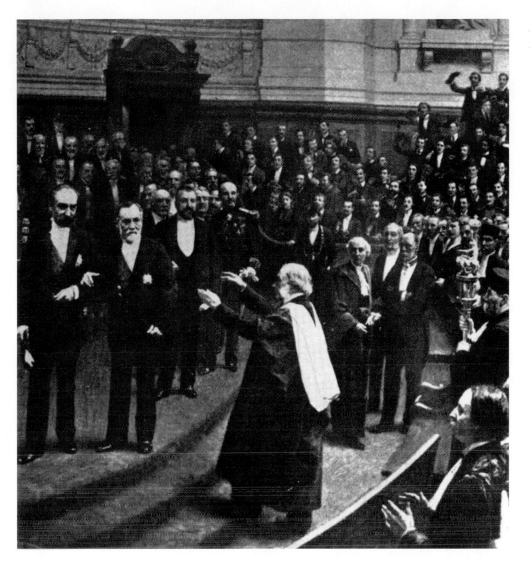

Joseph Lister (in white hood) joins a hallful of eminent scientists hailing Louis Pasteur (second from left) at the Sorbonne on December 27, 1892, during festivities marking Pasteur's 70th birthday

Lancet. Between 1865 and 1869, the mortality rate at Glasgow's Male Accident Ward dropped from 45% to 15%. Yet the response to his work continued to be mixed, especially in Britain, France, and the United States, partly as a result of continued reluctance to accept the germ theory of disease.

In an 1883 speech, Lister made the point that surgeons didn't need to believe in the germ theory to try his antiseptic method:

> *... First, as to theory, we do not require any scientific theory to enable us to believe in antiseptic treatment. You need not believe in germ theory at all ... All that you have to believe is that there are such things as putrefaction and other septic agencies, and that our wounds are liable to these, and that they are very pernicious, and that these things come from without, and that we have the means of preventing them by various chemical agencies ... anybody who knows the present state of surgical practice must admit these to be truisms ...*
>
> *And then to practice; it is not a very difficult thing to wash your hands in a carbolic solution, and have your instruments in their carbolic solution for a quarter of an hour before you operate. It is not a very difficult thing to wrap around the limbs a suitable envelope of antiseptic material. What I believe to be one of the most important things of all is ... when we change a*

dressing, invariably first to cover the wound with something pure; not to wash the surrounding parts with antiseptic solution, and then, after that has been done, put a dressing on the wound; but before we begin to defile the lotion at all, put on the wound what is pure, and last thing of all, wash the surrounding parts, which, though they look the same to our eyes, are different ... The edges of the dressing are septic; that wound, if it is as it ought to be, is aseptic ...[22]

Lister's insistence on the need to prevent wounds from coming in contact with contaminated surfaces was one of the most important contributions in the history of medicine and laid the foundation for modern surgery.

Progress in medicine continued at a fast pace. On December 27, 1892, the great theater of the Sorbonne was filled to capacity to honor Louis Pasteur on his 70th birthday. Lister, who represented the Royal Medical Societies of London and Edinburgh, said in his speech: "You have raised the veil which for centuries had covered infectious diseases; you have discovered and demonstrated the microbian pattern"[23]

Among those who eventually came to support the germ theory of disease during this period was Florence Nightingale. Although she had always emphasized the importance of maintaining cleanliness in hospitals, she now promoted specific germicidal measures, such as disinfecting linens by boiling them in a solution containing carbolic acid, having nurses wash their hands frequently with chlorinated soda, and using three sets of towels (for hands, bedpans, and basins). In a lengthy article on nurses' training that she wrote for *A Dictionary of Medicine*, published in 1894, she said: "The nurse must be taught the nature of contagion and infection, and the distinctions between deodorants, disinfectants, and antiseptics ... and that cuffs and sleeves and stuffed dresses are possible carriers of contagious matter."[24]

1893 World's Fair

The 1893 World's Fair in Chicago, officially known as the World's Columbian Exposition, was hailed as one of the most spectacular international world's fairs ever. It exhibited the latest technological achievements, such as electricity, the linotype, Pullman cars, the expansion engine, structural steel, and the first Ferris wheel.

Two features of this event received worldwide attention, although they weren't in the original plans. The first was a series of worldwide congresses on all aspects of society, such as government, law, and education, which included a nursing congress. The second was that, for the first time, women played a conspicuous and responsible role at an international event. President Benjamin Harrison had appointed a Board of Lady Managers to help plan many aspects of the fair and to coordinate local, national, and international participation of women.

The board planned to set up a special exhibit on the progress of women for the last 400 years. Lady Angela Burdett Coutts, the prominent philanthropist and one of the British planners, asked Nightingale to contribute a paper:

[As] the President of the British Philanthropic Section of the Woman's Auxiliary of the World's Columbian Exposition, to be held next year at Chicago, I am desirous of obtaining particulars of all philanthropic work initiated or carried on by women.

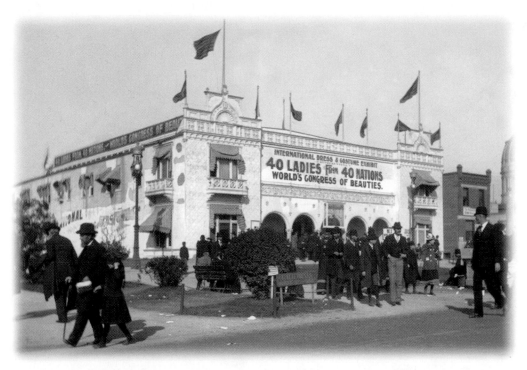

The particular object of my Section is to collect concise and well-written reports upon all philanthropic work in which women are immediately concerned, or which owes its genesis or its success to their co operation.

May I ask if you will kindly give me any information you can as to the work of women in connection with the Organization of which you are the head?

I shall also be very glad to receive your advice as to what are, in your opinion, the most practical and successful philanthropic efforts that have been, or are being, made by women ...[25]

Nightingale contributed a remarkable paper, "Sick-Nursing and Health-Nursing," which was read at the nursing congress. In this paper, she proclaimed that the "art of health-nursing" — by which she meant cultivating and maintaining good health — was as important as the "art of sick-nursing." In emphasizing the importance of illness prevention, which has become a major topic at the end of the 20th century, Nightingale was again more than a century ahead of her time. And in calling attention to nature's role in the healing process, she laid the foundation for the modern holistic nursing movement:[26]

... A new art and a new science has been created since and within the last forty years. And with it a new profession — so they say; we say, calling ... the art of nursing the sick. Please mark — nursing the sick; NOT nursing the sickness ...What is health nursing? ... the cultivation of health ...What is Sickness ... Nature's way of getting rid of the effects of conditions which have interfered with health. It is nature's attempt to cure. We have to help her ... What is health? Health is not only to be well, but to use well every power we have ... What is nursing? Both kinds of nursing are to put us in the best possible conditions for Nature to restore or preserve health ...[27]

At the same congress, Mrs. Dacre Craven (the former Florence Lees), a Nightingale disciple who had served as superintendent of the model training program for district

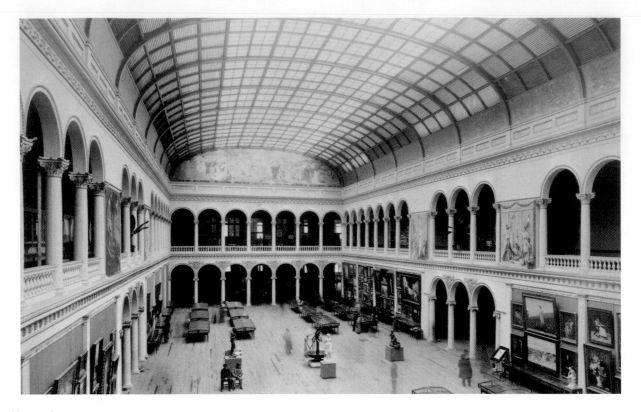

The Woman's Building at the 1893 World's Fair in Chicago, designed by a woman architect, Sophia Haydon. The building was the scene of a nursing congress to which Nightingale contributed an important paper, "Sick-Nursing and Health-Nursing."

nurses, presented a paper that laid the foundation for today's public health nursing and nursing the sick poor in their homes.

Mrs. Bedford Fenwick of the British Nurses' Association was one of the distinguished guests on the podium during opening ceremonies for the Woman's Building, where the exhibit on women's progress was held. The building itself, designed by a young woman who had won an architectural competition, was hailed as a "celebration of women." Fenwick's award-winning exhibit promoted nursing as a profession, and she used the occasion to strongly voice the need for nursing registration.

During her stay in the United States, Fenwick met with the American nursing leader Isabel A. Hampton (later Robb), nursing superintendent at Johns Hopkins Hospital in Baltimore. The two visionaries discussed plans for a nursing congress to be held within the framework of the upcoming international congress focusing on charities, correction, and philanthropy. Hampton, who was to spearhead the nursing congress, began a correspondence with Nightingale, receiving advice and recommendations.

At the World's Fair nursing congress, Hampton presented a paper on the need for uniform standards of nursing education. Many hospitals had established their own nursing programs, not to provide a sound nursing education but to help lower hospital costs. In Chicago, Hampton brought together 18 nursing superintendents who were interested in establishing a universal standard of training and education. In 1894, these superintendents became the first group of nurses to officially organize, calling themselves the American Society of Superintendents of Training Schools for Nurses.[28]

A number of hospital exhibits at the World's Fair, which featured miniature models of clean wards complete with patients and nurses, were very well received because Nightingale and other nursing leaders, such as Dorthea Dix, Clara Barton, and Mary

Ann Bickerdyke, had helped raise public awareness about deplorable hospital conditions. The Illinois Woman's Hospital Pavilion had a model hospital emergency treatment center that provided care for nearly 3,000 people during the fair.[29]

The historic nursing congress at the 1893 World's Fair marked the beginning of formal international collaboration among nurses and paved the way for all future national and international nursing conventions. While in Chicago, Fenwick also helped promote interest in a meeting to be held in London in 1899 of the International Council of Women, the first international organization of professional women.[30]

Reaping the fruit

Despite the below-average quality of some of its early graduates, Nightingale's secular nurses training program was a landmark achievement in the history of nursing. Because the program was so far ahead of its time, for the first 30 or 40 years there weren't enough educated women to become nurse tutors, so most lecturers were male doctors. Those who trained the early probationers didn't understand the public health needs of the general population. Because training occurred alongside developments in medicine, with nurses under the rule of doctors and hospital administrators, the emphasis was mostly on technical aspects of treatment, and a separate philosophy of the art and science of nursing did not develop as fully as Nightingale would have wished.

However, the concept of modern nursing was well established as the 19th century drew to a close. On April 25, 1893, the first Florence Nightingale Pledge was adminis-

NIGHTINGALE PLEDGE

I solemnly pledge myself before God and in the presence of this assembly:

To pass my life in purity and to practice my profession faithfully.

I will abstain from whatever is deleterious and mischievous, and will not take or knowingly administer any harmful drug.

I will do all in my power to maintain and elevate the standard of my profession, and will hold in confidence all personal matters committed to my keeping and all family affairs coming to my knowledge in the practice of my profession.

With loyalty will I endeavor to aid the physician in his work, and devote myself to the welfare of those committed to my care.

The Nightingale pledge, written under the leadership of Lystra E. Gretter, principal of the Farrand Training School for Nurses at Harper Hospital, Detroit, Michigan, in 1893

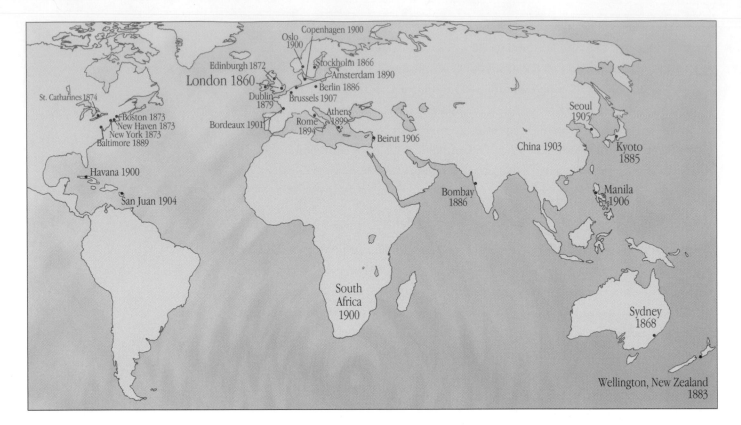

The map shows nurse training programs with locations and dates:

St. Catharines 1874
Boston 1873
New Haven 1873
New York 1873
Baltimore 1889
Havana 1900
San Juan 1904
Edinburgh 1872
London 1860
Dublin 1879
Bordeaux 1901
Oslo 1900
Copenhagen 1900
Stockholm 1866
Amsterdam 1890
Berlin 1886
Brussels 1907
Rome 1894
Athens 1899
Beirut 1906
South Africa 1900
Bombay 1886
China 1903
Seoul 1905
Kyoto 1885
Manila 1906
Sydney 1868
Wellington, New Zealand 1883

By 1910, the year Nightingale died, nurse training programs based on her system had been established in 20 countries.

tered to the graduating class at Farrand Training School for Nurses at Harper Hospital in Detroit, Michigan, under the chairmanship of the principal, Mrs. Lystra E. Gretter, later director emeritus of the Detroit Visiting Nurses Association. She had helped write the pledge, which expressed the art and science of nursing, along with two other nurses, a physician, and a clergyman.

By 1910, there were 1,000 nurse training programs in the United States alone, and programs based on the Nightingale model had been established in 20 countries. From the small seeds of Nightingale's first position as Lady Superintendent at Harley Street (1853), to Superintendent of Nurses in Turkey and the Crimea (1854-1856), and the opening of the Nightingale School of Nursing (1860), Florence Nightingale inspired women (and now men) around the world who would carry modern nursing forward as both an art and a science.

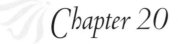

Chapter 20

Union with the Divine

Remember not, Lord (Perfect Wisdom, Perfect Love) Our offenses ... Oh could we but relinquish all Our earthly props and simply fall on thy Almighty arms.

—Florence Nightingale, Private Note, August 9, 1898[1]

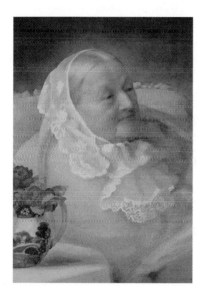

A watercolor of Florence
Nightingale at age 87
(detail of painting on page 405)

Like many aging mystics, Nightingale became more serene and pleasant as she grew older. Her quest for spiritual perfection and a greater understanding of God's love had always been her first concern. Now she could look back on her long life with the knowledge that she had responded to her Call and performed her worldly duties with fierce determination; having wrestled with her personal demons, she had passed through her "Dark Night of the Soul" and now emerged into a less demanding way of life and a place of tranquility. The main source of her serenity was not her concrete achievements, which were many, but a sense of her oneness with God, the final stage of the mystic's path.

In the late 1880s and 1890s, Nightingale was still working on various projects, but on a much smaller scale than in the past. Although she still often felt frustrated when the changes she sought were not achieved as quickly as she wanted, she never wavered from her profound conviction that her work and her life were for God. She took a great interest in the lives of her young nieces and nephews, and they in turn adored her and sought her advice. Her inner peace and acceptance of death are revealed in her letters and private notes, which, as usual, address a wide range of interests. Her most intimate correspondent continued to be her dear friend Benjamin Jowett, Master of Balliol College, Oxford.

Last years with Benjamin Jowett

As Nightingale and Jowett grew older, their mutual devotion deepened. They wrote each other often, and Jowett would stay with her once or twice a year either at South Street or Claydon. On December 31, 1886, he wrote her the following New Year's greeting:

Many happy returns of the New Year to you & to your work. May you live to complete it!
Most persons are engaged in feasting & holiday making amid their friends & relations. You

are alone in your room, devising plans for the good of the native of India or of the English sol-dier, as you have been for the last thirty years, and always deploring your failures as you have been doing for the last thirty years, though you have had a far greater & more real success in life than any other lady of your time. I think that you have chosen the better part.[2]

During a visit to South Street late in 1887, Jowett suffered a heart attack. Although many people wanted to visit him, Nightingale conspired with their mutual friend, the poet Robert Browning, to minimize the excitement of visitors. After Jowett returned to Oxford, Nightingale was in continuous correspondence with him or his housekeeper to inquire about his health and urge him to rest. On December 30, 1887, Jowett wrote her a note celebrating the silver anniversary of their long friendship:

"I hope this note will reach you on New Year's day: I cannot let the beginning of the year pass without wishing you every good & blessing on your labours.

Do you know that it is more than twenty five years since we became acquainted? I may venture, perhaps, to call ours a silver friendship. It has been a great blessing to me: one of the best things in my life.

I do not believe in going down hill; the truer, the safer, the better years of life are the later ones. We must find new ways of using them, doing not so much but in a better manner. Economising because economy has become necessary: for bodily strength obviously grows less. That is the will of God & cannot be escaped or denied ..."[3]

Jowett and Nightingale continued to discuss philosophical and spiritual matters, and they often recommended books to each other. One of their favorites was the Hindu classic the *Bhagavad Gita,* translated by Sir Edwin Arnold as "The Song Celestial." Both felt that this epic describing the battle between the forces of light and the forces of dark-ness expressed some of the most profound thoughts of the human heart: How easy it was not to fight, not to engage in battle for the things that mattered, and yet how neces-sary and right to do so. In her copy, Nightingale marked the following passage:

Abstaining from attachment to the work,
Abstaining from rewardment in the work,
While yet, one doeth it faithfully,
Saying, "Tis right to do!" — that is true act
And abstinence! Who doeth duties so,
Unvexed if his work fail, if it succeed
Unflattered, in his own heart justified
Quit of debates and doubts, his is "true" act.[4]

The primary motivation for all of Nightingale's reform efforts, including nurses' training, was spiritual, as revealed in the following letter to Jowett in 1889:

You say that "mystical or spiritual religion is not enough for most people without outward form." And I may say I can never remember a time when it was not the question of my life. Not so much for myself but for others. For myself the mystical or spiritual religion as laid down by St. John's Gospel, however imperfectly I have lived up to it, was and is enough. But the two thoughts which God has given me all my whole life have been – First, to infuse the mystical religion into the forms of others (always thinking they would show it forth much better than I), especially among women to make them the "handmaids of the Lord." Secondly, to give them an organization for their activity in which they could be trained to be the "handmaids of the Lord" ... When very many years ago I planned a future, my one idea was not organizing a Hospital, but organizing a Religion.[5]

Applied statistics at Oxford

Since 1890, Nightingale had been trying to establish a professorship in applied statistics at Oxford. For 30 years, she had been proclaiming that statistics was the one science essential to all political and social administration and to all education, yet no university in England taught the subject. For Nightingale, statistics was not merely a method of analyzing human behavior, of giving exact results of human experience, but also a way of understanding God's thoughts, for statistics were the measure of his purpose.

Among the social issues that Nightingale felt applied statistics should address were the deterrent effects of punishment on criminals; the impact of charity on workhouses; ways to prevent poverty in general; and whether the lives of children — especially girls — were improved or worsened by being in workhouses. She also wanted to investigate the best education for delinquent children, the type and amount of learning retained from night schools and secondary schools, and the types of university education that were best retained and those that were wasted after schooling.

Nightingale for years had been irritated by government officials' inability or unwillingness to make use of the excellent statistics that were available to them. She complained that they used such data only as ammunition for verbal battles with the opposition in Parliament. In her annual New Year's greeting to Jowett on January 3, 1891, she wrote:

> *... I thought our chief point was that the enormous amount of Statistics at this moment at their disposal ... is almost absolutely useless. Why? Because the Cabinet Ministers, the army of their subordinates, the House of Parliament, the large majority of whom have received a University education, have received no education whatever on the point upon which all legislation & all administration must — to be progressive & not see-saw-y — ultimately be based. We do not want a neat arithmetical sum. We want to know what we are doing. We want experience & not experiment ... What we want first is, not so much an accumulation of facts ... but to teach the men who are to govern the country what are the uses of facts, of "Statistics" ...*[6]

Nightingale and Jowett offered to contribute £2000 each to jointly endow a Chair in Applied Statistics at Oxford, with Jowett insisting that the professorship be named after Nightingale. To build support for the idea, the two approached Jowett's Oxford colleagues, Alfred Marshall and Arthur Balfour; Francis Galton, the noted statistician; and Arnold Toynbee, the Balliol tutor whom Jowett had previously assigned to students interested in Indian affairs. The authorities at Oxford were dubious about the proposal because the subject wasn't covered in university examinations, a major criterion for deciding which subjects to teach. In 1892, Nightingale revoked her £2,000 bequest by codicil because she feared the money would be used to sponsor a statistical essay contest rather than to teach statistics.

Death of Jowett

In the midst of this project, Jowett had another heart attack and became very ill. He had been losing stamina ever since his first heart attack in 1887. Nightingale, who had been staying at Claydon, considered going to Oxford, but her own health precluded the trip. In a letter of concern, she chided her old friend for having ignored his health:

> ... You live on your head for years. You entirely ignore the effect on the nerves, & the effect of the strained nervous system on the action of the heart and on sleep ... Nature sends in her bill. And that bill always has to be paid ... But if God wishes one to live, surely one ought to do all one can & all one knows to cooperate with Him. Else it is a kind of suicide ...[7]

By now, Nightingale and Jowett, both in their 70s, often reflected on old age, as in this prayer she wrote in a letter to him in October 1891: "O Father, God of childhood & youth & middle age, but more especially God of old age & of what we can do in old age, teach us to do all in Thy name & for Thy sake."[8] On May 6, 1892, he wrote to her to acknowledge all her support through the years:

> You are never out of my mind for long. I remember your extraordinary kindness to me during my long illness and before when I was ill five years ago & for more than thirty years before that. You have taken an interest in the College & my work. I have never come to you for sympathy & failed to receive it. And how little or nothing have I done in return for all this! I want to hold fast to you, dear friend, as I go down the hill. You and I are agreed that the last years of life are in a sense the best and that the most may be made of them even at the time when health & strength seem to be failing. I have ... left many things undone which I still hope to finish, or if I do not finish them to be resigned to the will of God.[9]

A note on September 18, 1893, included another tribute: "How greatly am I indebted to you for all your affection. How large a part has your life been of my life."[10] On October 1, Jowett died following another severe bout of illness. Nightingale penned a simple and profound tribute that she sent with flowers: "In loving remembrance of Revd Jowett, the Genius of Friendship among many trials, Above all the Friend of God who has now received the crown of life. Florence Nightingale Oct. 6, 1893."[11]

Nightingale received many letters after her friend's death, and two that touched her greatly were from Lord Lansdowne, who had been Jowett's favorite student at Balliol. Lansdowne was now Viceroy of India — the fifth viceroy Nightingale had educated on sanitation in the army stations in India. He wrote with affection about their mutual friend, who had influenced the lives of so many men in public affairs:

> Our dear old friend is, as far as his bodily presence in our midst is concerned, lost to us. It is a real sorrow to me. I had no more constant friend, and I cannot express the gratitude with which I look back to his unfailing interest in all that befell me and to his help and guidance at times when they were most needed. His saying that he meant to get better "because he had yet so much to do" is touching and characteristic. He was one who would never have sate [sat] down and said that his task was done, or that he was entitled to rest from toil for the remainder of his days. It would, however, be very far from the truth to think that his work was at an end because he is no longer here to carry it on with his own hands.[12]

On October 25, Lansdowne sent her another letter:

Of all the true and appreciative words which you have written of him, none seem to me truer than those in which you speak almost impatiently of the shallow fools who thought that he had "no religion." His religion always seemed to me nearer to that which The Master taught his followers than that of any other man or woman whom I have met, and I doubt whether any one of our time has done so much to spread true religion and Christianity in the best sense of the word.[13]

More old friends fall away

Sir Edwin Chadwick, the noted sanitary reformer with whom Nightingale had corresponded since 1857, died in 1890. Her faithful colleague, Dr. John Sutherland, died in 1891 after a serious illness. Sutherland had worked with her almost daily for 34 years, helping her compile and edit her many reports, and had served on the permanent Army Sanitary Commission until his retirement in 1888. On hearing of his illness, Nightingale had sent him a message. According to Mrs. Sutherland, when she told him about the letter, he roused himself to read it and said, "Give her my love and blessing" — these were almost his final words.[14]

In February 1894, Nightingale's brother-in-law, Sir Harry Verney, died at the age of 93. With the deaths of Jowett, Sutherland, and now Verney, Nightingale had lost her three main pillars of support. "I have lost the three nearest to me in twelve months," she wrote in a private note, and added of Verney that she felt the loss of "his courage, his courtesy, his kindness."[15]

In August 1894, William Shore Smith ("my boy Shore") died, and his younger son, Louis, inherited the Nightingale name and property. Shore's elder son, Samuel, had died the year before. Sam had served as a volunteer doctor in Bombay, prompting his aunt to remark that "the age of chivalry is come where people volunteer not to kill but to cure."[16] Lea Hurst had been rented out for a decade, and Nightingale never returned there after her mother's death. Her last visit to Embley came in August 1891, and the property was sold in 1896. Her final visit to Claydon, the Verney estate, was in January 1895, a year after Verney's death.

Sir Robert Rawlinson, the last surviving member of the Sanitary Commission, whom she had met during the Crimean War, died in 1898. The next year, her loyal friend and colleague Sir Douglas Galton, died; she wrote a detailed note about his work and how he had opened his ears and heart to the needs of the people with proper sanitation. Then, in 1902, came the death of philanthropist William Rathbone, founder of the Liverpool Workhouse Infirmary. Rathbone had worked closely with Nightingale on various nursing projects over the years, including the fight against nurses' registration in 1886 and 1887. He had supplied her room with flowers every week without fail since her birthday on May 12, 1865, and had once written of her, "In any matter of nursing Miss Nightingale is my Pope and I believe in her infallibility."[17] Nightingale sent a wreath to the Rathbone family inscribed "In remembrance and humblest love of one of God's best and greatest sons."

Final years

In honor of Nightingale's 70th birthday on May 12, 1890, a flood of congratulations poured in from royalty, distinguished politicians and friends, and nursing schools and societies all over the world. A greeting from Japan, praising her work, noted that the Japanese Nursing Society now numbered 1,500. In England, sending birthday letters to Florence Nightingale became a favorite exercise of school children.

On July 30, 1890, 12 years after Thomas Edison invented the phonograph, his assistant in London, Colonel George Gouraud, made a 41-second recording of Nightingale's voice at her home on South Street. Her recorded words reveal that her Crimean War experiences were never far from her mind: "When I am no longer even a memory, just a name, I hope my voice may perpetuate the great work of my life. God bless my dear old comrades of Balaclava and bring them safe to shore. Florence Nightingale."[18]

Nightingale continued to suffer from insomnia and during the long sleepless hours often wrote notes reflecting on her abundant life, her work for God, and her friends, most of whom she had by now outlived. She continued to mark the special dates on her spiritual journey, as in this 1892 private note:

Calls to work? to holiness.

Lea Hurst Shore's door	*Behold the handmaid of the Lord.*
Embley Feb. 7, 1837	*The way to do good*
Lea Hurst 1848	*On my knees in middle hours:*
	not going to Hamburg.
Alexandria 1850	*To throw my body in the breach.*
Bridge Hills 1844	*Call to hospital work.*

Which have I followed? [19]

A private note written the following year expressed gratitude and peace:

November 3-4, 1893. Thirty-nine years ago arrival at Scutari. The immense blessings I have had — the longings of my heart accomplished — and now drawn to Thee by difficulties and disappointments. Homeward bound. I have entered in.[20]

Nightingale's activities may have been curtailed in the 1890s, but her keen powers of observation and playful wit were undiminished, as revealed in a letter to Norman Bonham Carter, one of Henry's sons, on August 2, 1895:

... I learn the lesson of life from a little kitten of mine, one of two. The old cat comes in and says, very cross, "I didn't ask you in here, I like to have the Missis to myself!" And he runs at them. The bigger and handsomer kitten runs away, but the little one stands her ground, and when the old enemy comes near enough kisses his nose, and makes the peace. That is the lesson of life, to kiss one's enemy's nose, always standing one's ground ... [21]

Though she began to complain to her doctors of a new symptom in September 1895 — "want of memory" — she told her cousin Henry Bonham Carter: "I have my hands full, and am not idle, though people naturally think that I have gone to sleep or am dead."[22]

A plague of biographers

In 1895 and 1896, most of Nightingale's nonpersonal correspondence was with her nurses and matrons, who by this time were working at hospitals all over the world. However, she was also plagued by requests from biographers for copies of her letters and from other correspondents for her picture and "a few words." In numerous letters, she complained to Lady Margaret Verney, wife of Sir Harry's eldest son, Edmund:

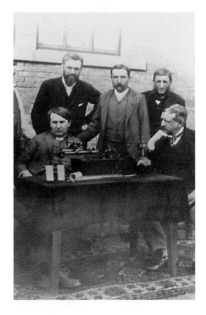

Thomas Edison (seated left), who sent his assistant, Colonel George Gouraud (seated right), to Nightingale's London home on July 30, 1890, to record her voice

> *My dear, I am a fool, but was there ever such a fool in the world as these American ladies suppose me? I have just had a … letter asking me to write a short "life" of myself for her and I have sometimes 19 similar letters by one mail … then they want a photograph … I cannot read her name. F for Fool.[23]*

When Benjamin Jowett's biographer, Evelyn Abbott, asked for her last letters to Jowett, Nightingale said she couldn't find them though there were enough letters in her drawers "to cover Australia."[24] She finally did cooperate with Abbott, however, and appreciated the fact that he let her review parts of the manuscript for which she had supplied information.

A proposed biography of Sidney Herbert was more distressing. When Nightingale learned that Herbert's widow, Elizabeth, had given the biographer all of her letters to Herbert without her consent, she expressed her irritation in a letter to Margaret:

> *Dearest Blessed Margaret … Honour has departed from the face of the earth in the matter of Biographies. Well might Sir Cornwall Lewis say: "A new terror is added to death." The only gentleman left is Mr. Evelyn Abbott, the biographer of Mr. Jowett's. Every page of which I have supplied the materials has passed thru' my hands & no extract has been printed without my sanction …*
>
> *The third veil has fallen upon me: it must be one of Dante's Purgatories. Gladstone and Lady Herbert have asked Lord Stanmore to write Sidney Herbert's life, S. Herbert whom he did not know & whom he is quite incapable of appreciating. And Lady Herbert with whom I was as intimate as with her husband, <u>without my knowledge or consent</u> has lent the whole of my letters to S. Herbert to Lord Stanmore!! who now coolly writes & asks me for all Sidney Herbert's!! letters to me!!! My letters to S. Herbert include all the time of the two Royal Sanitary Commissions of which he was President & during a time when he called every day while he was in London, upon me; & I wrote to him upon the matter of those confidential conversations … [25]*

Shortly thereafter, Stanmore asked her to review which of her joint works with Herbert had endured. She noted that the Army Sanitary Commission was still in existence; the military hospitals were being maintained; the Army Medical School had been moved to Netley; the School of Cookery at Aldershot was in the Queen's Regulations; the army's medical statistics were still published annually; and the Barracks Subcommission's recommendations of 1861 (including improved barrack construction and the addition of recreation and reading rooms) had been implemented.

Commemorating the Crimean War

In October 1895, Reverend T. G. Clark, from Birmingham, the Honorary Secretary of the Balaclava Anniversary Celebration, asked her to write a few words marking the battle's 40th anniversary. Her reply was:

> *You ask me to say a few words for the anniversary of the Balaclava Charge to your veterans. I am often speaking to them in my heart, but I am much overworked. And what I speak in my heart is something like this — The soldier has such good stuff in him ... He really "loves" his comrade "as himself" when he himself returns safe out of gunshot and he finds his comrade or his officer missing, he goes back to bring him off. How many have lost (or rather "gained") their lives in this way ...*
>
> *At one great battle which had to be fought in the defensive, and won, the men stood firm as rocks till they fell not a man stirred. They did not fight for glory. Where would England be but not for them? And may we say not, Where will England be if her men do not stand firm like rocks to the right, and the true, and the holy, and the loving?*
>
> *Is England better than she was for me? Let each man ask himself this question? Sometimes he forgets that we may fight the good fight — the good fight against the enemy — in common for home life as well as in the field ...*
>
> *Fight the good fight, never forget that you are the brave soldiers of God who loves you. You are fighting for Him and His England now.*
>
> *God bless you and He will bless you. Such are the thoughts for the old soldiers [from] their faithful servant.*[26]

Close ties to the younger generation

In the final decades of her life, Nightingale became very close to the Verney family — Sir Harry's children and grandchildren — as well as to some of the children of her cousins, whom she called her nieces and nephews. These young people felt that "Aunt Florence" understood them better than any other adult and often came to her with their problems, confident that she would have some marvelous solution. She responded with unfailing generosity, understanding, and affection.

Among her favorites in the younger generation were her frequent correspondent Margaret Verney (whom she often referred to as "blessed Margaret"); her goddaughter, Ruth Florence Verney, Margaret's daughter; Frederick Verney, Sir Harry's youngest son; and Rosalind Nash, daughter of William Shore Smith. She depended on these young nieces and nephews to help her with personal and work-related matters, thus taking some of the burden off her cousin Henry Bonham Carter.

In 1896, Nightingale made out her will and appointed Henry Bonham Carter the executor. By this time, he was managing all of her private affairs as well as the Nightingale School of Nursing. Although she never left South Street after 1896, her daily notes continued to be full of talk about daily life at South Street and at the homes of her relatives, including such topics as who was attending balls at Claydon or going to

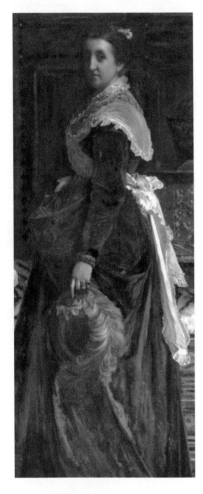

Margaret Verney, one of Nightingale's favorite relatives in the final years of her life

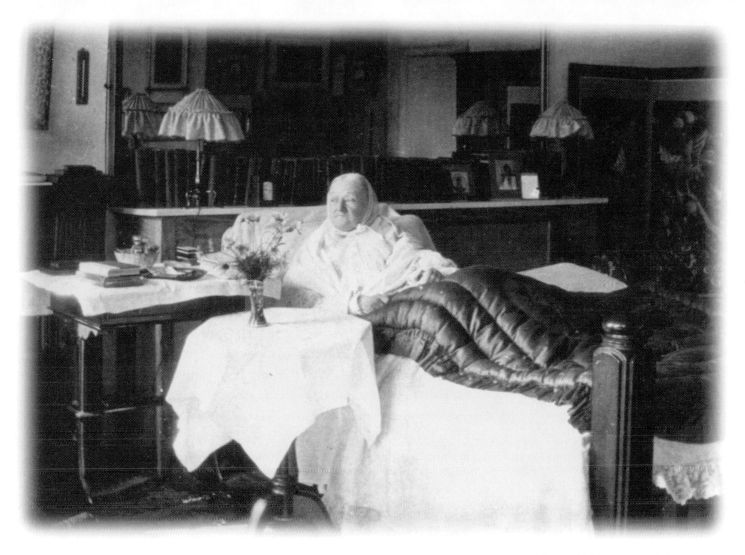

Florence Nightingale, age 86, in her London bedroom in a photo taken by her nurse, Elizabeth Bosanquet, c. 1906

London for business or the theatre. When Margaret Verney's daughter Ellin had her first child, Nightingale tried mightily in a volley of letters to convince her to name the baby girl "Balaclava" — to her one of the most beautiful names in the world.[27]

Many of her letters to Verney relatives contained reminiscences of Sir Harry and others who were now gone:

> *Dearest Blessed Margaret, Indeed I do think of dear old Sir Harry (old and Sir Harry no more) on this day and of your memorable words: "By his gentlemanship and courtesy he kept the command of himself and his room till the last moment." and of your making his last years so happy — happier than my father's ... My father has been dead 23 years and yet do you know I often find myself calling out to him, as if he were there, tho in all my life, I never can remember him caressing me.[28]*

With her eyesight failing, Nightingale now had books, newspapers, Blue Books, and other materials read to her. Among her favorite books was Theodore Roosevelt's *A Strenuous Life* and Browning's *The Ring and the Book*. It is easy to understand her enjoyment of Browning's book, which explored the power that one soul can wield over another. She wrote her favorite short poems and Bible verses on large cards that she read with difficulty. She would often recite favorite passages from Milton and Shelley as well as favorite selections of Italian and French verses in a vibrant voice that was said to fill the room.

Diamond Jubilee exhibition

In 1897, planning was underway for Queen Victoria's Diamond Jubilee celebration. In the proposed Victorian Era Exhibition, one section was to be devoted to nursing. Lady Wantage, an old friend, asked Nightingale for some of her personal mementoes from the Crimean War as well as her photographs, autographs, and the bust of her by Sir John Steell. Though Nightingale had little patience for such requests, she could not refuse this lady, of whom she was very fond. Yet, in a letter to Edmund Verney, Nightingale made clear that the true legacy of the Crimean War was not to be found in such "relics":

> ... About the bust by Steell of Edinburgh which is the one, I believe, at Claydon ... it was given me by the soldiers after the Crimean War; and I sat for it — it is left in my Will back to the soldiers, if it were not given back to them during my life — and enquiries have already been made where soldiers would like it best to be, whether at Aldershot, or where.
>
> I do not know who told Lady Wantage of this bust ... When she, Lady Wantage, came to me, she knew about it. And it was impossible for me to decline lending it to them for the ... Exhibition. (I have such a respect for Lady Wantage. She sometimes just reminds me a little of Margaret.) So I did promise it her. You perhaps know that I had previously refused all solicitations to give them "relics" of "me & the Crimean War," on the grounds that the real "relics" were:
>
> 1. Sidney Herbert's R. Commission & 4 Sub-Commissions which laid the imperishable seed of the great improvements in the soldier's daily life — direct & indirect.
>
> 2. the training of Nurses both in character and technical skill & knowledge. The untrained Nurses sent out to the Crimean War were — well, it is unspeakable what they were.
>
> 3. the Hygiene & Sanitation the want of which in the Military & Medical authorities caused Lord Raglan's death & that of thousands of our men from disease.
>
> That frightful lesson really, thanks to Dr. Sutherland, Sir Douglas Galton, Sir Robert Rawlinson & others, began & continued the enormous strides which have since been made in (Civil & Military) science of Life and Death ... [29]

Nightingale finally allowed the sculpted marble bust by Sir John Steell and her old Crimean carriage (found in pieces in a farmhouse loft at Lea Hurst) to be put on display. One of her friends justified the decision on the grounds that the people needed something to love, and they could not love a Royal Commission. When she heard that the bust was strung with flowers and that an old Crimean soldier was seen to have kissed it, she was highly irritated. In a private note, she revealed her own more modest perspective on her accomplishments in the war: "How inefficient I was in the Crimea! Yet He has raised up Trained Nursing from it!"[30]

Queen Victoria invited Nightingale to watch the Diamond Jubilee procession from the forecourt of Buckingham Palace. She declined the invitation but did purchase seats for several of her nurses.

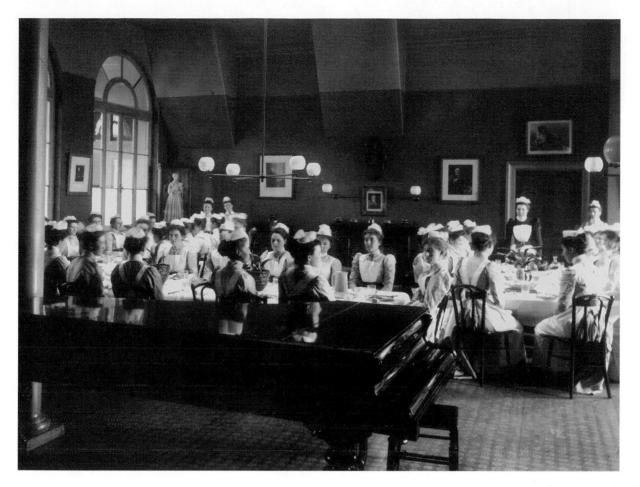

Nightingale School probationers in the dining room of the nurses' residence, c. 1900

Physical decline

After 1898, Nightingale had only a few visitors each week, mainly her close nieces and nephews and a few of her former nursing students. She could still carry on lively, fact-filled conversations, and still possessed her characteristic sense of humor. Visitors described her as robust and vigorous. With her needs tended to by a housekeeper and a cook, she still did a lot of corresponding. Her handwriting was still very legible, and she wrote most of her letters with a brand of pencil that had been supplied to her for years by an old friend at the War Office.

Nightingale always made it a point to correspond with old Crimean War veterans, and she was still concerned about the health of British soldiers, particularly during the Boer War in South Africa from 1899 to 1902. When her former nursing students were sent out to South Africa, she contributed £100 to the Scottish Hospital there.

As Nightingale celebrated her 80th birthday on May 12, 1900, congratulatory letters arrived from all over the world. A week later, she wrote one of her last addresses to the Nightingale School probationers, thanking them for their birthday greetings and gifts and still exhorting them to do honor to their profession:

> *My dear children, You have called me your Mother-Chief, it is an honour to me — & a great honour, to call you my children. Always keep up the honours of this honourable profession — I thank you — may I say our Heavenly Father thanks you for what you do!*

The old Romans were in some respects I think superior to us. But they had no idea of being good to the sick and weak. That came in with Christianity. Christ was the author of our profession. We honour Christ when we are good nurses. We dishonour Him when we are bad or careless nurses. We dishonour Him when we do not do our best to relieve suffering — even in the meanest creature. Kindness to sick man, woman & child came in with Christ. They used to be left on the banks of the great rivers to starve or drown themselves. Lepers were kept apart — the nation did not try to avert or to cure leprosy ... Now it is a thing almost if not quite unknown.

There have been great, I may say, discoveries in Nursing: *... The change in the treatment of Pneumonia ... is complete. I myself saw a Doctor take up a child sufferer, which seemed as if it could hardly breathe — carry it to the window, open the window at the top, & hold it up there. The nurse positively yelled with horror. He only said: "When my Patient can breathe but little air, I like that little good." The child recovered & lived to old age.*

Nursing is become a profession. Trained Nursing no longer an object but a fact. But, oh, if home Nursing could become an every day fact here in this big city of London, the biggest in the world in ... the smallest inhabited island in the world. But here in London in feeding — a most important branch of it — if you ask a mother who has perhaps brought you a sick child to "look at" [and you ask]: "What have you given it to eat?" she answers triumphantly, "O, it has the same as we have?(!). Yes, often including the gin ...

Now, will you let me try to thank you, tho' words cannot express my thankfulness for all your kind thoughts, for your beautiful books & basket of flowers & kind wishes, all. God bless you all and me your Mother Chief as you are good enough to call me, My dear children.

Florence Nightingale[31]

By 1901, Nightingale's eyesight had failed and her letters were being read to her by her relatives, but she still wrote a few short letters in large, legible script. She continued to receive letters from all over the world, including from some of her favorite former students, such as Angelique Pringle, Rachel Williams Norris, and Maria Machin Redpath. Still very alert, Nightingale revised her will three times, the last time on June 7, 1901.

For some years now, Nightingale had been receiving most of her medical care from a woman doctor, May Thorne. In 1902, she finally reached the point where she needed round-the-clock care, but she still had to be persuaded by the family. Alice Cochrane, who was hired to care for her, reported that after she tucked Nightingale in for the night, Nightingale would get out of bed and go next door to tuck *her* in.[32] After Cochrane married in 1904, Elizabeth Bosanquet was employed to care for her. Bosanquet was referred to as a "lady housekeeper" because Nightingale never took kindly to having to be cared for by a nurse.

Nightingale still maintained an active interest in family and community matters, such as the founding of the new public library and village hall near Claydon. In October 1904, when she received word that one of her original nurses in the Crimea had been living in a workhouse for 22 years, she arranged for the woman to move to a comfortable home and receive an annual pension. She continued to receive papers on India until 1906, when her secretary informed the India Office that she could no longer read them.

One of her last messages, written with great difficulty, was to the nursing staff of the Edinburgh Royal Infirmary on New Year's Day, 1905: "I pray with all my heart that God will bless the work abundantly in Edinburgh Infirmary, and enable the workers to

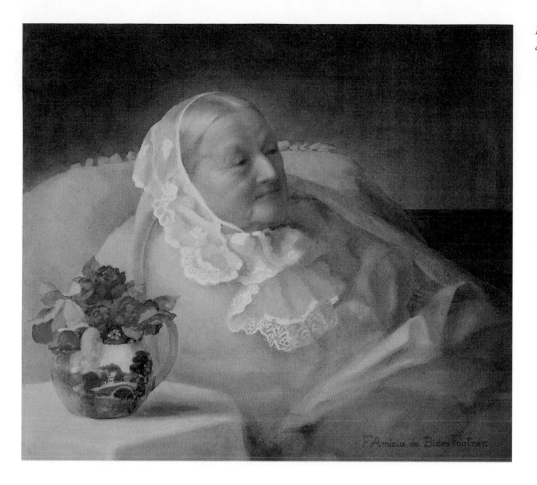

do it for Him, in the love which we owe Him."[33] In her final message, to the Crimean War veterans on their 1905 anniversary celebration, she referred to herself in the third person: "The anniversaries celebrated by the Veterans have always been marked days to her also."[34]

A slew of honors

Nightingale's last years were graced with some official — though belated — honors. In 1904, King Edward VII conferred upon her the title of a Lady of Grace of the Order of St. John of Jerusalem. On November 28, 1907, she became the first woman to receive the Order of Merit "in recognition of invaluable services to the country and humanity." The king's emissary delivered the medal to Nightingale on December 5. Although her mind had begun to fail and she wasn't fully capable of understanding the exact nature of the award, she was aware that some kindness had been bestowed upon her and replied, "Too kind, too kind."[35]

King Edward VII had created the Order of Merit in 1902 "as the Monarch's personal reward for especially eminent service."[36] Other well-known winners subsequently included Winston Churchill and Dwight Eisenhower, but no other woman received the award until 1965.

Hundreds of congratulations poured in from England, the Dominions, the United States, and elsewhere. Flowers, illuminated cards, and various presents, such as needlework and pictures, were sent by Crimean War veterans, school children, girls named

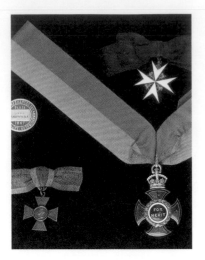

Florence, royalty, and Nightingale societies. The Mayor of Florence, Italy, sent congratulations; the Patriotic Society of Bologna bestowed upon her the Companion of Honour; and German Emperor Wilhelm II, who had been staying near the New Forest not far from Embley, her old home, sent his regards and flowers.

On June 8, 1907, the International Conference of Red Cross Societies held its eighth International Congress in London. Queen Alexandra sent a message referring to "the pioneer of the first Red Cross Movement, Miss Florence Nightingale, whose heroic efforts on behalf of suffering humanity will be recognized and admired by all ages as long as the world shall last."[37]

On February 13, 1908, Nightingale was awarded the Freedom of the City of London. She was the second woman to receive this honor; the first had been Lady Angela Burdett-Coutts, the philanthropist. Louis Shore Nightingale, the son of William Shore Smith, attended the ceremony at the Guildhall in London on Nightingale's behalf and accepted a copy of the Resolution, which read as follows:

> *At a Court of Common Council, 13 February, 1908, it was resolved unanimously: That the Honorary Freedom of this City, in a Gold Box of the value of one hundred Guineas, be presented to Miss Florence Nightingale, in testimony of this Court's appreciation of her philanthropic and successful efforts for the improvement of hospital nursing and management, whereby invaluable results have been attained for the alleviation of human suffering."[38]*

Order of Merit awarded to Florence Nightingale "in recognition of invaluable services to the country and humanity" by King Edward VII on November 28, 1907. No other woman received this honor until 1965.

BELOW: *Scroll of the Freedom of the City of London, one of several major awards Nightingale received in the last decade of her life*

When Nightingale heard about the gold box, she asked if the money that would have been spent on the box could instead be given to the Institution for the Care of Sick Gentlewomen in Distressed Circumstances on Harley Street, the scene of her first nursing position, and 100 guineas was duly gifted to the hospital. This institution was later renamed the Florence Nightingale Hospital for Gentlewomen. On March 16, Nightingale received a beautiful oak box engraved with the words "Crimea," "Inkerman," and "Sevastopol" that contained her scroll. Shortly thereafter, the city's Roll of Honor was brought to No. 10 South Street and Nightingale signed her initials with great difficulty.

In 1907, when Mary Adelaide Nutting became the first professor of nursing in the world at Teachers College, Columbia University, New York, she recognized Nightingale for her impact on nurses' training. In May 1910, a commemoration in honor of the

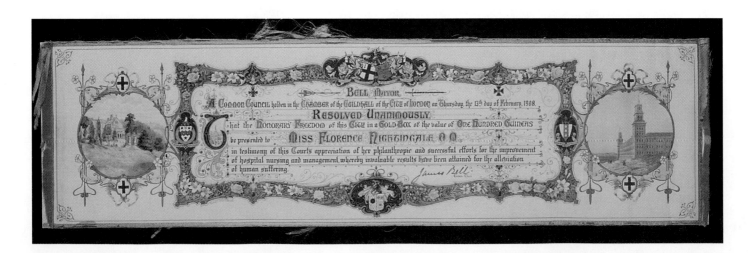

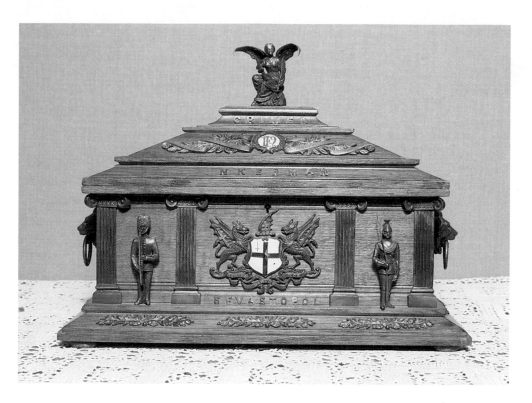

Death & burial

Jubilee of the Nightingale School of Nursing took place at Carnegie Hall in New York. The public orator Joseph Choate delivered an address "testifying to the admiration of the entire American people for Miss Florence Nightingale's great record and noble life."[39]

In the last few years of her life, Nightingale had trouble remembering which of her friends were dead; she frequently called for Sir Harry Verney and was puzzled when he didn't respond. She was unable to follow a story when being read to, but she liked to hear the old familiar hymns. The last person outside of the family to visit her was Angelique Pringle in February 1910. Pringle found Nightingale sitting up by the fire with a peaceful expression, seemingly reviewing memories in her mind; from time to time, she uttered a few words of contentment.

On August 13, 1910, Nightingale fell asleep at noon and did not wake again. She died 2½ hours later. Her death certificate recorded the cause of death as old age and heart failure. (This document was filled out by Dr. Louisa Garrett Anderson, the daughter of Dr. Elizabeth Garrett Anderson, the first Englishwoman to obtain a medical degree in England and who had sparred with Nightingale on the issue of women doctors.) Nightingale had lived 90 years and 3 months.

The British government offered to have an elaborate state funeral and burial in Westminster Abbey, but Nightingale's family honored her request for a simple burial, devoid of trappings, with no memorial to mark the place of her "mortal coil." Nightingale had wanted her body to be used for "medical science," but the family did not honor this request. At a tribute held in her honor at Westminster Abbey the following day, the minister spoke words with which Nightingale would no doubt have agreed : "No one has ever done anything great or useful by listening to the voices from without."[40]

On August 15, the London *Times* ran a four-column obituary that summarized her life and work under the headings "The Crimean War," "Arrival at the Front," "Criticism at Home," "Growth of the Work," "The End of the War," "Later Reform," "District Nursing," and "Writings." The last section, "Closing Years," said:

> *In these various ways one sees how Florence Nightingale, though a bedridden invalid, and well advanced in years, was still ready, as she had been throughout life, to devote her energies to promoting the practical well-being of her fellow creatures. What with writing papers, pamphlets, and letters, receiving reports concerning the many movements in which she was interested, and dealing with communications from Government authorities, and others all the world over, she was, even in the closing years of her life, essentially a hard-working woman. How great, indeed, were the demands made upon her time as well shown by a letter addressed by her on October 21, 1895, to the Rev. T. G. Clark, curate of St. Philip's, Birmingham, and local secretary of the Balaclava Anniversary Commemoration. In the course of this letter she said: — "I could not resist your appeal, though it is an effort to me, who know not what it is to have a leisure hour, to write a few words"; and she added: — " I generally resist all temptations to write, except on very pressing business. I am often speaking to your Balaclava veterans in my heart, but I am much overworked."[41]*

On August 20, huge crowds of mourners came to pay their respects at the memorial service at London's St. Paul's Cathedral. Over 2,500 people beseiged the War Office for tickets; many were turned away. The Nightingale School probationers traveled to the service in double-decker buses. Alderman Sir James Richie, acting for the Lord Mayor, drove in state to the service, attended by the Swordbearer, the Mace-bearer, and the City Marshall. The War Office and the army sent official representatives, as did most London hospitals and nursing societies.

Copy of Florence Nightingale's death certificate, signed by the daughter of the first English-woman to be listed in the British Medical Register

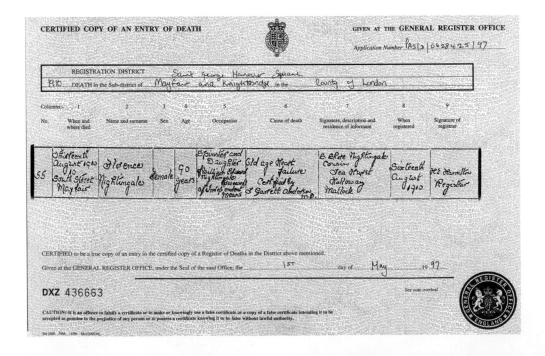

UNION WITH THE DIVINE

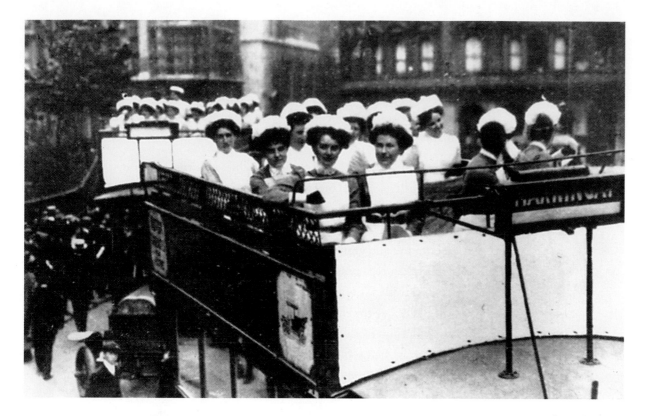

As the band of the Coldstream Guards played, the crowd swelled, overflowing into the space under the dome and into the choir galleries. To honor Nightingale's wishes, the service did not include a military ceremony, but the many officers and soldiers who attended wore their military uniforms. Seated along the south side of the dome were about 50 Crimean War veterans with their medals glittering. Some could walk only with sticks and crutches, and some had lost limbs; all were pensioners from the Chelsea Hospital for old and disabled soldiers, led by their Adjutant. Near the Chelsea pensioners were several contingents of nurses: the women representing the Territorial Forces Nursing Service, wearing short scarlet capes over their uniforms; the representatives of Queen Alexandra's Imperial Military Nursing Service in gray and scarlet capes; and the representatives of the Royal Naval Nursing Services.

Facing the altar were the representatives of King George V and Queen Mary, who were at Balmoral, the Queen Mother, the Duke of Connaught, and the Princess Christian; as well as the Prime Minister and other notables. Behind them sat numerous senior officers in brilliantly colored uniforms.

The inscription on the coffin was simple: "Florence Nightingale, Born May 12, 1820, Died Aug. 13, 1910."

After the national tribute at St. Paul's, Nightingale's coffin was taken by a special funeral train to the Nightingale family church, St. Margaret's in East Wellow, Hampshire, for burial. At the train station at Romsey, the coffin was placed on a funeral carriage. Nine men from units that had fought in the Crimea — the Grenadiers, the Coldstream Guards, and the Scots Guards — were chosen to shoulder the coffin.

The coffin was covered with Nightingale's white cashmere shawl and surrounded by many wreaths. At its foot lay Queen Alexandra's cross of mauve orchids fringed with

Nightingale nurses en route to St. Paul's Cathedral, London, for the memorial service in honor of Florence Nightingale

BELOW: *Announcement of the memorial service held at St. Paul's on August 20, 1910*

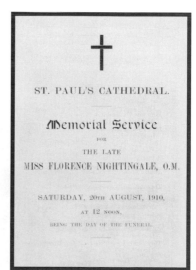

✝

ST. PAUL'S CATHEDRAL.

Memorial Service

FOR

THE LATE

MISS FLORENCE NIGHTINGALE, O.M.

SATURDAY, 20TH AUGUST, 1910,

AT 12 NOON,

BEING THE DAY OF THE FUNERAL.

white roses and lilies. Attached to it was a black-edged card with an inscription in the Queen Mother's handwriting:

> *To Miss Florence Nightingale. In grateful memory of the greatest benefactor to suffering humanity, by founding the Military Nursing Service in the year 1853* by her own individual exertions and heroism — August 20, 1910. From Alexandra [*Print error, should have been 1854-1856]*

Behind the hearse, five coaches carried the chief mourners. Among them were William Shore Smith's widow, Louisa; his son Louis and daughter Rosalind Nash and their spouses; Arthur Hugh Clough's son Arthur and his wife; Aunt Mai's daughter, Bertha Coltman, and her husband; Henry Bonham Carter's two children; and Sir Harry Verney's son Edmund and grandson Frederick.

As the funeral cortège passed slowly through Romsey's narrow streets, shopkeepers and villagers came to their doors and bowed their heads. The Union Jack flew at half-mast from the old Abbey tower, and the tolling of the church bells was heard for miles. The procession continued out of Romsey; past Broadlands, Lord Palmerston's estate; and along the narrow, hedge-bordered road between Romsey and East Wellow. When it reached the boundary of Embley Park, the Nightingales' old winter estate, it went through the main gate up the drive, past the front of the grand house, and left by another gate into the lane that led to the church. Only a few followed the funeral procession on foot to the church. Farm workers had left the fields to join many villagers and district people, and all were waiting at the churchyard to pay their respects to "Miss Florence," the woman whom their parents and grandparents had known.

As the procession reached the church, the warm late-August sunshine changed to a heavy rain. The guardsmen carried the coffin up the steep path to the church, where umbrella-covered onlookers stood three and four deep. In front of the coffin walked six former servants from Embley who had known Nightingale as children; behind followed

Nightingale's funeral carriage crossing the bridge over the River Test after leaving Romsey en route to St. Margaret's Church in East Wellow

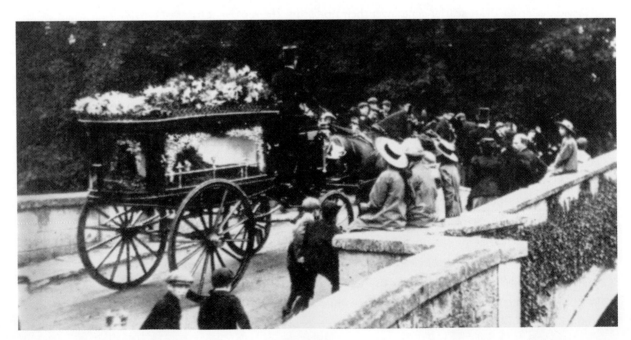

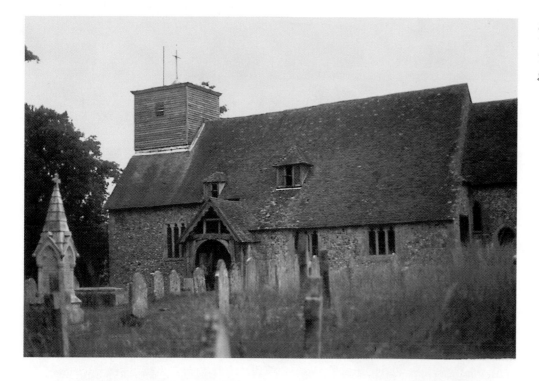

the family mourners. Under the church porch stood Private John Kneller, an 84-year-old Crimean War veteran who had lost an eye during the battle of Sebastopol and had lain for 3 months in the Barrack Hospital under Nightingale's care.[42]

In the 13th-century St. Margaret's Church, which was filled to capacity, the mourners recited the 90th Psalm and sang the hymns "On the Resurrection Morning" and "Now the Labourer's Task Is O'er." After the service, the coffin was carried to the grave by military pallbearers drawn from various regiments of the British Army.

Nightingale was buried next to her father and mother in the beautiful churchyard. As her body was lowered to the grave, mourners sang one of her favorite hymns — "The Son of God Goes Forth to War" — whose lyrics she often quoted:

> The Son of God goes forth to war,
> kingly crown to gain;
> His blood-red banner streams afar,
> Who follows in his train?
> Who best can drink his cup of woe,
> Triumphant over pain;
> Who patient bears his cross below,
> He follows in his train.

At the end of her autobiographical essay, "Cassandra," Nightingale had written, "Let neither name nor date be placed on her grave, still less the expression of regret or of admiration, but simply the words, 'I believe in God.'" In keeping with her wishes not to be glorified, the family grave marker was engraved with only a simple small cross and the words "F. N. Born 12 May 1820. Died 13 August 1910." This simple epitaph was consistent with the mystic's desire to leave behind the Self and to become one with the Absolute.

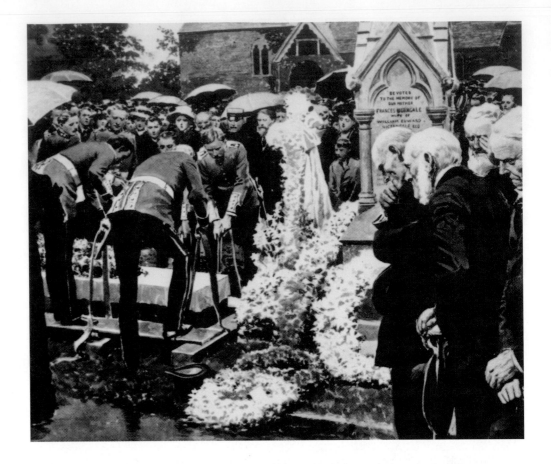

Lining the churchyard path lay some 500 wreaths from dignitaries, nursing associations, and ordinary people from all around the world, ranging from the American Ambassador and members of the Royal Army Medical Corps to the wife of Peter Grillage, the Russian orphan whom Nightingale had brought from the Crimea and taken into service. One wreath was from a 7-year-old girl, who wrote: "To dear Miss Nightingale. please may my wreath be put with the other flowers? I picked the heather and made it myself."[43]

Final bequests

The executors of Nightingale's will were Henry Bonham Carter, Louis Shore Nightingale, and Arthur Clough (the son). Nightingale's estate totaled £32,384 (approximately £2,000,000 and US$3,000,000 in current values[44]). The will bequeathed amounts ranging from £20 to £250 to several organizations and approximately 45 different relatives and friends, including her last messenger, cook, horseman, house maid, parlor maid, and a temporary servant. She bequeathed her cats and a parrot to one of her maids and another woman. Her valuables were distributed to individuals she had named. She bequeathed all of her other possessions along with her letters, papers, and manuscripts to Henry Bonham Carter.

To Sir William Wedderburn, who worked with Nightingale on India reform, she bequeathed £250 "for some Indian object[ive]."[45] Wedderburn and Rosalind Nash added to this amount and established the Florence Nightingale Fund for village sanitation. After the death of Indian nationalist Gopal Krishna Gokhale in 1915, Wedderburn proposed that the fund be used to endow a Gokhale Scholarship for an Indian female student to receive training in sanitary science.[46]

In accordance with Nightingale's wishes, her Crimean War decorations, the Order of Merit, the bracelet presented to her by the Sultan, the brooch given to her by Queen Victoria, and the marble bust commissioned by the soldiers were later placed in the Museum of the United Service Institute, where the soldiers could see them.

At the request of Nightingale's executors, Rosalind Nash, Nightingale's last housekeeper Elizabeth Bosanquet, and Mrs. Henry Toynbee were engaged to arrange, index, and classify all of Nightingale's letters and documents. The executors also commissioned Sir Edward T. Cook to write her biography, which was published in two volumes in 1913.

World memorials

Memorials were soon set up all over the world. Shortly after Nightingale's death, Mrs. Bedford Fenwick, President of the International Council of Nurses, initiated an international memorial to further nursing education throughout the world. The English community in Florence, Italy, set up a memorial in the Cloisters of Santa Croce. British army nurses established a memorial window in the chapel of the Military Hospital at Millbank. In Derby, a statue was commissioned by Countess Feodora Gleichen.

A National Memorial Fund was set up to collect money for a statue. At the Crimean War Memorial in Waterloo Place, London, where a memorial to Sidney Herbert was already in place, a statue of Florence Nightingale was erected on February 24, 1915, as a memorial to her great and lasting achievements. The sculptor, A.G. Walker, depicted Nightingale walking the hallway at Scutari. At the base of the statue are four panels. Three depict scenes from her life, and the fourth bears a simple inscription: "Florence

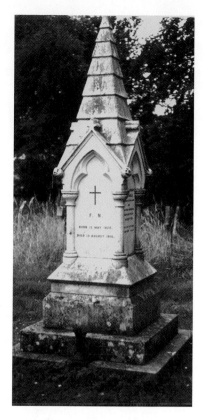

Nightingale's simple inscription on the family grave marker at St. Margaret's Church reads: "F.N., Born 12 May 1820, Died 13 August 1910."

BELOW: *Various medals, including the Order of Merit (bottom center), bestowed upon Nightingale*

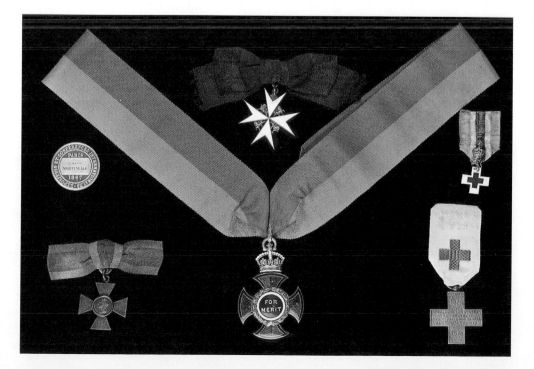

Crimean War Memorial at Waterloo Place in London, with statues of Florence Nightingale (center) and Sidney Herbert (right)

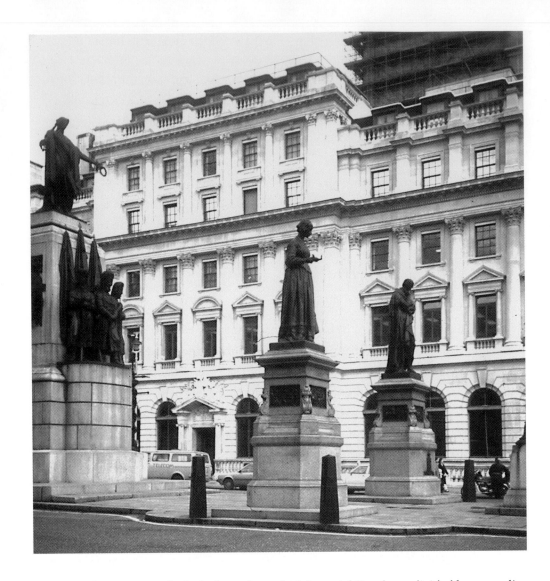

Nightingale 1820-1910." The balance from the Memorial Fund was divided between district nursing and the Nurse's Pension Fund.

Nightingale's memory continues to be celebrated in many places even today. Every year on her birthday, services are held at Westminster Abbey and St. Margaret's Church in Hampshire, and a wreath is laid at her statue in Waterloo Place. Many Anglican and Episcopal churches and cathedrals have Nightingale stained-glass windows and hold services in her memory. In 1915, her executors commissioned a bronze bust cast from the original 1862 marble bust by John Robert Steell, which now sits in the Florence Nightingale Museum in London.

Gandhi's tribute

The great Indian nationalist leader Mohandas K. Gandhi recognized Nightingale's immense achievements in 1915. Gandhi had returned to India from South Africa in 1914 and began writing a column in *Indian Opinion* to inspire his readers by sharing examples of great men and women, such as Tolstoy, Lincoln, Mazzini, and others. Gandhi wrote the following article on Florence Nightingale, which was published in *Indian Opinion* on September 9, 1915:

We have in an earlier issue of the journal published an account of the career of the benevolent lady, Elizabeth Fry. Just as she brought about an improvement in the condition of prisoners and devoted her life to their service, so also Florence Nightingale sacrificed herself in the service of the men in the army. When the Great Crimean War broke out in 1851 [actually 1853], the British Government was as usual not alive to the situation. There was no preparation. And just as in the Boer War, so in the Crimean War, too, they committed blunders in the beginning and suffered a crushing defeat.

Fifty years ago, the various facilities for nursing the wounded which are available today did not exist. People did not come out to render aid in large numbers as they do now. Surgery was not as efficacious then as it is today. There were in those days very few men who considered it an act of mercy and merit to succour the wounded. It was at such a time that this lady, Florence Nightingale, came upon the scene and did good work worthy of an angel descended from heaven. She was heart-stricken to learn of the sufferings of the soldiers.

Born of a noble and rich family, she gave up her life of ease and comfort and set out to nurse the wounded and the ailing, followed by many other ladies. She left her home on October 21, 1854. She rendered strenuous service in the battle of Inkerman. At that time there were neither beds nor other amenities for the wounded. There were 10,000 wounded under the charge of this single woman. The death rate among the wounded which was 42 per cent, before she arrived, immediately came down to 31 per cent, and ultimately to 5 per cent. This was miraculous, but can be easily visualized. If bleeding could be stopped, the wounds bandaged and the requisite diet given, the lives of many thousands would doubtless be saved. The only thing necessary was kindness and nursing, which Miss Nightingale provided.

It is said that she did an amount of work which big and strong men were unable to do. She used to work nearly twenty hours, day and night. When the women working under her went to sleep, she, lamp in hand, went out alone at midnight to the patients' bedside, comforted them, and herself gave them whatever food and other things were necessary. She was not afraid of going even to the battle-front, and did not know what fear was. She feared only God. Knowing that one has to die some day or other, she readily bore whatever hardships were necessary in order to alleviate the sufferings of others.

This lady remained single all her life, which she spent in good work. It is said that, when she died, thousands of soldiers wept bitterly like little children, as though they had lost their own mother.

No wonder that a country where such women are born is prosperous. That England rules over a wide empire is due not to the country's military strength, but to the meritorious deeds of such men and women.[47]

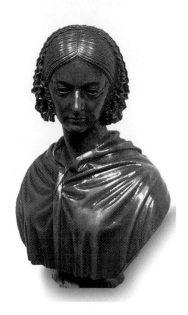

Bronze bust of Florence Nightingale commissioned by the executors of her will in 1915. It was cast from the original 1862 marble bust commissioned by veterans of the Crimean War.

A final word

Florence Nightingale was a giant in her time, a genius who achieved greatness against immense odds and in spite of a chronic illness. As we enter a new millennium, we can each weave her legacy of social conscience into our work as we strive to serve the greater community.

Nightingale would challenge each of us to identify our "must," as she referred to her work. If we listen well to her voice, we can feel within ourselves her wisdom, which embodies the vision and possibility of healing. She would describe this as "a lifelong journey toward harmony and balance — remembering what has been forgotten about connection, unity, and interdependence among all things living and nonliving."[48] She is a powerful guide in how to deepen our inner life by exploring our own spiritual awareness in the face of change. Change has always been the rule in society, and the radical changes that are occurring today provide us with a great opportunity to integrate caring and healing into all areas of our lives.

Like many remarkable humans, Florence Nightingale forged her own path. If her genius, her temperament, and her chronic illness made it difficult for others to understand her, this doesn't detract from her accomplishments. Florence Nightingale remains an icon for all of humanity. We are blessed that she walked before us and led the way. Our challenge is to carry on her vision of service to others with the same courage that she demonstrated. That vision remains her enduring gift.

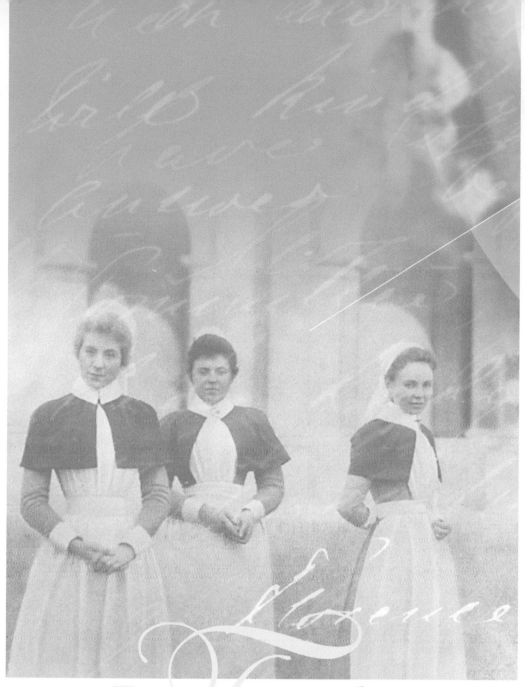

Appendices

*Pilgrimage to Scutari**

On a cool evening in early November, 1995, I arrived in Istanbul. I was finally going to explore the area where Florence Nightingale had arrived on November 4, 1854 as part of my historical research.[1] My thoughts were focused on what it would feel like to walk down the great halls of the Selimiye Barracks, which became know as the Barrack Hospital. Built between 1794 and 1799, the Turkish authorities turned it over to the British during the Crimean War, 1854-1856.

Traveling from the airport by taxi, my husband Larry and I passed primitive roads and small, shack-like wooden houses. Moving from the outskirts into Istanbul proper, streetlights shed a yellow glow onto this sprawling, modern, yet otherworldly city.

As we drove along a four-lane highway, we passed signs advertising cell phones and computers, and I thought about how different it was for Florence Nightingale to arrive here more than 140 years earlier. In her first note home to her family, after an arduous 2-week trip starting in London to Paris and a voyage from Marseille (**Fig. 1**) on the steamship *Vectis*, she wrote:

> *staggering on deck to look at the plains of Troy, the tomb of Achilles, the mouths of the Scamander, the little harbor of Tenedos, between which and the mainshore our Vectis, with steward's cabins and galley torn away, blustering, creaking, shrieking, storming, rushed on her way. It was in a dense mist that the ghosts of the Trojans answered my cordial hail, through which the old Gods, nevertheless, peered down from the hill of Ida upon their old plain. My enthusiasm for the heroes though was undiminished by wind and wave. We ... reached Constantinople* this morn in a thick and heavy rain, through which the Sophia, Sulieman, the Seven Towers, the walls, and the Golden Horn looked like a bad daguerreotype washed out.[2]*

[Note: the city's name was changed to Istanbul in 1930; ancient name Byzantium]

Istanbul is unique in that it literally rests on two continents, Europe and Asia, and is cleaved by the Bosphorus Strait (**Fig. 2**). We arrived at our hotel, situated on the European side; before settling into our room we rushed out onto the tenth-floor balcony to see what the night sky and the strait might reveal. The hotel was right next to the water, and we could hear the mournful fog horns of passing freighters and see their blinking signals, but we could see little else, save for a faint amber light in the hotel courtyard.

The next morning I awoke and again went out onto the balcony. The bright sunshine sparkling off the azure, white capped Bosporus and the busy waterway with huge freighters, barges, fishing boats, and ferries scurrying about and just barely missing one another was a sight to behold. On both sides of the strait were houses and buildings of

*Note: "Pilgrimage to Scutari" is © Barbara Dossey, Santa Fe. Reprinted with permission. The author thanks Nancy Ramsey for her excellent suggestions and edits on this essay.

Route (1854-1856) of Florence Nightingale and British Troops

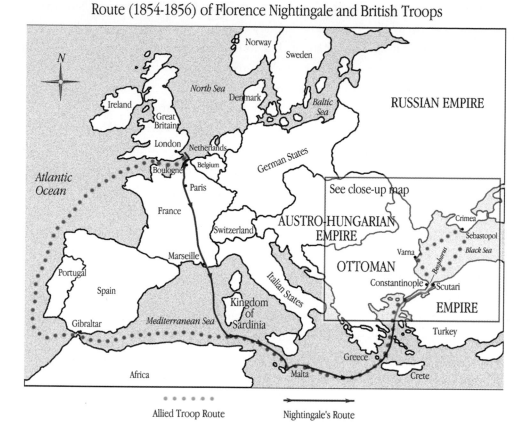

Allied Troop Route   Nightingale's Route

Figure 1. Routes taken by
Florence Nightingale and
British troops to Turkey and the
Crimea (Close-up of this map,
see Fig.2)

Constantinople and Scutari

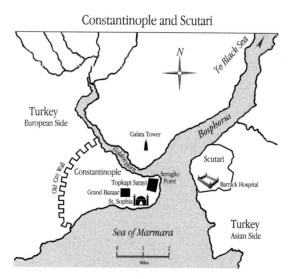

Figure 2. Map showing
Constantinople with its Grand
Bazaar, and Scutari, the site of
the Barrack Hospital, where
Nightingale served as
superintendent of nurses
throughout the Crimean War
(1854–1856)

cement, brick, and wood painted in every color of the rainbow. People were bustling off to work, crossing streets clogged with traffic and on sidewalks lined with palaces and mosques, many dating back two millennia.

It was a bright sunny day with the temperature in the mid-50s. From the balcony, I could see about 4 miles on a diagonal line across the Bosporus and onto the Asian side of the city, where the sprawling Selimiye Barracks sat. It was huge, as I had thought it would be, and I followed the sunlight off its long white walls and red tile roof until I found the northwest tower, where Nightingale had lived. "There it is! There it is!" I called out to my sleeping (not for long) husband, who knew exactly what I was talking about because it was the last thing I had mumbled before falling off to sleep the night before. As much as I wanted to walk the corridors of the barracks immediately, we decided to wait a few days and become completely rested after our 24 hours of travel from Santa Fe, New Mexico via Dallas, Texas and London to Istanbul.

By noon we were about to set off sightseeing. The weather had changed dramatically. It was now overcast and a light snow was falling. We decided that we would hire a taxi to take us to some of the most famous sites in old Istanbul. The oldest part of the city is situated on Seraglio Point, and its most famous landmark is the Hagia Sophia, an 800-year-old structure that for most of its life was the largest covered space in the world. At its apex, its dome is as high as a 15-story building. Next to it is the Blue Mosque, named for its beautiful, cobalt blue tiles; across the square is the splendid Topkapi Palace, built by Sultan Mehmet II after he conquered Constantinople in 1453.

But of course the minute we paid our driver and got out of the taxi, all I wanted to do was look at the Selimiye Barracks from this new perspective. I thought of Nightingale and her troop of 38 nurses anchored off Seragalio Point, "waiting for our fate whether with our heterogeneous mass, we should prefer." Looking north, I saw the Golden Horn, which she had written looked "like a bad daguerreotype washed out." Here three waterways converged, the Golden Horn, the Bosphorus, and the Sea of Marmora; they are the busiest, most exciting waterways I have ever seen.

As we made our way toward the Topkapi Palace, we passed modern department stores, sitting right next to small shops made of wood or stone or simply tin sheets braced together — each proprietor sitting cross-legged on carpets by the entrance. Right on the street merchants were selling food, leather goods, and books. Many local Turkish people in western dress headed to 10- and 15-story high office buildings; many men and women dressed in farm-style dress and traditional turbans and caftans and some women in veils were headed off to the local markets. And, of course, tourists in casual dress tried to take in every sight. But as if all these people were not enough to absorb, my mind's eye settled on the soldiers in uniform 140 years ago and waterways filled with steamships and the Sultan's elaborate caiques, the gondola-like rowing boats once used for transport from one shore to the other.

We walked up the long walkway, lined by stately, 50-foot-tall deciduous trees, to the Topkapi Palace, which stands on the highest point of the tip of the peninsula, exactly where the ancient acropolis had been. Now dusted with snow, the moorish-style buildings were breathtakingly beautiful. It is truly a feast for the eyes with its magnificent treasures: elaborate gold and silver embroidered satin and velvet robes and dresses worn by the emperors and their entourage; their crown jewels — two uncut emeralds, 8 pounds each, the dazzling emerald dagger seen in the movie *Topkapi*, the 84-carat spoonmaker diamond, which, according to the legend, a pauper found and traded for three spoons.

With each room revealing more and more jewels and relics of Ottoman splendor, I found myself nevertheless making a beeline to the window, peering out to take in yet another view of the Barrack Hospital across the water (**Fig. 3**). Nightingale's work and legacy

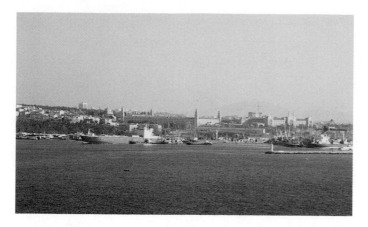

Figure 3. Selimiye Barracks, Uskadar (formerly Scutari, now part of greater Istanbul, Turkey; currently the Selimiye Barracks serves as the Turkish First Army Headquarters

filled my mind as I began wandering through the Topkapi Palace. I was struck by the contrast of the opulent residence and lifestyle of the sultan during the Crimean War, and just a mile and a quarter across the Bosporus, was the Barrack Hospital where Nightingale, a wealthy English lady, had entered the barren, filthy corridors, which she described shortly after her arrival as *Dante's Inferno.*

Over the next few days we wandered through the streets of Istanbul, which reflect a myriad of cultures — Turkish, Russian, European, Chinese, Japanese, American, and more. The city is immense, and it is easy to get lost. One of the many delights of traveling with Larry is that he always has his compass and is an excellent map reader; his frequent, "trust me, we need to go this way" comments were welcome when we'd come to yet another maze of nameless streets going off at all angles. The streets gave me a personal feeling for the meaning of "byzantine." We walked across the Galata Bridge, now lined with men and boys fishing, eventually coming to the ancient Galata Tower, where we climbed some stairs and then took an elevator to the top. While eating a late lunch, we looked down and around, and saw a vast panorama of wooden houses, mosques, and commercial buildings that seemed a motionless fleet moored on these historic waterways.

As we continued to walk the streets, it was easy to imagine the Crimean period Nightingale knew. Istanbul, although a modern city of more than 9 million people, still vibrates with ancient energies. Alongside modern cars, buses, trucks, and motor scooters are caravans of donkeys, horse-drawn wagons, and farmers herding sheep and carrying chickens. On foot are Turkish men in traditional dress and groups of veiled women coming and going on their daily shopping. The men carried baskets full of gorgeous red tomatoes, green peppers, yellow and green squash, asma kabah (a vegetable several feet long), nuts, fruits, spices and herbs — mint, scallions, parsley, dill, curry, coriander, cinnamon, and nutmeg. And the place to buy all these is the Grand Bazaar, located just behind Topkapi Palace.

Guidebooks cannot possibly convey what awaits here, and, amazingly, no sounds from inside the covered structure seep out. The bazaar is an immense stone structure, and the walls are 5-feet thick. Shoulder to shoulder with hundreds of people, we passed through the entrance, a wide, wooden archway. Despite the throng of people, there was an unexpected politeness about the crowd, and on several occasions a push from a person was quickly followed by a nod of apology. Once inside, it seemed our five senses went into overdrive: spices and herbs sprinkled on meat, sausage, falafel, fish, and bread created aromas that were at once sweet and pungent. Bright colors, fabrics, carpets, cushions, pillows, brocades, silks, and jewelry were everywhere. Rug dealers and their helpers moved in and out of shops quickly, carrying, literally, hundreds of pounds of carpets on their heads and shoulders. It was by far the grandest, most majestic, and most outrageous bazaar we had ever seen.

The bazaar goes on for miles. Rounding each corner there would be another maze of streets, narrow alleys and shops with products stacked, hanging, and piled to the ceiling. In each direction, as far as you can see, hundreds of merchants and vendors hawked their goods shouting and gesturing to us all at once to enter their shops and stalls — Miss, Mrs., Mr., Monsieur, Signore, Caballero, Senorita. Once inside, they'd quickly decide whether you were a good candidate for tea at the back of the shop, where, it just so happened, more expensive carpets and jewels were stored in locked chests. Some merchants sat cross-legged on their gorgeous carpets, while others lured us into their shops with their intriguing black marble eyes and friendly smiles and gestures. We had tea in one shop; thick, fragrant, Turkish coffee in the next. And of course, we knew never to accept the first price offered to us, and, much to our surprise, enjoyed the bargaining for a few rugs and beads we just happened to take home!

It seemed there was nothing that could not be found in this labyrinth of arcades, streets, cubicles, and stalls. I found myself looking for the socks, shirts, flannels, plates, knives, forks, spoons, scrubbing brushes, towels, soap, and lanterns that Nightingale's assistants had been sent to find. All were there! All of my senses were wildly overstimulated, and I felt dizzy and stunned with open-mouthed wonder, laughing and shaking my head at the cacophony of sounds and activities. That evening before falling asleep I read my husband several of Nightingale's long letters during November and December 1854 at the Barrack Hospital that was fascinating to him.

After a few days of sightseeing and with some afternoon naps, we were now rested and ready to venture to the Selimiye Barracks. The barracks (**Fig. 4**; also see page 124 for an 1854 depiction) is in the large suburb of Uskudar, located on the Asian shore. Today, the Selimiye Barracks serve as the Turkish First Army Headquarters and is a training facility; tall chain-linked fences mounted with barbed wire for security surround it. Two of

Figure 4. Exterior of Selimiye Barracks, Uskadar, Turkey

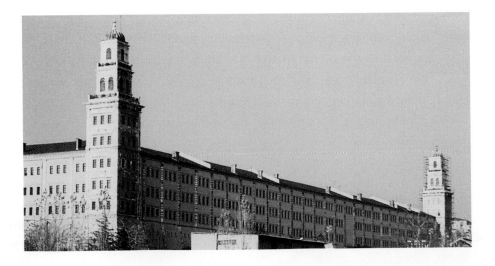

the sides have huge, barren cement parking lots with miles of parking places, with tanks and trucks sitting ready for military maneuvers.

By taxi once again, we crossed a large, modern bridge to Uskudar to the Asian side. Uskudar is a smaller-scale Istanbul, with many covered bazaars, mosques, and palaces. I compared our travel in a comfortable, heated taxi to that of Nightingale, who had arrived at the Barrack Hospital on a cold, wet, day in an uncomfortable open caique. Weaving our way through the narrow streets crowded with traffic and pedestrians oblivious to the moving cars was a challenge. Several times we had to stop, once to let a farmer with his donkey-drawn wagon pass, and another time to allow a man carrying a caged rooster and a teenage boy coaxing his three goats along to cross. And finally, after a 45-minute ride, we stopped on a high hill near the Selimeyi Barracks, so that we might see the entire, gigantic structure.

Continuing along to the entrance, we saw the ancient mosque that sits adjacent to the northwest tower. Loudspeakers located on the serefiye, or galleries high on the minarets, were calling worshippers to prayer. Before modern times muezzins would climb to the top of the minarets to give vocal call to prayer five times a day. The call's haunting monotone almost demands that you stop and listen as the echoing sounds resonate throughout the city, and seem to vibrate into every cell of your body. They echo for miles and can even penetrate a closed, modern hotel room. There is no doubt that Nightingale heard the call to prayer from the Barrack Hospital.

Tears filled my eyes as I thought about Nightingale's own "Call" to be of service in her teens, her conviction of religious tolerance, and the core of her spiritual philosophy: that the universe is the embodiment of a Transcendent God, and that all human beings can experience the underlying divinity of themselves and the world by a shift in consciousness. Although she emphasized Christian values and studied the medieval Christian mystics, Christian mysticism, and Eastern spiritual traditions, she argued "you must go to Mahometanism, to Buddhism, to the East, to the Sufis & Fakirs, to Pantheism, for the right growth of mysticism."[3] I stood on the curb for a few moments, needing to be still and silent within myself before entering the building because I felt shaky with excitement. My dear husband noticed and simply smiled and waited, knowing how much this visit meant to me.

Entering the Selimiye Barracks we went through a security gate where three military guards inspected my purse and our briefcases. We were asked a few simple questions and had to show our passports and state the reason for our visit. On stepping into the main entrance, I shivered with excitement.

Although the Barrack Hospital Tower, where Nightingale lived, is open to the public at different hours, I had called ahead so that I might meet an officer in the Turkish Army Protocol Department that could answer some specific questions I had. A male officer greeted us and introduced himself to us in English and led us down the main hallway toward the northwest tower. When we reached the end of the main corridor, I looked to my left and saw another of the great hallways. Before entering the large room that joins the northwest tower, I looked back down this immense corridor behind me (in 1854, **Fig. 5**) and was speechless, for here was one of the wide, empty corridors where Nightingale had worked (**Fig. 6**). These corridors are now painted white and have glossy,

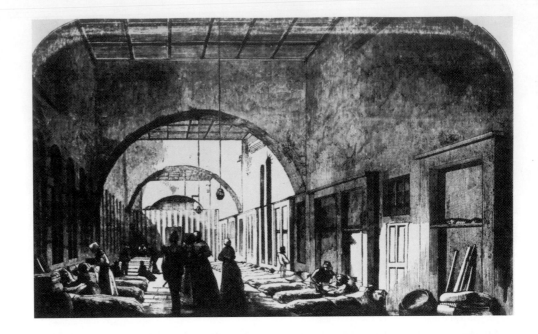

Figure 5. Hallway of the Barrack Hospital, showing some of the 4 miles of beds that were hastily assembled to make room for the thousands of causalities from the Crimea.

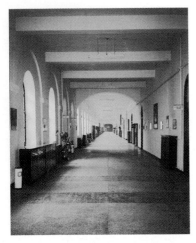

Figure 6. One of the great hallways today within the Selimiye Barracks tower where Florence Nightingale and her nurses cared for wounded soldiers during the Crimean War

waxed tile floors with an occasional institutional-type heater cabinet, a few plants, and medals and certificates hanging on the walls.

But that's not what I saw. I started walking down this empty corridor instead of heading toward the northwest tower and saw Florence Nightingale as she carried her lantern down this great hall; her shadow was cast on the wall, and was experience by the wounded soldiers as healing presence. I started reciting one of the most famous known poems of the American poet, Henry Wadsworth Longfellow, "Santa Filomena," that fixed the image of Nightingale and her lamp firmly in the public mind [published in November 1857 in the first issue of the *Atlantic Monthly*]:

> *... The wounded from the battle-plain*
> *In dreary hospitals of pain,*
> *The cheerless corridors,*
> *The cold and stony floors*
>
> *Lo! In that house of misery*
> *A lady with a lamp I see*
> *Pass through the glimmering gloom,*
> *And flit from room to room*
>
> *And slow, as in a dream of bliss,*
> *The speechless sufferer turns to kiss*
> *Her shadow, as it falls*
> *Upon the darkening walls...*

I saw her as she stopped at bed after bed to tend the sick and wounded soldiers — young men lying prostrate on their beds, suffering from battle wounds, high fevers, dysentery, typhoid, and typhus. I heard the soldiers moaning, crying in pain, and calling for help. I smelled their foul, infected wounds, and the stench of blocked sewage. I saw soldiers salute her when she passed, and I heard her as she talked to the soldiers and cheered them with her calm voice, her warm smile, and her gentle touch saying, "Never be ashamed of your wounds, my friend." I couldn't get enough of this corridor, and I walked a long way down the center of this empty corridor. As I turned around, Larry lovingly smiled at me, knowing that in my mind I was walking where Nightingale had walked.

We next walked from the corridor into an empty room that was part of Nightingale's and the nurses' living space, and I was seeing in my mind Nightingale's own floor plan sketch from her letters (**Fig. 7**). At the back was a narrow wooden staircase leading to the first-floor room and at the back of that was a staircase leading up to another small room to the top of the tower. We climbed the staircase and entered Nightingale's sitting room,

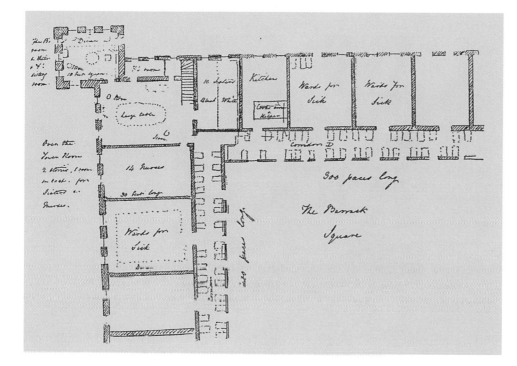

Figure 7. Nightingale's hand-drawn floor plan of the nurses' tower at the Barrack Hospital, showing where she and her party of nurses lived

smaller than I had imagined. Within the small northwest tower were a collection of a few of her letters, pictures, and newspaper clippings hanging on the wall, but the first thing that caught my attention was a Turkish lantern (**Fig. 8**) like the one she used on her night rounds sitting on a marble top side table! It was thrilling.

Then to slowing walk and take in the other period treasures such as a table and chairs with a Turkish urn (**Fig. 9**), and writing desk with an old oil lamp and inkwell (**Fig. 10**). As I looked at the inkwell, I imagined Nightingale writing her voluminous letters, making her notes and lists, meeting with the doctors, nurses, orderlies, and numerous others, and watching her pet turtle, Jimmy, as he crawled along the tiles. [In 1954, 100 years after the start of the Crimean War, the Turkish Nurses' Association, with the cooperation of the Turkish First Army, organized this Florence Nightingale Museum in the northwest tower].

I opened the window and leaned slightly out to take a photograph of the southwest tower (**Fig. 11**), a sight Nightingale had often seen. Again I felt overwhelmed with

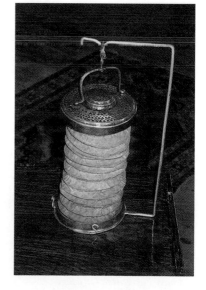

Figure 8. Close-up of the Turkish lantern that Florence Nightingale carried during her rounds in the Barrack Hospital

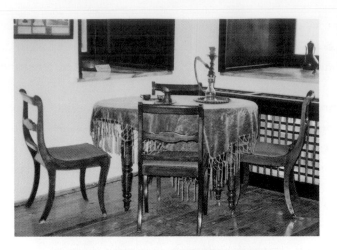

Figure 9. Chair, table, and 19th century Turkish pots in window and on table in the Florence Nightingale Museum in the Selimiye Barracks

Figure 10. Desk, chair, and oil lamp in the Florence Nightingale Museum in the Selimiye Barracks

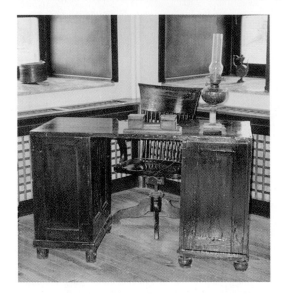

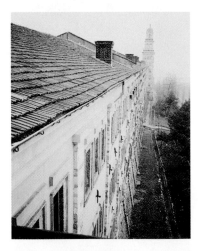

Figure 11. The view from the Selimiye Barracks tower where Florence Nightingale and the nurses lived during the Crimean War

immense gratitude for her visionary, spiritual work, and was thinking of her volumes of letters, memos, and meetings that came from this little tower that changed the course of medical and nursing history throughout the world. I felt deeply grateful to be involved in my chosen work of nursing.

During my research, I had often imagined what it would have been like to work with Nightingale during the Crimean War. Standing here in the Barrack Hospital, I could almost hear her, giving directions in her properly enunciated words to my imagined colleagues and me. I compared the abysmal working conditions of the Barrack Hospital to my various nursing experiences — to the modern, pristine, critical care units staffed with superbly competent colleagues working with the latest technology, to state-of-the-art universities and hospitals where I have taught the "art and science" of nursing. I thought back to my days with the Texas Air National Guard Air Force Reserve, setting up the field hospital to maintain our readiness in case our unit was sent to Viet Nam and to my experience in leading nursing organizations in which we continue to evolve the profession of nursing, and create strategies in how we can carry forth Nightingale's message and work. To think that the foundation of modern nursing started here, where I stood, in the midst of previous human agony and primitive conditions!

Leaving the Barrack Hospital, the bright shining sun was out and the blue sky above was welcome after the overcast sky when we had begun our visit. We next took a 10-minute drive, weaving our way once again through the streets of Uskudar, arriving at the gates of the Haydarpasa Cemetery where the dead of the Crimean War and two World Wars are buried.

Anticipating that there would be thousands of grave markers, I had brought with me a copy of an 1856 lithograph (**Fig. 12**) of the British military cemetery in Scutari, two specific grave markers in the foreground with a Turkish gravedigger kneeling on his

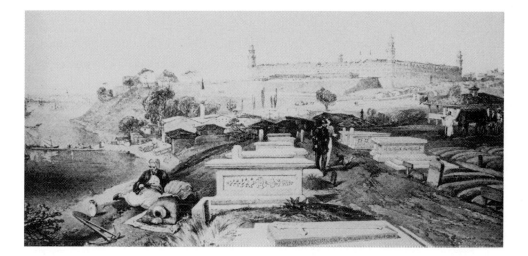

Figure 12. An 1856 lithograph of the British military cemetery in Scutari, with a Turkish gravedigger kneeling on his prayer rug, and the Barrack Hospital in the background

prayer rug, the Barrack Hospital in the background, and the Bosphorus on the left. The first was a 5-foot-high, white marble marker, elaborately carved; the second a 4-foot elongated, three-tiered, white marble marker with a large ornate cross on it. Entering the cemetery was a bit overwhelming at first. It was very crowded and there were thousands of markers everywhere. There were no people here except us, and as I looked around the beautifully terraced landscape filled with deciduous and evergreen trees, 40- to 60-feet tall, I steadied myself and then knew that we could find the Crimean markers. I was looking, for my mind's eye was back in 1854-1856, to the open fields and Turkish gravediggers burying the dead British soldiers.

We strolled a while, looking for grave markers dating back to the Crimean War years — without success. Then we saw an older Turkish gentleman cleaning a newer area of the grounds some distance away. When he saw us coming toward him he bowed, and we smiled. He spoke no English, so I showed him my lithograph, but he did not recognize anything in it. Today, with the modern, tall buildings in the sprawling city of Uskudar between the cemetery and the Selimiye Barracks, it was a very hard to gain the perspective during 1854-1856.

I was persistent and wrote the numbers "1856," on the margin of this picture and pointed to the gravestones and the Selimiye Barracks in the background. He scratched his head, and after a few moments he gestured that he understood and motioned for us to follow him. We walked a short distance to a tall hedge and found ourselves on a

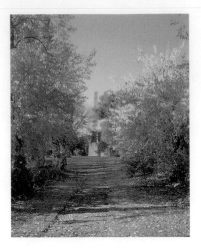

Figure 13. Walking up the path to the Scutari Cemetery, now contained within the Haydarpasa Cemetery, Uskadar, Turkey

narrow dirt path. In the distance and in the opposite direction from the Bosporus, I saw a large, solitary granite obelisk standing alone and I knew immediately that it was the obelisk (**Fig. 13**) that Nightingale had requested to be built; it fit precisely her description and design. We were now closer to identifying the two grave markers in the picture.

Very few graves date from 1854 to 1856, because many of the men and women, the wives and lovers of the soldiers who had accompanied them to war, who died from cholera and fevers, were all buried quickly to decrease the spread of infection. Haunted by the more than 5, 000 dead, Nightingale firmly believed that they needed their own monument. She had recorded in letters her walks through the cemetery that was between the Barrack Hospital and the General Hospital, another facility for wounded and sick British soldiers. As we walked a little further through the fallen leaves off the tree-lined path, I felt I was walking where Nightingale had walked many times, and it seemed sacred. I felt the spirit of Nightingale with me as I recalled a letter that she wrote to her family in which she talked about having the spirit of her deceased pet owl, Athena, with her:[4]

> *I saw Athena last night. She came to see me. I was walking home late from the Gen'l Hospt'l round the cliff, my favorite way, & looking, I really believe for the first time, at the view — the sea glassy calm & of the purest sapphire blue — the sky dark deep blue — one solitary bright star rising above Constantinople — our whole fleet standing with sails idly spread to catch the breeze which was none — including a large fleet of Sardinians carrying up Sardinian troops — the domes & minarets of Constantinople sharply standing out against the bright gold of the sunset — the transparent opal of the distant hills, (a color one never sees but in the East) which stretch below Olympus always snowy & on the other side the Sea of Marmora when Athena came along the cliff quite to my feet, rose upon her tiptoes, bowed several times, made her long melancholy cry, & fled away — like the shade of Ajax. I assure you my tears followed her.*

[Note. Ajax, the strong brave Greek warrior of the Trojan War who killed himself when Achilles' armor was given to Odysseus].

This walk was one of the few where she could be in solitude and contemplate her work of service for God and the soldiers. And when she heard the muezzins sound the call to prayer and watched the gravediggers stopping to kneel and pray, she undoubtedly said her own prayers.

As we walked toward the monument, I thought about a letter Queen Victoria had written to Sidney Herbert, Secretary at War. The Queen had asked if she personally might do anything to assist Nightingale. As I walked up to the monument, I again was struck by how Nightingale could focus on an idea and act on it quickly. After receiving word from Herbert that the Queen wished to help her, Nightingale replied within days that she would like an obelisk erected as a memorial to the dead and that it should be placed in a lovely spot overlooking the Sea of Marmora. Not long after, the British government was in correspondence with Sultan Aldulmecid, and the sultan granted approval for the British military cemetery at Scutari on March 5, 1855. Three days later, Nightingale wrote to her sister:[5]

> *... Please put yourself at once in communication, dear Pop [Parthenope], with the Chaplain-General Gleig, to get us working drawings for our Public Monument & Private Chapel in the*

British burial ground now to be enclosed on the cliff looking over Sea of Marmora — ... I should like "Wingless Victory" for Chapel — one single solitary column for monument to greet first our ships coming up the Sea of Marmora. It is such a position — high o'er the cliffs ... Five thousand & odd brave hearts sleep there — three thousand, alas! dead in Jan. & Feb. alone — here. But what of that? they are not there — But, for once, even I wish to keep their remembrance on earth — for we have been the Thermopylae* of this desperate struggle, when Raglan & cold & famine have been the Persians, our own destroyers — We have endured in brave Grecian silence ... We have folded our mantles about our faces & died in silence without complaining ...

[Note: Thermopylae is in ancient Greece; a mountain pass in Locris, near an inlet of the Aegean Sea; scene of a battle (480 BC) in which the Persians under Xerxes destroyed a Spartan army under Leonidas.]

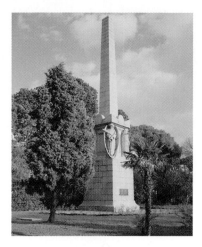

Figure 14. Crimean British Soldiers Memorial, Haydarpasa Cemetery, Uskadar, Turkey. Erected in 1857 due to Florence Nightingale requesting permission from Queen Victoria to establish and begin the design and secure the site with the British Secretary of Foreign Affairs and the Turkish sultan

And here I was, standing in front of this obelisk erected in 1857, a year after the Crimean War had ended (**Fig. 14** and **Fig. 15**). The plaque had the name of the Italian designer Baron Marochetti and an epitaph by the great English historian and statesman, 1st Baron Thomas Babington Macaulay of Rothley:

To the memory of the British soldiers and sailors, who during the years 1854 and 1855 died far from their country in defense of the liberties of Europe, this monument is erected by the gratitude of Queen Victoria and her people 1857.

And below that:

To Florence Nightingale Whose Work Near This Cemetery A Century Ago Relieved Much Human Suffering And Laid The Foundation For The Nursing Profession, 1854-1954. This Tablet Cast in the Coronation Year of Her Majesty Queen Elizabeth II, Has Been Raised By The British Community In Turkey in Her Memory.

According to the plaque on the obelisk, shortly after it was erected, families of the deceased soldiers began requesting that individual grave markers be placed nearby. Although I had found the monument to the more than 5,000 soldiers and others, I still wanted to identify the individual markers in the lithograph that I carried. I was thinking about Nightingale's philosophy and how she saw each and every soldier as a human being to be treated individually, and this underlying philosophy is the cornerstone of holistic nursing.

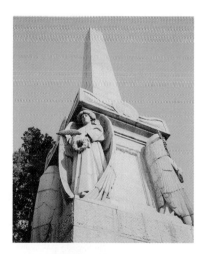

Figure 15. Florence Nightingale was responsible for the details of the massive granite memorial (erected in 1857) for the British officers and men who died in the Crimean War that is in the Haydarpas Cemetery, Uskadar, Turkey

I again pointed to the two distinct monuments to the Turkish gentleman, but he kindly gestured with a shrug of his shoulders and upturned hands that he did not know its location. But, wishing to help us, he picked up a fallen tree branch and began to sweep leaves from very small, simple, flat grave markers, many of which had no engraving left from years of harsh weather. There are hundreds of old gravestones, some standing and some flat, in this area that covers several acres. How I wanted to identify the grave markers in the drawing! We couldn't see the Selimiye Barracks over the tall buildings of the modern Uskudar, so I walked in a straight line from the monument, about one long city block, as far as I could to the edge of the cemetery and placed myself in the position at the cliff edge where the Turkish workers were praying in my 1854 picture. I peered through the 45-foot high hedge and looked straight down the steep cliffs from the edge of the cemetery, about one-quarter mile, and saw old houses and buildings. They were clinging to the steep cliffs that drop further down to a train station and neighboring freighter docks situated at the junction of the Bosporus Strait and the Sea of Marmora. Next, I turned in the direction of the Selimiye Barracks. Before long I recognized the grave markers I had been searching for, and screamed with joy (**Fig. 16**). The raised carvings are still on the markers, but the words have all disappeared from the years of harsh weather. I also wanted to find some of the smaller flat grave markers that the soldiers' families were responsible for placing here. Very quickly I did find 50 or so that were weathered, and only a few have remaining letters that are visible (**Fig. 17**):

Major C.S. Glazebrook, 49th Reg. on Foot, Died at Scutari, The 18th December 1854, of Wounds Received Before Sebastopol, on the 17th Nov. 1854.

Nightingale's wisdom, humanitarianism, and compassion, still ring true and are timeless, and can guide us. And we can ask ourselves, will an epoch of awakening to

Figure 16. Turkish worker sweeping leaves off of a Crimean grave markers in Haydarpas Cemetery, Uskadar, Turkey

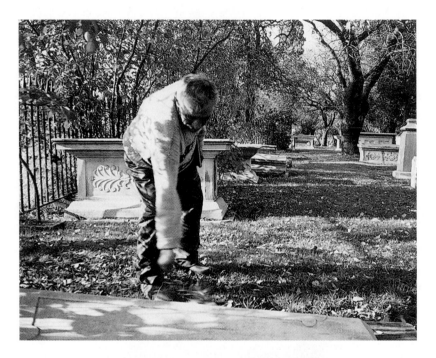

Figure 17. A grave marker from the Crimean War, Haydarpasa Cemetery, Uskadar, Turkey

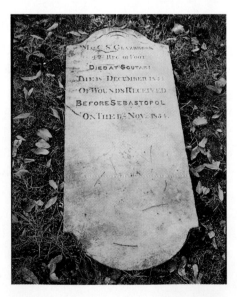

healing, leading, and global-vision arrive, as so many people today hope, or will illiteracy, poverty, religious intolerance, spiritual cynicism, and materialism of our age continue? Will we learn to live in harmony with nature and in unity with one another, as Nightingale encouraged us?

The burning flame of light represents healing. What kind of pattern will nurses and others cast in the dark shadows of health care? What light will we shed? This human quality of light is at the core of the human spirit. Sometimes human suffering is experienced as the "dark night of the soul" as expressed in the great spiritual mystic literature. Yet, with stillness and reflection, clarity often emerges, and we find our inner strengths to weave new patterns in our tapestry of healing. Each person can use her or his own light to return to the ultimate experience of unity and connection with all that is. Each nurse is a touchstone for patients, their family and friends, and colleagues.

As I looked around the huge cemetery and thought about our visit to the nearby Selimiye Barracks, I was filled with a profound sense of peace and joy. I thought about the work of Florence Nightingale — mystic, visionary, and healer — and reflected on her profound life's work that has had and will continue to have implications for generations upon generations. And driving out of the cemetery, Nightingale's words that had captivated me for a long time came forth from her last great 1893 paper, "Sick-Nursing" and "Health-Nursing."[6]

> *In the future which I shall not see, for I am old, may a better way be opened! May the methods by which every infant, every human being will have the best chance at health — the methods by which every sick person will have the best chance at recovery, be learned and practiced. Hospitals are only an intermediate stage of civilization, never intended, at all events, to take in the whole sick population.*
>
> *May we hope that when we are all dead and gone, leaders will arise who have been personally experienced in the hard, practical work, the difficulties and the joys of organizing nursing reforms, and who will lead far beyond anything we have done! May we hope that every nurse will be an atom in the hierarchy of ministers of the Highest! But then she [he] must be in the hierarchy, not alone, not an atom in the indistinguishable mass of thousands of nurses. High hopes, which will not be deceived!*

Family Tree

Nightingale family

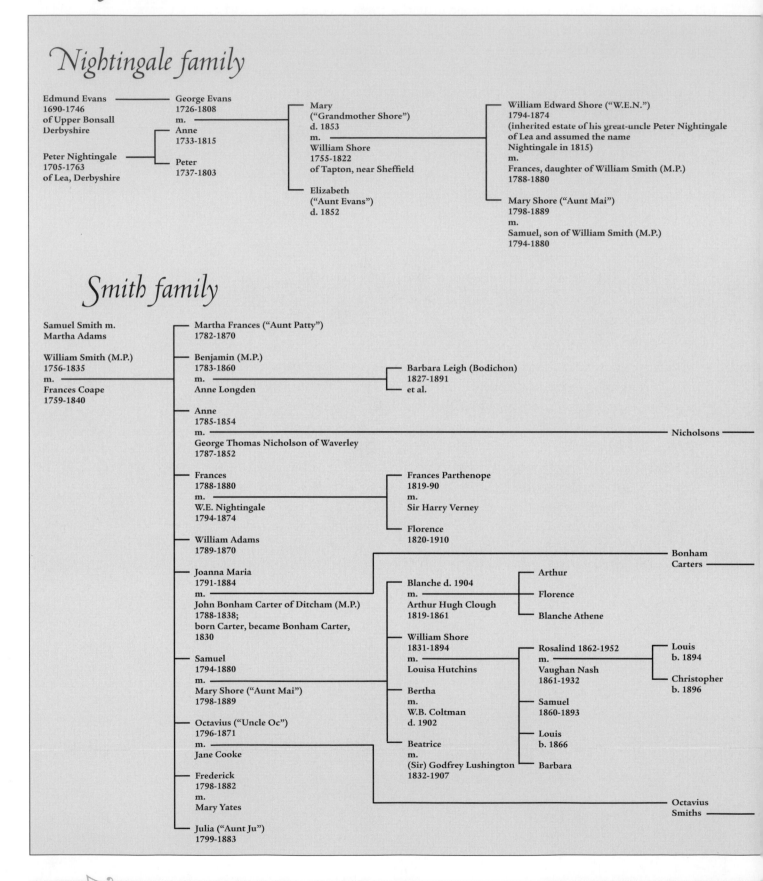

Edmund Evans
1690-1746
of Upper Bonsall
Derbyshire ———— George Evans
1726-1808
m.
Anne
1733-1815

Peter Nightingale
1705-1763
of Lea, Derbyshire ———— Peter
1737-1803

Mary
("Grandmother Shore")
d. 1853
m.
William Shore
1755-1822
of Tapton, near Sheffield

Elizabeth
("Aunt Evans")
d. 1852

William Edward Shore ("W.E.N.")
1794-1874
(inherited estate of his great-uncle Peter Nightingale
of Lea and assumed the name
Nightingale in 1815)
m.
Frances, daughter of William Smith (M.P.)
1788-1880

Mary Shore ("Aunt Mai")
1798-1889
m.
Samuel, son of William Smith (M.P.)
1794-1880

Smith family

Samuel Smith m.
Martha Adams

William Smith (M.P.)
1756-1835
m.
Frances Coape
1759-1840

Martha Frances ("Aunt Patty")
1782-1870

Benjamin (M.P.)
1783-1860
m.
Anne Longden

Barbara Leigh (Bodichon)
1827-1891
et al.

Anne
1785-1854
m.
George Thomas Nicholson of Waverley
1787-1852 ———————————————————————— Nicholsons

Frances
1788-1880
m.
W.E. Nightingale
1794-1874

Frances Parthenope
1819-90
m.
Sir Harry Verney

Florence
1820-1910

William Adams
1789-1870

Joanna Maria
1791-1884
m.
John Bonham Carter of Ditcham (M.P.)
1788-1838;
born Carter, became Bonham Carter,
1830

Blanche d. 1904
m.
Arthur Hugh Clough
1819-1861

Arthur

Florence

Blanche Athene ———————— Bonham Carters

William Shore
1831-1894
m.
Louisa Hutchins

Rosalind 1862-1952
m.
Vaughan Nash
1861-1932

Louis
b. 1894

Christopher
b. 1896

Samuel
1794-1880
m.
Mary Shore ("Aunt Mai")
1798-1889

Bertha
m.
W.B. Coltman
d. 1902

Samuel
1860-1893

Octavius ("Uncle Oc")
1796-1871
m.
Jane Cooke

Beatrice
m.
(Sir) Godfrey Lushington
1832-1907

Louis
b. 1866

Barbara

Frederick
1798-1882
m.
Mary Yates ————————————————————————————————————— Octavius
Smiths

Julia ("Aunt Ju")
1799-1883

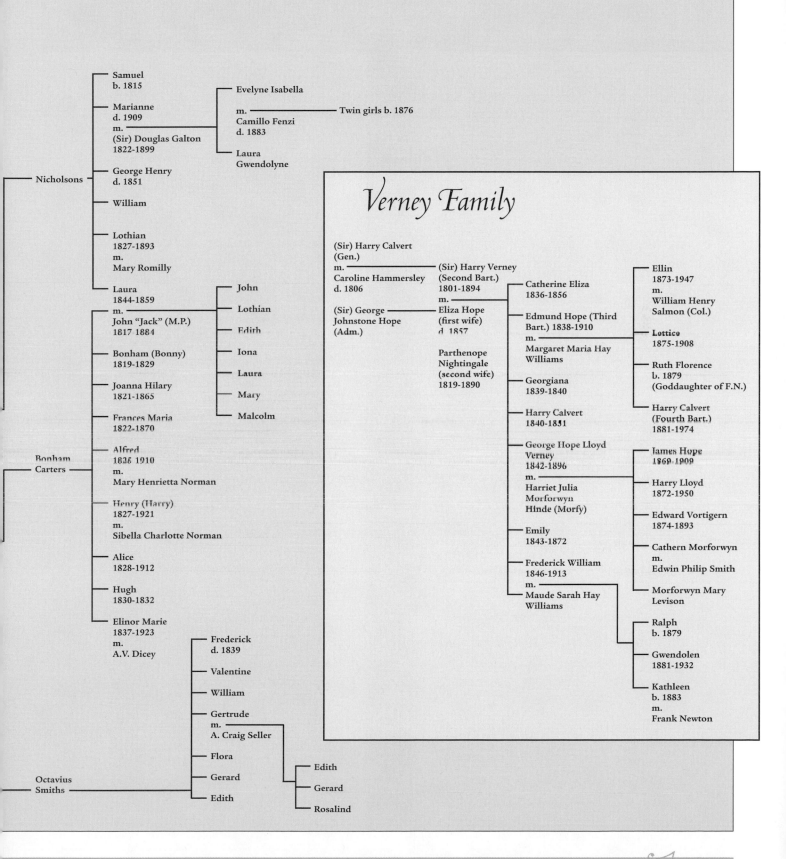

Nicholsons

Samuel
b. 1815

Marianne
d. 1909
m.
(Sir) Douglas Galton
1822-1899

Evelyne Isabella
m.
Camillo Fenzi
d. 1883 ——— Twin girls b. 1876

Laura
Gwendolyne

George Henry
d. 1851

William

Lothian
1827-1893
m.
Mary Romilly

Laura
1844-1859
m.
John "Jack" (M.P.)
1817-1884

John

Lothian

Edith

Iona

Laura

Mary

Malcolm

Bonham (Bonny)
1819-1829

Joanna Hilary
1821-1865

Frances Maria
1822-1870

Bonham
Carters

Alfred
1825-1910
m.
Mary Henrietta Norman

Henry (Harry)
1827-1921
m.
Sibella Charlotte Norman

Alice
1828-1912

Hugh
1830-1832

Elinor Marie
1837-1923
m.
A.V. Dicey

Frederick
d. 1839

Valentine

William

Gertrude
m.
A. Craig Seller

Flora

Gerard

Edith

Edith

Gerard

Rosalind

Octavius
Smiths

Verney Family

(Sir) Harry Calvert
(Gen.)
m. ———
Caroline Hammersley
d. 1806

(Sir) George ———
Johnstone Hope
(Adm.)

(Sir) Harry Verney
(Second Bart.)
1801-1894
m.

Eliza Hope
(first wife)
d. 1857

Parthenope
Nightingale
(second wife)
1819-1890

Catherine Eliza
1836-1856

Edmund Hope (Third
Bart.) 1838-1910
m.
Margaret Maria Hay
Williams

Georgiana
1839-1840

Harry Calvert
1840-1851

George Hope Lloyd
Verney
1842-1896
m.
Harriet Julia
Morforwyn
Hinde (Morfy)

Emily
1843-1872

Frederick William
1846-1913
m.
Maude Sarah Hay
Williams

Ellin
1873-1947
m.
William Henry
Salmon (Col.)

Lettice
1875-1908

Ruth Florence
b. 1879
(Goddaughter of F.N.)

Harry Calvert
(Fourth Bart.)
1881-1974

James Hope
1869-1909

Harry Lloyd
1872-1950

Edward Vortigern
1874-1893

Cathern Morforwyn
m.
Edwin Philip Smith

Morforwyn Mary
Levison

Ralph
b. 1879

Gwendolen
1881-1932

Kathleen
b. 1883
m.
Frank Newton

Timeline

Early years (1820-1854)

Nightingale's major life events and work		Related events
	1818	William Edward Nightingale (W.E.N.) and Frances (Fanny) Smith marry.
	1819	Frances Parthenope Nightingale born in Naples, Italy.
May 12. Florence Nightingale born at Villa Colombaia in Florence, Italy. **July 4.** Baptized in Florence.	1820	
	1821	On return from Italy, W.E.N. begins new home at Lea Hurst, Matlock, Derbyshire.
Shows independence at an early age; nurses her sick dolls.	1825	W.E.N. purchases Embley, near Romsey, Hampshire.
Sick much of winter.	1826	
	1827	Aunt Mai marries Uncle Sam; Miss Christie becomes Florence's governess.
	1828	Edwin Chadwick conceives the "sanitary idea," basic concept of modern public health.
Begins her autobiography "La Vie de Florence Rossignol." Makes notes on types of illness among villagers at Lea Hurst.	1829	W.E.N. High Sheriff for Hampshire. Cousin Bonham (Bonny) Carter dies in childhood.
Compiles first lists and tables.	1830	
Begins to be tutored by father.	1831	First cholera epidemic in England and Europe (1831-1832). William Shore Smith ("my boy Shore") born.
	1832	First Reform Bill passes in Parliament. Uncle John Bonham Carter and Sidney Herbert elected to Parliament.
	1833	First Reform Parliament abolishes slavery in British possessions. Lord Ashley begins work on Ten Hours Bill.
Translates Latin and Greek.	1835	W.E.N. fails in bid for Parliament because he refuses to bribe voters. Grandfather William Smith dies. Adolphe Quetelet publishes *Essai de Physique Sociale* in Belgium.
	1836	Adolphe Quetelet develops field of social statistics (demography). Pastor Theodore Fliedner establishes Institution of Deaconesses at Kaiserswerth, Düsseldorf, Germany.
February 7. Receives first Call from God at Embley. **September.** Departs with family for European tour. Begins collecting information on hospitals and charitable institutions.	1837	Enlargement and remodeling of Embley started. Queen Victoria begins reign. Smallpox and typhus fever epidemic in England.
Travels with family to Italy, Geneva, and Paris; meets Sismondi in Geneva and Mary Clarke in Paris.	1838	William Farr appointed Compiler of Abstracts in Registrar General's office. Poor Law commissioners write letter to Home Secretary calling for "removal of causes of disease."
Nightingales return to England. Presented to society before Queen Victoria. Learns firsthand of Ashley's reform work. Studies mathematics with cousin Henry Nicholson. Travels by railroad for first time.	1839	Embley remodeling completed. Lord Palmerston marries Lord Ashley's mother-in-law. Cousin Fred Smith dies in Western Australia on Grey expedition.
Aunt Mai convinces Nightingales to let Florence be tutored in mathematics. Nurses Aunt Jane at Thames Bank.	1840	Queen Victoria and Prince Albert marry in February. Grandmother Smith dies. Aunt Julia active in world antislavery convention in London. Health of Towns Report.
Interest grows in theology and women's issues. Stage manager for family Christmas theatrical at Waverley Abbey.	1841	Quetelet organizes Belgium's Central Statistical Bureau.
Nurses Aunt Julia. Meets von Bunsen. Introduced to Richard Monckton Milnes.	1842	Baron Christian von Bunsen becomes Prussian Envoy to England. Chadwick issues report on *Sanitary Conditions of Labouring Classes*. W.E.N. active in fund raising and elections for Whig party.
Comforts Helen Richardson after sister's death in childbirth.	1843	Grandmother Shore and Aunt Evans lose much money in bank failures. Oliver Wendell Holmes points out contagiousness of puerperal fever. Farr publishes life-table. John Stuart Mill's *A System of Logic* published.
Becomes ill at Waverley; begins close friendship with Aunt Hannah Nicholson. Asks Dr. Howe his opinion of her idea to study nursing. Declines Henry Nicholson's marriage proposal.	1844	Dr. Samuel Gridley Howe and his wife, Julia Ward Howe, visit Embley. Report of Health of Towns Commission. Metropolitan Health of Towns Association (London) founded. Society for Improvement of the Condition of the Laboring Classes (London) founded.
First attempt to train as nurse at Salisbury Hospital is thwarted. Mill's book reinforces her logical approach to speculation about God's laws. Nurses Grandmother Shore at Tapton and poor people at Wellow village.	1845	Sidney Herbert appointed Secretary at War under Peel. Selina Bracebridge becomes dear friend

Nightingale's major life events and work		Related events
Receives hospital reports from Mary Clarke in Paris and yearbook of Institution of Deaconesses at Kaiserswerth from von Bunsen.	1846	Corn Laws repealed; Peel government falls; Lord Palmerston becomes Foreign Secretary. Ashley becomes chairman of Ragged School Union.
Travels to Rome with Bracebridges; meets Madre Santa Colomba, Sidney and Elizabeth Herbert, Rev. Henry Manning, and Mary Stanley.	1847	Ten Hours Bill passes. Mary Clarke marries Julius Mohl. Elizabeth Blackwell admitted to medical school in Geneva, New York. Semmelweis discovers pathogenesis of puerperal fever but is ignored. Sir James Young Simpson discovers anesthetic use of chloroform.
Learns discipline of comtemplative prayer and meditation from Madre Santa Colomba during 10-day retreat at Trinità de Monti Convent, Rome. Returns to England in April.	1848	English Public Health Act of 1848. Queen's College for Women founded. J.S. Mill's *Political Economy* published. Second cholera epidemic (1848-1849) in England.
Inspects hospitals in London; teaches in Ragged Schools. Declines Richard Monckton Milnes's marriage proposal after 7-year courtship. Leaves for Egypt and Greece with Bracebridges in November. Receives second Call from God while in Egypt.	1849	Elizabeth Blackwell graduates as first woman doctor in America. Julius Mohl begins frequent correspondence with Florence on politics, literature, philosophy, and religion. John Snow publishes views on water-borne spread of cholera. Revolutions defeated in Europe.
May 12. On her 30th birthday in Athens, privately records her spiritual vow of obedience and chastity. **July-August.** First visit to Institution of Deaconesses at Kaiserswerth for a fortnight; writes 32-page pamphlet on the institute. After return to England, required by parents to devote 6 months to Parthe.	1850	Epidemiological Society (London) founded. Cousin Henry Nicholson drowns in Spain. Hilary Bonham Carter studies art in Paris and lives with the Mohls.
Frequently visits the Herberts at Wilton House. Meets Dr. Elizabeth Blackwell, first woman doctor in the United States. **July-October.** Trains at Institution of Deaconesses at Kaiserswerth.	1851	Lord Ashley becomes seventh Earl of Shaftesbury upon his father's death. Richard Monckton Milnes marries Annabel Crewe. Marianne Nicholson marries Captain Douglas Galton.
Accompanies W.E.N. to Umberslade for water cure. Completes *Suggestions for Thought*, which includes her feminist essay, "Cassandra." Begins plans to break free from family and begin her work. **May 2.** Experiences Call from God to be a "savior."	1852	Parthe has nervous breakdown in summer; Sir James Clark tells Nightingales that Parthe must learn to live without Florence. Aunt Evans dies. Farr reports on cholera epidemic of 1848-1849. Sidney Herbert appointed Secretary at War in Lord Aberdeen's cabinet.
Collects data on hospitals and charitable institutions on Paris visit. Nurses Grandmother Shore during her final illness. Receives annual allowance of £500 from W.E.N. Returns briefly to Paris for more nurse's training, but contracts measles. **August 12.** Superintendent at the Institute for the Care of Sick Gentlewomen in Upper Harley Street, London.	1853	Queen Victoria uses chloroform in childbirth for first time. Quetelet founds International Statistical Congress. Farr publishes second English life-table. Turkey declares war on Russia in October.
Recommended for superintendent of nurses at reorganized King's College Hospital. Volunteers to nurse cholera patients at Middlesex Hospital. Leaves Harley Street after 1 year, 2 months as superintendent.	1854	Florence's reputation spreads quickly in medical and professional circles. England and France declare war on Russia in March. Cousin Blanche Smith marries Arthur Hugh Clough. Cholera epidemic strikes London; John Snow's famous map finds focus of epidemic as Broad Street pump.

Crimean War years (1854-1856)

October 14. Reads war reports in the *Times* and volunteers to nurse the wounded in Turkey. **October 15.** Officially invited to become Superintendent of Female Nursing Establishment of the English Hospitals in Turkey by Herbert. **October 16.** Meets with Herbert to discuss plans for Scutari. **October 21.** Leaves for Scutari with 38 volunteers and the Bracebridges. **November 4.** Arrives at Barrack Hospital at Scutari. Finds supplies nonexistent; uses *Times* Fund to purchase supplies from Grand Bazaar in Constantinople, delegates tasks to nurses and orderlies, cleans wards, introduces extra kitchens and laundry facilities. **December.** Continues sending detailed letters to Herbert about army mismanagement. Hires 200 Turkish workers to rebuild wing of Barrack Hospital.	1854	**September 20.** Battle of the Alma. **October 13.** Sir Robert Peel opens the *Times* Fund. Dr. John Hall, Inspector-General of Hospitals for Crimean campaign, inspects Barrack Hospital and declares it satisfactory. **October 17.** Siege of Sebastopol begins. **October 17.** Nurse selection begins at Herbert's home; 38 women selected. **October 25.** Charge of the Light Brigade during the the Battle of Balaclava. **November 5.** Battle of Inkerman. **November 9.** Sick and wounded from Balaclava flood into Scutari; doctors finally ask nurses for assistance. **November 14.** Hurricane sinks supply ship *Prince;* winter supplies lost. **December 15.** Mary Stanley and second party of nurses arrive at Scutari.
January-February. Heaviest volume of new patients at Scutari. **March 8.** Begins planning of memorial for British Military Cemetery. **April.** Mortality rate at Scutari begins to fall. **May.** First visit to Crimea. **May 12.** Has severe case of Crimean fever; out of danger in 2 weeks. **July.** Goes to Therapia to recuperate. **August.** Returns to Scutari. **September.** Establishes "Inkerman Cafe" for soldiers; begins collecting soldiers' money to send home to their families. **October.** Returns to Crimea and is hospitalized for severe sciatica; returns to Scutari as new outbreak of cholera occurs. **November.** Awarded a brooch from Queen Victoria in appreciation of her work.	1855	**January 19.** 800 sick and wounded soldiers arrive in Scutari from Crimea; death rate of soldiers dramatically increases. **January 26.** M.P. John Roebuck calls for investigation of army conditions in Turkey. Lord Aberdeen's government falls; Herbert out of office. **February.** Lord Palmerston becomes Prime Minister; Lord Panmure becomes Secretary of State for War. Panmure sends Sanitary and Commissariat Commissions to Turkey to investigate conditions in hospitals and supply problems. Alexis Soyer, Reform Club chef, arrives in Scutari to reorganize army kitchens. **March 5.** Sultan of Turkey grants approval for British Military Cemetery at Scutari. **March.** Mary Stanley returns to England due to strain. **May 24.** Lord Raglan visits Nightingale during her recuperation; dies 1 month later. **July.** Bracebridges return to England. **September 9.** Russians begin to leave Sebastopol. Aunt Mai arrives to take Bracebridges' place. **November 29.** Formation of Nightingale Fund announced.

Nightingale's major life events and work		Related events
February 25. Finally receives General Orders confirming that she is in charge of all nurses in the British army. **March 16.** Returns to Crimea; writes final reports on all 229 nurses who served in military hospitals. **July 28.** Leaves for England, an international heroine at age 36.	**1856**	**January.** McNeill-Tulloch Report on findings of Commissariat Commission published. **March 30.** Treaty of Paris ends Crimean War. **June 20.** Nightingale Fund closes, having collected £44,039; Nightingale given power to direct all funds.

Post-war years (1856-1861)

August 7. Arrives home at Lea Hurst after 20 months in the East. Preoccupied with memories of the Crimean dead. **September 21.** Successful meeting at Balmoral with Queen Victoria and Prince Albert. **October.** Meets with Panmure and suggests creation of a Royal Commission. **November.** Moves into Burlington Hotel, London, where her quarters become known as the "Little War Office."	**1856**	Chelsea Board whitewashes McNeill-Tulloch Report. Sidney Herbert named chairman of army sanitary commission. Her loyal band of fellow reformers include Sidney Herbert, Dr. William Farr, and Dr. John Sutherland.
Analyzes her Crimean data with help from Farr. Invents her famous wedge diagrams to illustrate mortality statistics. "Little War Office" starts working nonstop in May. Completes *Notes on Matters Affecting the Health, Efficiency, and Hospital Administration of the British Army.* Introduces Parthe to Sir Harry Verney. Severe chronic illness continues; declares herself an invalid in September. Feels near death in November.	**1857**	Royal Warrant for army sanitary commission officially issued in May. Indian Mutiny breaks out; called the First War of Independence by Indian nationalists. Sidney Herbert writes Army Sanitary Commission Report based primarily on Nightingale's data. Sir Harry Verney, liberal member of House of Commons, is a frequent visitor. Aunt Mai comes to the Burlington Hotel in September to help Nightingale. Arthur Clough helps with transcription and secretarial work. Sidney Herbert receives directions for Nightingale Fund in case of her death.
Inducted into London Statistical Society (later the Royal Statistical Society)		
Daily meetings and correspondence on army reform. Pressure of work on Nightingale Fund increases. Revises *Suggestions for Thought* and compiles *Notes on Hospitals.* Privately prints her anonymous *Mortality of the British Army.*	**1858**	Palmerston's government falls; Panmure out of office. Sir Harry Verney and Parthe marry in June. Harriet Martineau writes articles and book using Nightingale's official report. Government of India Act passed; Lord Stanley becomes first Secretary of State for India.
Continuous work on health of army and civilian populations. Drafts *Circular of Enquiry* for 200 military stations in India. Severe symptoms with chronic illness in summer. Begins plans for Nightingale Fund nurses' training program. Works on model hospital statistical forms with Farr. *Notes on Hospitals* published in October.	**1859**	Arthur Clough appointed first secretary of Nightingale Fund. Farr publishes Healthy District Life Table. Palmerston becomes Prime Minister again in June. India Sanitary Commission established. Uncle Sam Smith and family ask Aunt Mai to return home. Sidney Herbert becomes Secretary for War.
Publishes *Notes on Nursing* in January. First edition (15,000) sells out in a month. Privately publishes *Suggestions for Thought.* Negotiations between Nightingale Fund and St. Thomas's Hospital completed for Nightingale School of Nursing. **July 9.** Nightingale School of Nursing opens with 11 probationers. Severe symptoms of chronic illness continue. Meets Adolphe Quetelet for first time and entertains other attendees of International Statistical Congress. Model hospital admission and census forms are presented at International Statistical Congress in London in July.	**1860**	Pasteur demonstrates presence of "dusts" in air. Benjamin Jowett, J.S. Mill, and Sir John McNeill review *Suggestions for Thought.* Her spiritual mother, Madre Santa Colomba, dies; Aunt Mai goes home in March. Mrs. Wardroper appointed Head Matron of Nightingale School of Nursing; Mr. Whitfield appointed lecturer. Hilary Bonham Carter takes Aunt Mai's place at Burlington Hotel in May. Herbert diagnosed with kidney disease; Clough's health begins to fail.
Becomes a consultant to Union side in American Civil War. Declines Queen Victoria's offer of apartment in Kensington Palace. Seriously ill for 4 weeks after Sidney Herbert's death in August. Grieves over November death of Arthur Clough. Consults on Canadian military expedition with Lord de Grey in December.	**1861**	Harriet Martineau popularizes *Notes on Nursing* in *Daily News.* Sir Harry Verney becomes chairman of Nightingale Fund and remains in post until his death at age 94. Sidney Herbert dies in August; Arthur Clough dies in November. Indian Sanitary Commission begins work. Semmelweis publishes classic paper on puerperal fever.
Analyzes data from military stations in India: completes first draft of India Sanitary Commission Report. Opposes Chadwick's proposed "Continental System" calling for inspection and regulation of prostitutes by police. Meets Benjamin Jowett for the first time when she asks him to come to London and administer the sacraments to her.	**1862**	Sir Bartle Frere appointed Governor of Bombay. Nightingale Fund starts midwifery training program at King's College Hospital. Mary Jones appointed Superintendent of Midwifery Training Program at King's College.
Asks Lord Palmerston and Harriet Martineau to agitate for appointment of Lord de Grey as Secretary of State for War. Completes India Sanitary Commission Report; prints condensed version known as "The Red Book." Briefs Sir John Lawrence on sanitary reform in India; her political influence in India Office grows.	**1863**	Palmerston reads Nightingale's letter in support of Lord de Grey to the queen; Harriet Martineau agitates for public support of de Grey. Lord de Grey appointed Secretary of State for War. Cholera epidemic in England. Sir John Lawrence appointed Viceroy of India. Jane Shaw Stewart named first superintendent of nurses at Royal Victoria Hospital.
Completes *Suggestions in Regard to Sanitary Works Required for the Improvement of India.* Drafts instructions for British delegates to Geneva Convention.	**1864**	William Rathbone writes to Nightingale for advice on Liverpool Workhouse Nursing. Contagious Disease Act passed. Lawrence sends copies of *Suggestions on Sanitary Works* to all Indian military stations. Representatives from 12 nations meet in Geneva to establish guidelines for the Red Cross, founded by Henri Dunant. *Times* reports on boy's death from neglect at Holborn Workhouse sparks public outcry for workhouse medical and nursing reform.

Reform years (1862-1879)

Nightingale's major life events and work		Related events
Meets with Charles Villiers, President of Poor Law Board, on workhouse and nursing reform. Works on plans for Liverpool Workhouse Infirmary. Moves permanently to 35 South Street (later renumbered 10). **July 28.** Records another Call from God.	1865	Agnes Jones becomes superintendent of Liverpool Workhouse Infirmary. Hilary Bonham Carter dies of cancer; Lord Palmerston dies.
Develops ABCs of workhouse medical and nursing reform for Metropolitan Poor Bill.	1866	First Women's Suffrage Committee presents petition to Parliament.
Continues to lobby for sanitary reform and public health service for India. Refuses Mill's request that she serve on board of National Society for Woman's Suffrage because she can't devote enough time to it. **May 7.** Reflects on her 30 years of service to God.	1867	Midwifery program at King's College closed due to high mortality rate. Sir Bartle Frere visits South Street to be briefed on Indian affairs. Cholera outbreak in India; catastrophic death rate. Lister presents first paper on antiseptic surgery. Sanitary Committee created in London's India Office; Frere named head. National Society for Women's Suffrage founded. Metropolitan Poor Act passed.
Visited often by Sir Bartle Frere at her own "little India Office." Anonymously writes and publishes "Una and the Lion" as a eulogy to Agnes Jones. Joins National Society for Women's Suffrage. Communicates almost daily with Sutherland for the next 20 years on army sanitation reform.	1868	Agnes Jones, superintendent of Liverpool Workhouse Infirmary, dies of fever.
Urges India Office to begin a sanitation survey in all military stations and nearby villages. Continues *India Annual Report*; recognized as most knowledgeable person for statistical data and historical perspective on India.	1869	Lawrence's term as Viceroy ends. J.S. Mill's *The Subjection of Women* published. Women obtain right to vote in municipal elections. Captain Douglas Galton, Nightingale's last direct contact at the War Office, retires. Royal Sanitary Commission established (Great Britain). Jane Shaw Stewart forced to resign as superintendent of Royal Victoria Hospital at Netley; succeeded by Jane Deeble. Lord Napier of Magdela appointed Commander-in-Chief of army in India.
Advisor to Army Medical Services in Franco-Prussian War (1870-1871). Advisor to National Society for Aid to the Sick and Wounded (later British Red Cross Society). Submits tract to Indian village elders on sanitary reform; elected honorary member of Bengal Social Science Association. Begins to focus on Nightingale School of Nursing, but chronic illlness prevents active participation.	1870	Franco-Prussian War (test of vaccination). Metropolitan Asylums Board established. Metropolitan Fever Hospitals established in London. England signs Treaty of Geneva.
Interviews nurse probationers to learn more about St. Thomas's and the Nightingale training program. Continues work with Henry Bonham Carter on Nightingale Fund and nurses' training program. Awarded Bronze Cross by French Société de Secours aux Blessés. Visited by Crown Princess of Prussia. Publishes *Notes on Lying-In Institutions*.	1871	St. Thomas's Hospital moves to new location in Lambeth in June.
Critiques portions of Benjamin Jowett's *Dialogues of Plato*, 2nd ed.; chooses stories for his Children's Bible; helps with his sermons and lectures. Awarded Prussian Cross of Merit by Emperor William I. Begins writing *Notes on Devotional Authors of the Middle Ages*.	1872	Whitfield resigns as lecturer at St. Thomas's; is replaced by Dr. John Croft, who improves the curriculum. Lord Mayo assassinated; Lord Northbrook becomes next Viceroy of India. Metropolitan Water Act, calling for piping of water to London, is passed. Charles Bracebridge dies. Infant Life Protection Act (England). Henri Dunant, founder of Red Cross, credits Nightingale as his inspiration.
Writes articles on Indian and theological topics; continues writing about the mystics.	1873	J.S. Mill dies. Boards of Health organized in 134 American cities.
Becomes honorary member of American Statistical Association. Contributes to Paulina Irby's fund for missionary work in Bosnia and Herzegovina.	1874	W.E.N. dies in January at age 80; Selina Bracebridge dies at age 74. Quetelet, Lord Panmure, and Mother Mary Clare Moore die. London School of Medicine founded by Sophia Jex-Blake.
Continues work on Indian sanitation. Spends more time with mother at Lea Hurst after father's death.	1875	Mary Crossland becomes Home Sister to nurse probationers at St. Thomas's. English Public Health Act. English Sale of Food and Drugs Act.
Engaged in various areas of nursing reform.	1876	Harriet Martineau dies. Physiological Society of London founded.
Promotes district nursing in London. Troubled by Indian famines and peasants' inability to get out of debt to large landowners.	1877	Julius Mohl dies. William Rathbone urges Nightingale to extend Liverpool Infirmary Nursing to London.
Asked to be a consultant on possible war with Russia.	1878	Women allowed to pursue degrees at University of London and to attend lectures at Oxford for first time.
Writes various papers on India.	1879	Sir John Lawrence dies. Koch publishes paper identifying six different bacteria, conclusively proving germ theory of disease.

Nightingale's major life events and work		Related events
Becomes closer to Parthe and Sir Harry; goes for extended visits to Claydon House. Concerned about army medical hospital service in India, South Africa, Egypt, and Sudan.	1880	Fanny dies in February at age 92. Pasteur identifies streptococci responsible for causing erysipelas, puerperal fever, and scarlet fever. Lord Ripon (Lord de Grey) appointed Viceroy of India. Uncle Sam Smith dies.
Reconciles with Aunt Mai after 20 years.	1881	Pasteur develops vaccine against anthrax. Koch introduces solid cultures for growing bacteria. Government Animal Vaccination Establishment begins.
Inspects Nightingale School of Nursing at St. Thomas's for first time.	1882	Married Women's Property Act amended. Koch discovers tubercle bacillus. Mary Clarke Mohl and Dr. William Farr die.
Receives Royal Red Cross medal from Queen Victoria. Much correspondence on proposed Ilbert Bill.	1883	Sir John McNeill dies. Discovery of bacilli responsible for cholera, diphtheria, and conjunctivitis.
Briefs Lord Dufferin before he goes to India as Viceroy. Writes pamphlet for health missionaries in towns and villages in India.	1884	Compromise Ilbert Bill passes. Sir Bartle Frere dies.
Very interested in First Indian National Congress.	1885	Richard Monckton Milnes (Lord Houghton) dies.
Receives many governement officials and visitors from India.	1886	Royal Institute of Public Health (London) founded.
Her Jubilee Year — 50 years since her first Call from God. Begins battle against registration of nurses (lasts 7 years). Nurses Benjamin Jowett when he becomes ill during a visit. Meets Sir William Wedderburn. Has another severe bout of illness; is treated by Dr. Brunton.	1887	Queen Victoria's Jubilee; bulk of Jubilee Fund used for district nursing. Mrs. Wardroper retires as matron of St. Thomas's Hospital after 27 years. Bruce identifies *Brucella melitensis*, organism that causes Crimean fever (today known as Malta or Mediterranean fever).
Advocates sanitary education for Indian villagers. Briefs Lord Lansdowne before he goes to India as new Viceroy. Becomes involved with curriculum for Health Missioner program.	1888	Dr. Sutherland retires after 34 years of working with Nightingale. Government establishes a Sanitary Board with executive and independent authority in each province in India Local Government Act provides money for health missioners.
Vehemently opposed to the British Nurses Association Charter.	1889	Aunt Mai dies. Bombay Village Sanitation Act passed. British Nurses Association applies for charter to register nurses. Queen Victoria's Jubilee Institute for Nurses chartered.
Fame rekindled on occasion of 70th birthday. Urges establishment of a Chair in Applied Statistics at Oxford to be funded by herself and Jowett.	1890	**May 12.** Parthe dies at age 81 on Florence's birthday. Thomas Edison's assistant records Nightingale's voice at South Street. Sir Edwin Chadwick dies.
Presents petition against British Nurses Association. Helps organize Indian delegation at International Health Congress.	1891	Sutherland dies.
Continues opposition to British Nurses Association plan for registration; wants nurses registered by individual schools.	1892	Dr. Croft resigns as lecturer for Nightingale School of Nursing. Hospital Board Council Committee hears from British Nurses Association and Nightingale and her allies about the pros and cons of registration.
Tries to restore good will between the factions for and against nurses' registration. Nightingale's final nursing text, "Sick-Nursing and Health-Nursing," read at nurse's congress at Chicago World's Fair; this meeting establishes beginning of formal international collaboration among nurses.	1893	Nightingale Pledge first administered at a Detroit nursing school. Charter granted to British Nurses Association, stipulating that it may keep a list of nurses but not officially call themselves "chartered" or "registered." Benjamin Jowett, last intimate friend, dies in October.
Works on syllabus for Dr. George De'ath's rural health missioners.	1894	Sir Harry Verney dies at age 93. William Shore Smith, heir to Nightingale estate, dies at age 63.
Last visit to Claydon.	1895	Mary Crossland retires after 21 years as Home Sister at Nightingale School; 600 nurses completed their probationary course under her care.
Makes out her will; appoints Henry Bonham Carter the executor. Never leaves South Street again.	1896	Embley is sold.
Meets with Sir William Wedderburn, Gopal Krishna Gokhale, and other Indian nationalists before the Royal Commission on Indian Expenditure.	1897	Queen Victoria's Diamond Jubilee; bulk of women's jubilee gift devoted to district nursing.
	1898	Army's Medical Department reorganized into the Royal Army Medical Corps. Sir Robert Rawlinson dies.
Expresses her thoughts on the Boer War in South Africa.	1899	Sir Douglas Galton dies.
	1902	William Rathbone dies; Alice Cochrane employed to care for Nightingale.
Receives Lady of Grace of the Order of St. John of Jerusalem from King Edward VII.	1904	Elizabeth Bosanquet hired to care for Nightingale after marriage of Alice Cochrane.
Receives Order of Merit from King Edward VII; first woman to receive honor.	1907	Mary Adelaide Nutting becomes first Professor of Nursing in the world at Teachers College, Columbia University, New York City.
Granted Freedom of the City of London (second woman to receive award).	1908	Meeting in honor of the Jubilee of Nightingale School of Nursing held at Carnegie Hall, New York City (1,000 nursing training programs now established in the United States and in 20 other countries).
August 13. Dies at age 90; family refuses offer of burial in Westminster Abbey. Buried at St. Margaret's Church, East Wellow, Hampshire.	1910	

Significant Family, Friends, and Correspondents

Bracebridge, Selina (1800-1874) (pp. 58, 130 No. 3): confidante; met in 1845 through Mary Clarke; with her husband Charles, took Nightingale to Rome in 1847, to Egypt and Greece in 1849-1850, and arranged for her first visit to Kaiserswerth on the return home, accompanied her to Scutari in 1854; until her death Nightingale called her "more than a mother to me"; (see Charles Bracebridge).

Bracebridge, Charles Holte (-1872) (p. 130 No. 4): liberal with many political and social connections; as a young man took part in the bloody Greek revolution against the Turks; Nightingale Fund trustee; provided Nightingale with personal hand reports of Nightingale School after his visits and gave her advice on training scheme, and matron; (see Selina Bracebridge).

Bowman, M. D., (Sir) William (1816-1892) (p. 96): distinguished ophthalmic surgeon and anatomist-physiologist; described the striated muscle, basement membrane, ciliary regions of the eye, the capsule (Bowman's capsule) around the renal glomerulus and the urinary tubules, advanced his theory of urinary secretion (1842), and scientific treatment of lacrimal disorders; met Nightingale at Harley Street in 1853 where she assisted him during a difficult eye surgery using chloroform; encouraged her to become the nursing superintendent at the reorganized King's College Hospital, but she was invited to head a group of nurses to serve in the Crimean War; original member of Nightingale Fund Council; assisted Nightingale and the Nightingale Fund Council to establish the Midwifery School at King's College Hospital; made many visits to the Nightingale Training Program at St. Thomas's and gave her many reports following his visits.

Bunsen, Christian Carl Josias von (1791-1860) (p. 50): wealthy Prussian theologian, scholar of ancient and oriental languages who applied his knowledge to the study of scriptures; entered diplomatic service in Rome under Prussian Ambassador, historian, Barhold Niebuhr (1817); met Richard Monckton Milnes and many English intellectuals who questioned the Church's teachings on the scriptures; introduced Max Müller and his scholarly *Sacred Books of the East* to Oxford; did much to further discussion and understanding of eastern thought and religion in England; became Ambassador to the Court of St. James (1842); met Nightingale through her parents who became good friends with him and his wife; first suggested to Nightingale that she study nursing at Kaiserswerth and sent her the Kaiserswerth Institute Annual Report.

Carter, Henry Bonham (1827-1921) (p. 300): first cousin of Nightingale, brother of Hilary; Unitarian, educated at Trinity College, Cambridge, called to the Bar, 1853; Managing Director, Guardian Life and Fire Assurance Company; Secretary of Nightingale Fund 1861-1899, continued on Council until 1914; became an authority on nursing and his involvement was a major reason for the accomplishments and success in the Nightingale Training School at St. Thomas's Hospital; had 11 sons and one daughter, many with distinguished careers.

Carter, Hilary Bonham (1821-1865) (p. 55): favorite first cousin and confidante of Nightingale during her early years; a gifted artist, stayed with the Mohls in Paris (1849-1850); gave her time to her family rather than her art; after Aunt Mai returned to her family, came to assist Nightingale (1860-1862).

Chadwick, (Sir) Edwin (1800-1890) (p. 232): protégé of Jeremy Bentham, Utilitarian philosopher, and leading sanitary reformer; secretary of the Poor Law Commission (1834-1846); his major Bluebook Report, *The Sanitary Conditions of the Labouring Population of Great Britain* (1842), was read by Nightingale; worked with her on Poor Law issues and many other sanitary matters; rejected germ theory early on because it threatened the focus on improved sanitation and sanitary principles.

Clark, M. D., (Sir) James (1788-1870) (p. 189): personal physician to the Nightingales in the 1820s-1850s; gave Nightingale advice about Parthe's detrimental dependence and attachment to her, which was a major factor in Nightingale seeking independence from her family in 1853; personal physician to Queen Victoria; responsible for arranging Nightingale's visit with the Queen after her return from the Crimea in September, 1856; worked with Nightingale in writing the curriculum and selections of professors for the first Army Medical School; served on the Nightingale Fund Council for many years.

Clough, Arthur Hugh (1819-1861) (p. 241): poet and scholar; took a keen interest in the theological controversies of the time, regarded Anglican doctrines as imperfect, coined the phrase the 'Broad Church'; married Blanch Smith (1854), daughter of Nightingale's Aunt Mai and Uncle Sam Smith; assisted Nightingale with correspondence 1857-1860; encouraged her to revise *Suggestions For Thought*; introduced Benjamin Jowett to her work; became the first secretary of the Nightingale Fund (1860); his health began to fail in 1859, and he died of malarial fever in Florence in 1861.

Farr, M. D., (Sir) William (1807-1891) (p. 195): pioneering medical statistician; Compiler of Abstracts for General Register Office; Assistant Commissioner for Censuses (1851, 1861), Commissioner for Census (1871) and wrote majority of each census report; spent much time in formulation of life tables for insurance purposes and general statistics; resigned his office when he was not appointed Registrar-General (1879); worked with Nightingale in the development and statistical analysis of her Scutari and Crimean Army hospital data, and India data; corresponded with her on nursing and many other topics; active member of the Statistical Society, serving as treasurer (1855-1867), vice-president (1869-1870), and president (1871-1872).

Frere, (Sir) Bartle (1815-1884) (p. 285): respected civil servant in India (1834-1856); member of the governor-general Council (1859-1860); governor of Bombay (1862); returned to England (1867) and given a seat on the Indian Council in London; Captain Galton arranged his first meeting with Nightingale to discuss problems in India, a frequent correspondent, referred to Nightingale's South Street residence as "the little India Office", became a frequent visitor with his wife to the Nightingales at Embley.

Galton, (Sir) Douglas (1822-1899): Captain, Royal Engineers; married Marianne Nicholson (1851), Nightingale's first cousin; member of the Royal Commission on the Sanitary Condition of the Barracks and Hospitals; Nightingale brought his engineering expertise to the attention of the War Office and persuaded them to secure his appointment as Assistant Under-Secretary of State for War (1862) in charge of health and sanitation of the Army; served on Army Sanitation Subcommission until 1865; retired from the War Office in 1869 and transferred to Director of Public Works until his retirement.

Herbert, Elizabeth (1821-1911) (pp. 61, 111): married Sidney Herbert in 1846; met Nightingale in Rome in 1847 through the Bracebridges; quickly recognized her as an authority on hospitals and sanitation, and a focused person with a desire to be of service; as a governing committee member of the Harley Street Institute recommended Nightingale for her first nursing position as Superintendent, Institute for Gentlewomen in Distressed Circumstances in 1853; supported her husband, Sidney, to invite Nightingale to head a party of nurses out to the Turkish hospitals in Scutari during the Crimean War; with Lady Canning, helped interview and hire all nurses who were sent; a supporter of Nightingale in her intense labors of army medical reform with her husband; converted to Catholicism in 1865; (see Sidney Herbert.)

Herbert, Lord Sidney Herbert of Lea (1810-1861) (p. 59, 113, 203): second son of George, 11th Earl of Pembroke; Secretary at War under Peel (1845-1846); Secretary at War under Aberdeen (1854-1855); Honorary Secretary of the Nightingale Fund (1855) and driving force of this movement; wrote official invitation to Nightingale to serve as Superintendent of Nurses in Turkey during the Crimean War; Chair, Royal Commission on the Health of the Army (1857-1861), Chair of the four subcommissions on army sanitary matters (1857-1861), Secretary for War under Palmerston (1859-1861), the Indian Royal Commission (1859-1861); gave up seat in House of Commons (1860) due to failing health, created Lord Herbert of Lea (1860); died of Bright's disease (1861). (See Elizabeth Herbert.)

Jowett, Benjamin (1817-1893) (p. 330): liberal theologian and university reformer; educated at Balliol College, Oxford; began tutorship at Balliol (1842), became Regis Professor of Greek (1855), Master of Balliol (1870); vice-chancellor (1882-1886); met Nightingale through Arthur Hugh Clough (1860) when he was given Nightingale's *Suggestions for Thought* to critique; *their* first face-to-face meeting occurred when she asked him to come to London to give her the Sacraments (1862) due to severe illness and feeling that she might die soon; after he gave her the Sacraments became a frequent visitor; their correspondence over 33 years is a remarkable portrait of friendship.

Lawrence, (Sir) John (1811-1879) (p. 279): Viceroy of India (1863-1869), was first recognized by his outstanding civilian service during the Indian Mutiny (1857) and various military roles and maneuvers; on appointment as Viceroy to India (1863), he visited Nightingale to receive her "historical perspective" and perceptions on the most urgent sanitary and medical reforms for India; Nightingale's favorite Viceroy who made many improvements in municipal and military sanitation, railroads and road construction, canals and irrigation, although she felt that he should have accomplished more.

Manning, (Cardinal) Henry Edward (1808-1892): educated at Balliol College, Oxford and a fellow of Merton; an authoritarian leader in the High Church movement until he joined the Church of Rome in 1851; met Nightingale in Rome in 1848 when she had many discussions about the Roman Catholic Church and its doctrine; became Archdeacon of Westminster (1865) and Cardinal of Westminster (1875) with a mission to expand parochial school education.

Martineau, Harriet (1802-1876) (p. 216): from a prominent Unitarian family, her father a Norwich manufacturer, and her brother a well-known minister and writer; her sister taught Hilary Bonham Carter; prolific writer and most noted woman journalist of her day; regular contributor to the *Daily News* and the *Edinburgh Review*; Nightingale provided her with governments reports, facts, and letters to help shape public opinion on politics, nursing, military, War Office, and India Office reform; deaf from an early age, used an ear-trumpet; in poor health, took to her bed for 5 years and was cured by mesmerism; in 1855 told that she had heart disease, but lived 20 more years.

McNeill, M. D., (Sir) John (1797-1883) (p. 152): doctor and diplomat in the East India Company; minister plenipotentiary to Persia; head of Poor Law board in Scotland; met Nightingale when sent with Colonel Alexander Tulloch to inquire into the management of the Commissariat in the Crimea (1855); the final McNeill-Tulloch report confirmed allegations of army and government mismanagement but the Chelsea Board (1856) whitewashed report; Nightingale roused politicians and her friends to honor McNeill and Tulloch and the findings of their official report; on her return from the Crimea, Nightingale frequently consulted with him on formation of the Royal Commission as well as other matters and areas of reform; original member of Nightingale Fund Council and trustee; he deeply understood Nightingale's lifelong grief over deaths of Herbert and Clough from his own personal loss from the deaths of two wives and all his children but one daughter.

Mill, John Stuart (1806-1873) (p. 317): philosopher, author, liberal M. P. for Westminster (1865-1869); critiqued Nightingale's *Suggestions for Thought* (1860) and encouraged her to publish it with revisions; a great supporter of women's rights, published *The Subjection of Women* (1869); corresponded with her on poor law and women's rights.

Milnes, (Lord Houghton) Richard Monckton (1809-1885) (p. 52): poet, educated at Trinity College, Cambridge, became M. P. (1838); met

Nightingale in 1842 and their courtship lasted until 1849 when she broke it off, but they remained lifelong friends; married Annabel Crewe (1851), named a daughter Florence and asked her to be a godparent to their son; active in various committees for Juvenile Boys' Reformatories, British Museum trustee, and Nightingale Fund trustee; gave her advice after the Crimea to widen her circle of advisors such as meeting Lord Stanley on Indian affairs; supported many people in their endeavors, Keats scholar, traveled widely and known to collect erotica; created Lord Houghton (1863).

Mohl, Julius (1800-1876) (p. 56): German aristocrat and leading Orientalist, translated oriental classics into a European language, known primarily for his translations of Firdausi's Persian epic *Shah Nameh* (Book of Kings); through him (and von Bunsen) Nightingale became more familiar with German theologians and historians, and knowledgeable about the spiritual legacy of the Near and Far East such as Buddhism, Hinduism, Islam, Zoroastrianism, and ancient Egyptian religions; became a French citizen to be near Mary Clarke whom he married (1847); President of the Asiatic Society and the Académie des Inscriptions; corresponded with Nightingale, circulated her hospital statistics form in Paris, was interested in her work until his death. (See Mary Clarke Mohl.)

Mohl, Mary Clarke (1793-1883) (pp. 41, 56): created the leading intellectual salon of her day in Paris; a friend of the renown Madame Récamier, social leader in intellectual and literary circles; Nightingale met "Clarkey" in 1838, and was a major influence on Nightingale's awareness of gaining her independence and freedom from her family; married Julius von Mohl (1847); Madame Mohl became a lifelong correspondent and Nightingale wrote some of her most personal feelings on family and women to her. (See Julius Mohl.)

Moore, Mother Mary Clare (1814-1874) (pp. 130 #8, 327): began Sisters of Mercy Convent in Dublin (1831) and had much experience working with cholera patients and the poor (1832-1838); became Mother Superior of Sister of Mercy Convent of Bermondsey (1839) in one of London's poor district; Mother Mary Clare and four of her nurses accompanied Nightingale to the Crimea in 1854, one of her most important nurses and supporters during this period; remained correspondents until her death about spiritual ideas, exchanging books on the medieval mystics, and their mutual work and service for God and humanity.

Nightingale, Frances Smith (1778-1880) (pp. 3, 7, 207): daughter (one of 10 children) of William Smith, a M. P. for more than 40 years and a leader for religious freedom, humanitarian reform for the disenfranchised and poor, a stalwart in the anti-slavery movement with the leading abolitionist William Wilberforce; beautiful, social, enjoyed entertaining her very elite, politically influential friends; Nightingale had much conflict with her mother in her earlier years, but in older life, she and her mother were more cordial.

Nightingale, Parthenope (Lady Verney) (1819-1890) (pp. 3, 44, 207, 208, 215): Nightingale's older sister called Parthe; much sibling rivalry during early years; Nightingale had great concern for her sister's welfare and happiness and introduced her to Sir Harry Verney whom she married (1858), they had no children together; the life of a Lady suited her well; took a great interest in the Verney family and responsibilities of the Claydon House Mansion; wrote five novels, essays on agriculture, and memoirs on the Verney family during the English Civil War; had severe, crippling rheumatoid arthritis last years of her life; became very close to Nightingale after her marriage as seen in correspondence from 1860 until near her death; she died on May 12, Nightingale's birthday. (See Sir Harry Verney.)

Nightingale, William Edward (1794-1874) (pp. 30, 208, 263): Nightingale's father, born William Shore, changed his name to Nightingale on inheritance of the wealthy (lead mines and other holdings) Lea property in Derbyshire from his uncle Peter Nightingale, called W. E. N. by friends and family; went to Trinity College, Cambridge; married Frances Smith (1818); High Sheriff of Hampshire (1829), lost bid for Parliament (1835) because he refused to bribe voters; educated his daughters at home in a classical education; provided Nightingale with £500 allowance per annum (1853) to be on her own; was interested in politics and theosophical ideas and frequent discussed and corresponded with his daughter on these topics.

Palmerston, (Lord) Henry John Temple (1784-1865) (p. 187): great British statesman and politician. He was Secretary at War (1809-1828), Foreign Secretary (1830-1834, 1835-1841, 1846-1851), Home Secretary (1852-1855), Prime Minister, (1855-1858, 1859-1865). A pragmatist who judged every question on its merits, he pledged himself to no party, as his early Tory affiliation evolved to Whig and then Liberal, although he always upheld the rights of the aristocracy; one of the first politicians to realize and utilize the emerging power of public opinion and mass newspapers; a master of the subject matter and personalities in governance and foreign policy; friend and neighbor (Embley) of the Nightingales; a key supporter of Nightingale's work and ideas.

Panmure, (Lord) Fox Maule (1801-1874) (p. 193): native of Scotland, served 12 years and retired as Captain of 79th Highlanders in 1832; M. P. from 1835-1852, when his father's death raised him to the peerage; Secretary at War 1846-1852; Secretary of War (office reformed to combine Secretary at War and Secretary for War) under Lord Palmerston, 1855-1858; personally and professionally receptive to Nightingale's recommendations for Army reform, his effectiveness was limited by his easygoing approach to his administrative responsibilities.

Pringle, Angelique Lucille (1846-1920) (p. 304): Trained at St. Thomas's, 1868; Nightingale affectionately called her "The Pearl" and "Little Sister"; appointed Lady Superintendent of Nurses at Edinburgh Royal Infirmary (1873-1887); converted to Roman Catholicism (1889) and had to give up her nursing position; continued to be a frequent visitor and was the last person outside of the family to visit Nightingale before her death.

Quetelet, Lambert Adolphe Jacques (1796-1874) (p. 229): Belgium mathematician and scientist; considered founder of social statistics and was the first person in Europe to record social statistics, i.e., education, marriage, work, deaths, to predict outcome of social conditions; organized the Commission Central de Statistique (1841), that led to the International Statistical Congress (1853) of which Nightingale was a member; first published his work as *Essai de Physique Sociale* (1835); Nightingale saw his work as "a revelation of the Will of God," and felt that Quetelet's science was essential to all political and social administration; after he gave her his revised *Physique Sociale* (1869; two volumes), she treated it like a new book.

Ripon, (Lord) George Frederick Samuel Robinson (1827-1909) (p. 361): held the title of Lord Ripon after his father death (1833) and then a joint title Lord de Grey after his uncle's death (1859); greatly influenced by the Christian socialist movement; he served as Under-Secretary for War in Lord Palmerston's second administration (1859), Secretary for War (1863), Secretary for India (1866), Viceroy for India (1880-1884); asked Nightingale to consult with the War Office (1861) when it appeared that England and the northern states of America were on the brink of war; frequent consultant to and with her on India affairs from 1865-1882.

Rathbone, William (1819-1902) (p. 294): philanthropist, reformer, and wealthy merchant, appalled by conditions at the Brownlow Hill Workhouse; provided funds to bring trained nurses to the Liverpool Workhouse Infirmary and to start the Training School for Nurses in Liverpool in 1865; to commemorate the opening of the Liverpool Workhouse Infirmary, he sent Nightingale a plant stand for her bedroom and supplied her with flowers or plants weekly until his death; was involved with Nightingale in fight against nurses registration in 1886.

Shaftesbury, Lord (1801-1885) (p. 48): earlier years held title of Lord Ashley; noted English humanitarian and reformer; his example of translating his religious beliefs into social reform through political action was a formative influence on Nightingale; he was first to suggested that she study the government documents, called the "Blue Books," on hospital statistics and sanitary reform.

Smith, Mary Shore (1798-1889) (pp. 10, 46, 81): W. E. Nightingale's only and younger sister, called "Aunt Mai"; married Fanny Nightingale's younger brother Samuel (1827); their son, Shore (1832) whom Nightingale called "my boy Shore," became the heir to the Nightingale property; was responsible for Nightingale's private tutor for study of mathematics; helped her work through her religious and theosophical treatise, *Suggestions for Thought*, "the Stuff" as they called it; was also influential in pressing for Nightingale to have her own annual allowance to pursue her nursing and independence; came out to Scutari when the Bracebridges returned to England in 1855 and stayed with her until the end of July, 1856; assisted Nightingale after the Crimean War 1856-1859 when her family requested that she return home. (See Samuel Smith.)

Smith, Samuel (1794-1880) (p. 10): during the Crimean War, Nightingale sent Uncle Sam the soldiers' pay in order to purchase money bonds to be sent to the soldiers' families; assisted Nightingale after the Crimea with settling bills, paying the nurses for their service in the Crimea, and miscellaneous administrative tasks and correspondence; kept order to Nightingale's personal bank account and paid her personal bills. (See Mary Shore Smith.)

Sutherland, M. D., John (1808-1891) (pp. 151, 258): doctor and authority on sanitation; head of the 1855 Sanitary Commission sent to the Crimea with full executive power to implement needed reform that had been identified by Nightingale and specific military officers and doctors; was Nightingale's medical advisor, chief daily advisor on Army and sanitation matters, helped her compile and edit her voluminous reports from 1857-1888; active in the Royal Commission on the Health of the Army and the Royal Commission on the State of the Army in India; only member with a paid position on the permanent Army Sanitary Commission until his retirement (1888).

Tulloch, (Colonel) Alexander (1801-1864) (p. 152): Army internal affairs investigator and collaborator in the McNeill-Tulloch Report. A native of Scotland, he was trained in the law, but joined the army in 1826 and was posted to India as lieutenant; a reformer at heart, he took up the causes of unsuitable food for enlisted men, salary payment to soldiers in depreciated silver coin, and inadequate canteen arrangements, all before his return to England in 1831; on his own, published (1835) tables on army mortality at various stations in India; was then assigned to a three-man committee to fully report on army mortality, which was published in four volumes in 1840; uncovered fraud in army pensioners' payments, which led to reform and creation of a pensioner corps with administrative controls; published "the Crimean Commission and the Chelsea Board" in 1857, which clarified in public debate his and Sir John McNeill's roles, resulting in a knighthood for Tulloch and privy councilor for McNeill; introduced Nightingale to Dr. William Farr; able member of Nightingale's circle of reformers.

Verney, (Sir) Harry (1801-1894) (pp. 214, 347, 349, 351): wealthy, liberal M. P from Buckinghamshire, widower with seven children, owner of the historic Claydon House Mansion; first elected to parliament in 1832 and held position till 1884; reformer and pioneer in improvements for rural health, sanitation, and education; after first wife died, married Parthenope Nightingale (1858); very supportive of Nightingale's reforms, became known as the "M.P. for Miss Nightingale"; was Chairman of Nightingale Fund Council (1861-1893), beginning in 1872 read many of Nightingale's annual addresses to nurse probationers at St. Thomas's Hospital; in later years Nightingale spent much time at Claydon and was attached to many of the Verney family calling them her nieces and nephews, as they called her their aunt. (See Parthenope Nightingale Verney.)

Williams, Rachel (Norris) (1840-1908) (p. 304): Trained as a 'Free-Special' at St. Thomas's, 1871-1872; Nightingale affectionately called her "The Goddess"; later Matron of St. Mary's Hospital; served in the Egyptian campaign (1876) where she met Daniel Norris and later married.

Nightingale & the Western Tradition of Mysticism

A *mystic* is a person who has, to a greater or lesser degree, had a direct experience of God.[1] The life of such a person is focused not merely on religious practice or belief, but on first-hand personal knowledge — the Divine Reality — of God.[2] For the mystic, God ceases to be an object and becomes a deeply personal experience.

Mysticism is a universal experience spanning both the East and West. In the West, popular misconceptions about the lives of well-known mystics commonly obscure the real accomplishments and divine motivation of these men and women.

Western mystical activism

The lives of Western mystics and saints are generally not sweet, gentle stories, but tumultuous, complex sagas because most of these talented and chosen individuals took up the cause of reform. In many cases, their mission was to revitalize or reform a church that had grown worldly, lax in religious practice, corrupt, and oppressive. As a result, many of these reformers found themselves battling political authority and taking on the role of political and social activist.

The Western mystic is not comfortable with the world as it is, but envisions what it can and should be. This call to personal action is an element in the spiritual development of all mystics; it is not an externally imposed task, but an inner compulsion that the mystic can only refer to as his or her true vocation and destiny.

Mystics are not perfect human beings. Because they are so committed to carrying out what they see as the Divine Will, they often experience tortured relationships with family, friends, and colleagues. This was certainly the case with Florence Nightingale — from her early struggles to break free from her conventional upper-class family and the restraints imposed upon women in Victorian society, to her decades of work from her sickbed, when she pushed herself and all those around her to give their all for the army, nursing, and India reforms that she felt were her mission.

Like the writings of the great mystics and saints, many of Nightingale's private notes, diaries, and letters — particularly those that touch on God, perfection, and mysticism — are emotional and passionate. Some authors have erroneously asserted that this emotionalism resulted from hysteria, exaggeration, the Victorian penchant for melodrama, psychopathology, low self-esteem, the need to manipulate and control others, frustration, rage, anger, and so forth. It is very easy to peruse the work of a person who wrote 14,000 letters in her lifetime, select passages out of context, and render uninformed judgments.

Evelyn Underhill's classic text, *Mysticism*,[3] published in 1911, contained no information on Nightingale, because the official Nightingale biography by E.T. Cook was not released until 1913. However, in *Practical Mysticism*,[4] published in 1915, Underhill obviously had read or been provided with information from the biography because she makes three references to Nightingale's spiritual development, calling her "one of the most balanced contemplatives of the nineteenth century."[5]

Five phases of spiritual development

In *Mysticism*, Underhill proposed five recognizable phases in the spiritual development of a mystic: (1) awakening, (2) purgation, (3) illumination, (4) surrender, and (5) union.[6] The process is not necessarily an orderly one, with discrete stages; rather, it is similar to an upward spiral, in which the aspirant progresses only to sometimes drop back, then move forward again. It is important to remember that the descriptions of the five stages that follow are a composite. Like nearly all other mystics, Nightingale did not necessarily fit neatly into each stage.

Awakening. In this first phase of the mystic's spiritual development, the individual experiences a conversion of the ego-oriented Self to a higher Self, which leads to consciousness of a Divine Reality within. This shift in awareness may be abrupt and is typically accompanied by feelings of joy and exaltation. Florence Nightingale's awakening came on February 7,

1837, at age 16, when she received a Call from God to be of service. Nightingale always marked this date as her awakening to a higher reality.

Purgation. The second phase of spiritual development involves great pain and effort. The Self becomes increasingly aware of Divine Beauty as contrasted with its own imperfection and finiteness. For Nightingale, this phase took place during her teens and twenties, when she struggled against her "dreaming" and strove to separate herself from her love of worldly success and acclaim. By the end of her trip to Egypt and Greece in 1850, she had given away most of her possessions and taken a vow of chastity, determined to be a handmaid of the Lord.

Illumination. This third phase is characterized by the spiritual "betrothal," wherein the mystic contemplates a profound union with the Absolute. Underhill says that mystics want to heal the disharmony between the actual (their perceptions of daily life) and the real (Divine Perfection). They are able to work for this healing with a singleness of purpose and an invincible optimism denied to the ordinary person.

From 1850 to 1853, Nightingale alternated between the Purgation and Illumination stages. She broke free from family restraints, completed her *Suggestions for Thought*, and began her professional career at Harley Street. The same fire that drew St. Catherine of Siena from contemplation to politics, and that compelled Joan of Arc to fight to save France, drove Florence Nightingale to battle the deplorable conditions at Scutari day and night for 20 months and to devote her total being to reform of the army Medical Department upon her return to England.[7] Underhill reminds us that the two women who have left the deepest mark on the military history of France and England —Joan of Arc and Florence Nightingale— both acted under mystical compulsion.[8]

Surrender. In this fourth phase of spiritual development, also called the "Dark Night of the Soul" or the "Great Desolation," the mystic further dissociates himself or herself from all thoughts of personal happiness and moves to a deeper level in service to God. All great mystics search for the inner significance of every aspect of life. In an hour of such self-examination, Nightingale exclaimed, "I must strive to see only God in my friends, and God in my cats."[9]

Nightingale's "Dark Night of the Soul" began after her 6 years of intense work at Harley Street, in the Crimean War, and on army medical reform. Her chronic ill health combined with stress, overexertion, and the deaths of her soulmates, Sidney Herbert and Arthur Clough, brought her to a low point until she realized that God was taking all human help away from her "in order to compel me to lean on Him alone."[10] During this period, she was often self-critical, impatient, and demanding because she felt that her own death was imminent and she had not a moment to waste.

Union. The fifth phase, Union with the Absolute, is the ultimate goal of the mystic's quest. It is a state of equilibrium characterized by peace, joy, enhanced powers, and intense certitude. An examination of Nightingale's writings in the last decades of her life shows that she manifested the characteristics of the unitive state. She saw "God in all things, and all things in God."[11] No longer pushing herself and others to the limit, she appreciated her blessings — "the longings of my heart accomplished — and now drawn to Thee by difficulties and disappointments. Homeward bound. I have entered in."[12]

Conclusion

Florence Nightingale's life embodied social action and a profound spiritual calling and purpose, which our world sorely needs. Nightingale's life has been analyzed by hundreds of scholars. Why have so many individuals been captivated by her for more than a century and a half? Perhaps we sense in her the wisdom that is demonstrated by the great mystics throughout history. We are drawn to her because we can identify with the problems she faced and the challenges she overcame. We, like her, are involved in our own search for meaning and purpose. By her shining example, she invites us to explore our own spiritual development.

The Case for Brucellosis

Florence Nightingale paid a heavy personal price for her achievements in nursing and public health: She fought a decades-long struggle with a debilitating disease contracted during the Crimean War. This illness, which first struck her on May 12, 1855, was known at the time as Crimean fever. Nightingale's symptoms included fever, extreme fatigue, delirium, and inability to eat or walk. Crimean fever was one of six recognized fevers (including typhoid and typhus) that killed soldiers on both sides far more efficiently than bullets and shells. Although Nightingale recovered from the initial episode in 2 weeks, she had to be hospitalized a few months later for severe sciatica. For the rest of her stay in Turkey, she experienced dysentery, earaches, laryngitis, and insomnia.

Upon her return to England, Nightingale had several severe attacks of symptoms, which included palpitations, dyspnea, syncope, weakness, and indigestion. After a second severe fever episode in September 1857, she officially declared herself an "invalid" to lessen the demands on her time and physical strength. For the next three decades, she would be forced at various times to take to her bed for long periods and to isolate herself from coworkers and visitors in order to complete her heavy workload. Because she felt her death was imminent, especially between 1857 and 1861, she was often impatient and demanding with her family and fellow reformers. In December 1887, she had another severe episode of joint pain. In the late 1880s, Nightingale's symptoms gradually subsided,

Over the years, some of Nightingale's critics have viewed her invalidism as merely another unfortunate aspect of her strong-willed personality, characterizing her as "neurotic" or a "recluse." Others have attributed her chronic illness to such causes as neurasthenia,[1] stress-induced anxiety neurosis,[2,3] malingering,[4] chronic lead poisoning,[5] chronic fatigue immune deficiency syndrome,[6] systemic lupus erythematosus,[7] stress and job burnout,[8] and posttraumatic stress disorder.[9]

In 1995, D.A.B. Young, a former scientist at the Wellcome Foundation in London, proposed that Nightingale's Crimean fever was actually Mediterranean fever, otherwise known as Malta fever; this disease is included under the generic name brucellosis.[10]

Early studies of Crimean fever

During the Crimean War, the British army encountered six recognized forms of fever: typhoid fever, typhus, remittent fever, intermittent fever, simple continued fever, and relapsing fever. The commonest and most fatal was typhoid, followed by typhus. Army doctors on the scene were able to differentially diagnose typhoid and typhus, and they distinguished these from remittent fever, which became known as Crimean fever.

The characteristic features of remittent fever were nervous irritability, fever, delirium, and prolonged gastric irritation. The disease had two distinct phases from which its name is derived: two periods of exacerbation (morning and evening) followed by complete remission in 24 hours.[11] Relapse was very common; the resulting chronic, debilitating condition followed an extremely protracted and irregular course that required months of convalescence.

In his 1863 report on Malta fever in the army, J.A. Marston added more details to previous reports of remittent fever, describing its greater prevalence during the spring with tachycardia, depression, and restlessness.[12] Most patients developed some form of neuralgia or rheumatism, and an apparent recovery was typically followed by a sudden excruciating attack of sciatica, just as Nightingale experienced. In 1887, David Bruce, a surgeon in the Army Medical Service, along with his wife, Mary, identified the causative agent of Crimean fever as the bacterium *Brucella melitensis*, which had been isolated from the spleens of several British army personnel who died of Malta fever.[13] The first monograph on Malta fever was written in 1897 by M.L. Hughes, a British officer who worked with Bruce. Hughes emphasized the symptoms of anemia, breathlessness, debility, cachexia (general physical wasting and malnutrition), and aging that followed the initial illness. He found the incubation period of Malta fever to be between 10 days and one month.[14]

In 1905, T. Zammit identified goats as the reservoir for *Brucella melitensis*.[15] With this discovery, goat's milk and all milk products were prohibited in all British government facilities, thus dramatically reducing the incidence of Malta fever among army troops compared with the civilian population. In 1906, B. Bang established that a related organism, *B. abortus,* was the causal agent of abortion fever in cattle in Denmark.[16]

Brucellosis did not receive full recognition as a human disease until 1918, when Alice Evans, a distinguished bacteriologist, established the close association between the causal agents of Malta fever in humans and abortion fever in cattle.[17] Evans became infected while working with cultures of *B. melitensis* and suffered for nearly 6 years with a diagnosis of neurasthenia before the organism was cultured from her blood. She suffered from recurrent chronic brucellosis for the next 17 years.[18]

What we know about brucellosis

Brucellosis is an acute febrile illness transmitted to humans from animals by consumption of contaminated unpasteurized milk and milk products or undercooked meat and by direct contact with infected animals or their secretions and excretions. It's most common among farmers, stock handlers, butchers, and veterinarians.

The disease is caused by gram-negative, nonmotile, coccobacilli of the genus *Brucella.* The four species pathogenic for humans are *B. melitensis* from goats, *B. abortus* from cows, *B. suis* in pigs, and *B. canis* in dogs.[19] *B. melitensis* and *B. suis* are the most virulent forms for humans.[20] Once the pathogens enter the bloodstream, they localize in the lymph nodes, spleen, liver, and bone marrow. The kidneys and central and peripheral nervous systems may also be involved.

Clinical features

Brucellosis is a systemic infection that can involve all major organs and tissues. Symptoms generally occur within 2 to 3 weeks of inoculation.[21] Osteoarticular manifestations, which include arthralgias, arthritis, spondylitis, osteomyelitis, tenosynovitis, bursitis, and sacroilitis, occur in up to 85% of patients.[22] These symptoms are more common in patients infected with *B. melitensis.* Bone and joint involvement is the most common complication of brucellosis, occurring in 40% of cases.

A majority of patients with brucellosis, regardless of the infection route, experience intestinal complaints, such as appetite loss, weight loss, nausea, vomiting, and abdominal discomfort. Mental fatigue and depression are also common complaints; however, central nervous system involvement occurs in less than 2% of patients.[23]

Clinical course and classification

The clinical course of the disease varies, depending on the causative species. *B. melitensis* is usually the most virulent and invasive.[24] The resulting illness may be followed weeks, months, or even years later by serious complications.[25] Brucellosis can be classified according to its clinical presentation as acute, relapsing, or chronic. *Chronic brucellosis,* referring to illness lasting more than a year, can take two forms: specific and nonspecific.[26] The specific form has long been recognized; the nonspecific form is more controversial and sometimes disputed because it has no distinctive symptoms and can be complicated by neurosis.

In the *specific* form, the patient manifests distinct signs and symptoms that can be attributed to the late effects of brucellosis. Nervous and skeletal system symptoms are the most significant, particularly in *B. melitensis.* Symptoms of neurobrucellosis include myelitis, neuralgia, radiculitis, sciatica, and vasomotor disturbances. Autonomic and central nervous system symptoms are probably the most significant features of the disease. Bone and joint involvement includes arthralgia (most frequently of the large joints of hip, knee, and sacroiliac); spondylitis often results in permanent disability, usually involving lumbar vertebrae and leading to radiculoneuritis and severe paraparesis.

In the *nonspecific* form, symptoms aren't as distinct, making differential diagnosis extremely difficult. General complaints include anorexia, nausea at sight of food, indigestion, anemia, insomnia, nervousness, depression, palpitations, syncope, dyspnea, weakness, nervous tremors, headaches, and flushing. Severe depression and nervousness (gross tremors of hands and fingers, irritability, emotional instability) aren't distinctive symptoms, although they are related to neurobrucellosis. When the disease is active for a long period of time and in people with neurotic tendencies, brucellosis may have serious personality repercussions.

Nightingale's chronic illness

Nightingale's letters and private notes from 1855 to the late 1880s (integrated within Parts 2 to 5 of this biography) clearly document that she suffered a variety of significant symptoms that are consistent with the specific form of chronic brucellosis discussed above. Her severe spinal pain, today called spondylitis, is a complication of chronic brucellosis that is said to be one of the most painful maladies that can affect humans.[27] At other times, her nonspecific symptoms were probably due to bacteremic episodes that presented much like her initial feverish episode.[28]

Because the incubation period of Crimean fever is 2 to 3 weeks, Nightingale appears to have been infected in the Scutari area in April 1855. The most likely source of infection was contaminated food, such as meat or raw milk, cheese, or butter. She and others had reported a high incidence of Crimean fever and contaminated food during April and May.

Conclusion

Although it's obviously impossible to make a specific diagnosis in retrospect with absolute certainty, Florence Nightingale's debilitating, chronic symptoms over a 32-year period are certainly compatible with a diagnosis of chronic brucellosis.

If Nightingale were alive today, she almost certainly would have received a proper diagnosis. Because she became ill in an area where brucellosis was endemic, she would have been tested for this pathogen. Her initial febrile episode would have been treated with antibiotics, and her chronic, severe pain and disability would have been managed more successfully. We must consider clearly and carefully the evidence of chronic brucellosis as the cause of Nightingale's debilitating, chronic illness and not be misled by the various interpretations of her invalidism and work style that have surfaced from time to time.

Nightingale's Personality Type

A retrospective analysis of Florence Nightingale's personality type using the Myers-Briggs Type Indicator® (MBTI®) instrument sheds new light on some areas of her life that have been misinterpreted or misunderstood: her spiritual development and social action as a practicing mystic, her responses to the challenges of chronic illness, and her strategies for achieving success against great odds. In a 6-year study of hundreds of Nightingale's letters, reports, and other writings, the author used the MBTI psychometric test to determine that Nightingale had an INTJ (Introverted, Intuition, Thinking, Judging) personality type.

The MBTI instrument, based on Carl Jung's descriptions of personality types, is a widely used personality assessment tool for nonpsychiatric populations. It was developed in 1942 by Isabel Briggs Myers and her mother, Katharine Cook Briggs, and was refined by Myers over the next four decades.

Jung suggested that human behavior is powerfully shaped by three sets of preferences humans have: for orienting themselves in the world (*extravert or introvert*), for collecting information (*sensing or intuition*), and for making decisions (*thinking or feeling*).[1] Myers and Briggs added a fourth category — the manner in which people prefer to live their lives (*judging or perceiving*).[2]

Myers's contribution was in developing a questionnaire that identifies a person's attitudes, feelings, perceptions, and behaviors — thereby revealing his preference, and strength of preference, in each of the four sets of opposites. These sets of opposites interact to produce a matrix of 16 personality types, as described in the MBTI. The pairs of opposites are summarized as follows:

• *Extraversion or Introversion (EI).* The EI scale indicates whether a person derives his energy from the outer or inner world. People who focus on the outer world of people, activities, or things are extraverts (E). Those who prefer to focus on their inner world of ideas, emotions, or impressions are introverts (I).

• *Sensing or Intuition (SN).* The SN scale indicates how a person acquires information. People who use their five senses to gather information about objects, events, and facts of daily life are sensing (S). Those who focus internally on meanings, possibilities, and patterns and relationships among things — who have a "sixth sense" or just "get it" — are intuitive (N).

• *Thinking or Feeling (TF).* The TF scale shows how a person makes decisions. People who make decisions in an objective and impersonal way, based on logical analysis, are thinking (T) types. Those who make decisions using a process of personal valuing — considering the emotions of themselves and others — are feeling (F) types.

• *Judging or Perceiving (JP).* The JP scale describes the manner in which people live their lives. People who prefer to have their daily lives planned, organized, and settled have a judging (J) attitude. Those who value a spontaneous and flexible lifestyle and who like to keep their options open have a perceiving (P) attitude.

The existence of these pairs of opposites was nothing new, as Jung himself pointed out. However, Jung's insight was that an initial choice between the basic opposite pairs determines the line of development for how a person gathers information and makes decisions. This insight has profound consequences in the field of personality, for it makes possible a coherent explanation for a variety of simple human differences, complexities of personality, and widely different satisfactions and motivations. The concept of personality type also sheds light on the things that people value most, on their personal communication and work styles, and on their behavior patterns.[3]

What the analysis shows

Based on what we know about Nightingale from her thousands of letters (14,000 in two major collections), notes, and published works, it appears evident that her dominant preferences were Introversion, Intuition, Thinking, and Judging — the INTJ personality type. The INTJ type is described as original, visionary, private, independent, logical, critical, theoretical, systems-minded, firm, and demanding[4] — all qualities that epitomize Nightingale from her earliest days to the end of her life. Furthermore, her personal history indicates that she had a strong preference for each choice — which helps us understand her qualities of determination, perseverance, and single-mindedness.

Introversion. As an introverted, practicing mystic, Nightingale found her inner spiritual life far more compelling than trivial external events. She continually rejected the external demands of family, friends, and other acquaintances in favor of following her inward path. Much has been made of the solitary manner in which she chose to live as an invalid. Limiting visitors and setting appointments was a strategy to manage her pain and preserve her compromised physical stamina.[5] She chose to meet with others only when necessary as the best way for her to maximize her talents, satisfy the needs of her introversion, and at the same time most efficiently achieve the group's objectives.

Intuition. Nightingale's greatest gifts came from her intuition — her flashes of inspiration, her insight into the relationships of ideas and their meanings, her ability to envision things that others couldn't see, and her realization that she could accomplish more by working behind the scenes. Her intuitive, administrative, organizational, and systems genius allowed her to form models in her mind; all she needed was an opportunity for action to create new realities. Because she was by nature an initiator and promoter of ideas, her complete confidence in the validity of her intuition rendered her impervious to the influence of outside judgment.

Thinking. Nightingale had strong conceptual and organizational skills, dating back to childhood. She was tough-minded and task-oriented; in her drive to accomplish her goals, she often appeared unfeeling, extremely critical of others, and unconcerned with the effect of her actions and criticisms on others. This perception of her as an abrasive and unfeeling person has led to much criticism over the years. Nightingale is an excellent example of how the thinking type of personality, sensitive to injustice and inefficiency, can use logic and analysis to achieve goals and unfairly get a reputation for being heartless.

Judging. A judging person prefers having a system, a routine, a plan of action in work and daily life; does things in a decisive, settled, and orderly way; and seeks closure on one thing before beginning another. Throughout her life, Nightingale was an inveterate note-taker, planner, and organizer, working tirelessly and methodically to accomplish her tasks. She was a master of what today is called time management.

Conclusion

Florence Nightingale was the epitome of the INTJ personality type — visionary, independent, individualistic, and single-minded. For Nightingale, as for most INTJs, the world was a place to create things; abstract models were as real and objective to her as oak trees and mountains are to others.

INTJs are the most intellectual of all personality types and can see farther into the unknown, as it were, than most people. In contemporary MBTI samples, many INTJs are research scientists and design engineers.[6] Nightingale's great accomplishments in the fields of nursing, sanitation, and statistics reflect the strong conceptual and design skills — supported by exhaustive and accurate research — she brought to all her endeavors.

It's easy to imagine Nightingale, had she been born 150 years later, as a great feminist and scholar, author, policy maker, or leader. Instead, as a woman born at the beginning of the Victorian era, she worked alone in her bedroom for decades. Her unrelenting efforts helped achieve groundbreaking improvements in health, sanitation, nursing, and many other aspects of society — initially for the British soldier but, in the end, for all of England and India and, indeed, all of humankind. She was a modern mystic in an extraverted world of business and politics, and her introversion was her cloister.

Written Works

Below is a chronological list of Florence Nightingale's most significant written works, spanning nearly 50 years.

1850s

The Institution of Kaiserswerth on the Rhine, for the Practical Training of Deconesses, under the Direction of the Rev. Pastor Fliedner, Embracing the Support and Care of a Hospital, Infant and Industrial Schools, and a Female Penitentiary. London: Printed by the inmates of the London Ragged Colonial Training School, Westminster, 1851. Published anonymously.

Letters from Egypt (1849 and 1850). London: A. and G.A. Spottiswoode,1854.

Report upon the State of the Hospitals of the British Army in the Crimea and Scutari, 1855, Nightingale's evidence at pp. 330-331, 342-343.

Statements Exhibiting the Voluntary Contributions Received by Miss Nightingale for the Use of the British War Hospitals in the East, with the Mode of their Distribution, in 1854, 1855, 1856. London: Harrison, 1857.

Notes on Matters Affecting the Health, Efficiency, and Hospital Administration of the British Army Founded Chiefly on the Experience of the Late War. Presented by Request to the Secretary of State for War. London: Harrison & Sons, 1858.

Mortality of the British Army, at Home and Abroad, and During the Russian War, as Compared with the Mortality of the Civil Population in England. Illustrated by Tables and Diagrams. (Reprinted from the *Report of the Royal Commission Appointed to Enquire into the Regulations Affecting the Sanitary State of the Army.*) London: Harrison & Sons, 1858.

A Contribution to the Sanitary History of the British Army during the Late War with Russia. Illustrated with Tables and Diagrams. London: Harrison & Sons, 1859.

Notes on Hospitals: Being Two Papers Read before the National Association for the Promotion of Social Science, at Liverpool, in October 1858. With Evidence given to the Royal Commissioners on the State of the Army in 1857. London: John W. Parker & Son, 1859.

1860s

Notes on Nursing: What it is and what it is not. London: Harrison & Sons, 1860.

Notes on Nursing: What it is and what it is not. London: Harrison & Sons, Revised edition late 1860.

"Hospital Statistics" and "Proposal for a Uniform Plan of Hospital Statistics." Proceedings of the International Statistical Congress, Fourth Session, 1860, pp. 65-71.

Suggestions for Thought to the Searchers after Truth among the Artizans of England. London: Eyre & Spottiswoode, 3 vols, 1860.

Notes on Nursing for the Labouring Classes. London: Harrison & Sons, 1861 (Reprinted in 1865, 1868, 1876, 1883, 1885, 1888, 1890, 1894, 1898).

Report of the Royal Commission on the Sanitary State of the Army in India, 1863. 2 vols. Nightingale's contributions in vol. I, pp. 347-70, illustrations; pp. 371-462.

Observations on the Evidence Contained in the Stational Reports Submitted to the Royal Commission on the Sanitary State of the Army in India. London: Edward Stanford, 1863. (Reprint of above.)

"Proposal for Improved Statistics of Surgical Operations." Paper presented at the International Statistical Congress, Berlin, December 1863.

Note on the Supposed Protection Afforded against Venereal Disease by Recognizing Prostitution and Putting it under Police Regulation, 1863.

Notes on Hospitals. (3ed.) London: Longmans, 1863.

Suggestions in Regard to Sanitary Works Required for Improving Indian Stations, Prepared by the Barrack and Hospital Improvement Commission, 1864.

Remarks by the Barrack and Hospital Improvement Commission on a Report by Dr. Leith on the General Sanitary Conditions of the Bombay Army. Parliamentary Paper, No. 329, 1865.

Memorandum on Measures Adopted for Sanitary Improvements in India up to the End of 1867; Together with Abstracts of the Sanitary Reports Hitherto Forwarded from Bengal, Madras, and Bombay. Printed by the order of the Secretary of State for India in Council, 1868.

"A Note on Pauperism," *Fraser's Magazine,* March 1869, pp. 281-290.

1870s

Report on Measures adopted for Sanitary Improvements in India from June 1869 to June 1870; together with Abstracts. London, 1870.

Introductory Notes on Lying-in Institutions. Together with a Proposal for Organising an Institution for Training Midwives and Midwifery Nurses. London: Longmans, Green & Co., 1871.

"Address from Miss Nightingale to the Probationer Nurses in the "Nightingale Fund" School at St. Thomas's Hospital, 1872, 1873, 1874, 1875, 1876, 1878, 1879, 1881, 1883, 1884, 1886, 1888, 1897, 1900.

"A 'Note' of Interrogation," *Fraser's Magazine,* May 1873, pp, 567-577,

"A 'Sub-Note of Interrogation.' What Will our Religion Be in 1999?" *Fraser's Magazine,* July 1873, pp. 25-36.

"The People of India," *Nineteenth Century,* August 1878, pp. 193-221.

"A Missionary Health Officer in India," *Good Words,* July, August, September 1879, pp. 492-496, 565-571, 635-640.

1880s

"The Dumb Shall Speak, and the Deaf Shall Hear; or, the Ryot, the Zemindar, and the Government," paper read at a meeting of the East India Association. Printed in its Journal, July 1883, pp. 163-211.

"Our Indian Stewardship," *Nineteenth Century,* August 1883, pp. 329-338.

1890s

"Sick-Nursing and Health-Nursing," in *Woman's Mission: a Series of Congress Papers on the Philanthropic Work of Women by Eminent Writers.* Arranged and edited by the Baroness Burdett-Coutts. London: Sampson Low, Marston & Co., 1893.

"Training of Nurses," in *A Dictionary of Medicine, Including General Pathology, General Therapeutics, Hygiene, and the Diseases of Women and Children,* R. Quain, ed. London: Longmans, Green & Co., 1894, p. 237-244.

"Village Sanitation in India," paper read at 8th International Congress of Hygiene and Demography at Budapest. London: 20 August 1894.

Chapter Notes & References

Key to abbreviations

BL Add. MSS = British Library Additional Manuscripts (London)

f = folio

LDFNM = Florence Nightingale Museum (London)

LMA = London Metropolitan Archives (formerly Greater London Record Office [GLRO])

Wellcome MSS = Wellcome Institute Library Manuscripts (London)

Chapter 1

1. A. Sticker, *Florence Nightingale: Curriculum Vitae* (Düsseldorf, Germany: Diakoniewert, 1965), pp. 3-4.

2. E. Haldane, *Mrs. Gaskell and Her Friends* (Freeport, N.Y.: Books for Libraries Press, 1970), p. 102.

3. Equivalents supplied by Federal Reserve Bank, Dallas. Available online at: http://web.calstatela.edu/faculty/btm/lor/globalfd.htm. Accessed January 1999.

4. Florence Nightingale to Mrs. Nightingale, [No date], Wellcome MSS 8993:f31.

5. E.T. Cook, *The Life of Florence Nightingale* (London: Macmillan Publishing Co., 1913), vol. I, p. 9.

6. I.B. O'Malley, *Florence Nightingale, 1820-1856: A Study of Her Life Down to the End of the Crimean War* (London: Thornton Butterworth, 1931), p. 17.

7. Ibid., p. 19.

8. Florence Nightingale to Grandmother Shore, 30 March 1828, Wellcome MSS 8991:f6.

9. Florence Nightingale to Mrs. Nightingale, 1 April 1828, Wellcome MSS 8991:f7.

10. Florence Nightingale to Mr. and Mrs. Nightingale, after 19 February 1829, Wellcome MSS 8991:f25.

11. O'Malley, *Florence Nightingale, 1820-1856*, p. 22.

12. Ibid.

13. Florence Nightingale to Parthe Nightingale, 4 April 1828, Wellcome MSS 8991:f8.

14. Cook, *The Life of Florence Nightingale*, vol. I, p. 14.

15. O'Malley, *Florence Nightingale, 1820-1856*, p. 32.

16. Florence Nightingale to Miss Brydges, June 1829, Wellcome MSS 8991:f30.

17. Haldane, *Mrs. Gaskell and Her Friends*, p. 90.

18. O'Malley, *Florence Nightingale, 1820-1856*, p. 24.

19. Florence Nightingale to Mrs. Nightingale or governess, January 1830, Wellcome MSS 8991:f42.

20. Florence Nightingale to Parthe with a note to Mrs. Nightingale, 24 February 1830, Wellcome MSS 8991:f44.

21. Florence Nightingale to Mr. and Mrs. Nightingale and Parthe, 18 February 1830, Wellcome MSS 8991:f43.

22. Florence Nightingale to Mrs. Nightingale with a note to Parthe, 28 March 1830, Wellcome MSS 8991:f52.

23. Florence Nightingale to Mrs. Nightingale, 12 July 1830, Wellcome MSS 8991:f55.

24. Ibid.

25. Ibid.

26. Cook, *The Life of Florence Nightingale*, vol. I, p. 11.

27. O'Malley, *Florence Nightingale, 1820-1856*, p. 35.

28. Ibid.

29. Ibid., p. 34.

30. Sticker, *Curriculum Vitae*, p. 3.

31. Haldane, *Mrs. Gaskell and Her Friends*, p. 91.

32. C. Woodham-Smith, *Florence Nightingale* (New York: McGraw Hill, 1951), p. 11.

33. David Chapman, Head Master, Embley Park School, Romsey, Hampshire, letter to author, September 1998.

34. J.R. Martin, *Reclaiming a Conversation: The Ideal of the Educated Woman* (New Haven: Yale University Press, 1985), p. 28, cited in V.E. Slater, "The Educational and Philosophical Influences on Florence Nightingale, An Enlightened Conductor," *Nursing History Review* 2:140, 1994.

35. B. Jowett, *The Dialogues of Plato*, 3rd ed. (Oxford: Oxford University Press, 1892), vol. III, p. 227.

36. Dugald Stewart, *Elements of the Philosophy of the Human Mind* (Boston: James Monroe and Company, 1842), pp. 20-26, cited in V. E. Slater, "The Educational and Philosophical Influences on Florence Nightingale, An Enlightened Conductor," *Nursing History Review* 2:141-42, 1994.

37. *Dictionary of National Biography* (London: Oxford University Press, 1917), vol. II, p. 270.

38. R. Altick, *Victorian People and Ideas* (New York: W.W. Norton & Co., Inc., 1973), pp. 118-119.

39. J. Moore, *A Zeal for Responsibility: The Struggle for Professional Nursing in Victorian England, 1868-1883* (Athens, Ga.: University of Georgia Press, 1988), p. xii.

40. Cook, *The Life of Florence Nightingale*, vol. I, p. 12.

41. A. Briggs, *A Social History of England* (New York: Viking Press, 1984), p. 154.

42. Altick, *Victorian People and Ideas*, p. 31.

43. O. Chadwick, *The Victorian Church* (New York: Oxford University Press, 1966), p. 3.

44. Ibid., pp. 80-81.

45. Ibid., p. 5.

46. E. Halévy, *A History of the English People in the Nineteenth Century* (London: Ernest Benn Limited, Bouvie House, 1922), pp. 163-164.

47. *Dictionary of National Biography*, vol. XVIII, p. 557.

48. G. Trevelyan, *British History in the Nineteenth Century* (New York: Longmans, Green & Co., 1928), p. 63.

49. Florence Nightingale, Address to the Probationer Nurses in the "Nightingale Fund" School at St. Thomas's Hospital, 26 May 1875, p. 4, LDFNM:0727.

50. Trevelyan, *British History*, p. 51.

51. J. Pollock, *William Wilberforce: A Man Who Changed his Times* (Burke, Va.: The Trinity Forum, 1996), p. 14.

52. *Dictionary of National Biography*, vol. XVIII, p. 559.

53. Florence Nightingale to Mrs. Nightingale, 19 May 1832, Wellcome MSS 8991:f64.

54. J. Simon, *English Sanitary Institutions* (London: Cassell and Company, 1890), p. 172.

55. Chadwick, *The Victorian Church*, p. 36.

56. A.J. Youngson, *The Scientific Revolution in Victorian Medicine* (New York: Holmes & Meier, 1979), pp. 21-22.

57. Ibid., pp. 22-23.

58. Simon, *English Sanitary Institutions*, p. 170.

59. Ibid., p. 175.

60. Youngson, *The Scientific Revolution*, p. 76.

61. F.F. Cartwright, *Disease and History* (New York: Barnes and Noble, 1972), p. 159.

62. E.W. Gilbert, "Pioneer Maps of Health and Disease in England," *Geographical Journal* 124(1958):173.

63. Ibid., p. 175.

64. Simon, *English Sanitary Institutions*, p. 167.

65. Haldane, *Mrs. Gaskell and Her Friends*, p. 99.

66. Sticker, *Curriculum Vitae*, p. 7.

67. R. Strachey, *The Cause: A Short History of the Women's Movement in Great Britain* (Port Washington, N.Y.: Kennikat, 1969), p. 13.

68. Florence Nightingale to Mrs. Nightingale, [No date] 1834, Wellcome MSS 8991:f73.

69. Altick, *Victorian People and Ideas*, p. 25.

70. Equivalents supplied by Federal Reserve Bank, Dallas. Available online at: http://web.calstatela.edu/faculty/btm/lor/globalfd.htm. Accessed January 1999.

71. Florence Nightingale to Parthe Nightingale, 12 January 1837, Wellcome MSS 8991:f80.

72. Ibid., f81.

73. Ibid., f80.

74. Florence Nightingale to Marianne Nicholson and Parthe, 12 February 1837, Wellcome MSS 8991:f86.

75. Cook, *The Life of Florence Nightingale*, vol. I, p. 15.

Chapter 2

1. Florence Nightingale to Aunt Hannah Nicholson, 24 September 1846, BL Add. MSS 45794:ff39-40.

2. E. Underhill, *Mysticism: A Study in the Nature and Development of Man's Spiritual Consciousness* (1911; New York: E.P. Dutton, 1961), p. 198.

3. Cook, *The Life of Florence Nightingale*, vol. I, p. 15.

4. Strachey, *The Cause*, p. 18.

5. W. Churchill, *A History of the English-Speaking Peoples* (New York: Dodd, Mead. & Company, 1958), vol. 4, p. 55.

6. Ibid.

7. O'Malley, *Florence Nightingale, 1820-1856*, p. 48.

8. Ibid., p. 50.

9. Ibid.

10. Haldane, *Mrs. Gaskell and Her Friends*, p. 99.

11. F.B. Artz, *Reaction and Revolution: 1814-1832* (New York: Harper & Row, 1934), p. 145.

12. Florence Nightingale to Grandmother Shore, 15 May 1838, Wellcome MSS 8991:f99.

13. Ibid.

14. Ibid.

15. Florence Nightingale to Grandmother Shore, 6 October 1838, Wellcome MSS 8991:f97.

16. Youngson, *The Scientific Revolution*, p. 10.

17. Cook, *The Life of Florence Nightingale*, vol. I, p. 17.

18. Florence Nightingale to Grandmother Shore, 6 October 1838, Wellcome MSS 8991:f97.

19. Cook, *The Life of Florence Nightingale*, vol. I, pp. 20-21.

20. Ibid., p. 22.

21. Florence Nightingale to Grandmother Shore, 10 May 1839, Wellcome MSS 8991:f102.

22. Florence Nightingale to the Nightingales, Spring 1840, Wellcome MSS 8992:f10.

23. Woodham-Smith, *Florence Nightingale*, p. 27.

24. Florence Nightingale to the Nightingales, Spring 1840, Wellcome MSS 8992:f10.

25. L.M. Osen, *Women in Mathematics* (Boston: Colonial Press, 1974), p. 100.

26. Ibid., p. 104.

27. Florence Nightingale, Address to the Nurses and Probationers Trained Under the "Nightingale Fund," June 1897, p. 15, LDFNM:0277.

28. Florence Nightingale to Mrs. Nightingale, [No date], Wellcome MSS 8992:f35.

29. O'Malley, *Florence Nightingale, 1820-1856*, pp. 84-85.

30. Ibid., p. 87.

31. M.D. Calabria and J.A. Macrae, *Suggestions for Thought by Florence Nightingale: Selections and Commentaries* (Philadelphia: University of Pennsylvania Press, 1994), pp. xxiv-xxv.

32. Woodham-Smith, *Florence Nightingale*, p. 30.

33. Florence Nightingale to Mrs. Nightingale, 15 May 1843, Wellcome MSS 8992:ff37-38.

34. Cook, *The Life of Florence Nightingale*, vol. I, p. 46.

35. Florence Nightingale to Aunt Hannah Nicholson, 10 July 1844, BL Add. MSS 45794:ff6-8.

36. J.W. Howe, *Reminiscences 1818-1899* (Boston: Houghton Mifflin, 1899), p. 108.

37. O'Malley, *Florence Nightingale, 1820-1856*, p. 93.

38. Ibid.

39. M.P. Donahue, *Nursing: The Finest Art* (St. Louis: Mosby–Year Book, Inc., 1985), p. 213.

40. O'Malley, *Florence Nightingale, 1820-1856*, p. 109-110.

41. Ibid., pp. 60, 63.

42. Ibid., pp.44-45.

43. Florence Nightingale to Aunt Hannah Nicholson, 24 September 1846, BL Add. MSS 45794:f38.

44. Cook, *The Life of Florence Nightingale*, vol. I, p. 64.

45. Ibid., p. 101.

46. Ibid., pp. 66-67.

47. Florence Nightingale to Aunt Hannah Nicholson, October 1847, BL Add. MSS 45794:ff64-66.

48. O'Malley, *Florence Nightingale, 1820-1856*, p. 132.

49. Ibid., p. 133.

50. Cook, *The Life of Florence Nightingale*, vol. I, pp. 71-72.

51. O'Malley, *Florence Nightingale, 1820-1856*, pp. 144-145.

52. Cook, *The Life of Florence Nightingale*, vol. I, p. 74.

53. Ibid., pp. 82-83.

54. Ibid., pp. 100-101.

Chapter 3

1. Florence Nightingale, private note, May 1850, BL Add. MSS 43402:f38.

2. Florence Nightingale to the Nightingales, 2 November 1849, Wellcome MSS 8993:f26.

3. Florence Nightingale, private notes, 10-21 March 1850, BL. Add. MSS 45846:f21, cited in M.D. Calabria, *Florence Nightingale in Egypt and Greece* (Albany, N.Y.: State University of New York Press, 1997), pp. 45-49.

4. Cook, *The Life of Florence Nightingale*, vol. I, p. 95.

5. A. Sattin, *Florence Nightingale, Letters from Egypt: A Journey on the Nile 1849-1850* (New York: Grove Press, 1987), p. 208.

6. Cook, *The Life of Florence Nightingale*, vol. 1, p. 89.

7. Calabria, *Florence Nightingale in Egypt and Greece*, p. 57.

8. Ibid.

9. Ibid., p. 59.

10. Ibid., p. 60.

11. Ibid., p. 64.

12. Ibid., p. 72.

13. Ibid., p. 81.

14. Sticker, *Curriculum Vitae*, 1851, p. 12.

15. Anonymous, *The Institution of Kaiserwerth on the Rhine for the Practical Training of Deaconesses under the Direction of the Rev. Pastor Fliedner, Embracing the Support and Care of a Hospital, Infant and Industrial Schools, and a Female Penitentiary*, pp. 8-10.

16. Florence Nightingale, private note, 1857, BL Add. MSS 43402:ff178-187.

17. Florence Nightingale, private note, 30 December 1850, BL Add. MSS 43402:f55.

18. Florence Nightingale, private note, 1851, BL Add. MSS 43402:ff79-83.

19. Ibid.

20. Ibid.

21. Ibid.

22. Florence Nightingale, private note, 7 January 1851, BL Add. MSS 43402:f79.

23. E. Blackwell, *Pioneer Work in Opening the Medical Profession to Women* (London: Longmans, Green & Co., 1895; New York: Source Book Press, 1970), p. 73.

24. Ibid., p. 154.

25. Ibid., p. 176

26. Ibid., p. 185.

27. Florence Nightingale, private note, 8 June 1851, BL Add. MSS 43402:f68.

28. Sticker, *Curriculum Vitae*, 1851, pp. 4-7.

29. Florence Nightingale, Kaiserswerth notes, 4-10 August 1851, Wellcome MSS 9025:f77.

30. Ibid., f70.

31. Ibid.

32. Florence Nightingale, private note, 7 December 1851, BL Add. MSS 43402:f66.

33. Florence Nightingale to Mrs. Nightingale, 8 January 1852, Wellcome MSS 8993:f70.

34. Ibid., f71.

35. Florence Nightingale to Mrs. Nightingale, April 1852, Wellcome MSS 8993:f82.

36. W.E. Nightingale to Mrs. Nightingale, 8 January 1852, Wellcome MSS 8993:f71.

37. Chadwick, *The Victorian Church*, p. 325.

38. Calabria and Macrae, *Suggestions for Thought by Florence Nightingale*, p. 64.

39. O'Malley, *Florence Nightingale, 1820-1856*, p. 193.

40. Strachey, *The Cause*, p. 396.

41. Ibid., pp. 407-408.

42. Ibid., pp. 417-418.

43. Underhill, *Mysticism*, pp. 169, 233.

44. Florence Nightingale to Mr. Nightingale, 12 May 1852, cited in M. Vicinus and B. Nergaard, *Ever Yours, Florence Nightingale* (London: Verago Press, 1989) p. 57.

45. Florence Nightingale to the Rev. Henry Manning, [No date] 1852, cited in Vicinus and Nergaard, *Ever Yours*, pp. 60-61.

46. O'Malley, *Florence Nightingale, 1820-1856*, p. 198.

47. Ibid., p. 201.

Chapter 4

1. Florence Nightingale to Lady Charlotte Canning, 29 April 1853, LDFNM:0281.

2. Equivalents supplied by Federal Reserve Bank, Dallas. Available online at: http://web.calstatela.edu/faculty/btm/lor/globalfd.htm. Accessed January 1999.

3. Cook, *The Life of Florence Nightingale*, vol. I, p. 138.

4. Ibid., p. 130.

5. W.F. Neff, *Victorian Working Women* (New York: Columbia University Press, 1929), pp. 11-16.

6. Strachey, *The Cause*, p. 97

7. Florence Nightingale to Lady Charlotte Canning, 29 April 1853, LDFNM:0281.

8. Cook, *The Life of Florence Nightingale*, vol. I, p. 133.

9. Florence Nightingale to Lady Charlotte Canning, 5 June 1853, BL Add. MSS 45796:f39.

10. Cook, *The Life of Florence Nightingale*, vol. I, pp. 134-135.

11. Ibid., pp.138-139.

12. H. Verney, *Florence Nightingale at Harley Street: Her Reports to the Governors of her Nursing Home 1853-1854* (London: J. M. Dent & Sons, 1970), pp. 1-2.

13. Ibid., pp. viii-ix.

14. Florence Nightingale to Lady Charlotte Canning, 13 September 1853, Lord Canning Papers, 177(Z)5, cited in Vicinus and Nergaard, *Ever Yours*, p. 72-73.

15. Ibid., p. 73.

16. Ibid., p. 73.

17. Florence Nightingale to Mrs. Nightingale, 29 October 1854, Wellcome MSS , cited in Vicinus and Nergaard, *Ever Yours*, p. 72.

18. F. Nightingale, "Superintendent's Quarterly Report," 14 November 1853, cited in Verney, *Florence Nightingale at Harley Street*, pp. 1-7.

19. Florence Nightingale to Mr. Nightingale, 3 December 1853, BL Add. MSS 45790:f152.

20. Florence Nightingale to Hannah Nicholson, 11 January 1854, BL Add. MSS 45794:f72.

21. F. Nightingale, "Superintendent's Quarterly Report," 20 February 1854, cited in Verney, *Florence Nightingale at Harley Street*, pp. 11-19.

22. F. Nightingale, "Superintendent's Quarterly Report," 15 May 1854, cited in Verney, *Florence Nightingale at Harley Street*, pp. 21-28.

23. F. Nightingale,. "Superintendent's Quarterly Report," 7 August 1854, cited in Verney, *Florence Nightingale at Harley Street*, pp. 33-36.

24. Cook, *The Life of Florence Nightingale*, vol. I, p. 141.

25. P.B. Hoeber, *Source Book of Medical History* (New York: Harper & Row, 1942), p. 374.

26. Youngson, *The Scientific Revolution*, p. 70.

27. E. Longford, *Queen Victoria: Born to Succeed* (New York: Harper & Row, 1964), p. 234.

28. Haldane, *Mrs. Gaskell and Her Friends*, p. 93.

29. Hoeber, *Source Book of Medical History*, p. 469.

30. Cartwright, *Disease and History*, p. 161.

31. Haldane, *Mrs. Gaskell and Her Friends*, pp. 100-101.

32. Cook, *The Life of Florence Nightingale*, vol. I, p 141.

Chapter 5

1. Sidney Herbert to Florence Nightingale, 15 October 1854, cited in E. T. Cook, *The Life of Florence Nightingale*, vol. I, p. 153.

2. A. Summers, *Angels and Citizens: British Women as Military Nurses 1854-1914* (London: Routledge & Kegan Paul, 1988), p. 30.

3. Florence Nightingale, "Evidence Given to the Royal Commissioners on the State of the Army in 1857," in

Notes on Hospitals (London: John Parker and Son, 1859), p. 39.

4. E. Grey, *The Noise of Drums and Trumpets* (London: Butler & Tanner, 1971), p. 31.

5. *The Times* (London), 12 October 1854, p. 8, col. A.

6. *The Times* (London), 13 October 1854, p. 8, col. A.

7. Florence Nightingale to Elizabeth Herbert, 14 October 1854, BL Add. MSS 43396:f11.

8. M. Nutting and L. Dock, *A History of Nursing* (New York: G. P. Putnam's Sons, 1907), vol. II, pp. 68-69.

9. Third Report from the Select Committee on the Army Before Sebastopol 1855, "Parliamentary Papers, 1854-55," vol. 34, p. 132, cited in S.M. Goldie, *I Have Done My Duty: Florence Nightingale in the Crimean War, 1854-1856* (Manchester, England: Manchester University Press), p. 22.

10. Ibid.

11. Ibid.

12. Sidney Herbert to Florence Nightingale, 25 October 1854, cited in E. T. Cook, *The Life of Florence Nightingale*, vol. I, pp. 151-154.

13. Sr. M.T. Austin Carroll, *Leaves from the Annals of the Sisters of Mercy* (New York: H.J. Hewitt, 1881) vol. II, p. 134, cited in M.A. Bolster, *The Sisters of Mercy in the Crimean War* (Cork, Ireland: Mercier Press, 1964), p. 13.

14. O'Malley, *Florence Nightingale, 1820-1856*, p. 220.

15. Bolster, *The Sisters of Mercy*, p. 21

16. Cook, *The Life of Florence Nightingale*, vol. I, p. 160

17. Ibid, p. 161.

18. Ibid.

19. Ibid.

Chapter 6

1. Florence Nightingale to Caroline Fliedner, December 1854, cited in Sticker, *Curriculum Vitae*, pp. 15-16.

2. Florence Nightingale to the Nightingales, 4 November 1854, Wellcome MSS , cited in Goldie, *I Have Done My Duty*, p. 33.

3. *The Times* (London), October 12, 1854, p. 9.

4. Mrs. Rebecca Lawfield, speech, 5 November 1854, cited in Goldie, *I Have Done My Duty*, p. 36.

5. Florence Nightingale to Dr. William Bowman, 14 November 1855, cited in Goldie, *I Have Done My Duty*, pp. 36-37.

6. Cook, *The Life of Florence Nightingale*, vol. I, p. 221.

7. Ibid., pp. 230-231.

8. Florence Nightingale to the Nightingales, 4 December 1854, Wellcome MSS , cited in Vicinus and Nergaard, *Ever Yours*, p. 92.

9. Florence Nightingale to Sidney Herbert, 25 November 1854, BL. Add. MSS 43393:f13.

10. Cook, *The Life of Florence Nightingale*, vol. I, p. 207.

11. Ibid., p. 215.

12. Ibid.

13. Ibid., p. 216.

14. Bolster, *The Sisters of Mercy*, p. 49.

15. Ibid., p. 64.

16. Ibid.

17. Ibid., p. 52.

18. Cook, *The Life of Florence Nightingale*, vol. I, p. 191.

19. Florence Nightingale to Sidney Herbert, 15 December 1854, BL Add. MSS 43393:f34.

20. Florence Nightingale to Sidney Herbert, 25 December 1854, BL Add. MSS 43393:f45.

21. Bolster, *The Sisters of Mercy*, p. 111.

22. Ibid., p. 112.

23. Ibid., pp. 113-114.

24. "The Bridgeman Diary," p. 18, cited in Bolster, *The Sisters of Mercy*, pp. 115-116.

25. *The Times* (London), 1 February 1855, p. 10, col. B.

26. Florence Nightingale to Sidney Herbert, 28 Janaury 1855, BL Add. MSS 43393:ff126-136.

27. Florence Nightingale to Mrs. Nightingale, 5 February 1855, Wellcome MSS , cited in Goldie, *I Have Done My Duty*, pp. 86-87.

28. W.H. Russell, *The British Expedition to the Crimea* (London: Routledge, 1858), p. 182.

29. Ibid., p. 158.

30. Elizabeth Hoet, *The Crimean War* (East Sussex, England: Wayland, 1974), p. 83.

31. Florence Nightingale to Sidney Herbert, 8 January 1855, BL Add. MSS 43393:f75.

32. Florence Nightingale to Sidney Herbert, 4 January 1855, BL Add. MSS 43393:f60.

33. Florence Nightingale to Sidney Herbert, 18 March 1855, BL Add. MSS 43393:f192.

34. Florence Nightingale to Sidney Herbert, 19 February 1855, BL Add. MSS 43393:f164.

Chapter 7

1. Florence Nightingale to the Nightingales, 5 May 1855, Wellcome MSS , cited in Goldie, *I Have Done My Duty,* p. 126.

2. Lord Stanmore, *Sidney Herbert, Lord Herbert of Lea: A Memoir* (London: John Murray, 1906), vol. I, p. 250.

3. *Memoir of the Right Hon. Sir John McNeill, G.C.B. and of his Second Wife, Elizabeth Wilson* (London: John Murray, 1910), p. 321.

4. G. Battiscombe, *Shaftesbury: The Great Reformer, 1801-1885* (Boston: Houghton Mifflin, 1975), p. 247.

5. Ibid., p. 248.

6. F. Nightingale, "Evidence Given to the Royal Commissioners on the State of the Army in 1857" in *Notes on Hospitals,* pp. 38-39.

7. Cook, *The Life of Florence Nightingale,* vol. I, p. 236.

8. Ibid., p. 239.

9. Ibid., p. 237.

10. Ibid., p. 238.

11. Ibid.

12. Bolster, *The Sisters of Mercy,* pp. 130-131.

13. Ibid., p. 154.

14. Stanmore, *Sidney Herbert,* vol. I, p. 412.

15. Florence Nightingale to the Nightingales, 5 March 1855, Wellcome MSS , cited in Vicinus and Nergaard, *Ever Yours,* pp. 110-111.

16. Florence Nightingale to Parthe, 8 March 1855, Wellcome MSS , cited in Vicinus and Nergaard, *Ever Yours,* p. 112.

17. Cook, *The Life of Florence Nightingale,* vol. I, p. 276.

18. Ibid., p. 257.

19. Goldie, *I Have Done My Duty,* p. 130.

20. Ibid., p. 130-131.

21. Ibid., p. 130.

22. Florence Nightingale to Sidney Herbert, 5 March 1855, BL Add. MSS 43393:f183.

23. A. Soyer, *Soyer's Culinary Campaign (*London: Routledge, 1857), cited in D.A.B. Young, "Florence Nightingale's Fever," *British Medical Journal* 311:1698, 1995.

24. G. Lawson, *Surgeon in the Crimea: The Experiences of George Lawson Recorded in Letters to His Family 1854-1855* (London: Constable, 1968), cited in Young, "Florence Nightingale's Fever," *British Medical Journal* 311:1698, 1995.

25. Florence Nightingale to Parthe, 9 July 1855, cited in Goldie, *I Have Done My Duty,* p. 133.

26. Cook, *The Life of Florence Nightingale,* vol. I, p. 295.

27. Ibid., p. 286.

28. Bolster, *The Sisters of Mercy,* p. 196.

29. D.A.B. Young, "Florence Nightingale's Fever," *British Medical Journal* 311:1698, 1995.

30. O'Malley, *Florence Nightingale, 1820-1856,* pp. 332-333.

31. Minutes of the NFC, LMA/NFC/27/1, 8 November 1855, cited in M. Baly, *Florence Nightingale and the Nursing Legacy* (London: Croom Helm, Ltd., 1986), pp. 8-9.

32. Cook, *The Life of Florence Nightingale,* vol. I, p. 269.

33. Ibid., p. 270.

34. Ibid., p. 269.

35. Florence Nightingale to Fanny Nightingale, 29 November 1855, BL Add. MSS 43402:f156.

36. Yildiz Dagdalen, Mimar Sinan University, Istanbul, Turkey, letter to author, April 1996.

37. Cook, *The Life of Florence Nightingale,* vol. I, p. 274.

Chapter 8

1. Florence Nightingale to Sidney Herbert, 21 February 1856, BL Add. MSS 43393:f224.

2. Bolster, *The Sisters of Mercy,* p. 247.

3. Ibid., p. 249.

4. Florence Nightingale to Sidney Herbert, 6 January 1856, Herbert Papers, Wilton House, cited in Baly, *Florence Nightingale and the Nursing Legacy,* p. 11.

5. Florence Nightingale to Charles Bracebridge, 31 January 1856, BL Add. MSS 43397:f179.

6. Bolster, *The Sisters of Mercy,* p. 236.

7. Equivalents supplied by Federal Reserve Bank, Dallas. Available online at: http://web.calstatela.edu/faculty/btm/lor/globalfd.htm. Accessed January 1999.

8. Florence Nightingale to Reverend Mother Mary Clare Moore, 29 April 1856, Wellcome MSS , cited in Vicinus and Nergaard, *Ever Yours,* p. 156.

9. I. Palmer, *Florence Nightingale and the First Organized Delivery of Nursing Services* (Washington, D.C.: American Association of Colleges of Nursing, 1983), pp. 7-9.

10. Florence Nightingale to Parthenope Nightingale, 22 April 1856, Wellcome MSS , cited in Goldie, *I Have Done My Duty,* p. 261.

11. Florence Nightingale to Reverend Mother Mary Clare Moore, 7 July 1856, BL Add. MSS 45789:f1.

Chapter 9

1. Florence Nightingale, private note, 1857, BL Add. MSS 43402:ff178-187.

2. Cook, *The Life of Florence Nightingale,* vol. I, p. 304.

3. Florence Nightingale, private note, 1856, BL Add. MSS 43402:f166.

4. Parthenope Nightingale to Elizabeth Herbert, 13 August 1856, BL Add. MSS 43396:ff48-49.

5. Parthenope Nightingale to Elizabeth Herbert, August 1856, BL Add. MSS 43396:ff50-52.

6. Florence Nightingale to Mother Mary Clare Moore, January 1857, BL Add. MSS 45789:f7.

7. Goldie, *I Have Done My Duty,* p. 283.

8. Florence Nightingale, *Notes on Hospitals* (London: John Parker and Son, 1859), p. 89, Note F.

9. Cook, *The Life of Florence Nightingale,* vol. I, p. 318.

10. *Memoir of the Right Hon. Sir John McNeill,* p. 396.

11. Florence Nightingale to Sir John McNeill, 1 March 1857, LMA H1/ST/NC3/SU/75.

12. Cook, *The Life of Florence Nightingale,* vol. I, pp. 322-323.

13. Ibid., p. 324.

14. J.M. Eyler, *Victorian Social Medicine: The Ideas and Methods of William Farr* (Baltimore: Johns Hopkins University Press, 1979), p. 103.

15. F.G. Garrison, *History of Medicine,* 4th ed. (Philadelphia: W.B. Saunders Co., 1929), p. 662.

16. Cook, *The Life of Florence Nightingale,* vol. I, p. 328.

17. E. Underhill, *Practical Mysticism,* (New York: E.P. Dutton, 1915), pp. 161-162.

18. Florence Nightingale, private note, 1856, BL Add. MSS 43402:f166.

19. Cook, *The Life of Florence Nightingale,* vol. I, p. 341.

20. Equivalents supplied by Federal Reserve Bank, Dallas. Available online at: http://web.calstatela.edu/faculty/btm/lor/globalfd.htm. Accessed January 1999.

21. Cook, *The Life of Florence Nightingale,* vol. I, pp. 342-343.

22. Ibid., p. 335.

23. Ibid., p. 336.

24. Florence Nightingale to Sir John McNeill, 11 March 1857, LMA H1/ST/NC3/SU/75, cited in Vicinus and Nergaard, *Ever Yours,* p. 174

25. Cook, *The Life of Florence Nightingale,* vol. I, p. 316.

Chapter 10

1. F. Nightingale, "Answers to Written Questions to the Commissioners Appointed to Inquire into the Regulations Affecting the Sanitary Conditions of the Army," *Report of the Royal Commission 1857,* cited in Nightingale, *Notes on Hospitals,* p. 24.

2. Cook, *The Life of Florence Nightingale,* vol. I, p. 357-58.

3. Ibid., p. 312.

4. Ibid., p. 358.

5. Dr. William Farr to Florence Nightingale, 21 May 1857, BL Add. MSS 43398:ff10-12.

6. Dr. William Farr to Florence Nightingale, 11 November 1857, BL Add. MSS 43398:f14.

7. Florence Nightingale to Sidney Herbert, 25 December 1857, BL Add. MSS 43394:ff210-214.

8. Cook, *The Life of Florence Nightingale,* vol. I, pp. 359-360.

9. Woodham-Smith, *Florence Nightingale,* p. 199.

10. Florence Nightingale, private note, 1857, BL Add. MSS 43402:ff178-187.

11. Mai Smith to Mr. and Mrs. W.E. Nightingale, August 1857, Wellcome MSS . 9041:f25.

12. Cook, *The Life of Florence Nightingale,* vol. I., p. 368-369.

13. Ibid., p. 369.

14. Dr. John Sutherland to Florence Nightingale, 7 September 1857, BL Add. MSS 45751:ff42-43.

15. Cook, *The Life of Florence Nightingale,* vol. I, pp. 371-72.

16. During Nightingale's lifetime, some of her critics dismissed her complaints as evidence of neurosis and hypochondria. Today, however, these recurrent episodes of fever and debilitating symptoms are recognized as a classic clinical picture of chronic brucellosis. For more information see "The Case for Brucellosis" in the appendices and the following articles: B.M. Dossey, "Florence Nightingale's Crimean Fever and Chronic Illness," *Journal of Holistic Nursing* 16(2):168-196, 1998; D.A.B. Young, "Florence Nightingale's Fever," *British Medical Journal* 311:1697-1700, 1995; and E.J. Young, "An Overview of Human Brucellosis," *Clinical Infectious Disease* 21:283-290, 1994.

17. Florence Nightingale to Sidney Herbert, 2 November 1857, BL Add. MSS 43394:ff190-94.

18. Cook, *The Life of Florence Nightingale,* vol. I, p. 374.

19. Ibid., pp. 380-381.

20. Ibid., p. 498-99.

21. H. Martineau, *Harriet Martineau's Autobiography* (London: Smith Elder, 1877), vol. II, p. 180.

22. Florence Nightingale to Harriet Martineau, 4 December 1858, BL Add. MSS 45788:ff5-6.

23. Florence Nightingale to Harriet Martineau, 23 January 1859, BL Add. MSS 45788:ff29-31.

24. Florence Nightingale to Harriet Martineau, 16 January 1859, BL Add. MSS 45788:f29.

25. Florence Nightingale to Harriet Martineau, 3 March 1859, BL Add. MSS 45788:f35.

26. Cook, *The Life of Florence Nightingale,* vol. I, p. 387.

27. Ibid., p. 392.

28. Florence Nightingale to Aunt Hannah Nicholson, 24 September 1846, BL Add. MS. 45794:f41.

29. Cook, *The Life of Florence Nightingale,* vol. I, p. 399.

Chapter 11

1. Florence Nightingale to Sir John McNeil, 13 August 1860, LMA HI/ST/NC1/SU132, cited in Baly, *Florence Nightingale and the Nursing Legacy,* p. 23.

2. Florence Nightingale to Sidney Herbert, 24 May 1859, Herbert Papers vol. 1859, Wilton House, cited in Baly, *Florence Nightingale and the Nursing Legacy,* p. 31.

3. Z. Cope, *Florence Nightingale and the Doctors* (Philadelphia: Lippincott Williams & Wilkins, 1958), pp. 108-110.

4. Ibid., p. 111.

5. "First Report of the Nightingale Fund Council," June 1861, LMA HI/ST/NTS/AI/3, cited in Baly, *Florence Nightingale and the Nursing Legacy,* p. 35.

6. Florence Nightingale to Sir John McNeil, December 1859, LMA HI/ST/NC3/SU123, cited in Baly, *Florence Nightingale and the Nursing Legacy,* p. 34.

7. "First Report of the Nightingale Fund Council," June 1861, LMA A/NFC5/1, cited in B. Howlett, *The Origins of the Nightingale School* (London: The Florence Nightingale Museum), p. 6.

8. Baly, *Florence Nightingale the Nursing Legacy,* p. 38.

9. F. Nightingale, "Hospital Statistics" in *Programme of the Fourth Session of the International Statistical Congress* (London:

Eyre and Spottiswoode for HMSO, 1860), p. 66, cited in D.J. Speigelhalter, "Surgical Audit: Statistical Lessons from Nightingale and Codman," paper presented to the Royal Statistical Society Conference, University of Surrey, England, 1996.

10. Florence Nightingale to Dr. William Farr, 21 April 1860, BL Add. MSS 43398:f175.

11. Florence Nightingale to Dr. William Farr, 8 April 1861, BL Add. MSS 43399:ff10-12.

12. Florence Nightingale to Dr. William Farr, 23 February 1874, BL Add. MSS 43400:f276.

13. Florence Nightingale to Hilary Bonham Carter, 17 July 1860, BL Add. MSS 45794:ff159-162.

14. D.J. Boorstin, *The Discoverers* (New York: Random House, 1983), p. 673.

15. Ibid.

16. Florence Nightingale's annotation in Adolphe Quetelet's *Physique Sociale,* p. 62, cited in M. Diamond and M. Stone, "Nightingale on Quetelet II, The Marginalia," J.R. Statistical Society A: 1981, Part 2, 144:181-182.

17. Ibid., p. 177.

18. Ibid., p. 204.

19. Florence Nightingale to Benjamin Jowett, 3 January 1891, BL Add. MSS 45785:f144-145.

20. Florence Nightingale's annotation in Quetelet's *Physique Sociale, cited* in Diamond and Stone, "Nightingale on Quetelet II, The Marginalia," J.R. Statistical Society A: 1981, Part 1, 144:72.

Chapter 12

1. Florence Nightingale to Harriet Martineau, 29 July 1860, BL Add. MSS 45788:ff91-92.

2. J. G. Widerquist, "Sanitary Reform and Nursing: Edwin Chadwick and Florence Nightingale," *Nursing History Review* (5).149-160, 1997.

3. Edwin Chadwick to Florence Nightingale, 6 December 1858, BL Add. MSS 45770:ff89-91.

4. Youngson, *The Scientific Revolution,* p. 166.

5. Ibid., p. 186.

6. Nightingale, *Notes on Hospitals,* p. 23.

7. Ibid., p. 100.

8. R. Morris, *Cholera, 1832: The Social Response to an Epidemic* (New York: Holmes & Meier, 1976), p. 176.

9. Ibid.

10. Youngson, *The Scientific Revolution,* p. 137.

11. Nightingale, *Notes on Hospitals,* pp. 6-7.

12. Cook, *The Life of Florence Nightingale,* vol. I, p. 417.

13. Nightingale, *Notes on Hospitals,* Preface.

14. Ibid., p. 159.

15. Ibid., p. 2.

16. Ibid., p. 171.

17. Dr. John Sutherland to Florence Nightingale, 12 February 1859, BL Add MSS 45751:ff125-126.

18. F. Nightingale, *Notes on Nursing,* p. 1.

19. Cook, *The Life of Florence Nightingale,* vol. I, p. 448.

20. Maria Weston Chapman to Harriet Martineau, March 1860, BL Add. MSS 45788:f69.

21. Harriet Martineau to Florence Nightingale, 11 June 1860, BL Add. MSS 45788:ff73-75.

22. Edwin Chadwick to Florence Nightingale, 23 August 1861, BL Add. MSS 45770:f245.

23. Harriet Martineau, review of *Notes on Nursing, Quarterly Review* 107:393, 19 June 1860, BL Add. MSS 45788:f79.

24. Arthur Hugh Clough, *The Poetical Works of Arthur Hugh Clough* (New York: Thomas Y. Crowell, 1897), pp. vii-x.

25. Calabria and Macrae, *Suggestions for Thought by Florence Nightingale,* p. xxxi.

26. *Plutarch's Lives.* Dryden Edition, Introduction by A.H. Clough (London: J.M. Dent and Sons, 1910), pp. vii-xxvii.

27. "Florence Nightingale as a Leader in the Religious and Civic Thought of Her Time," *Hospitals,* 1836, p. 78.

28. Ibid., p. 79.

29. Benjamin Jowett to Florence Nightingale, 17 November 1861, cited in V. Quinn and J. Prest, *Dear Miss Nightingale: A Selection of Benjamin Jowett's Letters to Florence Night-*

ingale (1860-1893) (Oxford: Clarendon Press, 1987), p. 13.

30. Ibid., p. 14.

31. Sir John McNeill to Florence Nightingale, BL Add. MSS 45768:f120.

32. In 1845, Henry Bence Jones discovered a special protein in the urine of patients with myelopathic albumosuria or proteinuria; he is memorialized in the urine test called the Bence Jones protein determination.

33. Florence Nightingale to Elizabeth Herbert, 13 December 1860, BL Add. MSS 43396:ff97-102.

34. Elizabeth Herbert to Florence Nightingale, 12 August 1861, BL Add. MSS 43396:f153.

35. Florence Nightingale to Mr. Nightingale, 21 August 1861, BL Add. MSS 45790:ff217-221.

36. Florence Nightingale to Harriet Martineau, 24 September 1861, BL Add. MSS 45788:ff133-145.

37. Cook, *The Life of Florence Nightingale,* vol. I, p. 408.

38. Florence Nightingale to Mary Clarke Mohl, 13 December 1861, cited in Vicinus and Nergaard, *Ever Yours,* p. 231.

39. Cook, *The Life of Florence Nightingale,* vol. I, p. 412.

40. Arthur Hugh Clough, *The Poetical Works* (New York: Thomas Y. Crowell, 1897), pp. xlix-li.

41. Florence Nightingale to Sir John McNeill, 18 November 1861, LMA H1/ST/NC/ SU 143.

42. Sir John McNeill to Florence Nightingale, 19 November 1861, BL Add. MSS 45968:f169.

43. Florence Nightingale to Madame Mohl, 13 December 1861, Wellcome MSS, cited in Vicinus and Nergaard, *Ever Yours,* p. 229.

44. Harriet Martineau to Florence Nightingale, 20 September 1861, BL Add. MSS 45788:ff125-26.

45. Florence Nightingale to Harriet Martineau, 24 September 1861, BL Add. MSS 45788:ff127-30.

46. Among the volunteer nurses who served in the Civil War were Dorothea Dix (Superintendent of Female Nurses for the Union Army), Clara Barton (a Patent Office clerk who organized a supply effort for the troops and years later started the American Red Cross), the author Louisa May Alcott, Mary Ann Bickerdyke (head of nursing services with General Grant's armies), and the poet Walt Whitman.

Chapter 13

1. Florence Nightingale to Mrs. Nightingale, 7 March 1862, BL Add. MSS 45790:ff253-64.

2. Florence Nightingale to Mary Clarke Mohl, 21 December 1861, Woodward Memorial Biomedical Library, University of British Columbia, cited in Vicinus and Nergaard, *Ever Yours,* p. 233.

3. Florence Nightingale to Mrs. Nightingale, 7 March 1862, BL Add. MSS 45790:ff253-64.

4. Florence Nightingale, private note, 5 November 1864 BL Add. MSS 45844:f72.

5. Cook, *The Life of Florence Nightingale,* vol. II, p. 303.

6. Florence Nightingale to Samuel Smith, 23 June 1863, BL Add. MSS 45793:ff29-30.

7. Florence Nightingale to Mrs. Nightingale, 7 March 1862, BL Add. MSS 45790:ff253-64.

8. Cook, *The Life of Florence Nightingale,* vol. II, p. 206.

9. Ibid, p. 207.

10. Ibid. p. 206.

11. Ibid. p. 207.

12. Florence Nightingale to Hilary Bonham Carter, January 1862, BL Add. MSS 45794:f174.

13. Hilary Bonham Carter to Florence Nightingale, January 1862, BL Add. MSS 45794:f175.

14. Florence Nightingale to Hilary Bonham Carter, 18 January 1863, BL Add. MSS 45794:f208.

15. Florence Nightingale to Hilary Bonham Carter, 20 May 1863, BL Add. MSS 45794:ff209-210.

16. Florence Nightingale to Hilary Bonham Carter, 11 August 1863, BL Add. MSS 45794:f220.

17. Cook, *The Life of Florence Nightingale,* vol. II, p. 93.

18. Ibid., p. 92.

19. Florence Nightingale to Elizabeth Herbert, 14 February 1863, BL Add. MSS 43396:ff188-189.

20. Florence Nightingale to Elizabeth Herbert, 2 August 1865, BL Add. MSS 43396:f195.

21. Florence Nightingale to Elizabeth Herbert, 12 January 1869, BL Add MSS 43396:f215.

22. Florence Nightingale to Madame Mohl, 30 July 1864, BL Add. MSS 43397:ff319-310.

23. Cook, *The Life of Florence Nightingale,* vol. II, p. 89.

24. Florence Nightingale to Selina Bracebridge, January 1864, BL Add. MSS 43397:f195.

25. Florence Nightingale to Henry Bonham Carter, 25 June 1864, BL Add. MSS 4598:f243.

26. Cook, *The Life of Florence Nightingale,* vol. II, p. 89.

27. Florence Nightingale to Julius Mohl, [No date], BL Add. MSS 46385:ff15-17.

28. Ibid.

29. Florence Nightingale to Elizabeth Herbert, 12 January 1869, BL Add. MSS 43396:f206.

30. Cook, *The Life of Florence Nightingale,* vol. I, p. 503.

31. Ibid.

32. Cook, *The Life of Florence Nightingale,* vol. II, p. 163.

33. Florence Nightingale to Elizabeth Herbert, 8 January 1874, BL Add. MSS 43396:f220.

34. Woodham-Smith, *Florence Nightingale,* p. 331.

35. Equivalents supplied by Federal Reserve Bank, Dallas. Available online at: http://web.calstatela.edu/faculty/ btm/lor/globalfd.htm. Accessed January 1999.

36. Cook, *The Life of Florence Nightingale,* vol. II, p. 311.

37. Florence Nightingale to Sir Harry Verney and Lady Verney, 17 September 1874, Wellcome MSS 9006:f124.

38. Florence Nightingale to Elizabeth Herbert, 3 February 1874, BL Add. MSS 43396:f223.

39. Cook, *The Life of Florence Nightingale,* vol. II, p. 236.

40. Probate of the Will of Florence Nightingale, LDFNM.

41. Florence Nightingale to Dr. William Farr, 23 February 1874, BL Add. MSS 43400:f276.

42. Woodham-Smith, *Florence Nightingale,* p. 333.

43. Florence Nightingale to May Coape Smith, 8 January 1876, LDFNM 1.0278.

44. Woodham-Smith, *Florence Nightingale,* p. 339.

45. F. Nightingale, *How People May Live and Not Die in India,* 2nd ed. (London: Longmans Publishing, 1864), flyleaf.

Chapter 14

1. Cook, *The Life of Florence Nightingale,* vol. II, p. 20.

2. Ibid.

3. Ibid., vol. I, p. 339.

4. Ibid., p. 272.

5. Florence Nightingale to Hilary Bonham Carter, 4 September 1862, BL Add. MSS 45794:ff183-185.

6. Equivalents supplied by Federal Reserve Bank, Dallas. Available online at: http://web.calstatela.edu/faculty/ btm/lor/globalfd.htm. Accessed January 1999.

7. F. Nightingale, *Observations on the Evidence Contained in The Stational Reports Submitted to Her by the Commission of the Sanitary State of the Army in India,* 1863, p. 4.

8. Ibid., p. 27.

9. Cook, *The Life of Florence Nightingale,* vol. II, p. 18.

10. Ibid., p. 36.

11. F. Nightingale, *Observations on the Evidence,* pp. iii-iv.

12. Woodham-Smith. *Florence Nightingale,* p. 274.

13. Cook, *The Life of Florence Nightingale,* vol. II, pp. 37-38.

14. Ibid., p. 38.

15. Florence Nightingale to Harriet Martineau, 16 April 1863, BL Add. MSS 45788:f174.

16. *Dictionary of National Biography,* vol. XI, p. 714.

17. Ibid., p. 712.

18. Cook, *The Life of Florence Nightingale,* vol. II, p. 44.

19. Ibid., p. 46.

20. Ibid., p. 49.

21. Ibid., p. 50.

22. Ibid., p. 53.

23. Florence Nightingale to Dr. J. Pattison Walker, 3 June 1864, BL Add. MSS 45781:ff219-22.

24. Equivalents supplied by Federal Reserve Bank, Dallas. Available online at: http://web.calstatela.edu/faculty/btm/lor/globalfd.htm. Accessed January 1999.

25. Florence Nightingale to Harriet Martineau, 20 February 1865, BL Add. MSS 45788:ff288.

26. Florence Nightingale to Sir John Lawrence, 26 September 1864, BL Add. MSS 45777:f49-53.

27. Cook, *The Life of Florence Nightingale*, vol. II, p. 57.

28. Florence Nightingale, "Note on the Aboriginal Races in Australia," paper read at the annual meeting of the National Association for the Promotion of Social Science in York, England, 1864, p. 3.

29. Sir John Lawrence to Florence Nightingale, 7 February 1867, cited in Cook, *The Life of Florence Nightingale,* vol. II, p. 156.

30. Florence Nightingale to Sir Stafford Northcote, 28 September 1867, BL Add. MSS 45779:f114-19.

31. Cook, *The Life of Florence Nightingale*, vol. II, p. 147.

32. Ibid., p. 148.

33. Ibid., p. 150.

34. Ibid., p. 151.

35. Ibid., p. 181.

36. Sir Bartle Frere to Florence Nightingale, 5 July 1869, cited in Cook, *The Life of Florence Nightingale,* vol. II, p. 181.

37. Cook, *The Life of Florence Nightingale*, vol. II, p. 158.

38. Ibid., p. 160.

39. Sir Bartle Frere to Florence Nightingale, 11 December 1869, BL Add. MSS 45780:ff174-77.

40. Florence Nightingale to Julius Mohl, 1 April 1870, LMA H1/ST/NC1/70/4.

41. Cook, *The Life of Florence Nightingale*, vol. II, pp. 178-79.

42. Sir Bartle Frere to Florence Nightingale, 18 June 1870, BL Add. MSS 45780:ff199-200.

43. Quinn and Prest, *Dear Miss Nightingale*, pp. 167-68.

Chapter 15

1. B. Abel-Smith, *A History of the Nursing Profession* (London: Heinemann, 1960), p. 25.

2. B. Abel-Smith, *The Hospitals 1800-1948: A Study in Social Administration in England and Wales* (London: Heinemann, 1964), p. 46.

3. Ibid.

4. Ibid., p. 55.

5. Florence Nightingale to Reverend Mother Mary Clare Moore, 3 September 1864, BL Add. MSS 45789:ff27-28.

6. Cook, *The Life of Florence Nightingale*, vol. II, p. 127.

7. F. Nightingale, "Una and the Lion," *Good Words,* June 1868, p. 362.

8. Abel-Smith, *The Hospitals 1800-1948,* p. 71.

9. Ibid., pp. 50-55.

10. Ibid., p. 55.

11. Ibid., p. 57.

12. Ibid., p. 72.

13. Florence Nightingale to Edwin Chadwick, 9 July 1866, BL Add. MSS 45771:ff102-10.

14. Ibid.

15. Florence Nightingale to Henry Bonham Carter, 4 June 1867, BL Add. MSS 47714:f203.

16. *The Report of the National Association for Providing Trained Nurses for the Sick and Poor,* 13 June 1876. LMA H1/ST/NC15.

17. *Nightingale Fund Council Annual Reports* 1876-1878.

18. Baly, *Florence Nightingale and the Nursing Legacy,* p. 131.

19. Florence Nightingale, private note [No date], BL Add. MSS 45841:f30.

20. Baly, *Florence Nightingale and the Nursing Legacy,* p. 53

21. Address from Florence Nightingale to the Probationer Nurses in the "Nightingale Fund" School at St. Thomas's Hospital, 23 July 1874, LDFNM:0256.

22. Address from Florence Nightingale to the Probationer Nurses in the "Nightingale Fund" School at St. Thomas's Hospital, 26 May 1875, LDFNM:0727.

23. Florence Nightingale to Matron, Home Sister, and Nurses at St. Thomas's Hospital, New Year's Day 1878, LDFNM:0728.

24. Cook, *The Life of Florence Nightingale,* vol. II, p. 194.

25. Florence Nightingale to Harriet Martineau, 24 September 1861, BL Add. MSS 45788:ff131-132.

26. F. Nightingale, *Introductory Notes on Lying-in Institutions Together with a Proposal for Organising an Institution for Training Midwives and Midwifery Nurses* (London: Longmans, Green & Co., 1871), p. 9-10.

27. Nightingale, *Notes on Nursing,* p. 53. Hand washing and donning clean gowns became more of a practice protocol around 1890; rubber gloves weren't introduced into surgery until 1891.

28. Nightingale, *Introductory Notes on Lying-in Institutions,* p. 67.

29. Cope, *Florence Nightingale and the Doctors,* p. 121.

30. Strachey, *The Cause,* p. 15.

31. Ibid.

32. S. Mitchell, *Victorian Britain: An Encyclopedia* (New York: Garland Publishing, 1988), p. 85.

33. Strachey, *The Cause,* p. 75.

34. Ibid., p. 71

35. J.S. Mill, *The Subjection of Women,* 2nd ed. (London: Longmans, Green & Co., 1869), p. 75.

36. Florence Nightingale to John Stuart Mill, 11 August 1867, BL Add. MSS 45787:ff38-42.

37. F. Nightingale, *Opinions of Women on Women's Suffrage.* (Manchester: A. Ireland, 1878), p. 1.

38. Mitchell, *Victorian Britain,* p. 414.

39. Ibid., p. 82.

40. Florence Nightingale to Sir Harry Verney, 16 April 1867, cited in Vicinus and Nergaard, *Ever Yours,* p. 277-82.

41. Ibid.

42. Florence Nightingale to Sir Henry Acland, 19 April 1876, cited in M. Baly, *As Miss Nightingale Said,* 2nd ed. (London: Balliere Tindall, 1997), p. 72.

43. Florence Nightingale to Dr. T. Longmore, 31 August 1864, BL Add. MSS 45773:ff173-174.

44. *The Times* (London), 7 August 1872.

Chapter 16

1. F. Nightingale, *Notes from Devotional Authors of the Middle Ages Collected, Chosen, and Freely Translated by Florence Nightingale,* BL Add. MSS 45841:ff1-87.

2. Ibid., ff11-28.

3. Florence Nightingale to Mother Mary Clare Moore, 21 October 1863, BL Add. MSS 45789:ff11-12. The entire collection of letters between Nightingale and Mother Mary Clare Moore can be found in *The Friendship of Florence Nightingale and Mary Clare Moore,* Mary C. Sullivan, ed. Philadelphia: University of Pennsylvania Press, 1999.

4. Florence Nightingale, Religious Essay [No date], BL Add. MSS 45843:f63.

5. Florence Nightingale to Mother Mary Clare Moore, 24 December 1863, BL Add. MSS 44789:ff13-16.

6. Florence Nightingale to Mother Mary Clare Moore, 15 December 1863, BL Add. MSS 45789:ff13-16.

7. Florence Nightingale to Mother Mary Clare Moore, 24 December 1863, BL Add. MSS 45789:ff17-20.

8. Florence Nightingale to Mother Mary Clare Moore, 28 February 1865, BL Add. MSS 45789:ff43-44.

9. Florence Nightingale to Mother Mary Clare Moore, 1 September 1865, BL Add. MSS 45789:f34.

10. Florence Nightingale, private note, 7 May 1867, BL Add. MSS 45844:f6.

11. Florence Nightingale to Mother Mary Clare Moore, 8 September 1868, BL Add. MSS 45789:ff55-56.

12. M.A. Schimmelpenninck, *Narrative of the Demolition of the Monastery of Port Royal des Champs* (London: J. & A. Arch, 1816).

13. *Dictionary of National Biography,* vol. XXII, p. 925.

14. C. Sorabji, *India Calling* (London: Nisbet, 1934), pp. 31-32.

15. Florence Nightingale to Benjamin Jowett, 16 July 1862, BL Add. MSS 45783:ff3-12.

16. Benjamin Jowett to Florence Nightingale, 9 November 1862, BL Add. MSS 45783:ff14-15.

17. Calabria and Macrae, *Suggestions for Thought by Florence Nightingale,* p. xxxii.

18. Benjamin Jowett to Florence Nightingale, 3 December 1862, BL Add. MSS 45783:ff16-18.

19. Benjamin Jowett to Florence Nightingale, April 1864, BL Add. MSS 45783:ff19-20.

20. Florence Nightingale to Benjamin Jowett, 1 June 1867, BL Add. MSS 45783:ff112-13.

21. Florence Nightingale to Benjamin Jowett, 7 August 1871, BL Add. MSS 45783:ff237-50.

22. Florence Nightingale to Benjamin Jowett, 17 August 1871, BL Add. MSS 45783:ff255-64.

23. Ibid., ff265-75.

24. Benjamin Jowett to Florence Nightingale, 31 October 1872, cited in Quinn and Prest, *Dear Miss Nightingale,* p. 235.

25. Florence Nightingale to Benjamin Jowett, 17 August 1871, BL Add. MSS 45783:ff255-264.

26. Cook, *The Life of Florence Nightingale,* vol. II, p. 224-25.

27. Quinn and Prest, *Dear Miss Nightingale,* p. 332.

28. Ibid., p. 229.

29. Florence Nightingale to Benjamin Jowett, 9 August 1872, BL Add. MSS 45783:ff96-99.

30. Calabria & Macrae, *Suggestions for Thought by Florence Nightingale,* p.114.

31. Florence Nightingale's Bible, Florence Nightingale Museum, London. LDFNM:1.0343. A team of scholars led by Dr. Lynn McDonald of the University of Guelph in Ontario, Canada, is currently gathering material for the collected works of Florence Nightingale, which will include all of her works, both published and unpublished, in electronic form, with selected works to be published in print, beginning in 2000, by Wilfred Laurier University Press, Waterloo, Ontario, Canada.

32. Benjamin Jowett to Florence Nightingale, 28 February 1871, BL Add. MSS 45783:ff232-36.

33. F. Nightingale, "A Sub-Note of Interrogation: What Shall Our Religion Be in 1999," *Fraser's Magazine* (July): 25-36, 1873.

34. Cook, *The Life of Florence Nightingale,* vol. II, p. 220.

35. Ibid., p. 229.

36 . Quinn and Prest, *Dear Miss Nightingale,* p.226.

37. Florence Nightingale to Benjamin Jowett, [No date], BL Add. MSS 45784:f123.

38. Underhill, *Mysticism,* p. 437.

39. Calabria and Macrae, *Suggestions for Thought by Florence Nightingale,* p. xiii.

40. Nightingale, *Notes from Devotional Authors,* BL Add. MSS 45841:f73.

41. Ibid., ff11-28.

Chapter 17

1. Florence Nightingale to Sir Harry Verney, 12 May 1889, Wellcome MSS 9012:f192.

2. Cook, *The Life of Florence Nightingale,* vol. II, p. 323.

3. Florence Nightingale to Sir Harry Verney, 2 February 1880, Wellcome MSS 9008:f7.

4. Florence Nightingale to Lady Verney, 6 February 1880, Wellcome MSS 9008:f11.

5. Florence Nightingale to Sir Harry Verney, 13 February 1880, Wellcome MSS 9008:f16.

6. Florence Nightingale to Lady Verney, 16, February 1880, Wellcome MSS 9008:f19.

7. Florence Nightingale to Lady Verney, 26 March 1880, Wellcome MSS 9008:f37.

8. Henry Bonham Carter to Florence Nightingale, 24 April 1880, Wellcome MSS 9008:f49.

9. Florence Nightingale to Lady Verney, 19 April 1880, Wellcome MSS 9008:f46.

10. F. Verney, *Stone Edge* (London: Smith Elder, 1868).

11. F. Verney, *Essays and Tales* (London: Simplin Marshall Hamilton, 1891).

12. F. Verney, *Memoirs of the Verney Family during the Civil*

War (London: Longmans, Green & Co., 1892).

13. Florence Nightingale to Sir Harry Verney, 8 January 1881, Wellcome MSS 9008:f106, f110.

14. Florence Nightingale to Sir Harry Verney, 17 November 1880, Wellcome MSS 9008:f98.

15. It's interesting to note that 1887, the year that Nightingale sought another medical opinion about her chronic symptoms, was the same year that Sir David Bruce, a surgeon in the Army Medical Services, and his wife, Mary, a microscopist, isolated the organism responsible for Nightingale's original bout of Crimean fever, *Brucella melitensis*. Today, Crimean fever is properly called Malta fever or Mediterranean fever and is the general disease classified as brucellosis. The Bruces' original slides and photographs of their pioneering work can be seen at the Wellcome Institute of Medicine in London. Wellcome RAMC 1242 Box D/ Appendix D Sir David Bruce.

16. J.L. Thornton, "Sir Thomas Lauder Brunton, 1844-1916." *St. Bartholomew's Journal*, August 1967, pp. 289-93.

17. Florence Nightingale to Dr. Thomas L. Brunton, 18 December 1887. (This letter is on loan to the Florence Nightingale Museum.)

18. Thornton, "Sir Thomas Lauder Brunton, 1844-1916," pp. 289-293.

19. A. Stille, et al. "Potassii bromidum and Spiritus chloroformi," *The National Dispensatory*, 5th ed. (Philadelphia: Lea Brothers, 1894), pp. 1282, 1502.

20. Florence Nightingale to Lady Verney, 28 April 1888, Wellcome MSS 9012:f24.

21. Florence Nightingale to Lady Verney, 4 April 1888, Wellcome MSS 9012:f14.

22. Florence Nightingale to Lady Verney, 19 April 1888, Wellcome MSS 9012:f20.

23. Florence Nightingale to Lady Verney, 25 December 1888, Wellcome MSS 9012:f71.

24. Cook, *The Life of Florence Nightingale*, vol. II, p. 388.

25. Florence Nightingale, private note, 17 January 1889, BL Add. MSS 45793:f225.

26. Florence Nightingale, private note, 30 January 1889, Wellcome MSS 9012:f3.

27. Florence Nightingale to Sir Harry Verney, 18 January 1889, Wellcome MSS 9012:f188.

Chapter 18

1. Florence Nightingale to Sir William Wedderburn, September 1885, cited in S.K. Ratcliffe, *Sir William Wedderburn and the Indian Reform Movement* (London: George Allen & Unwin, 1923), pp. 123.

2. Florence Nightingale to Sir Harry Verney, 17 November 1880, Wellcome MSS 9008:f96.

3. M.J. Gilbert, "Florence Nightingale and the Indian National Congress" in *Interfacing Nations: Indo/Pakistani/Canadian Reflections on the 50th Anniversary of India's Independence*, R.C. Tremblay, et al., eds. (New Delhi: B.R. Publishing, 1998), p. 21.

4. Charles Gordon to Florence Nightingale, 30 April 1880, BL Add. MSS 45806:f146, cited in Gilbert, "Nightingale and the Indian National Congress," pp. 25-26.

5. Florence Nightingale to Lord Ripon, 14 April 1881, Wellcome MSS 9008:f138.

6. Ratcliffe, *Sir William Wedderburn and the Indian Reform Movement*, p. 121.

7. Cook, *The Life of Florence Nightingale*, vol. II, p. 344.

8. Ibid., p. 345.

9. Quinn and Prest, *Dear Miss Nightingale*, p. 309.

10. B. Misra, *The Administrative History of India 1834-1947: General Administration* (Bombay: Oxford University Press, 1970), p. 41.

11. Florence Nightingale to Sir William Wedderburn, September 1885, cited in Ratcliffe, *Sir William Wedderburn and the Indian Reform Movement*, p. 123.

12. Florence Nightingale to P.K. Sen, 20 June 1879, in P.K. Sen, *Florence Nightingale's Indian Letters* (Calcutta: Mihir Kumar, 1937), cited in Gilbert, "Nightingale and the Indian National Congress," p. 22.

13. Ibid., 16 July 1881.

14. Florence Nightingale to Sir Harry Verney, 29 April 1888, Wellcome MSS 9012:f25.

15. B.R. Nanda. *Gokhale: The Indian Moderates and the British Raj* (Delhi: Oxford University Press, 1977), p. 92.

16. Florence Nightingale to Sir William Wedderburn, 13 August 1896, BL Add. MSS 45813:f227.

17. Nanda, *Gokhale*, p. 90.

18. Ibid., p. 59.

19. Ibid.

20. Ibid., p. 101.

21. Ibid., p. 97.

22. Quinn and Prest, *Dear Miss Nightingale*, p. 322.

23. Cornelia Sorabji to family, 16 February 1893, India Office Library and Records, European F Manuscripts 165:ff44-45, cited in Gilbert, "Nightingale and the Indian National Congress," p. 39.

24. C. Sorabji, *India Calling*, pp. 31-32.

25. B.R. Nanda, letter to author, 14 January 1999.

Chapter 19

1. F. Nightingale, "Sick-Nursing and Health-Nursing" in *Woman's Mission*, Baroness Burdett Coutts, ed. (London: Sampson, Low, Martson, 1893), pp. 198.

2. Cook, *The Life of Florence Nightingale*, vol. II, pp. 326-27.

3. Ibid., pp. 336-37.

4. Ibid., p. 336.

5. Florence Nightingale to Ella Pirrie, 14 October 1885, LDFNM, LMA: H1/ST/NCI/85/9.

6. Florence Nightingale to Henry Bonham Carter, 1 May 1894, BL Add. MSS 47726:f6.

7. Florence Nightingale to Sir Harry Verney, 29 May 1888, Wellcome MSS 9012:f30.

8. Florence Nightingale to Henry Bonham Carter, 4 December 1899, LMA H1/ST/NC18/15, cited in Baly, *Florence Nightingale and the Nursing Legacy*, p. 138.

9. In 1949, Queen Alexandra's Imperial Military Nursing Service was renamed Queen Alexandra's Royal Army Nursing Corps (QARANC). In 1992, male nurses were admitted to QARANC. Cited in P.W. Kirkby, *Royal Victoria Country Park, Netley*, Hampshire County Council, 1994.

10. Cope, *Florence Nightingale and the Doctors*, p. 146.

11. Florence Nightingale to Miss Ella Pirrie, 22 July 1889, LDFNM, LMA: H1/ST/NCI/89/10.

12. L. Hockey, "Feeling the Pulse. London: Queen's Institute of District Nursing, 1966," cited in Baly, *Florence Nightingale and the Nursing Legacy*, p. 136.

13. Equivalents supplied by Federal Reserve Bank, Dallas. Available online at: http://web.calstatela.edu/faculty/btm/or/globalfd.htm. Accessed January 1999.

14. Florence Nightingale to Henry Bonham Carter, May 1895, BL Add. MSS 47726:f158.

15. The Queen Victoria Jubilee Institute had 539 trained nurses in 1900 and eventually became the model for Britain's 20th-century District Nursing Service. Cited in M. Baly, *A New Approach to District Nursing* (London: Heinemann, 1981), p. 292.

16. Nightingale, "Sick-Nursing and Health-Nursing" in *Woman's Mission*, p. 203.

17. Cook, *The Life of Florence Nightingale*, vol. II, pp. 384.

18. B. Abel-Smith, *A History of the Nursing Profession* (London: Heinemann, 1960), p. 24.

19. G. Yeo, *Nursing at Bart's* (London: Alan Sutton, 1992), pp. 36, 58.

20. Address from Florence Nightingale to the Probationer Nurses in the "Nightingale Fund" School at St. Thomas's Hospital, 16 May 1888, LDFNM:0310.

21. Cope, *Florence Nightingale and the Doctors*, p. 137.

22. Youngson, *The Scientific Revolution*, p. 153.

23. R. Vallery-Radot, *The Life of Pasteur* (Garden City, N.Y.: Garden City Publishing, 1923), p. 449.

24. F. Nightingale, "Training of Nurses," in *A Dictionary of Medicine, Including General Pathology, General Therapeutics, Hygiene, and the Diseases of Women and Children*. R. Quain, ed. (London: Longmans, Green & Co., 1894), vol. II, pp. 241-42.

25. Nightingale, "Sick-Nursing and Health- Nursing" in *Woman's Mission*, p. 367.

26. B. Dossey, et al. *Holistic Nursing: A Handbook for Practice* (Gaithersburg, Md.: Aspen Publishers, 2000).

27. Nightingale, "Sick-Nursing and Health- Nursing" in *Woman's Mission*, pp. 184-205.

28. In 1912, this organization became the National League for Nursing Education, which was reorganized in 1952 as the National League for Nursing. At this 1874 meeting, nursing leaders Isabel A. Hampton, Adelaide Nutting, and Lavinia Dock conceived the idea for an American nursing organization to represent all graduate nurses in practice. In 1896, the Nurses' Associated Alumnae of the United States and Canada was formed. This organization was instrumental in beginning the *American Journal of Nursing* in 1900 and was the forerunner of the American Nurses Association, established in 1911.

29. E.R. Benson, "Ninteenth Century Women, The Neophyte Nursing Profession and the World's Columbian Exposition of 1893," cited in V. Bullough, et al., *Florence Nightingale and Her Era*, (New York: Garland Publishing, 1990), p. 119.

30. At this meeting, Fenwick called on the nursing leaders from around the world to organize and unite. The International Council of Nurses, founded in 1899, celebrated its 100th anniversary in London in June 1999. Today the ICN, based in Geneva, Switzerland, is a federation of 120 nurses' associations representing 1.5 million nurses. Its mission is to provide leadership and assistance in resolving present and future health care needs. Cited in B.L. Brush and J.E. Lynaugh, *Nurses of All Nations: A History of the International Council of Nurses 1899-1999* (Philadelphia: Lippincott Williams & Wilkins, 1999), p. xii.

Chapter 20

1. Florence Nightingale, private note, 9 August 1898, LDFNM:0852.

2. Quinn and Prest, *Dear Miss Nightingale*, p. 301.

3. Ibid., p. 308.

4. Cook, *The Life of Florence Nightingale*, vol. II, p. 242.

5. Ibid., p. 366.

6. Florence Nightingale to Benjamin Jowett, 3 January 1891, BL Add. MSS 45785:f144-45.

7. Quinn and Prest, *Dear Miss Nightingale*, p. 319.

8. Ibid.

9. Ibid., p. 321.

10. Ibid., p. 323.

11. Florence Nightingale, private note, 6 October 1893, BL Add. MSS 45785:f204.

12. Cook, *The Life of Florence Nightingale*, vol. II, pp. 400-01.

13. Ibid., p. 401.

14. Ibid., p. 387.

15. Ibid., p. 399.

16. Florence Nightingale to Margaret Verney, 24 February 1898. Wellcome MSS 9015:f125.

17. Cook, *The Life of Florence Nightingale*, vol. II, p. 357.

18. Voice Recording of Florence Nightingale, National Park Service, Edison National Historic Site, West Orange, N.J.

19. Florence Nightingale, private note, 7 February 1892, BL Add. MSS 45844:f64.

20. Cook, *The Life of Florence Nightingale*, p. 415.

21. Ibid., p. 392.

22. Ibid., p. 404.

23. Florence Nightingale to Margaret Verney, 16 January 1897, Wellcome MSS 9015:f88.

24. Florence Nightingale to Margaret Verney, 27 May 1895, Wellcome MSS 9014:f45.

25. Florence Nightingale to Margaret Verney, 23 April 1896, Wellcome MSS 9015:f71.

26. Florence Nightingale to Rev. T.G. Clark, 1 October 1895, BL Add. MSS 68890:f92.

27. Woodham-Smith, *Florence Nightingale*, p. 364.

28. Florence Nightingale to Margaret Verney, 13 February 1897, Wellcome MSS 9015:f92.

29. Florence Nightingale to Edmund Verney, 10 March 1897, Wellcome MSS 9015:f96.

30. Cook, *The Life of Florence Nightingale,* vol. II, p. 410.

31. Florence Nightingale, Address to the Nurses and Probationers Trained Under the Nightingale Fund, 28 May 1900, LDFNM:0731.

32. Cook, *The Life of Florence Nightingale,* vol. II, p. 417.

33. Ibid., p. 458.

34. Ibid.

35. Ibid., p. 418.

36. Paul Heironymussen, *Orders and Decorations of Europe in Color* (London: Macmillan, 1967), pp. 137-38.

37. Cook, *The Life of Florence Nightingale,* vol. II, p. 420.

38. Freedom of the City of London, 13 February 1908. LDFNM:0683.1-2.

39. Cook, *The Life of Florence Nightingale,* vol. II, p. 421.

40. J. Montgomery, *Florence Nightingale* (London: Herron Books, 1970), p. 320.

41. *The Times* (London), 15 August 1910, p. 8.

42. Montgomery, *Florence Nightingale,* pp. 318-24.

43. Ibid., pp. 323-24.

44. Equivalents supplied by Federal Reserve Bank, Dallas. Available online at: http://web.calstatela.edu/faculty/btm/lor/globalfd.htm. Accessed January 1999.

45. Ratcliffe, *Sir William Wedderburn and the Indian Reform Movement,* p. 125.

46. Ibid., pp. 125-26.

47. M. Gandhi, "No. 80, Florence Nightingale" in *The Collected Works of Mahatma Gandhi,* vol. V, 1905-1906 (New Delhi: Publications Division, Ministry of Information & Broadcasting, Government of India, 1994), pp. 61-62. (Errata: Printed as September 9, 1905 in vol. 5, but actually published September 9, 1915.)

48. J. Achterberg, et al. *Rituals of Healing* (New York: Bantam, 1994), p. 10.

Appendices: Pilgrimage to Scutari

1. B.M. Dossey, *Florence Nightingale: Mystic, visionary, healer* (Philadelphia: Lippincott, William & Wilkins, 2000).

2. Florence Nightingale to the Nightingales, November 4, 1854. London: Wellcome Institute Library. Cited in Goldie, S. I have done my duty. (Iowa City, Iowa: University of Iowa Press), p. 33.

3. Florence Nightingale. Private note. March 2, 1853. Cited in M.D. Calabria and J.A. Macrae *Suggestions for thought by Florence Nightingale: Selections and commentaries* (Philadelphia: University of Pennsylvania Press, 1994), p. xiii.

4. M. Vicinus and B. Nergaard, *Ever yours, Florence Nightingale* (London: Virago Press, 1989), pp. 110-111.

5. M. Vicinus and B. Nergaard, B. Ever yours, Florence Nightingale (1989), p. 112.

6. F. Nightingale, Sick-nursing and health-nursing. In Burdett-Coutts, Baroness Lady Angela, *Woman's mission: A series of congress papers on the philanthropic work of women by eminent writers* (pp.184-205). (New York: Charles Scribner's Sons, 1893), p. 199.

Resources

1. *The Florence Nightingale Museum:* http://www.florence-nightingale.co.uk

2. *The Collected Works of Florence Nightingale (CWFN):* http://www.wlupress.wlu.ca

3. M. Bostridge, *Florence Nightingale: The Making of an Icon* (New York: Farrar, Straus and Giroux, 2008).

4. The Nightingale Declaration Campaign http://www.nightingaledeclaration.net

Appendices: Mysticism

1. E. Underhill, *Mystics of the Church* (Cambridge: James Clarke, 1925), pp. 9-10.

2. C.L. Flinders, *Enduring Grace* (San Francisco: Harper, 1993), p. xxii.

3. E. Underhill, *Mysticism: A Study in the Nature and Development of Man's Spiritual Consciousness* (New York: E.P. Dutton, 1911; reprint 1961), p. 439.

4. E. Underhill, *Practical Mysticism* (1915; reprint New York: E.P. Dutton & Co., 1943), pp. x, 102, 162.

5. Ibid., p. 102.

6. Underhill, *Mysticism,* p. 169-70.

7. Underhill, *Practical Mysticism,* pp. 161-62.

8. Ibid., p. x.

9. Ibid., p. 102.

10. E.T. Cook, *The Life of Florence Nightingale* (London: Macmillan, 1913), vol. II, p. 243.

11. Ibid., p. 245.

12. Ibid., p. 415.

Appendices: Brucellosis

1. E.T. Cook, *The Life of Florence Nightingale* (London: Macmillan, 1913), vol. I, p. 493.

2. Z. Cope, *Florence Nightingale and the Doctors* (London: Museum Press, 1958).

3. G. Pickering, *Creative Malady* (London: Allen and Unwin, 1974).

4. F.B. Smith, *Florence Nightingale: Reputation and Power* (London: Croom Helm, 1982).

5. H. Ference, "Lead at Lea," *Notes on Nursing Science* I:118, 1988.

6. S. Veith, "The Recluse: A Retrospective Health History of Florence Nightingale," in Bullough, V.L., et al., eds. *Florence Nightingale and Her Era,* pp. 75-89.

7. Ibid.

8. J.J. Brook, "Some Thoughts and Reflections on the Life of Florence Nightingale from a Twentieth-Century Perspective," in Bullough, V.L., et al., eds. *Florence Nightingale and Her Era,* pp. 23-39.

9. Ibid.

10. D.A.B. Young. "Florence Nightingale's Fever," *British Medical Journal* 311:1697-1700, 1995.

11. J.A. Marston, "Report on Fever (Malta)," in *Army Medical Department Reports,* vol. 3. London: HMSO, 1863: 486-521, cited in D.A.B. Young, "Florence Nightingale's Fever," *British Medical Journal* 311:1697-1700, 1995.

12. Ibid.

13. D. Bruce, "The Micrococcus of Malta Fever," *Practitioner* 40:241, 1888.

14. M.L. Hughes, *Mediterranean, Malta or Undulant Fever* (London: Macmillan, 1897).

15. T. Zammit, "A Preliminary Note on the Examination of the Blood of Goats Suffering from Mediterranean Fever," in *Reports of Royal Society of London. Mediterranean Fever Commission* (London: Harrison's and Sons [Part IV], 1905).

16. B. Bang, "The Etiology of Epizootic Abortion," *Journal of Comprehensive Pathology Therapies,* 19:91, 1906.

17. A.C. Evans, "Chronic Brucellosis," *Journal of the American Medical Association* 103:665-67, 1934.

18. Ibid.

19. I.Z. Trujillo, et al. "Brucellosis," *Infectious Disease Clinics of North America* 8:225-41, 1994.

20. E.J. Young, "An Overview of Human Brucellosis," *Clinical Infectious Disease* 21:283-90, 1994.

21. Ibid.

22. Trujillo, et al. "Brucellosis," *Infectious Disease Clinics of North America* 8:225-41, 1994.

23. E.J. Young, "An Overview of Human Brucellosis," *Clinical Infectious Disease* 21:283-90, 1994.

24. Trujillo, et al. "Brucellosis," *Infectious Disease Clinics of North America* 8:225-41, 1994.

25. Ibid.

26. D.A.B. Young, "Florence Nightingale's Fever," *British Medical Journal* 311:1697-1700, 1995.

27. W.W. Spink, *The Nature of Brucellosis* (Minneapolis: University of Minnesota Press, 1956).

28. B. Dossey, "Florence Nightingale's Crimean Fever and Chronic Illness," *Journal of Holistic Nursing* 16(2):168-196, 1998.

Appendices: Personality type

1. C.G. Jung, *Psychological Types: The Collected Works of C.G. Jung* (Princeton, N.J.: Princeton University Press, 1971), Bollingen Series XX, vol. 6.

2. I. Myers and P.B. Myers, *Gifts Differing* (Palo Alto, Calif.: Consulting Psychologists Press, Inc., 1980), pp. 22-24.

3. Ibid., pp. 27-51.

4. S.K. Hirsh and J.M. Kummerow, *Introduction to Type in Organizations,* 3rd ed. (Palo Alto, Calif.: Consulting Psychologists Press, Inc., 1998), p. 9.

5. B. Dossey, "Florence Nightingale's Crimean Fever and Chronic Illness," *Journal of Holistic Nursing* 16(2):168-96, 1998.

6. Myers & Myers, *Gifts Differing,* pp. 41-43.

Picture Credits

FNM; p. 46, 56, 58: HCRO; p. 48, 59: Wellcome; p. 49: HGLA; p. 50: Bildarchiv; p. 61, 62: Wilton. **Chapter 3** — p. 63: Graphic House/ Corbis; p. 64, 69, 71: FNM; p. 65: Birmingham Museum and Art Gallery, England; p. 68, 75, 76: Bildarchiv ; p. 73: Elizabeth Blackwell Center, Riverside Methodist Hospitals, Columbus, Ohio; p. 79: HGLA; p. 81: Appears in I. B. O'Malley *Florence Nightingale 1820-1856,* London: Thornton Butterworth, 1931; p. 83: National Trust, London; p. 84: Irene S. Palmer, San Diego. **Chapter 4** — p. 85: Author; p. 86, 87: FNM; p. 89: HGLA; p. 96: RSM; p. 97: New York Academy of Medicine; p. 98: Wellcome; p. 99: BL.

Part 2 — opener: FNM. **Chapter 5** — p. 103, 107, 108, 118, 119: FNM; p. 104 (left), 109: HGPC; p. 104 (bottom), 106: Crane, © Author; p. 105, 123, 143: FNM; p. 111: Wilton; p. 113: NPG; p. 120: Peninsular and Oriental Steam Navigation Co., London. **Chapter 6** — p. 121, 124, 126, 128, 129 (bottom), 130 (middle), 132, 141, 142, 145, 146: FNM; p. 122 (top): Crane, © Author; p. 122 (bottom), 129 (top): Tarih Vakfi Museum, Istanbul; p. 134, 139, 147: RAMC; p. 130 (top): NPG. **Chapter 7** — p. 149, 152 (top): RAMC; p. 151, 152 (bottom): HGPC; p. 153, 155, 157, 159, 160 (bottom), 161, 162, 164, 169, 170 (bottom): FNM; p. 158: Author; p. 160 (top), 167, 168: National Army Museum, London; 163: Fine Art Society, London; 163: Stapleton Collection, London; 166: Bridgeman/ Private Collection, London; **Chapter 8** — p. 169, 170 (bottom): FNM; p. 170: (top) Royal Artillery Institution, London.

Part 3 — opener: FNM. **Chapter 9** — p. 179, 180: National Trust, London; p. 182: Rev. George Biggs, Wellow Vicarage, St. Margaret's Church, East Wellow, England; p. 183

(top), 184, 185 (bottom), 188: FNM; p. 185 (top): Corbis/ Bettmann; p. 187, 190, 193: HGPC; p. 189, 195: Wellcome; p. 192: Windsor. **Chapter 10** — p. 201, 204, 208, 214: FNM; p. 203: HGLA; p. 205: Appears in Florence Nightingale, *Notes on Hospitals,* London: John W. Parker & Son (1859); p. 207: BL; p. 209: Corbis/Wild Country; p. 211, 216: HGPC; p. 215 (top): Courtauld; p. 215 (bottom): National Trust, London. **Chapter 11** — p. 219, 223, 224: FNM; p. 225 (top): Wellcome; p. 225 (bottom), 226: Appears in Florence Nightingale, *Hospital Statistics and Hospital Plans,* reprinted from the *Transactions of the National Association for the Promotion of Social Science* (Dublin Meeting, August 1861), London: Emily Faithful & Co. (1862); p. 229: Observatoire Royale de Belgique, Brussels. **Chapter 12** — p. 231, 239: Author; p. 232: Wellcome; p. 234: Appears in Florence Nightingale, *Notes on Hospitals,* London: John W. Parker & Son (1859); p. 236: HGLA; p. 237: Corbis/ Bettmann; p. 241: HGPC; p. 242: FNM; p. 244: RSM; p. 248: Irene S. Palmer, San Diego.

Part 4 — opener: FNM. **Chapter 13** — p. 253: HGPC; p. 255, 256: FNM; p. 258: Appears in I. B. O'Malley, *Florence Nightingale 1820-1856,* London: Thornton Butterworth, 1931; p. 263: HCRO. **Chapter 14** — p. 267, 268, 279, 285, 288: HGPC; p. 269: Crane, © Author; p. 271, 272: Corbis/Bettmann; p. 273, 274, 276: All appear in Florence Nightingale, *Observations on the Sanitary State of the Army in India,* London: Edward Stanford (1863); p. 278: Wellcome; p. 281: Corbis/ Christopher Cormack, New York; p. 286: Corbis/Michael Nicholson, New York; p. 290: Corbis. **Chapter 15** — p. 291, 295, 298, 300, 301, 302, 303, 304, 305, 314, 315: FNM; p. 293: The Mansell

Collection, London; p. 294, 323: Wellcome; p. 308: HGLA; p. 313: Appears in Florence Nightingale, *Introductory Notes on Lying-in Institutions,* London: Longmans, Green & Co. (1871); p. 316, 317: HGPC; p. 318: Corbis/Bettmann; p. 319: HGLA. **Chapter 16** — p. 325: HGLA; p. 326: Corbis/ Bettmann; p. 327: Sister M. Imelda Keena and Sister Theresa Green, Bermondsey Convent, London; p. 330, 333: HGPC; p. 335, 343: BL; p. 338: FNM.

Part 5 — opener: FNM. **Chapter 17** — p. 347, 349: FNM; p. 351: HGPC; p. 352: HGLA; p. 354: Louise C. Selanders, East Lansing, MI. **Chapter 18** — p. 355, 371 (bottom): Navajivan Trust, Ahmedabad, India; p. 359, 360, 370: B.R. Nanda, New Delhi; p. 361, HGPC; p. 362: Bridgeman/ Private Collection, London; p. 363, 371 (top): Corbis/ Bettmann; p. 373: BL. **Chapter 19** — p. 375, 379: Kirkby; p. 376, 378: FNM; p. 382, 387: HGLA; p. 383: The Queen's Nursing Institute, London; p. 384: St. Bartholomew's Archives, London; p. 389: Corbis/ Bettmann; p. 390: Corbis; p. 391: Author; p. 392: Crane, © Author. **Chapter 20** — p. 393, 401, 403, 405, 406 (bottom), 407, 409, 410, 412, 415: FNM; p. 400: Courtauld, Courtesy of Sir Ralph Verney and Sir Edmund Verney; p. 399: Edison National Historic Site, National Park Service; p. 406 (top), 413 (bottom): National Army Museum, London; p. 408: General Register Office, London; p. 411, 413 (top), 414: Louise C. Selanders, East Lansing, MI.

Appendices — p. 417: Kirkby.

Fig 1, Fig 2: Barbara M. Dossey and John Crane; Fig 3, Fig 4, Fig 6, Fig 8, Fig 9, Fig 10, Fig 11, Fig 13, Fig 14, Fig 15, Fig 16, Fig 17, Fig 18: Author; Fig 5, Fig 12: FNM; Fig 7: Wellcome

Acknowledgments

Few books are written in isolation, and I have received the assistance of many individuals, institutions, books, and documents during the development of this illustrated biography. First and foremost, very special thanks are due to Robert H. Craven, Jr., President, F. A. Davis Company and Joanne DaCunha, Acquisitions Nursing Editor for their excitement for publishing Florence Nightingale: Mystic, Visionary, Healer Commemorative Edition that is a dream come true. I wish to also thank the following F. A. Davis team members: to Kim DePaul for her attention to editorial details; to Cynthia Mondgock for her permissions work; to Sam Rondinelli, Book Production Manager; to Lisa Thompson, Project Editor; to Carolyn O'Brien for logo, book design, and production details; to Katharine Margeson, Illustration Coordinator; to Michael Torio, Marketing Team Manager; and to all others who have made this Commemorative edition a reality.

I wish to express my deepest gratitude to the marvelous creative team at my former publisher, Springhouse Corporation: project manager Doris Weinstock and book designer Mary Ludwicki — what a wonderful creative dance! Nancy Holmes and Peter Johnson for their excellent editing; Liz Schaeffer, who kept us on schedule; Kris Magyarits for his brilliant cover illustration and the rest of the design team, Jarrett Zigon and Donna S. Morris; Brenna Mayer, Priscilla DeWitt, and Pamela Wingrod for their excellent copy editing; Pat Schull and Trish Fischer for their early support; Judith McCann for her encouragement; Sarah Alderman and staff; Joanne DiNunzio and the marketing team.

I am also immensely grateful to my twin brother, Bo Montgomery, whose research and editorial assistance helped shape many of the ideas in this book.

My special thanks go to the following archives, picture collections, and libraries for their assistance on the first edition and the Commemorative Edition.

• The Florence Nightingale Museum, London, and the Florence Nightingale Museum Trust, whose mission is to preserve Florence Nightingale's legacy for the benefit of the present and future generations.
• Western Manuscripts, Wellcome Institute Library for the History of Medicine, London, Wellcome Medical Centre for Science, Photographic Department. The Claydon House Collection and London Metropolitan Archives, British Library. The Henry Bonham Carter Will Trust and its Radcliffe Solicitors.
• Convent of Our Lady of Mercy, St. Marie's of the Isles, Cork, Ireland; St. Margaret's Church, East Wellow, Romsey, Hampshire, England; The National Army Museum, London; Ottenheimer Library, University of Arkansas at Little Rock; Central Arkansas Library System, Little Rock; Royal Collection Enterprises, Windsor Castle, Berkshire, England; Embley Park School, Romsey, Hampshire; The National Portrait Gallery, London; Courtauld Gallery, London; Navajivan Trust, Ahmedabad, India; University of New Mexico Health Science Center Library, Albuquerque; St. Bartholomew's Hospital; London; Royal Society of Medicine, London; Academic Microforms, London; Convent of Mercy, Bermondsey, London; Royal Victoria Country Park, Netley, Southampton; Riverside Methodist Hospitals, Columbus, Ohio; The National Trust, Photographic Library, London; Hulton Getty Picture Collection Ltd., London; New York Academy of Medicine, New York; Observatoire Royale de Belgique, Brussels; Peninsular and Oriental Steam Navigation Co., London; The Queen's Nursing Institute, London; Bildarchiv PreuBischer Kulturbesitz, Berlin, Germany; Birmingham City Council and Birmingham Museums and Art Gallery, England; Royal Army Medical Corps Historical Museum, Keough Barracks, Aldershot, Hants; Hampshire County Record Office; Wilton House, Salisbury, England; Turkish Army Protocol

Department, Selimiye Barracks, Istanbul; Mimar Sinan University, Istanbul; Tarih Vakfi, Istanbul; Starline Printing, Albuquerque; Crane Digital Media, Santa Fe, N.M.; Thomas Alva Edison National Historic Site, West Orange, N.J.
• To the following Nightingale scholars for their important research: Monica E. Baly, Michael D. Calabria, O.P. Dwivedi, Sue M. Goldie, Helen M. Ference, Jocelyn Keith, Janet A. Macrae, Lynn McDonald, Lois Monteiro, Irene Sahelberg Palmer, Bea Nergaard, Louise C. Selanders, Victoria Slater, Mary C. Sullivan, Victor Skretowicz, Hugh Small, Reeta Chowdhari Tremblay, Martha Vicinus, Jo Ann G. Widerquist and Mark Bostridge.
• The Reverend Canon Ted Karpf, former Assistant to the Bishop, Episcopal Diocese of Washington, Washington National Cathedral, for his assistance to Louise C. Selanders and me in the reconsideration process of Florence Nightingale's inclusion in the Episcopal Church's Liturgical Calendar that was accepted July 2000.

And finally, my warmest thanks to my family: Boyd Montgomery, my dear Daddy, who loved history, read a portion of the first draft of the manuscipt, and gave his support and blessings on the project before he made his transition, and who is with me in spirit; Bette Montgomery, my sweet mother who read the first edition, who has made her transition and is with me in spirit, and Beverly Dunaway, my wonderful sister and twin brother Bo Montgomery, for their continuous encouragement; and my husband, Larry, with whom I continually weave the rich healing tapestry and bond of unity and oneness.

The Florence Nightingale Museum *is on the site of the former Nightingale Training School at St. Thomas's Hospital. It houses a unique collection of personal artifacts, Crimean mementos, and nursing history plus a temporary exhibition space, a shop, and a resource center and has a traveling exhibition.*

Florence Nightingale Museum,
2 Lambeth Palace Road, London SE1 7EW;
telephone: 020 7620 0374; fax: 020 7928 1760;
E-mail: <curator@florence-nightingale.co.uk>;
web site: <http:\\www.florence-nightingale.co.uk>.

The Collected Works of Florence Nightingale
(16 volumes) by Lynn McDonald, Ed (2001-2010) are all the
available surviving writing of Florence Nightingale.
See CWFN Project: sociology.uoguelph.ca/fnightingale

Wilfrid Laurier University Press:E-mail press@wlu.ca
Website: www.wlupress.wlu.ca

**The Nightingale Initiative for Global Health
(NIGH)** is a grassroots, nurse-inspired movement to
increase global public awareness about the priority of
human health. Our inclusive, collaborative, and syner-
gistic initiatives give nurses a voice and create new
opportunities for them to discover possibilities for their
unique contributions toward health and well-being for all.

We honor the legacy of Florence Nightingale and other
nurses, midwives, and healthcare workers, past and
present, who have shown by their example how personal
actions can make a significant difference. We seek to
engage the values and wisdom of millions of nurses
and concerned citizens and to act as a catalyst for the
transformation of individuals, communities, and
society for the achievement of a healthy world. See
http://www.nightingaledeclaration.net

Index

i indicates a page with an illustration; *q* indicates a page with a quotation.

i indicates a page with an illustration; *q* indicates a page with a quotation.

i indicates a page with an illustration; *q* indicates a page with a quotation.